国际经典内科学教科书

第10版

Cecil Essentials of Medicine
希氏内科学精要
中英双语版

原　著　Edward J. Wing, MD, FACP, FIDSA
Former Dean of Medicine and Biological Sciences
Professor of Medicine
Warren Alpert Medical School of Brown University, Providence, Rhode Island

Fred J. Schiffman, MD, MACP
Sigal Family Professor of Humanistic Medicine
Vice Chair, Department of Medicine
Warren Alpert Medical School of Brown University, Providence, Rhode Island

中英双语版　编辑委员会　主任委员　王　辰

———— 第 2 分册 ————

心血管疾病

主　译　郑金刚　任景怡

北京大学医学出版社

XISHI NEIKEXUE JINGYAO（DI 10 BAN） DI 2 FENCE　XINXUEGUAN JIBING（ZHONGYING SHUANGYU BAN）

图书在版编目（CIP）数据

希氏内科学精要：第 10 版 . 第 2 分册，心血管疾病：汉、英 /（美）爱德华·温（Edward J. Wing），（美）弗雷德·谢夫曼（Fred J. Schiffman）原著；郑金刚，任景怡主译 . -- 北京：北京大学医学出版社，2024. 11. -- ISBN 978-7-5659-3252-6（2025.4 重印）

Ⅰ. R5

中国国家版本馆 CIP 数据核字第 2024RY6477 号

北京市版权局著作权合同登记号：图字：01-2024-4518

Elsevier (Singapore) Pte Ltd.
3 Killiney Road, #08-01 Winsland House Ⅰ, Singapore 239519
Tel: (65) 6349-0200; Fax: (65) 6733-1817

Cecil Essentials of Medicine, Tenth Edition
Copyright © 2022 by Elsevier, Inc. All rights are reserved, including those for text and data mining, AI training, and similar technologies.
Publisher's note: Elsevier takes a neutral position with respect to territorial disputes or jurisdictional claims in its published content, including in maps and institutional affiliations.
Previous editions copyrighted 2016, 2010, 2007, 2004, 2001, 1997, 1993, 1990, and 1986.
ISBN-13: 978-0-323-72271-1

This translation of Cecil Essentials of Medicine, Tenth Edition by Edward J. Wing and Fred J. Schiffman was undertaken by Peking University Medical Press and is published by arrangement with Elsevier (Singapore) Pte Ltd.

Cecil Essentials of Medicine, Tenth Edition by Edward J. Wing and Fred J. Schiffman 由北京大学医学出版社进行翻译，并根据北京大学医学出版社与爱思唯尔（新加坡）私人有限公司的协议约定出版。

《希氏内科学精要（第 10 版） 第 2 分册　心血管疾病（中英双语版）》（郑金刚　任景怡　主译）
ISBN: 978-7-5659-3252-6
Copyright © 2024 by Elsevier (Singapore) Pte Ltd. and Peking University Medical Press.
All rights reserved. No part of this publication may be reproduced or transmitted in any form or by any means, electronic or mechanical, including photocopying, recording, or any information storage and retrieval system, without permission in writing from Elsevier (Singapore) Pte Ltd. and Peking University Medical Press.

注　意

本译本由北京大学医学出版社独立完成。相关从业及研究人员必须凭借其自身经验和知识对文中描述的信息数据、方法策略、搭配组合、实验操作进行评估和使用。由于医学科学发展迅速，临床诊断和给药剂量尤其需要经过独立验证。在法律允许的最大范围内，爱思唯尔、译文的原文作者、原文编辑及原文内容提供者均不对译文或因产品责任、疏忽或其他操作造成的人身及（或）财产伤害及（或）损失承担责任，亦不对由于使用文中提到的方法、产品、说明或思想而导致的人身及（或）财产伤害及（或）损失承担责任。

Published in China by Peking University Medical Press under special arrangement with Elsevier (Singapore) Pte Ltd. This edition is authorized for sale in the People's Republic of China only, excluding Hong Kong SAR, Macau SAR and Taiwan. Unauthorized export of this edition is a violation of the contract.

希氏内科学精要（第 10 版）　第 2 分册　心血管疾病（中英双语版）

主　　译：郑金刚　任景怡

出版发行：北京大学医学出版社

地　　址：（100191）北京市海淀区学院路 38 号　北京大学医学部院内

电　　话：发行部 010-82802230；图书邮购 010-82802495

网　　址：http://www.pumpress.com.cn

E-mail：booksale@bjmu.edu.cn

印　　刷：北京信彩瑞禾印刷厂

经　　销：新华书店

策划编辑：高　瑾

责任编辑：高　瑾　　责任校对：靳新强　　责任印制：李　啸

开　　本：889 mm×1194 mm　1/16　印张：22.75　字数：850 千字

版　　次：2024 年 11 月第 1 版　2025 年 4 月第 2 次印刷

书　　号：ISBN 978-7-5659-3252-6

定　　价：150.00 元

版权所有，违者必究

（凡属质量问题请与本社发行部联系退换）

中英双语版 编辑委员会

主任委员

王　辰

委　员（按姓氏笔画排序）

王　洁	王伊龙	王建祥	巴　一	代华平	宁　光	宁晓红	朱　兰
任景怡	刘海鹰	李小鹰	李梦涛	李雪梅	杨爱明	张福杰	郑金刚
房静远	赵　晶	赵明辉	郝　伟	姜　辉	栗占国	贾继东	夏维波
黄　慧	黄晓军	曹　彬	彭　斌	潘　慧			

第 1 分册　内科学概论·呼吸与危重症医学·术前和术后照护
　　　　　主译　王　辰　代华平　赵　晶　黄　慧

第 2 分册　心血管疾病
　　　　　主译　郑金刚　任景怡

第 3 分册　肾脏疾病
　　　　　主译　李雪梅　赵明辉

第 4 分册　胃肠疾病·肝脏与胆道系统疾病
　　　　　主译　房静远　杨爱明　贾继东

第 5 分册　血液疾病
　　　　　主译　黄晓军　王建祥

第 6 分册　肿瘤疾病
　　　　　主译　王　洁　巴　一

第 7 分册　内分泌疾病与代谢疾病·女性健康·男性健康·骨与骨矿物质代谢疾病
　　　　　主译　宁　光　朱　兰　姜　辉　夏维波　潘　慧

第 8 分册　肌肉骨骼与结缔组织疾病
　　　　　主译　栗占国　李梦涛

第 9 分册　感染性疾病
　　　　　主译　刘海鹰　张福杰　曹　彬

第 10 分册　神经疾病·老年医学·缓和医疗·酒精和物质使用
　　　　　主译　彭　斌　王伊龙　李小鹰　宁晓红　郝　伟

医学名词审定指导

任慧玲　李晓瑛　冀玉静　张燕舞　李军莲

中英双语版 序言

让我国医学生与国际医学生站在同一起跑线上的首要之事，是为其提供具有世界先进水平的标准教材。我们应争取使每一位医学生都能接触到内容经典、充分代表现代医学水平的国际权威原文教材并力求准确翻译，提供原文与中文双语对照版本，使医学生和医生在学习中形成双语医学词语、概念、概念间逻辑及由此构成的医学知识体系。在这样的思想驱动下，国际经典内科学教科书《希氏内科学精要（第10版）》中英双语版应运而生。

《希氏内科学》原著以其论述严谨准确、系统全面，被誉为"标准的内科学参考书"。自1927年首次出版以来，在内科学领域渐享世界级声誉，成为全球众多优秀医学院校，包括哈佛医学院、斯坦福大学医学院、约翰斯·霍普金斯大学医学院、牛津大学医学部、剑桥大学医学院、墨尔本大学医学院、新加坡国立大学医学院及多伦多大学医学院等普遍采用的内科学参考书。首版《希氏内科学精要》则诞生于1986年，旨在凝炼其全本的精华和要点，以最为简洁明确的方式向以医学生为主体的医学界精辟传达《希氏内科学》的核心信息，包括书中所体现出的人文精神。此后，每版精要本都力求凝炼地反映当时最新医学成果和医疗实践指南，愈来愈成为各国医学生、住院医师、专培医师及教师学习和传授内科学的主要教本，在世界医学教材体系中居引领地位。《希氏内科学》和《希氏内科学精要》两个版本不仅在英语国家被广泛使用，更被翻译为葡萄牙语、西班牙语、希腊语、意大利语、日语、简体中文版，为全球医学界广泛采用。

中国的医学生、住院医师、专培医师需要培养国际专业信息获取能力。将精要本原文引进并准确翻译，以中英文对照的形式呈现，便于读者进行双语对照阅读和学习，使之在学习理解国际标准医学内容的同时，学习好中英文医学词语，为国际医学交流打好基础。相信此举对于提高我国的医学教育水平，培养国际型医学人才至为有益。

《希氏内科学精要》精练地涵盖了内科学的所有主要领域，包括心血管疾病、呼吸疾病与危重症、消化疾病、肾脏疾病、内分泌和代谢疾病、风湿疾病、血液疾病、肿瘤、感染性疾病、神经与老年疾病等，构建了较为系统的知识体系。在翻译引进过程中，我们遵循将相关内容集中的原则，将原书按系统器官拆分为十个分册，使其更具有专科阅读的对应性，以更加灵活轻便的形式为读者提供多样化的阅读选择。

为确保译文质量，我们在译者遴选上采取了严谨的标准。从《希氏内科学（第26版）》翻译团队中择优选取责任心强、译文优质的译者，同时吸纳了临床医学专业"101"计划核心教材的编者团队。每个分册均由主译专家带领各自译者团队完成翻译、审校、交叉互审、通审四级审校工作。这些译者具备扎实的英语与专业能力，他们在翻译过程中，深入理解原文，准确阐述作者思想，并多角度审视译文的准确性、流畅性与风格一致性，确保译文的忠实性、规范性与可读性，在不同的语言和文化间架起坚实的桥梁。尤其值得称赞的是，对原著中疏漏或不够完善之处，译文中以"译者注"的形式加以适当解释和说明，使译文内容在忠实于原著的基础上更为准确。

本书读者定位于具有一定学习能力和基础的高等医学院校医学专业8年制、5年制学生以及相关医学专业人员，可作为医务人员的内科学参考书、住院医师规范化培训和专科医师规范化培训辅导教材、研究生入学考试辅导教材、内科学教师参考书、内科学各专科医师复习回顾其他专科知识的重要读本。

呼吸与危重症医学教授
中国医学科学院院长
北京协和医学院校长
2024年11月

对学习者，教科书重要。
对学医者，内科学重要。
世界上的内科学教科书，
首推《希氏内科学精要》。

中文是中国医生的主要执业用语。
英文是国际医学交流的主要文字。
学习医学，当以双语对应阅读为好。
如此，可获纵横国际之效。

本书力求有助于此。

In Memoriam

Thomas E. Andreoli, MD

Dr. Thomas Andreoli, along with Drs. Lloyd Hollingsworth (Holly) Smith, Jr., Fred Plum, and Charles C.J. Carpenter, was one of the four founding editors of *Cecil Essentials of Medicine*. He served as editor for editions one through eight before he passed away on April 14, 2009. Dr. Andreoli was born in the Bronx, New York, in 1935, attended Catholic primary and high schools, and graduated from St. Vincent College and the Georgetown School of Medicine. He trained as a resident at Duke University under legendary Chair of Medicine Dr. Eugene Stead, who recognized him as a brilliant physician and scientist and encouraged his research career. Dr. Andreoli received his research training at the NIH and then in the laboratory of Dr. Tosteson at Duke. His research focused on the biochemical and biophysical properties of renal tubular cell membranes and their role in water and electrolyte transport. He made fundamental discoveries on the normal renal physiology, illuminating the way to subsequent work by many others on renal health and disease. His research was recognized with numerous awards and election to honorific societies both in the United States and in Europe. Dr. Andreoli also served as editor of *The American Journal of Physiology: Renal Physiology* and Editor in Chief of *Kidney International*.

Tom's national prominence and leadership qualities were recognized early in his career when he became head of Nephrology at the University of Alabama in Birmingham. There he helped faculty and trainees develop outstanding research, organized clinical services, and created a hemodialysis program to build one of the outstanding Divisions of Nephrology in the country. In 1979, Dr. Andreoli was appointed Chair of the Department of Internal Medicine at the University of Texas, Houston, where he assembled an outstanding faculty focused on research, clinical care, and teaching. In 1988, he accepted the position as Chairman of Internal Medicine at the University of Arkansas School of Medicine, a position he held until his death. There he again assembled a distinguished faculty who were outstanding researchers but also dedicated to outstanding clinical care and teaching. Morning report and clinical rounds with Dr. Andreoli were rigorous and riveting, focusing on the individual patient, not only their diagnoses and treatment but also on each patient's personal concerns and well-being. Dr. Andreoli was revered by medical students, his house staff, faculty, and colleagues, and I (EJW) personally can attest to what he regarded as his most cherished role—the mentorship and education of the next generation of physicians.

One of Dr. Andreoli's great interests was *Cecil Essentials of Medicine*, for which he was the editor/chief editor for eight of its ten editions, an interest that reflected his commitment to the education of students, house staff, and other physicians in the "essentials" of Internal Medicine.

Dr. Andreoli was devoted to his family. He was married to Elizabeth Berglund Andreoli from 1987 until his death. He was previously married to Dr. Kathleen Gainor Andreoli, mother of his three children and their ten grandchildren. Being of Italian ancestry and from Bronx, New York, it is not surprising that Dr. Andreoli was a passionate fan of the New York Yankees, Italian opera, which he could sing in Italian, and Frank Sinatra.

Dr. Andreoli's legacy lives on in his numerous previous students, house staff, colleagues, and in this book.

缅 怀

托马斯·安德里奥利博士

托马斯·安德里奥利（Thomas E. Andreoli）博士携手李奥德·霍灵斯沃斯·史密斯［Lloyd Hollingsworth（Holly）Smith］博士、弗雷德·普拉姆（Fred Plum）博士和查尔斯·卡彭特（Charles C.J. Carpenter）博士同为《希氏内科学精要》的创始编者。他在2009年4月14日去世前，曾担任该书第1至第8版的编者。安德里奥利博士于1935年出生于美国纽约布朗克斯区，就读于天主教小学和中学，后毕业于圣文森特学院和乔治城大学医学院。他在杜克大学医学院接受住院医师培训期间师从著名内科主任尤金·斯特德（Eugene Stead）博士，后者将其视为杰出的医生和科学家，并鼓励他投身科研事业。安德里奥利博士在美国国立卫生研究院接受科研训练后，前往杜克大学托斯特森（Tosteson）博士的实验室继续深造。他重点研究肾小管细胞膜的生化和生物物理特性及其在水和电解质转运中所发挥的作用。他在正常肾脏生理学方面的重要发现为后续关于肾脏健康和疾病的研究铺平了道路。安德里奥利博士的研究工作荣获多个学术奖项，并入选美国和欧洲的多个荣誉学会。他还担任《美国生理学杂志：肾脏生理学篇》（The American Journal of Physiology: Renal Physiology）的编辑以及《国际肾脏杂志》（Kidney International）的主编。

安德里奥利博士担任阿拉巴马大学伯明翰分校肾脏病学系主任后不久，即因其杰出领导力而赢得全美业内声誉。他帮助本校师生们取得科研突破，负责临床业务的组织实施，并因开创血液透析业务而使该科跻身全美顶级肾脏内科之列。1979年，安德里奥利博士被任命为得克萨斯大学休斯敦分校内科学系主任，他在该系组建了一支科研、临床诊疗和教学并重的优秀教职团队。自1988年起，他担任阿肯色大学医学院内科学系主任，直至辞世。在这里他再次组建了一支卓越的教职团队，他们不仅科研工作出色，临床诊疗和教学工作也出类拔萃。安德里奥利博士带领的晨会报告和查房非常严谨而引人入胜，不仅尽心竭力于每位患者的诊断和治疗，还关注到他们每个人的个体情况和福祉。安德里奥利博士深受医学生、住院医师、教职人员和同事的崇敬，我（EJW）可以证明，他最珍视的角色当属培养和教育下一代医生。

安德里奥利博士对《希氏内科学精要》倾注了满腔热忱，先后担任了该书10版中8版的编者/主编，践行他为医学生、住院医师和其他各科医生们传授内科学"精要"的承诺。

安德里奥利博士高度重视家庭。他与第二任妻子伊丽莎白·伯格兰德·安德里奥利（Elizabeth Berglund Andreoli）的婚姻从1987年延续到辞世。他与第一任妻子凯瑟琳·盖娜·安德里奥利（Kathleen Gainor Andreoli）博士育有三个子女和十个孙辈。作为意大利裔和纽约布朗克斯人，安德里奥利博士是纽约洋基队、意大利歌剧（他能用意大利语演唱）和美国著名歌手、演员、主持人弗兰克·辛纳屈（Frank Sinatra）的忠实拥趸。安德里奥利博士将永远被他的众多学生、住院医师和同事怀念，并因本书而流芳百世。

In Memoriam

Charles C.J. Carpenter, MD

Dr. Charles C.J. Carpenter joined Drs. Thomas Andreoli, Lloyd Hollingsworth Smith, Jr., and Fred Plum as a founder of *Cecil Essentials of Medicine*. He served as editor for seven editions and was followed in that role by Dr. Ivor Benjamin and then Dr. Edward Wing. Sadly, Chuck passed away on March 19, 2020, surrounded by his wife and children. He was Professor Emeritus of Medicine at The Warren Alpert Medical School of Brown University and Physician-in-Chief Emeritus at The Miriam Hospital.

Chuck was born in Savannah, Georgia, on January 5, 1931. He attended college at Princeton and medical school at Johns Hopkins where he also did his house staff training, including chief residency, and then joined the Johns Hopkins faculty. With his young family, he travelled to Calcutta, India, where he carried out landmark studies for the treatment of cholera.

Before coming to Brown in 1986, he was Chair of Medicine at Baltimore City Hospital and Case Western Reserve University.

His contributions to medical science and clinical care were many. While in Calcutta, using basic scientific evidence coupled with practical approaches, Dr. Carpenter developed "oral rehydration therapy" to address the cholera epidemic there. This treatment has saved millions of lives. While at Case, one of his innovations was to develop the nation's first Division of Geographic Medicine because of his strong belief that all physicians should be medical citizens of the world. In 1987, as he became deeply involved in the clinical management of persons living with HIV, he initiated a unique program in which Brown University faculty and trainees assumed responsibility for all HIV care in the Rhode Island State prison system.

Dr. Carpenter served as Chairman of the American Board of Internal Medicine and President of the Association of American Physicians. He has been a member of the NIH AIDS Executive Committee, the National Advisory Allergy and Infectious Diseases Council, and the USPHS AIDS Task Force. He was Chair of the Antiretroviral Treatment Panel of the International AIDS Society-USA and authored their recommendations on antiretroviral treatment. He also served as Chair of the Treatment Committee to evaluate the President's Emergency Plan for HIV/AIDS Relief. He became the director of the Brown University International Health Institute and the director of the Lifespan/Brown Center for AIDS Research with several Boston hospitals.

Throughout his career, Dr. Carpenter was the recipient of many international, national, and regional awards, accepting each with characteristic humility. With both small and large groups of learners, Chuck made certain that every member of his team was well educated, and each felt that they contributed to the well-being of their patients. His ability to sit calmly at the bedside, hold the patient's hand, comfort them, and listen in a genuinely focused way, influenced so many physicians. He was truly grateful for the opportunity to care for those less fortunate than he, and the feeling of being privileged to do so was clearly transmitted to all. Dr. Carpenter was a wonderful blend of profound compassion combined with the adherence to scholarship and teaching. Sir William Osler wrote that physicians should "Do the kind thing and do it first." Chuck lived by this precept. Vigor and insight characterized his approach to clinical and ethical challenges, always with younger colleagues at his side. In a recent tribute to him, many emphasized that Dr. Carpenter dedicated his life to his patients, many of whom were the most vulnerable members of society. We hope that we will have some of his strength and use his example as our compass as we are challenged to reduce suffering and improve the health of all for whom we are responsible.

He is survived by his wife of 61 years, Sally; three sons, Charles, Murray, and Andrew; and seven grandchildren.

缅 怀

查尔斯·卡彭特博士

查尔斯·卡彭特（Charles C.J. Carpenter）博士与 托马斯·安德里奥利（Thomas E. Andreoli）博士、李奥德·霍灵斯沃斯·史密斯（Lloyd Hollingsworth Smith）博士和弗雷德·普拉姆（Fred Plum）博士共同开创了《希氏内科学精要》。他共担任了7版的编者，嗣后由艾弗·本杰明（Ivor Benjamin）博士和爱德华·温（Edward Wing）博士接任。查尔斯·卡彭特博士于2020年3月19日在妻子和子女们的陪伴下辞世。他曾担任布朗大学沃伦·阿尔珀特医学院的内科学系名誉教授和米里亚姆医院的名誉主任医师。

查尔斯·卡彭特博士于1931年1月5日出生于美国佐治亚州萨凡纳市。他在普林斯顿大学获得学士学位后进入约翰斯·霍普金斯大学医学院，并完成了包括住院总医师在内的住院医师培训，随后加入了约翰斯·霍普金斯大学的教职团队。他曾携妻子和年幼的孩子前往印度加尔各答，在当地对霍乱的治疗进行了具有里程碑意义的研究工作。

在1986年入职布朗大学之前，他曾担任巴尔的摩市医院和凯斯西储大学医学院的内科学主任。

他在医学科学研究和临床诊疗领域建树颇多。在加尔各答期间，基于基础科学证据及临床实践，查尔斯·卡彭特博士开创了"口服补液疗法"以遏制当地的霍乱疫情。这一疗法拯救了数百万人的生命。秉承医生无国界的世界公民理念，他在凯斯西储大学做了一项开创性工作，建立了美国首个地缘医学部（研究地理环境因素对人体健康和疾病影响的学科）。1987年，他深度参与人类免疫缺陷病毒（HIV）携带者的临床管理，并发起了一个独特的项目——由布朗大学教职团队和医学生们承担罗德岛州监狱系统内所有艾滋病相关诊疗工作。

查尔斯·卡彭特博士曾担任美国内科医师委员会主席和美国医师协会主席。他曾是美国国立卫生研究院艾滋病行政委员会、美国国家过敏与传染病咨询委员会以及公共卫生服务部艾滋病工作组的成员。他还曾担任国际艾滋病学会-美国分会抗逆转录病毒治疗组主席，并撰写了抗逆转录病毒治疗建议。他还担任过艾滋病治疗委员会主席，该委员会负责评估美国总统防治艾滋病紧急救援计划；曾担任布朗大学国际健康研究所所长，以及大学与多家波士顿当地医院合办的生命周期/布朗大学艾滋病研究中心主任。

查尔斯·卡彭特博士在职业生涯中获得过诸多国际性、全美和地区性奖项，同时展现其谦逊品格。无论学员人数多寡，查尔斯·卡彭特博士都会确保人人都能受到良好教育，并让他们感到自己也对患者的健康做出了贡献。他能够安静地坐在病床边，握住患者的手，安慰他们，并全神贯注地听取患者倾诉，这一举动深深地感染了许多医生。他十分珍视诊治不幸染病者的机会，并且能够将这种殊荣感传递给所有人。查尔斯·卡彭特博士完美地融汇了对患者的宅心仁厚与对学术和教学的坚守。威廉·奥斯勒（William Osler）爵士曾写道，医生应该"行善事，为人先"，而这正是查尔斯·卡彭特博士一生奉行的信条。他在面对临床和伦理挑战时充满活力和洞察力，始终重视提携年轻同事。许多人的悼词中都重点指出，查尔斯·卡彭特博士将毕生致力于患者福祉，其中许多人属于社会上最弱势群体。我们希望，在我们面临减少患者痛苦及改善其健康状况的挑战时，能够拥有他的力量，并以他为榜样获得指引。

查尔斯·卡彭特博士与妻子萨丽（Sally）共度了61年的婚姻时光，育有查尔斯（Charles）、穆雷（Murray）和安德鲁（Andrew）三子以及七个孙辈。

ABOUT THE EDITORS

Dr. Edward J. Wing was an editor of *Cecil Essentials of Medicine,* editions 8 and 9, and is the lead editor of edition 10. He graduated from Williams College in 1967 and from the Harvard Medical School in 1971. He was a resident in Internal Medicine at the Peter Bent Brigham and completed an Infectious Diseases Fellowship at Stanford University. Joining the faculty at the University of Pittsburgh in 1975, he focused his NIH-funded research on mechanisms of cell-mediated immunity as well as various clinical aspects of Infectious Diseases. From 1990 to 1998, the University and UPMC appointed him as Physician-in-Chief at Montefiore Hospital, then Chief of Infectious Diseases, and finally Interim Chair of Medicine.

In 1998, Dr. Wing became Chair of Medicine at Brown University (1998–2008) where he consolidated the department across hospitals, practice plans, and training programs. As Dean of Medicine and Biological Sciences at Brown University (2008–2013) he strengthened ties with affiliated hospitals (Lifespan and Care New England), increased research, and oversaw the construction of a new medical school building. International exchange programs with medical schools in Kenya, the Dominican Republic, and Haiti were established during his years as chairman and dean. Dr. Wing has cared for patients with HIV since the beginning of the epidemic in outpatient clinics. He continues to be active in research, clinical care, and teaching.

Dr. Fred J. Schiffman, who along with Dr. Edward Wing is editor of *Cecil Essentials of Medicine,* 10th edition, attended Wagner College and then the New York University School of Medicine, from which he graduated in 1973. He performed his early house staff training at Yale-New Haven Hospital and then spent two years at the National Cancer Institute. He returned to Yale as Chief Medical Resident followed by a hematology fellowship. He became Medical Director of Yale's Primary Care Center before coming to Brown University in 1983, where he has been a leader in the medical residency program as well as Associate Physician-in-Chief at The Miriam Hospital.

Dr. Schiffman holds The Sigal Family Professorship in Humanistic Medicine at The Warren Alpert Medical School of Brown University. His scholarly interests include the structure and function of the human spleen and the intersection of the arts and medical care. He has directed or championed many projects and programs, including those that encourage and reinforce wellness and resilience in patients, families, and caregivers. He began a novel program that places medical students and physicians with other nonmedical professionals as they share in the viewing of works of art in the Museum of the Rhode Island School of Design. Dr. Schiffman recently led a Brown University edX course entitled, "Artful Medicine: Art's Power to Enrich Patient Care," with worldwide participation. Dr. Schiffman has also edited texts on hematologic pathophysiology, consultative hematology, and the anemias.

原著主编

爱德华·温（Edward J. Wing）博士是《希氏内科学精要》第 8 版和第 9 版的编者，以及第 10 版的主编。他先后于 1967 年和 1971 年毕业于威廉姆斯学院和哈佛医学院。他曾在彼得·本特·布里格姆医院任内科住院医师，后在斯坦福大学完成了传染病学的专科医师（Fellowship）课程。自 1975 年加入匹兹堡大学医学院以来，他通过美国国立卫生研究院资助的研究项目，探索细胞介导免疫的机制以及传染病学各领域的临床诊疗工作。1990—1998 年期间，他先后被匹兹堡大学及其医学中心任命为蒙特菲奥里医院的主任医师、传染病科主任，后担任内科临聘主任。

1998 年起，温博士担任布朗大学医学院的内科主任（1998—2008 年）。在此期间，他在不同医院、实践计划和培训项目间对内科进行整合。在担任布朗大学医学与生物科学院院长（2008—2013 年）期间，他加强了与各附属医院（Lifespan 医院和 Care New England 医院）间的联系，提升了科研工作的水准，并为医学院建成了一座新楼。在担任主任和院长期间，他还建立了与肯尼亚、多米尼加共和国和海地的医学院的国际交流项目。温博士自艾滋病流行初期便在门诊诊治艾滋病患者，并始终工作在科研、临床和教学一线。

弗雷德·谢夫曼（Fred J. Schiffman）博士与爱德华·温（Edward Wing）博士共同担任《希氏内科学精要》第 10 版的主编。他就读于瓦格纳学院，随后进入纽约大学医学院，并于 1973 年毕业。他在耶鲁大学附属纽黑文医院接受早期住院医师培训，随后在美国国家癌症研究所工作了两年。回到耶鲁大学后，他担任住院总医师，然后完成了血液学专科医师课程，随后成为耶鲁初级保健中心医学主任。他于 1983 年入职布朗大学，领导医学住院医师项目并担任米里亚姆医院的副主任医师。

谢夫曼博士担任布朗大学沃伦·阿尔珀特医学院人文医学系的西格尔家庭医学教授。他的学术兴趣涵盖人体脾脏的结构和功能，以及艺术与医疗的交叉融合。他主持或参与了许多项目和计划，其中包括许多旨在鼓励和加强患者、家人和医护人员的福祉与康复能力的项目。他所创办的一个新项目可以让医学生和医生与其他非医学专业人士一起，共同欣赏罗德岛设计学院博物馆的艺术作品。谢夫曼博士近期还主持了布朗大学名为"艺术与医学：艺术赋能患者照护"的 edX 课程，此课程的参与者来自全球多个国家。谢夫曼博士还出版了有关血液病理生理学、血液科会诊和贫血的著作。

原著者名单

Jinnette Dawn Abbott, MD
Rajiv Agarwal, MD
Marwa Al-Badri, MD
Hyeon-Ju Ryoo Ali, MD
Jason M. Aliotta, MD
Khaldoun Almhanna, MD, MPH
Mohanad T. Al-Qaisi, MD
Zuhal Arzomand, MD
Akwi W. Asombang, MD, MPH
Su N. Aung, MD, MPH
Christopher G. Azzoli, MD
Christina Bandera, MD
Debasree Banerjee, MD
Mashal Batheja, MD
Jeffrey J. Bazarian, MD, MPH
Selim R. Benbadis, MD
Ivor J. Benjamin, MD, FAHA, FACC
Eric Benoit, MD
Marcie G. Berger, MD
Clemens Bergwitz, MD
Nancy Berliner, MD
Jeffrey S. Berns, MD
Pooja Bhadbhade, DO
Ratna Bhavaraju-Sanka, MD
Tanmayee Bichile, MD
Ariel E. Birnbaum, MD
Charles M. Bliss, Jr., MD
Andrew S. Blum, MD, PhD
Bryan J. Bonder, MD
Russell Bratman, MD
Glenn D. Braunstein, MD
Alma M. Guerrero Bready, MD
Richard Bungiro, PhD
Anna Marie Burgner, MD, MEHP
Jonathan Cahill, MD
Andrew Canakis, DO
Benedito A. Carneiro, MD, MS
Brian Casserly, MD
Abdullah Chahin, MD, MA, MSc
Philip A. Chan, MD
Kimberle Chapin, MD
William P. Cheshire, Jr., MD
Waihong Chung, MD, PhD
Emma Ciafaloni, MD

Joaquin E. Cigarroa, MD
Michael P. Cinquegrani, MD
Andreea Coca, MD, MPH
Harvey Jay Cohen, MD
Scott Cohen, MD, MPH
Beatrice P. Concepcion, MD, MS
Nathan T. Connell, MD, MPH
Maria Constantinou, MD
Roberto Cortez, MD
Timothy J. Counihan, MD, FRCPI
Anne Haney Cross, MD
Cheston B. Cunha, MD, FACP
Joanne S. Cunha, MD
Susan Cu-Uvin, MD
Noura M. Dabbouseh, MD
Kwame Dapaah-Afriyie, MD, MBA
Erin M. Denney-Koelsch, MD
Andre De Souza, MD
An S. De Vriese, MD, PhD
Neal D. Dharmadhikari, MD
Leah Dickstein, MD
Don Dizon, MD, FACP, FASCO
Robyn T. Domsic, MD, MPH
Kim A. Eagle, MD
Michael G. Earing, MD
Pamela Egan, MD
Wafik S. El-Deiry, MD, PhD, FACP
Mitchell S. V. Elkind, MD, MS
Tarra B. Evans, MD
Michael B. Fallon, MD
Dimitrios Farmakiotis, MD
Francis A. Farraye, MD
Ronan Farrell, MD
Panayotis Fasseas, MD, FACC
Mary Anne Fenton, MD
Fernando C. Fervenza, MD, PhD
Sean Fine, MD
Arkadiy Finn, MD
Timothy Flanigan, MD
Brisas M. Flores, MD
Andrew E. Foderaro, MD
Theodore C. Friedman, MD, PhD
Joseph Metmowlee Garland, MD, AAHIVM

Eric J. Gartman, MD
Abdallah Geara, MD
Raul Macias Gil, MD
Timothy Gilligan, MD, FASCO
Michael Raymond Goggins, MB BCh BAO, MRCPI
Geetha Gopalakrishnan, MD
Vidya Gopinath, MD
Susan L. Greenspan, MD, FACP
Osama Hamdy, MD, PhD
Johanna Hamel, MD
Sajeev Handa, MD, SFHM
Mitchell T. Heflin, MD, MHS
Robert G. Holloway, MD, MPH
Christopher S. Huang, MD
Zilla Hussain, MD
T. Alp Ikizler, MD
Iris Isufi, MD
Carlayne E. Jackson, MD
Paul G. Jacob, MD, MPH
Matthew D. Jankowich, MD
Niels V. Johnsen, MD, MPH
Jessica E. Johnson, MD
Rayford R. June, MD
Tareq Kheirbek, MD, ScM, FACS
Alok A. Khorana, MD, FACP, FASCO
Sena Kilic, MD
David Kim, MD
James Kleczka, MD
James R. Klinger, MD
Patrick Koo, MD, ScM
Pooja Koolwal, MD
Mary P. Kotlarczyk, PhD
Nicole M. Kuderer, MD
Awewura Kwara, MD
Jennifer M. Kwon, MD, MPH
Richard A. Lange, MD, MBA
Jerome Larkin, MD
Alfred I. Lee, MD, PhD
Daniel J. Levine, MD
David E. Lewandowski, MD
Kelly V. Liang, MD, MS
Kimberly P. Liang, MD, MS
David R. Lichtenstein, MD

扫描二维码了解更多信息

Douglas W. Lienesch, MD
Geoffrey S.F. Ling, MD, PhD
Ester Little, MD, FACP
Yi Liu, MD
Nicole L. Lohr, MD, PhD
John R. Lonks, MD, FACP, FIDSA, FSHEA
Gary H. Lyman, MD, MPH
Jeffrey M. Lyness, MD
Shane Lyons, MD, MRCPI, MRCP(UK)
Diana Maas, MD
Talha A. Malik, MD, MSPH
Sonia Manocha, MD
Susan Manzi, MD, MPH
Frederick J. Marshall, MD
F. Dennis McCool, MD
Russell J. McCulloh, MD
Kelly McGarry, MD, FACP
Eavan Mc Govern, MD, PhD
Robin L. McKinney, MD
Anthony Mega, MD
Shivang Mehta, MD
Douglas F. Milam, MD
Maria D. Mileno, MD
Abhinav Kumar Misra, MBBS, MD
Orson W. Moe, MD
Niveditha Mohan, MBBS
Larry W. Moreland, MD
Alan R. Morrison, MD, PhD
Steven F. Moss, MD
Christopher J. Mullin, MD, MHS
Sinéad M. Murphy, MB, BCh, MD, FRCPI
Sagarika Nallu, MD, FAAP, FAAN, FAASM
Javier A. Neyra, MD, MSCS
Ghaith Noaiseh, MD

Thomas A. Ollila, MD
Steven M. Opal, MD
Biff F. Palmer, MD
Jen Jung Pan, MD, PhD
Anna Papazoglou, MD
Aric Parnes, MD
Nayan M. Patel, DO, MPH
Ari Pelcovits, MD
Mark A. Perazella, MD
Michael F. Picco, MD, PhD
Kate E. Powers, DO
Laura A. Previll, MD, MPH
Nilum Rajora, MD
Adolfo Ramirez-Zamora, MD
John Reagan, MD
Rebecca Reece, MD
Harlan Rich, MD, AGAF, FACP
Jennifer H. Richman, MD
Lisa R. Rogers, DO
Ralph Rogers, MD
Michal G. Rose, MD
James A. Roth, MD
Sharon Rounds, MD
Jason C. Rubenstein, MD
Abbas Rupawala, MD
Jenna Sarvaideo, DO
Ramesh Saxena, MD, PhD
Fred J. Schiffman, MD, MACP
Ruth B. Schneider, MD
Kristin A. Seaborg, MD
Anil Seetharam, MD
Stuart Seropian, MD
Jigme Michael Sethi, MD
Sanjeev Sethi, MD, PhD
Elizabeth Shane, MD
Esseim Sharma, MD

Shani Shastri, MD, MPH
Barry S. Shea, MD
Lauren Shevell, MD, MPH
Joseph A. Smith, Jr., MD
Robert J. Smith, MD
Davendra P.S. Sohal, MD, MPH
Christopher Song, MD, FACC
Thomas Sperry, MD
Jeffrey M. Statland, MD
Emily M. Stein, MD
Jennifer L. Strande, MD, PhD
Rochelle Strenger, MD
Thomas R. Talbot, MD, MPH
Christopher G. Tarolli, MD, MSEd
Yael Tarshish, MD
Pushpak Taunk, MD
Philip Tsoukas, MD
Allan R. Tunkel, MD, PhD
Jeffrey M. Turner, MD
Zoe G.S. Vazquez, MD
Stacie A. F. Vela, MD
Paul M. Vespa, MD, FCCM, FAAN, FANA, FNCS
Wanpen Vongpatanasin, MD
Marcella D. Walker, MD
Eunice S. Wang, MD
Sharmeel K. Wasan, MD
Thomas J. Weber, MD
Brandon J. Wilcoxson, MD
Edward J. Wing, MD, FACP, FIDSA
Ellice Wong, MD
John J. Wysolmerski, MD
Rayan Yousefzai, MD
Thomas R. Ziegler, MD
Rebecca Zon, MD

ACKNOWLEDGMENTS

Dr. Schiffman and I wish to thank first of all, the authors of the 128 chapters that make up the tenth edition of *Cecil Essentials of Medicine*. They have worked diligently to compose the material for each chapter and apply their mastery as they added the newest information, in clear language, to the text. Their efforts are apparent in the excellence of the book, and we are immensely grateful for their work. We wish to also thank Marybeth Thiel, Jennifer Ehlers, and Dan Fitzgerald from Elsevier who guided and supported our work as editors and whose expertise has made this volume possible. Finally, we are always thankful to our wives, Dr. Rena Wing and Ms. Gerri Schiffman, without whose love, support, and especially humor, this book would not have happened.

致 谢

谢夫曼博士和我首先要致谢《希氏内科学精要》第 10 版全书 128 章的各位作者。感谢他们精益求精地撰写每一章节，并运用其专业知识，以简明的语言将前沿资讯呈现在书中。正是他们的辛勤努力确保了本书的卓越地位，对他们唯有由衷的感激。我们还要感谢爱思唯尔出版集团的玛丽贝丝·蒂尔（Marybeth Thiel）、詹妮弗·埃勒斯（Jennifer Ehlers）和丹·菲茨杰拉德（Dan Fitzgerald），他们对本书的编辑工作给予了指导和支持，其专业水准保障了本书的完稿。最后，要特别感谢我们的妻子——蕾娜·温（Rena Wing）博士和盖瑞·谢夫曼（Gerri Schiffman）女士，对她们的爱和支持，特别是积极乐观的心态始终心存感激，她们为本书的圆满完成发挥了不可或缺的作用。

总目录

第 1 分册

第 1 篇　内科学概论　Introduction to Medicine
第 2 篇　呼吸与危重症医学　Pulmonary and Critical Care Medicine
第 3 篇　术前和术后照护　Preoperative and Postoperative Care

第 2 分册

心血管疾病　Cardiovascular Disease

第 3 分册

肾脏疾病　Renal Disease

第 4 分册

第 1 篇　胃肠疾病　Gastrointestinal Disease
第 2 篇　肝脏与胆道系统疾病　Diseases of the Liver and Biliary System

第 5 分册

血液疾病　Hematologic Disease

第 6 分册

肿瘤疾病　Oncologic Disease

第 7 分册

第 1 篇　内分泌疾病与代谢疾病　Endocrine Disease and Metabolic Disease
第 2 篇　女性健康　Women's Health
第 3 篇　男性健康　Men's Health
第 4 篇　骨与骨矿物质代谢疾病　Diseases of Bone and Bone Mineral Metabolism

第 8 分册

肌肉骨骼与结缔组织疾病　Musculoskeletal and Connective Tissue Disease

第 9 分册

感染性疾病　Infectious Disease

第 10 分册

第 1 篇　神经疾病　Neurologic Disease
第 2 篇　老年医学　Geriatrics
第 3 篇　缓和医疗　Palliative Care
第 4 篇　酒精和物质使用　Alcohol and Substance Use

第2分册

心血管疾病

第 2 分册译者名单

主　译

郑金刚　任景怡

译　者（按姓氏笔画排序）

马业新　华中科技大学同济医学院附属同济医院	张　恒　中国医学科学院阜外医院
王　红　华中科技大学同济医学院附属同济医院	张　斌　中国医学科学院阜外医院
王　利　中国医学科学院阜外医院	陈改玲　中日友好医院
王婧莹　哈尔滨医科大学附属第一医院	周　强　华中科技大学同济医学院附属同济医院
石　静　哈尔滨医科大学附属第一医院	周益锋　中日友好医院
任景怡　中日友好医院	周晶亮　北京大学人民医院
刘　芃　中日友好医院	郑　哲　中国医学科学院阜外医院
刘　靖　北京大学人民医院	郑金刚　中日友好医院
刘嘉慧　北京大学人民医院	钟晓丹　华中科技大学同济医学院附属同济医院
刘震宇　中国医学科学院北京协和医院	耿嘉璐　北京大学人民医院
杨晓云　华中科技大学同济医学院附属同济医院	郭义龙　海南医科大学第二附属医院
李　悦　哈尔滨医科大学附属第一医院	唐思琪　中国医学科学院北京协和医院
李依珂　中日友好医院	盛兆雪　中日友好医院
李学斌　北京大学人民医院	曾和松　华中科技大学同济医学院附属同济医院
李宗哲　华中科技大学同济医学院附属同济医院	戴晨光　哈尔滨医科大学附属第一医院
里程楠　首都医科大学附属北京安贞医院	魏　荧　哈尔滨医科大学附属第一医院
吴永健　中国医学科学院阜外医院	

第 2 分册目录

心血管疾病　Cardiovascular Disease

1　Structure and Function of the Normal Heart and Blood Vessels, 4
　心血管系统的解剖结构与功能，5

2　Evaluation of the Patient With Cardiovascular Disease, 16
　心血管疾病患者的评估，17

3　Diagnostic Tests and Procedures in the Patient With Cardiovascular Disease, 44
　心血管疾病的诊断性检查和方法，45

4　Heart Failure and Cardiomyopathy, 82
　心力衰竭与心肌病，83

5　Congenital Heart Disease, 106
　先天性心脏病，107

6　Valvular Heart Disease, 124
　心脏瓣膜病，125

7　Coronary Heart Disease, 150
　冠心病，151

8　Cardiac Arrhythmias, 194
　心律失常，195

9　Pericardial and Myocardial Disease, 242
　心包和心肌疾病，243

10　Other Cardiac Topics, 258
　其他心脏疾病，259

11　Vascular Diseases and Hypertension, 274
　血管疾病与高血压，275

索引 Index，318

CECIL ESSENTIALS OF MEDICINE

Cardiovascular Disease

Cardiovascular Disease

1. Structure and Function of the Normal Heart and Blood Vessels, 4
2. Evaluation of the Patient With Cardiovascular Disease, 16
3. Diagnostic Tests and Procedures in the Patient With Cardiovascular Disease, 44
4. Heart Failure and Cardiomyopathy, 82
5. Congenital Heart Disease, 106
6. Valvular Heart Disease, 124
7. Coronary Heart Disease, 150
8. Cardiac Arrhythmias, 194
9. Pericardial and Myocardial Disease, 242
10. Other Cardiac Topics, 258
11. Vascular Diseases and Hypertension, 274

心血管疾病

1 心血管系统的解剖结构与功能，5

2 心血管疾病患者的评估，17

3 心血管疾病的诊断性检查和方法，45

4 心力衰竭与心肌病，83

5 先天性心脏病，107

6 心脏瓣膜病，125

7 冠心病，151

8 心律失常，195

9 心包和心肌疾病，243

10 其他心脏疾病，259

11 血管疾病与高血压，275

1

Structure and Function of the Normal Heart and Blood Vessels

Nicole L. Lohr, Ivor J. Benjamin

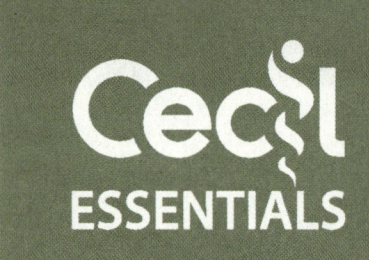

DEFINITION

The circulatory system comprises the heart, which is connected in series to the arterial and venous vascular networks. These vascular networks are arranged in parallel and connect at the level of the capillaries (Fig. 1.1). The heart is composed of two atria, which are low-pressure capacitance chambers that function to store blood during ventricular contraction (systole) and then fill the ventricles with blood during ventricular relaxation (diastole). The two ventricles are high-pressure chambers responsible for pumping blood through the lungs (right ventricle) and to the peripheral tissues (left ventricle). The left ventricle is thicker than the right, in order to generate the higher systemic pressures required for perfusion.

There are four cardiac valves that facilitate unidirectional blood flow through the heart. Each of the four valves is surrounded by a fibrous ring, or annulus, that forms part of the structural support of the heart. Atrioventricular (AV) valves separate the atria and ventricles. The mitral valve is a bileaflet valve that separates the left atrium and left ventricle. The tricuspid valve is a trileaflet valve that separates the right atrium and right ventricle. Thin, fibrous connective tissue (chordae tendineae) attaches the ventricular aspects of these valves to the papillary muscles of their respective ventricles for proper opening of the valves. Additional valves include the aortic valve that separates the left ventricle from the aorta, and the pulmonic valve that separates the right ventricle from the pulmonary artery.

A thin, double-layered membrane called the pericardium surrounds the heart. The inner, or visceral, layer adheres to the outer surface of the heart, also known as the epicardium. The outer layer is the parietal pericardium, which attaches to the sternum, vertebral column, and diaphragm to stabilize the heart in the chest. Between these two membranes is a pericardial space filled with a small amount of fluid (<50 mL). This fluid serves to lubricate contact surfaces and limit direct tissue-surface contact during myocardial contraction. A normal pericardium exerts minimal external pressure on the heart, thereby facilitating normal movement of the interventricular septum during the cardiac cycle. Too much fluid in this space (i.e., pericardial effusion) can cause impaired ventricular filling and abnormal septal movement. (Please refer to Chapter 68, "Pericardial Diseases," in ❖ *Goldman-Cecil Medicine*, 26th Edition).

CIRCULATORY PATHWAY

The purpose of the circulatory system is to bring deoxygenated blood, carbon dioxide, and other waste products from the tissues to the lungs for disposal and reoxygenation (see Fig. 1.1A). Deoxygenated blood drains from peripheral tissues through venules and veins, eventually entering the right atrium through the superior and inferior venae cavae during ventricular systole. Venous drainage from the heart enters the right atrium through the coronary sinus. During ventricular diastole, the blood in the right atrium flows across the tricuspid valve and into the right ventricle. Blood in the right ventricle is ejected across the pulmonic valve and into the main pulmonary artery, which bifurcates into the left and right pulmonary arteries and perfuses the lungs. After multiple bifurcations, blood reaches the pulmonary capillaries, where carbon dioxide is exchanged for oxygen across the alveolar-capillary membrane. Oxygenated blood then enters the left atrium from the lungs via the four pulmonary veins. Blood flows across the open mitral valve and into the left ventricle during diastole and is ejected across the aortic valve and into the aorta during systole. The blood reaches various organs, where oxygen and nutrients are exchanged for carbon dioxide and metabolic wastes, and the cycle begins again.

The heart receives its blood supply through the left and right coronary arteries, which originate in outpouchings of the aortic root called the *sinuses of Valsalva*. The left main coronary artery is a short vessel that bifurcates into the left anterior descending (LAD) and the left circumflex (LCx) coronary arteries. The LAD supplies blood to the anterior and anterolateral left ventricle through diagonal branches and to the anterior interventricular septum through septal perforator branches. The LAD travels anteriorly in the anterior interventricular groove and terminates at the cardiac apex. The LCx traverses posteriorly in the left AV groove (between left atrium and left ventricle) to perfuse the lateral aspect of the left ventricle (through obtuse marginal branches) and the left atrium. The right coronary artery (RCA) courses down the right AV groove to the *crux* of the heart, the point at which the left and right AV grooves and the inferior interventricular groove meet. The RCA gives off branches to the right atrium and acute marginal branches to the right ventricle.

The blood supply to the diaphragmatic and posterior aspects of the left ventricle varies. In 85% of individuals, the RCA bifurcates at the crux to form the posterior descending coronary artery (PDA), which travels in the inferior interventricular groove to supply the inferior left ventricle and the inferior third of the interventricular septum, and the posterior left ventricular (PLV) branches. This course is termed a *right-dominant circulation*. In 10% of individuals, the RCA terminates before reaching the crux, and the LCx supplies the PLV and PDA. This course is termed a *left-dominant circulation*. In the remaining individuals, the RCA gives rise to the PDA and the LCx gives rise to the PLV in a *co-dominant circulation*.

CONDUCTION SYSTEM

The sinoatrial (SA) node is a collection of specialized pacemaker cells, 1 to 2 cm long, located in the right atrium between the superior vena cava and the right atrial appendage (see Fig. 1.1B). The SA node is supplied by the SA nodal artery, which is a branch of the RCA in about 60% of the population and a branch of the LCx in about 40%. An

心血管系统的解剖结构与功能

郭义龙 译　王利 审校　任景怡 通审

基本概念

循环系统由心脏及与其串连的动、静脉血管网构成。动、静脉血管网大多平行分布且在毛细血管水平相互连接（图 1.1）。心脏由两个心房和两个心室组成；心房是低压容纳腔，它们的功能是在收缩期储存血液，并在舒张期将血液排入心室；心室是高压腔，右心室负责将血液排入肺部，而左心室则负责将血液输送至周围组织。左心室的心室壁比右心室厚，以至于前者能产生更高的体循环压，进而满足周围组织灌注的需求。

心脏内有 4 个瓣膜，它们的作用是引导血流以单一方向通过心脏。每个瓣膜周围都有纤维环包绕（纤维环也称为瓣环）；4 个瓣环是心脏支撑结构的重要组成部分。心房和心室由房室（AV）瓣分隔；其中，二尖瓣为双瓣叶结构，分隔左心房与左心室；三尖瓣为三瓣叶结构，分隔右心房与右心室。房室瓣的心室面通过薄的纤维结缔组织（腱索）与相应心室内的乳头肌连接，从而维持房室瓣的正常关闭（译者注：原文有误，"opening"应为"closing"）。此外，主动脉瓣分隔左心室与升主动脉，而肺动脉瓣则分隔右心室和肺动脉。

心脏表面被心包组织（双层薄膜结构）包绕。内层心包（脏层）又称心外膜，紧贴心脏外表面；外层心包又称壁层心包，附着于胸骨、脊柱和膈肌上，把心脏稳定在胸腔中。两层心包之间的腔隙为心包腔，其内含有少量心包液（< 50 ml）。心包液主要起润滑作用，它可以在心肌收缩时减少双层心包间的接触面积，降低表面摩擦力。正常心包组织对心脏的外压很低，有利于室间隔在心动周期中的正常运动。心包腔内液体增多（心包积液）可以导致心室充盈受损和室间隔运动异常（具体可参考 Goldman-Cecil Medicine 第 26 版第 68 章"心包疾病"）。

循环途径

循环系统将组织中的脱氧血液、二氧化碳等代谢废物运送至肺部，在肺内进行代谢废物清除和血液再氧合（图 1.1A）。周围组织中的脱氧血液通过微、小静脉逐级回流，并在收缩期经上、下腔静脉进入右心房。心脏本身的静脉血则经冠状静脉窦流入右心房。在心室舒张期，右心房的血液经三尖瓣口流入右心室。右心室的血液经肺动脉瓣排入主肺动脉，随后分别进入左、右肺动脉并灌注双侧肺组织。左、右肺动脉内的血液依次流经多级肺血管后进入肺毛细血管网，在此处通过肺泡-毛细血管膜进行二氧化碳和氧气交换。氧合后的血液经由四根肺静脉回流入左心房。左心房内的氧合血在舒张期经二尖瓣进入左心室，随后在收缩期经主动脉瓣进入主动脉。主动脉内的血液随后抵达不同组织器官，氧气和营养物质被交换为二氧化碳和代谢废物，血液循环再次开始。

心脏通过左冠状动脉和右冠状动脉接受血液供应，而左、右冠状动脉分别起源于主动脉根部向外突出的主动脉窦，又称为瓦氏窦（sinuses of Valsalva）。左冠状动脉主干是一条短的血管，其可发出左前降支（LAD）和左回旋支（LCx）。LAD 通过对角支给左心室前壁和前侧壁供血，同时还通过穿间隔支给前室间隔供血。LAD 沿前室间沟下行并终止于心尖部。LCx 沿左房室沟（左心房与左心室之间）向后走行并给左心室侧壁（通过钝缘支）和左心房供血。右冠状动脉（RCA）沿右房室沟下行，终止于左、右房室沟与后室间沟的交汇处（后十字交叉）。RCA 不仅给右心房供血，还通过锐缘支给右心室供血。

左心室膈面和后壁心肌供血方式存在差异。约有 85% 个体的 RCA 在心脏后十字交叉处发出后降支（PDA）和左室后支（PLV）；PDA 沿室间沟下行，给左室下壁及室间隔下 1/3 的心肌组织供血。这种冠脉供血模式被称为右优势循环（right-dominant circulation）。约有 10% 个体的 RCA 在抵达心脏后十字交叉点前便已终止，由 LCx 给 PLV 和 PDA 供血；这种冠脉供血模式被称为左优势循环（left-dominant circulation）。剩余个体的 PDA 由 RCA 发出，而 PLV 则由 LCx 发出；这种冠脉供血模式被称为均衡优势循环（co-dominant circulation）。

传导系统

窦房（SA）结由一群特殊的起搏细胞构成，长 1～2 cm，位于右心房中上腔静脉与右心耳之间的区域（图 1.1B）。窦房结的血供来源于窦房结动脉，其起源于 RCA（人群中占比 60%）或 LCx（人群中占比

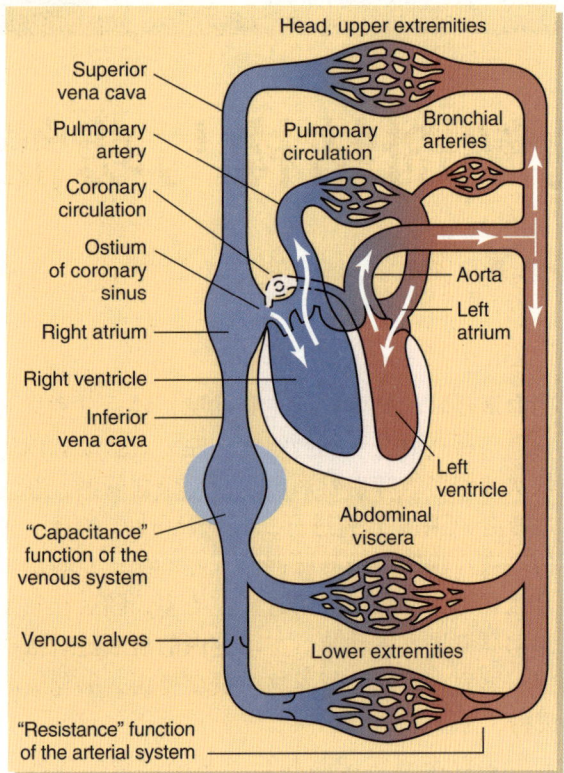

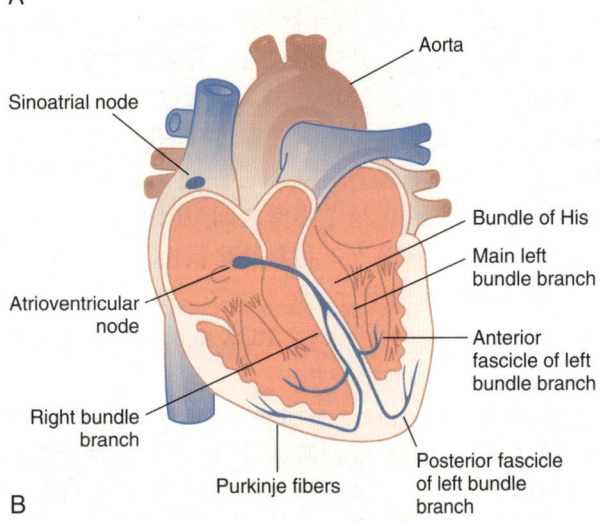

Fig. 1.1 (A) Schematic representation of the systemic and pulmonary circulatory systems. The venous system contains the greatest amount of blood at any one time and is highly distensible, accommodating a wide range of blood volumes (high capacitance). The arterial system is composed of the aorta, arteries, and arterioles. Arterioles are small muscular arteries that regulate blood pressure by changing tone (resistance). (B) A schematic representation of the cardiac conduction system.

electrical impulse originates in the SA and is conducted to the AV node by internodal tracts within the atria.

The AV node is a critical electrical interface between the atria and ventricles, because it facilitates electromechanical coupling. The AV node is located at the inferior aspect of the right atrium, between the coronary sinus and the septal leaflet of the tricuspid valve. The AV node is supplied by the AV nodal artery, which is a branch of the RCA in about 90% of the population and a branch of the LCx in 10%. Electrical impulse conduction slows through the AV node and continues to the ventricles by means of the His-Purkinje system. The increased impulse time through the AV node allows for adequate ventricular filling.

The bundle of His extends from the AV node down the membranous interventricular septum to the muscular septum, where it divides into the left and right bundle branches, finally terminating in Purkinje cells, which are specialized cells that facilitate the rapid propagation of electrical impulses. The Purkinje cells directly stimulate myocytes to contract. The right bundle and the left bundle are supplied by septal perforator branches from the LAD. The distal and posterior portion of the left bundle has an additional blood supply from the AV nodal artery (PDA origin); for that reason, it is more resistant to ischemia. Conduction can be impaired at any point, from ischemia, medications (e.g., β-blockers, calcium channel blockers), infection, or congenital abnormalities. (Please refer to Chapter 55, "Principles of Electrophysiology," in *Goldman-Cecil Medicine*, 26th Edition.) ❖

NEURAL INNERVATION

The autonomic nervous system is an integral component in the regulation of cardiac function. In general, sympathetic stimulation increases the heart rate (HR) (chronotropy) and the force of myocardial contraction (inotropy). Sympathetic stimulation commences in preganglionic neurons located within the superior five or six thoracic segments of the spinal cord. They synapse with second-order neurons in the cervical sympathetic ganglia and then propagate the signal through cardiac nerves that innervate the SA node, AV node, epicardial vessels, and myocardium. The parasympathetic system produces an opposite physiologic effect by decreasing HR and contractility. Its neural supply originates in preganglionic neurons within the dorsal motor nucleus of the medulla oblongata, which reach the heart through the vagus nerve. These efferent neural fibers synapse with second-order neurons located in ganglia within the heart that terminate in the SA node, AV node, epicardial vessels, and myocardium to decrease HR and contractility. Conversely, afferent vagal fibers from the inferior and posterior aspects of the ventricles, the aortic arch, and the carotid sinus conduct sensory information back to the medulla, which mediates important cardiac reflexes.

MYOCARDIAL STRUCTURE

The proper cellular organization of cardiac tissue (myocardium) is critical for the generation of efficient myocardial contraction. Disruptions in this structure and organization lead to cardiac dyssynchrony and arrhythmias, which cause significant morbidity and mortality. Atrial and ventricular myocytes are specialized, branching muscle cells that are connected end to end by intercalated disks. These disks aid in the transmission of mechanical tension between cells. The myocyte plasma membrane, or sarcolemma, facilitates excitation and contraction through small transverse tubules (T tubules). Subcellular features specific for myocytes include increased mitochondria number for production of adenosine triphosphate (ATP); an extensive network of intracellular tubules, called the *sarcoplasmic reticulum*, for calcium storage; and *sarcomeres*, which are myofibrils comprised of repeating units of overlapping thin actin filaments and thick myosin filaments and their regulatory proteins troponin and tropomyosin. Specialized myocardial cells form the cardiac conduction system (described earlier) and are responsible for the generation of an electrical impulse and

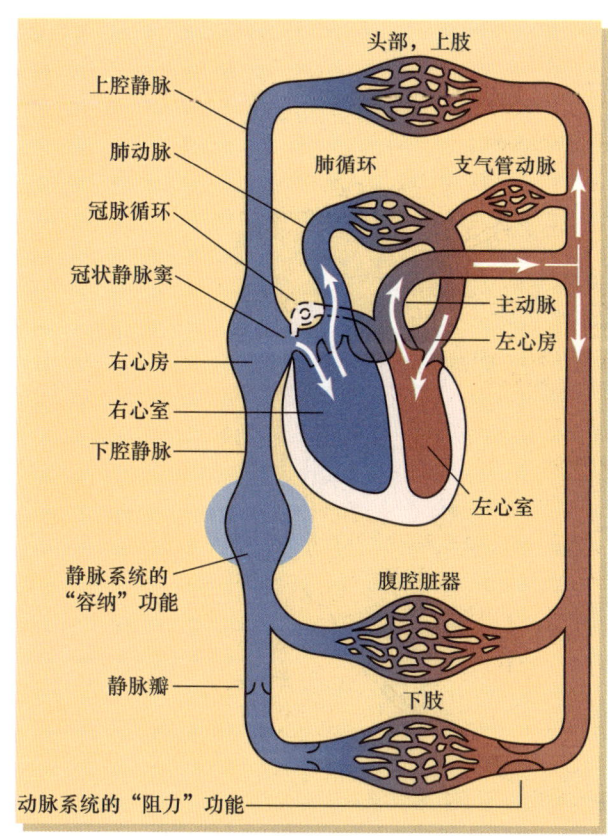

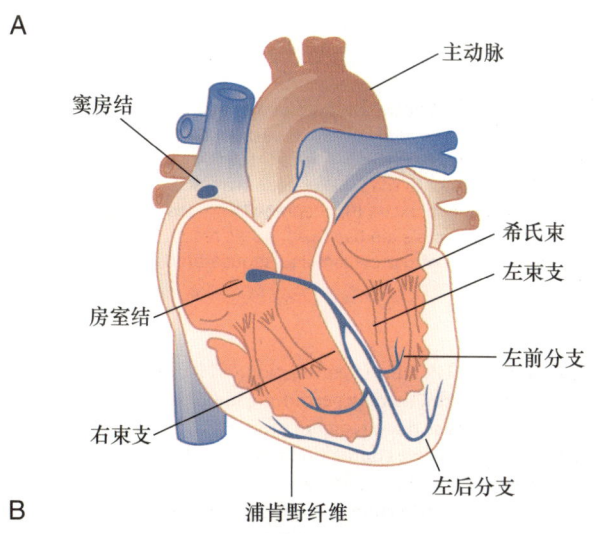

图 1.1 （A）体循环与肺循环示意图；静脉系统可随时高度扩张、最大程度地容纳血液，以此适应大范围的血容量波动（"容纳"功能）。动脉系统由主动脉、动脉和微动脉组成；微动脉具有肌性结构，可通过调节血管张力（"阻力"功能）调控血压。（B）心脏传导系统示意图

40%）。窦房结产生的心电冲动可沿心房内的结间束传导至房室结。

房室结是心电冲动由心房向心室传递的重要节点，有利于心脏的电-机械偶联。房室结位于右心房下方，冠状静脉窦与三尖瓣隔叶之间。房室结的血供来源于房室结动脉，其起源于 RCA（人群中占比约 90%）或 LCx（人群中占比约 10%）。心电冲动通过房室结减慢后由希氏束-浦肯野纤维系统传导全心室。房室结处心电冲动传导时间延长为心室充分充盈提供了必要条件。

希氏束起自房室结，经由室间隔膜部下行至室间隔肌部后分为左、右束支并终止于浦肯野细胞。浦肯野细胞是一种特殊分化的细胞，能快速传导心电冲动并直接刺激心肌细胞收缩。左、右束支由 LAD 发出的穿间隔支动脉供血。左束支的远端及后部还可额外接受房室结动脉（起源于 PDA）的血液供应；因此左束支更能耐受缺血损伤。心电冲动传导可能在任何时候受损，如缺血、药物干预（如 β 受体阻滞剂、钙通道阻滞剂）、感染和先天发育异常（具体可参考 Goldman-Cecil Medicine 第 26 版第 55 章"电生理机制"）。

神经分布

自主神经系统在心功能调节中发挥着不可或缺的作用。通常情况下，交感神经兴奋可以提高心率（变时性），增强心肌收缩力（变力性）。交感神经冲动起源于 T5、T6 胸髓节段的节前神经元。它们在颈交感神经节与二级神经元换元后通过心脏神经将神经冲动传递至窦房结、房室结、心外膜血管及心肌细胞。副交感神经具有负性调控作用，表现为减慢心率、降低心肌收缩力。副交感神经起源于延髓背侧运动神经核团的节前神经元，经迷走神经到达心脏；其传出神经纤维在心内神经节与二级神经元换元后将神经冲动传递至窦房结、房室结、心外膜血管和心肌细胞，从而减慢心率和降低心肌收缩力。同时，起自心室下壁、后壁、主动脉弓和颈动脉窦部的迷走神经传入纤维可将感觉信号传回延髓，并在一系列重要的心脏反射中发挥介导作用。

心肌结构

心肌细胞合适的细胞排布对心脏的有效收缩至关重要。心肌的组织结构破坏可导致心脏收缩不同步和心律失常，增加心脏疾病的发病率与死亡率。心房肌和心室肌细胞是特殊的、通过闰盘首尾相连的分叉肌细胞，闰盘有助于机械张力在心肌细胞之间传递。心肌细胞膜（肌纤维膜）能通过横管（T 管，T tubules）传导心电冲动并促成心肌细胞收缩。心肌细胞具有独特的亚细胞结构特征：包括线粒体数量增多，以生成更多的 ATP；大量的细胞内小管构成肌质网（sarcoplasmic reticulum），用以储存钙离子；由重叠的粗肌丝（肌球蛋白）、细肌丝（肌动蛋白）及调节蛋白（肌钙蛋白和原肌球蛋白）共同构成肌原纤维，随后由肌原纤维构成肌节（sarcomeres）。此外，由前文所述的特殊心肌

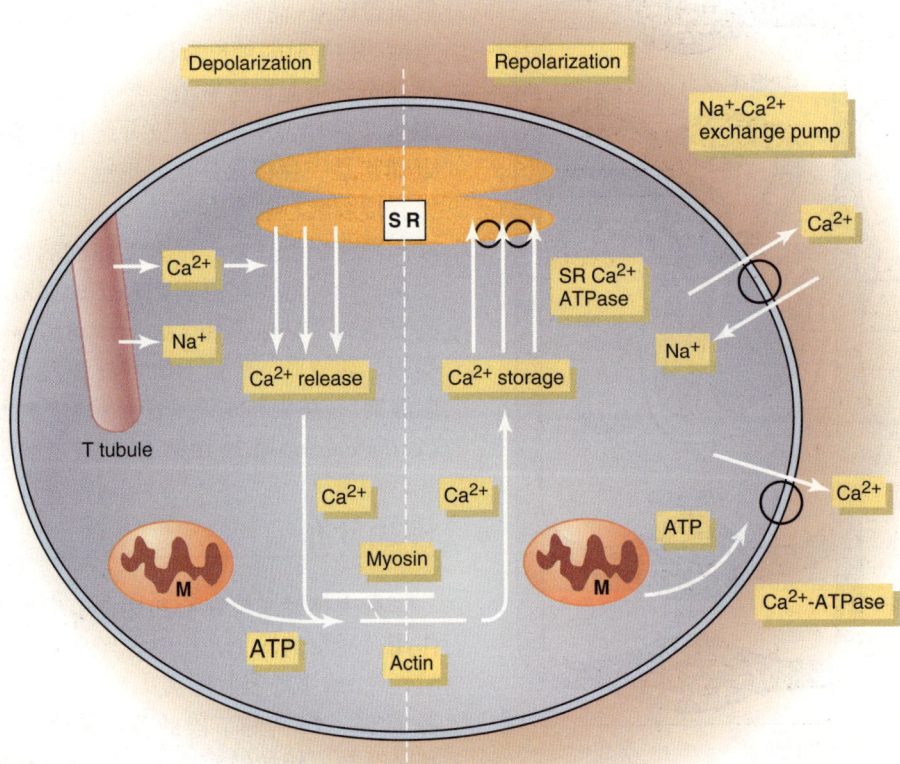

Fig. 1.2 Calcium dependence of myocardial contraction. (1) Electrical depolarization of the myocyte results in an influx of Ca^{2+} ions into the cell through channels in the T tubules. (2) This initial phase of calcium entry stimulates the release of large amounts of Ca^{2+} from the sarcoplasmic reticulum (SR). (3) The Ca^{2+} then binds to the troponin-tropomyosin complex on the actin filaments, resulting in a conformational change that facilitates the binding interaction between actin and myosin. In the presence of adenosine triphosphate (ATP), the actin-myosin association is cyclically dissociated as the thick and thin filaments slide past each other, resulting in contraction. (4) During repolarization, the Ca^{2+} is actively pumped out of the cytosol and sequestered in the SR. *ATPase*, Adenosine triphosphatase; *M*, mitochondrion.

organized propagation of that impulse to cardiac myocytes, which, in turn, respond by mechanical contraction.

MUSCLE PHYSIOLOGY AND CONTRACTION

Calcium-induced calcium release is the primary mechanism for myocyte contraction. When a depolarizing stimulus reaches the myocyte, it enters special invaginations within the sarcolemma called T tubules. These specialized channels open in response to depolarization, permitting calcium flux into the cell (Fig. 1.2). The sarcoplasmic reticulum closely proximates the T tubules, and the initial calcium current triggers the release of large amounts of calcium from the sarcoplasmic reticulum into the cell cytosol. Calcium then binds to the calcium-binding regulatory subunit, troponin C, on the actin filaments of the sarcomere, resulting in a conformational change in the troponin-tropomyosin complex. The myosin binding site on actin is now exposed, to facilitate binding of actin-myosin cross-bridges, which are necessary for cellular contraction. The energy for myocyte contraction is derived from ATP. During contraction, ATP promotes dissociation of myosin from actin, thereby permitting the sliding of thick filaments past thin filaments as the sarcomere shortens.

The force of myocyte contraction is regulated by the amount of free calcium released into the cell by the sarcoplasmic reticulum. More calcium allows for more frequent actin-myosin interactions, producing a stronger contraction. On repolarization of the sarcolemmal membrane, intracellular calcium is rapidly and actively resequestered into the sarcoplasmic reticulum, where it is stored by various proteins, including calsequestrin, until the next wave of depolarization occurs. Calcium is also extruded from the cytosol by various calcium pumps in the sarcolemma. The active removal of intracellular calcium by ATP ion pumps facilitates ventricular relaxation, which is necessary for proper ventricular filling during diastole.

Circulatory Physiology and the Cardiac Cycle

The term *cardiac cycle* describes the pressure changes within each cardiac chamber over time (Fig. 1.3). This cycle is divided into *systole*,

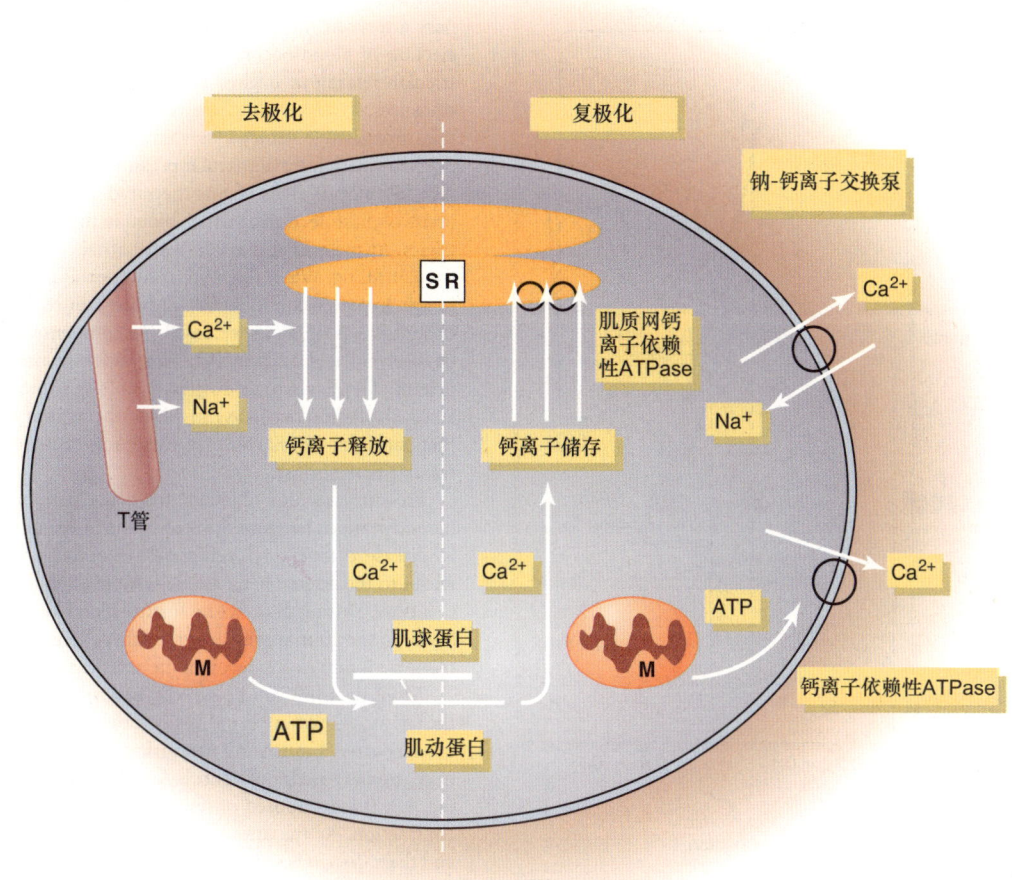

图1.2 钙离子依赖性心肌收缩。(1) 心肌细胞去极化诱导外源性钙离子通过 T 管上的离子通道流入心肌细胞；(2) 外源性钙离子进入心肌细胞后刺激肌质网（SR）释放大量内源性钙离子；(3) 钙离子与肌动蛋白丝上的肌钙蛋白-原肌球蛋白复合体结合，诱导后者构象改变，促使肌动蛋白与肌球蛋白结合。在三磷酸腺苷（ATP）的作用下，肌动蛋白-肌球蛋白复合体反复分离，粗、细肌丝相互滑动并实现心肌收缩；(4) 心肌细胞复极时胞质内的钙离子被主动泵出细胞外或被肌质网回收。ATPase：三磷酸腺苷酶；M：线粒体

细胞构成心脏传导系统，产生心电冲动并有组织地传导至心肌细胞，诱导心肌细胞产生机械收缩。

心肌生理特点与收缩

外源性钙离子诱导的心肌细胞内源性钙离子释放是心肌细胞收缩的主要机制。心肌细胞去极化可刺激肌纤维膜上特殊的凹陷性管道（T管），促使其上的钙离子通道开放并允许外源性钙离子经由该通道进入细胞内（图1.2）。肌质网与 T 管紧密相邻，外源性钙离子可以诱导肌质网向细胞质内释放大量内源性钙离子。钙离子与肌动蛋白丝（位于肌节上）的钙结合调节亚基（肌钙蛋白 C）结合，诱导肌钙蛋白-原肌球蛋白复合体构象改变，暴露肌动蛋白上的肌球蛋白结合位点，诱导心肌细胞收缩所必需的肌钙蛋白-肌球蛋白桥接形成。心肌细胞收缩的能量来源是 ATP。心肌细胞收缩时 ATP 促进肌球蛋白与肌动蛋白分离，诱导粗、细肌丝相向滑动，并最终使肌节缩短。

心肌细胞收缩强度取决于肌质网释放到细胞质中的游离钙离子总量。游离钙离子增多可诱导肌动蛋白与肌球蛋白间频繁的相互作用，促使心肌收缩力增强。当肌纤维膜复极时细胞质内的钙离子会被肌质网主动、迅速地回收，并且与肌质网内的多种蛋白结合（如钙隔离蛋白），直至下一次心肌细胞去极化。钙离子也可以通过肌纤维膜上的多种钙离子泵排到细胞外。ATP依赖性离子泵可主动清除细胞质内钙离子，诱导心室舒张，有利于心室在舒张期的自然充盈。

循环系统生理机制与心动周期

"心动周期（cardiac cycle）"是指心腔内压力随时间而产生的周期性变化（图1.3）。心动周期分为收缩期和舒张期：收缩期是心室肌收缩阶段，而舒张期则

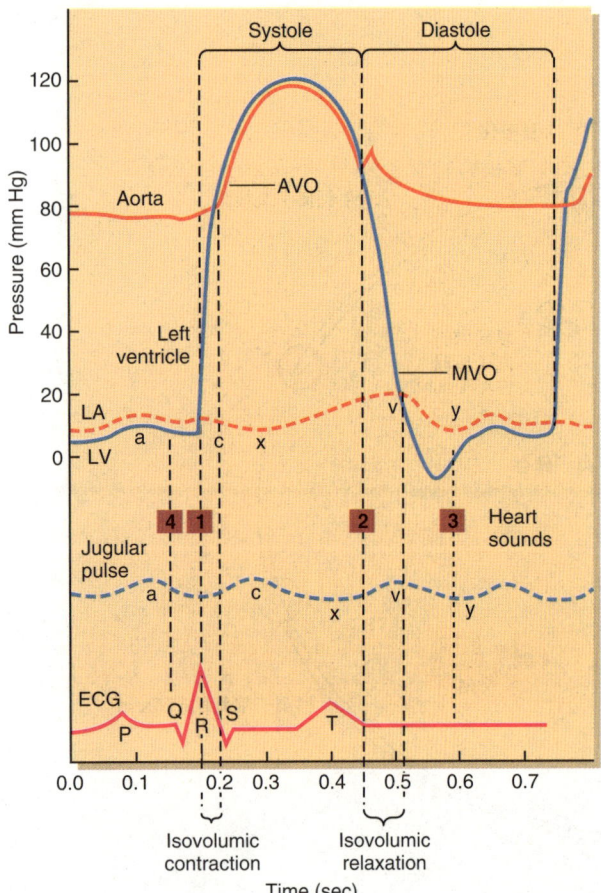

Fig. 1.3 Simultaneous electrocardiogram (ECG) and pressure tracings obtained from the left atrium (LA), left ventricle (LV), and aorta and the jugular venous pressure during the cardiac cycle. (For simplification, pressures on the right side of the heart have been omitted. Normal right atrial (RA) pressure closely parallels that of the LA, and right ventricular and pulmonary artery pressures are timed closely with their corresponding left-sided counterparts; they are reduced only in magnitude. Normally, closure of the mitral and aortic valves precedes closure of the tricuspid and pulmonic valves, whereas valve opening reverses this order. The jugular venous pulse lags behind the RA pulse.) During the course of one cardiac cycle, the electrical (ECG) events initiate and therefore precede the mechanical (pressure) events, and the latter precede the auscultatory events (heart sounds) that they themselves produce *(red boxes)*. Shortly after the P wave, the atria contract to produce the *a* wave. The QRS complex initiates ventricular systole, followed shortly by LV contraction and the rapid buildup of LV pressure. Almost immediately, LV pressure exceeds LA pressure, closing the mitral valve and producing the first heart sound. After a brief period of isovolumic contraction, LV pressure exceeds aortic pressure and the aortic valve opens (AVO). When the ventricular pressure once again falls to less than the aortic pressure, the aortic valve closes to produce the second heart sound and terminate ventricular ejection. The LV pressure decreases during the period of isovolumic relaxation until it drops below LA pressure and the mitral valve opens (MVO). See text for further details.

the period of ventricular contraction, and *diastole*, the period of ventricular relaxation. Each cardiac valve opens and closes in response to pressure gradients generated during these periods. At the onset of systole, ventricular pressures exceed atrial pressures, so the AV valves passively close. As myocytes contract, the intraventricular pressures rise initially, without a change in ventricular volume (isovolumic contraction), until they exceed the pressures in the aorta and pulmonary artery. At this point, the semilunar valves open, and ventricular ejection of blood occurs. When intracellular calcium levels fall, ventricular relaxation begins; arterial pressures exceed intraventricular pressures, so the semilunar valves close. Ventricular relaxation initially does not change ventricular volume (isovolumic relaxation). At the point at which intraventricular pressures fall below atrial pressures, the AV valves open. This begins the rapid and passive ventricular filling phase of diastole, during which blood in the atria empties into the ventricles. At the end of diastole, active atrial contraction augments ventricular filling. When the myocardium exhibits increased stiffness due to age, hypertension, diabetes, or heart failure, the early passive phase of ventricular filling is decreased. To compensate for the reduction in passive ventricular filling, there is reliance on atrial contraction to sufficiently fill the ventricle during diastole. A pathologic consequence of atrial fibrillation, a disease in which the atrium does not contract, is that patients often have worse symptoms because this additional ventricular filling is lost.

Pressure tracings obtained from the periphery complement the hemodynamic changes exhibited in the heart. In the absence of valvular disease, there is no impediment to blood flow moving from the ventricles to the arterial beds, so the systolic arterial pressure rises sharply to a peak. During diastole, no further blood volume is ejected into the aorta, so the arterial pressure gradually falls as blood flows to the distal tissue beds and elastic recoil of the arteries occurs.

Atrial pressure can be directly measured in the right atrium, but the left atrial pressure is indirectly measured by occluding a small pulmonary artery branch and measuring the pressure distally (the pulmonary capillary *wedge* pressure). An atrial pressure tracing is shown in Fig. 1.3. It is composed of several waves. The *a wave* represents atrial contraction. As the atria subsequently relax, the atrial pressure falls, and the *x descent* is seen on the pressure tracing. The x descent is interrupted by a small *c wave*, generated as the AV valve bulges toward the atrium during ventricular systole. As the atria fill from venous return, the *v wave* is seen, after which the *y descent* appears as the AV valves open and blood from the atria empties into the ventricles. The normal ranges of pressures in the various cardiac chambers are shown in Table 1.1.

Cardiac Performance

The amount of blood ejected by the heart each minute is referred to as the cardiac output (CO). It is the product of the stroke volume (SV), which is the amount of blood ejected with each ventricular contraction, and the HR:

$$CO = SV \times HR$$

The cardiac index is a way of normalizing the CO to body size. It is the CO divided by the body surface area and is measured in $L/min/m^2$. The normal CO is 4 to 6 L/min at rest and can increase fourfold to sixfold during strenuous exercise.

The main determinants of SV are preload, afterload, and contractility (Table 1.2). *Preload* is the volume of blood in the ventricle at the end of diastole; it is primarily a reflection of venous return. Venous return is determined by the plasma volume and the venous compliance. Clinically, intravenous fluids increase preload, whereas diuretics or venodilators such as nitroglycerin decrease preload. When the preload is increased, the ventricle stretches, and the ensuing ventricular contraction becomes more rapid and forceful, because the increased sarcomere length facilitates actin and myosin cross-bridge kinetics by means of an increased sensitivity of troponin C to calcium. This phenomenon is known as the Frank-Starling relationship. Ventricular filling pressure (ventricular end-diastolic pressure, atrial pressure, or

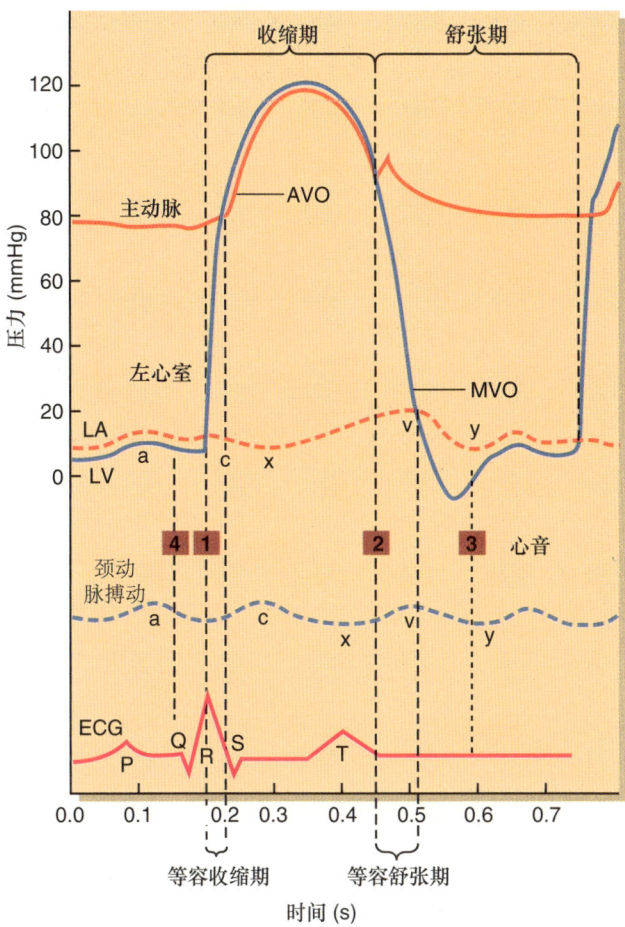

图 1.3 心电图（ECG）以及左心房（LA）、左心室（LV）、主动脉和颈静脉压力随心动周期的变化曲线。[为了简化图片，右侧心腔的压力变化已被省略。通常情况下，右心房（RA）压力与 LA 压力呈平行关系，右心室、肺动脉压力与左心室压力也具有相同的变化趋势，前两者较后者仅在压力数值上有所减小；二尖瓣、主动脉瓣关闭先于三尖瓣和肺动脉瓣，而瓣膜开放顺序则相反；颈静脉搏动滞后于 RA 搏动]。在单一心动周期中，心电（ECG）事件在时间上先于心腔内机械压力（pressure）变化，而机械压力变化又先于心脏听诊（心音）改变（红框标记处）。P 波后紧跟着由心房收缩产生的 a 波；QRS 复合波标志着心室收缩开始，在此期间可迅速出现 LV 收缩和 LV 压力升高。LV 压力迅速超过 LA 压力，诱导二尖瓣关闭并产生第一心音。经过短暂的等容收缩期后 LV 压力超过主动脉压力，诱导主动脉瓣开放（AVO）。当 LV 压力下降至低于主动脉压力时，主动脉瓣关闭并产生第二心音，LV 射血结束。等容舒张期 LV 压力持续下降，当 LV 压力小于 LA 压力时二尖瓣开放（MVO）。详见正文

是心室肌舒张阶段。各心腔内压力阶差随心动周期改变并诱导相应心脏瓣膜的开放与关闭。心室收缩早期，心室压高于心房压，房室瓣关闭；随后心室肌持续收缩，在心室内血容量无改变的情况下心室内压力迅速上升直至超过主动脉和肺动脉压力（等容收缩期）；此时，半月瓣（主动脉瓣和肺动脉瓣）开放，心室开始

射血。随后，心肌细胞内钙离子水平逐渐下降，心室进入舒张期，动脉压力超过心室内压力，半月瓣关闭。心室舒张早期，室内血容量无改变，这一时期称为等容舒张期。当心室压低于心房压时，房室瓣开放，心房内血液快速进入心室（心室快速充盈期）。舒张晚期，心房肌主动收缩增加心室充盈量。高龄、高血压、糖尿病或心力衰竭均可诱导心肌组织变僵硬，抑制心室快速充盈；此时，心房肌可通过加强自身收缩维持心室在舒张期足够的血液充盈量。心房颤动时心房肌的收缩功能消失，以至于患者常因心室充盈受损而导致临床症状加重。

外周血管压力描记结果可以补充显示心脏内的血流动力学变化。在无瓣膜疾病的情况下，心室内血液可顺畅地进入动脉血管网，动脉收缩压迅速升高至峰值；舒张期，由于不再有血液排入主动脉且动脉内血液逐渐流向周围组织，动脉压逐渐下降；与此同时会出现由动脉弹性回缩引起的压力波。

右心房压力可直接测得；左心房压力则需要间接测量，即阻塞一小段肺动脉分支血管并测量阻塞远端的肺动脉压力（肺毛细血管楔压，pulmonary capillary wedge pressure）。心房压描记结果见图 1.3。它由许多波型构成：a 波代表心房收缩；心房舒张时，心房内压力下降，出现下行的 x 波；x 降支波被一个小 c 波打断，这是由心室收缩导致房室瓣凸向心房所致。腔静脉血液充盈心房时出现 v 波；随后房室瓣开放，心房内血液排入心室并出现下行的 y 波；心动周期中各心腔内压力变化的正常值见表 1.1。

心功能

心脏每分钟的射血量定义为心输出量（CO）。它由每搏输出量（SV）乘以心率（HR）所得。SV 是指心脏每收缩一次向主动脉内的射血量。

$$CO = SV \times HR$$

心脏指数是利用体表面积对 CO 进行标准化所得的参数。它由 CO 除以体表面积所得，单位为 L/(min·m²)。休息时 CO 的正常值为 4~6 L/min，而剧烈运动时 CO 可上升 4~6 倍。

SV 的主要影响因素为心室前、后负荷及心肌收缩力（表 1.2）。前负荷是指舒张末期心室内的血容量，它主要体现的是静脉回流情况。静脉回流的主要影响因素为体内总体血容量及静脉血管的顺应性。临床上可通过静脉补液提高前负荷，或使用利尿剂、静脉扩张药（如硝酸甘油）降低前负荷。前负荷增加可以使心室扩张和心肌组织的肌节延长，诱导肌钙蛋白 C 对钙的敏感性升高，促进肌钙蛋白-肌球蛋白桥接形成，最终促使心室肌收缩变快、变强。这一生理现象称之为 Frank-Starling

TABLE 1.1 Normal Values for Common Hemodynamic Parameters	
Heart rate	60-100 beats/min
Pressures (mm Hg)	
Central venous	≤9
Right atrial	≤9
Right ventricular	
Systolic	15-30
End-diastolic	≤9
Pulmonary arterial	
Systolic	15-30
Diastolic	3-12
Pulmonary capillary wedge	≤12
Left atrial	≤12
Left ventricular	
Systolic	100-140
End-diastolic	3-12
Aortic	
Systolic	100-140
Diastolic	60-90
Resistance	
Systemic vascular resistance	800-1500 dynes-sec/cm^{-5}
Pulmonary vascular resistance	30-120 dynes-sec/cm^{-5}
Cardiac output	4-6 L/min
Cardiac index	2.5-4 L/min

TABLE 1.2 Factors Affecting Cardiac Performance
Preload (Left Ventricular Diastolic Volume)
Total blood volume
Venous (sympathetic) tone
Body position
Intrathoracic and intrapericardial pressures
Atrial contraction
Pumping action of skeletal muscle
Afterload (Impedance Against Which the Left Ventricle Must Eject Blood)
Peripheral vascular resistance
Left ventricular volume (preload, wall tension)
Physical characteristics of the arterial tree (elasticity of vessels or presence of outflow obstruction)
Contractility (Cardiac Performance Independent of Preload or Afterload)
Sympathetic nerve impulses
Increased contractility
Circulating catecholamines
Digitalis, calcium, other inotropic agents
Increased heart rate or post-extrasystolic augmentation
Anoxia, acidosis
Decreased contractility
Pharmacologic depression
Loss of myocardium
Intrinsic depression
Heart Rate
Autonomic nervous system
Temperature, metabolic rate
Medications, drugs

pulmonary capillary wedge pressure) is frequently used as a surrogate measure of preload.

Afterload is the force against which the ventricles must contract to eject blood. The main determinants of afterload are the arterial pressure and the dimensions of the left ventricle. As the arterial blood pressure increases, the amount of blood that can be ejected into the aorta decreases. Wall stress, a significant and often overlooked determinant of afterload, is directly proportional to the size of the ventricular cavity and inversely proportional to the ventricular wall thickness (Laplace's law). Diuretics reduce the increased wall stress associated with pathologic dilatation in cardiomyopathy by decreasing left ventricular volume and size. In addition, ventricular wall hypertrophy is a compensatory mechanism to reduce afterload caused by systemic hypertension. Drugs that treat hypertension, such as angiotensin-converting enzyme (ACE) inhibitors and hydralazine, reduce blood pressure (BP) and thereby reduce afterload.

Contractility, or inotropy, represents the force of ventricular contraction in the presence of constant preload and afterload. Inotropy is regulated at a cellular level through stimulation of catecholaminergic (epinephrine, norepinephrine, and dopamine) receptors, intracellular signaling cascades (phosphodiesterase inhibitors), and intracellular calcium levels (affected by levosimendan and, indirectly, by digoxin). Many antihypertensive medications (e.g., β-blockers, calcium channel antagonists) interfere with adrenergic receptor activation or intracellular calcium levels, which can decrease the strength of ventricular contractions. (Please refer to Chapter 47, "Cardiac and Circulatory Function," in *Goldman-Cecil Medicine*, 26th Edition.)

Physiology of the Coronary Circulation

The normally functioning heart maintains equilibrium between the amount of oxygen delivered to myocytes and the amount of oxygen consumed by them (myocardial oxygen consumption, or Mvo_2). If a myocyte works harder because it is contracting with increased frequency (HR), with increased intensity (contractility), or against an increased load (wall stress), then it will use more oxygen and its Mvo_2 will increase. In order to meet this increase in demand for more oxygen, the heart will have to either increase blood flow or increase its efficiency in extracting oxygen. The heart is unique in that its oxygen extraction is almost maximal at resting conditions. Therefore, increasing blood flow is the only reasonable means of increasing oxygen supply.

Microvascular blood flow in the coronary circulation is impaired during systole because the intramyocardial blood vessels are compressed by contracting myocardium. Therefore, most coronary flow occurs during diastole. Accordingly, the diastolic pressure is the major pressure driving flow within the coronary circulation. Systolic pressure impedes intramyocardial arterial blood flow but augments venous flow. On a clinical note, tachycardia is particularly detrimental because coronary flow is reduced when the diastolic filling time is abbreviated, and the Mvo_2 increases with increasing HR. In order to sustain constant perfusion to the myocardium, coronary blood flow is maintained constant over a wide range of pressures in a process called autoregulation.

In response to a change in Mvo_2, the coronary arteries dilate or constrict, which changes the vascular resistance and thereby appropriately changes flow. This regulation of arterial resistance occurs at the arterioles and is mediated by several factors. Adenosine, a metabolite of ATP, is released during contraction and acts as a potent vasodilator.

表 1.1 常见血流动力学参数的正常值	
心率	60～100 次/分
压力（mmHg）	
中心静脉	≤9
右心房	≤9
右心室	
收缩压	15～30
舒张末压	≤9
肺动脉	
收缩压	15～30
舒张压	3～12
肺毛细血管楔压	≤12
左心房	≤12
左心室	
收缩压	100～140
舒张末压	3～12
主动脉	
收缩压	100～140
舒张压	60～90
血流阻力	
体循环血流阻力	800～1500 dynes-s/cm^5
肺循环血流阻力	30～120 dynes-s/cm^5
心输出量	4～6 L/min
心脏指数	2.5～4 L/min

表 1.2 心功能的影响因素
前负荷（左心室舒张期容积）
总体血容量
静脉张力（受交感神经调控）
体位变化
胸腔和心包腔内压力
心房收缩
骨骼肌运动诱发的泵作用
后负荷（左心室射血需要克服的阻力）
周围血管阻力
左心室血容量（前负荷，室壁张力）
动脉血管网的生理特性（血管弹性、流出道受阻）
心肌收缩力（独立于心室前、后负荷的心功能影响因素）
交感神经兴奋
心肌收缩力增强
循环系统中儿茶酚胺水平
洋地黄、钙离子或其他正性肌力药
心率增快或期外收缩后心肌收缩力增强
缺氧、酸中毒
心肌收缩力下降
药物抑制
心肌细胞减少
原发性心肌收缩功能抑制
心率
自主神经系统
体温、代谢率
医疗措施、药物

定律。心室充盈压（心室舒张末压、心房压或肺毛细血管楔压）常被用做前负荷的替代测量指标。

后负荷是指心室收缩射血需要克服的阻力。后负荷的主要影响因素是主动脉压和左心室大小。主动脉压力升高则左心室的射血量减少。室壁应力是一个重要却常被忽视的后负荷影响因素；它与心室大小成正比，与室壁厚度成反比[拉普拉斯（Laplace）定律]。利尿剂可以减少左心室容量负荷及大小来减少心肌病中与病理性扩张相关的室壁应力增加。此外，心室壁肥厚是一种代偿机制，以减小因全身性高血压所导致的后负荷升高。降压药物[如血管紧张素转换酶（ACE）抑制剂和肼屈嗪]可以降低血压（BP），从而减小左心室后负荷。

收缩力或正性肌力是指在前、后负荷固定的情况下，心室肌的收缩力。正性肌力在细胞水平的调控方式有三种，分别是刺激儿茶酚胺能受体（肾上腺素、去甲肾上腺素和多巴胺受体）、调控细胞内信号级联（磷酸二酯酶抑制剂）和钙离子水平[左西孟旦、地高辛（间接调控）]。许多降压药物可以通过干扰肾上腺素受体活性或降低细胞内钙离子水平（如β受体阻滞剂和钙通道阻滞剂）以降低心室收缩力（具体可参考 Goldman-Cecil Medicine 第 26 版第 47 章"心脏与循环功能"）。

冠状动脉循环生理机制

正常的心功能可以维持心肌氧供与氧耗（心肌氧耗量，Mvo_2）之间的动态平衡。心率（HR）增快、心肌收缩力（contractility）增强或室壁应力（wall stress）增加均可使心肌作功增多，使其氧耗增加（Mvo_2 升高）；故而需要提高心肌供血量或增强心肌氧摄取效率以满足心肌氧耗升高的需求。心肌组织的特性在于其在休息状态下的氧摄取效率已基本达到最高值。因此，提高心肌供血量是增加心肌氧供的唯一合理方式。

分布于心肌组织中的冠脉循环微血管会被收缩的心肌组织压迫，以至于收缩期冠脉微循环中的血流量减少。因此，冠脉循环主要在舒张期供血，而且舒张压是驱动冠脉循环供血的主要动力。虽然心肌收缩可以阻碍心肌组织中的冠脉微循环血流，但它可以促进静脉血液回流。从临床角度看，心动过速危害较大：当舒张期充盈时间缩短时，冠脉血流减少，并且 Mvo_2 随着心率增加而增加。为了保证持续有效的心肌灌注，冠脉循环血流量可以在较大的血压波动范围内保持相对稳定，这一现象称之为自动调节。

Mvo_2 变化可调控冠脉舒张或收缩，以此调节冠脉血管阻力并诱导冠脉循环血流量相应的改变。上述动脉血管阻力调节现象出现于小动脉，且受多种因素影响。腺苷是 ATP 的代谢产物，仅在收缩期释放，是一种强力血管扩张剂。心肌代谢的其他结果，如氧分压降低、二

Other consequences of myocardial metabolism, such as decreased oxygen tension, increased carbon dioxide, hydrogen peroxide, acidosis, and hyperkalemia, also mediate coronary vasodilation. The endothelium produces several potent vasodilators, including nitric oxide and prostacyclin. Nitric oxide is released by the endothelium in response to acetylcholine, thrombin, adenosine diphosphate (ADP), serotonin, bradykinin, platelet aggregation, and an increase in shear stress (called *flow-dependent vasodilation*). Finally, the coronary arteries are innervated by the autonomic nervous system, and activation of sympathetic neurons mediates vasoconstriction or vasodilation through α- or β-receptors, respectively. Parasympathetic neurons from the vagus nerve secrete acetylcholine, which mediates vasodilation. Vasoconstricting factors, notably endothelin, are produced by the endothelium and may be important in conditions such as coronary vasospasm. (Please refer to Chapter 47, "Cardiac and Circulatory Function," in *Goldman-Cecil Medicine*, 26th Edition.)

Physiology of the Systemic Circulation

The normal cardiovascular system delivers appropriate blood flow to each organ of the body under a wide range of conditions. This regulation is achieved by maintaining BP through adjustments in cardiac output and tissue blood flow resistance by neural and humoral factors.

Poiseuille's law generally describes the relationship between pressure and flow in a vessel. Fluid flow (F) through a tube is proportional (proportionality constant = K) to the pressure (P) difference between the ends of the tube:

$$F = K \times \Delta P$$

K is equivalent to the inverse of resistance to flow (R); that is, K = 1/R. Resistance to flow is determined by the properties of both the fluid and the tube. In the case of a steady, streamlined flow of fluid through a rigid tube, Poiseuille found that these factors determine resistance:

$$R = 8 \eta L / \pi r^4$$

Where r is the radius of the tube, L is its length, and η is the viscosity of the fluid. Notice that changes in radius have greater influence than changes in length, because resistance is inversely proportional to the fourth power of the radius. Poiseuille's law incorporates the factors influencing flow, so that:

$$F = \Delta P / R = \Delta P \pi r^4 / 8 \eta L$$

Therefore, the most important determinants of blood flow in the cardiovascular system are ΔP and r^4. Small changes in arterial radius can cause large changes in flow to a tissue or organ. Practically, systemic vascular resistance (SVR) is the total resistance to flow caused by changes in the radius of resistance vessels (small arteries and arterioles) of the systemic circulation. The SVR can be calculated as the pressure drop across the peripheral capillary beds (mean arterial pressure – right atrial pressure) divided by the blood flow across the beds (i.e., SVR = BP/CO). It is normally in the range of 800 to 1500 dynes-sec/cm^{-5}.

The autonomic nervous system alters systemic vascular tone through sympathetic and parasympathetic innervation as well as metabolic factors (local oxygen tension, carbon dioxide levels, reactive oxygen species, pH) and endothelium-derived signaling molecules (NO, endothelin). Neural regulation of BP occurs by means of constitutive and reflex changes in autonomic efferent outflow to modulate cardiac chronotropy, inotropy, and vascular resistance.

The baroreflex loop is the primary mechanism by which BP is neurally modulated. Baroreceptors are stretch-sensitive nerve endings that are distributed throughout various regions of the cardiovascular system. Those located in the carotid artery (e.g., carotid sinus) and aorta are sometimes referred to as *high-pressure baroreceptors* and those in the cardiopulmonary areas as *low-pressure baroreceptors*. After afferent impulses are transmitted to the central nervous system, the signals are integrated, and the efferent arm of the reflex projects neural signals systemically through the sympathetic and parasympathetic branches of the autonomic nervous system. In general, an increase in systemic BP increases the firing rate of the baroreceptors. Efferent sympathetic outflow is inhibited (reducing vascular tone, chronotropy, and inotropy), and parasympathetic outflow is increased (reducing cardiac chronotropy). The opposite occurs when BP decreases. (Please refer to Chapter 47, "Cardiac and Circulatory Function," in *Goldman-Cecil Medicine*, 26th Edition.)

Physiology of the Pulmonary Circulation

Like the systemic circulation, the pulmonary circulation consists of a branching network of progressively smaller arteries, arterioles, capillaries, and veins. The pulmonary capillaries are separated from the alveoli by a thin alveolar-capillary membrane through which gas exchange occurs. The partial pressure of oxygen (Po_2) is the main regulator of pulmonary blood to optimize blood flow toward well-ventilated lung segments and away from poorly ventilated segments.

SUGGESTED READINGS

Berne RM, Levy MN: Physiology: part IV. The cardiovascular system, ed 7, St. Louis, 2017, Elsevier.

Guyton AC, Hall JE: Textbook of medical physiology, ed 13, St. Louis, 2015, Elsevier.

氧化碳分压升高、过氧化氢增多、酸中毒和高钾血症等均可引起冠脉扩张。血管内皮细胞可产生多种血管扩张剂，如一氧化氮和前列环素。内皮细胞受乙酰胆碱、凝血酶、二磷酸腺苷（ADP）、血清素、缓激肽、血小板聚集和血流剪应力增加（血流依赖性血管舒张，flow-dependent vasodilation）等因素刺激后可释放一氧化氮。冠状动脉还受自主神经系统的支配，交感神经激活可分别通过 α 或 β 受体诱导冠脉血管的收缩或舒张。迷走神经的副交感神经元可分泌乙酰胆碱，诱导冠脉血管舒张。由内皮细胞分泌的血管收缩因子（尤其是内皮素）在某些疾病如冠脉痉挛中，发挥着重要的作用（具体可参考 Goldman-Cecil Medicine 第 26 版第 47 章"心脏与循环功能"）。

体循环生理机制

心血管系统可以在多种条件下向机体各组织器官输送适量血液。该生理功能有赖于神经和体液因子对心输出量及周围组织血流阻力的调控，进而维持适当的 BP。

泊肃叶（Poiseuille）定律描述了血压与血管内血流量之间的关系。血流量（F）与血管两端的压力（P）阶差成正比（比例常数＝K）：

$$F = K \times \Delta P$$

K 等于液体流动阻力（R）的倒数，即 K = 1/R；液体流动阻力由液体性质及管道特性共同决定。泊肃叶定律指出，当稳定的线流液体在刚性管道内流动时，其液体流动阻力计算方法如下：

$$R = 8\eta L/\pi r^4$$

r 为管道半径，L 为管道长度，η 为流动液体的黏度。值得注意的是，由于液体流动阻力与管道半径的四次方成反比，因此管道半径对液体流动阻力的影响大于管道长度。依据泊肃叶定律，血管内血流量的计算公式如下：

$$F = \Delta P/R = \Delta P\pi r^4/8\eta L$$

因此，对心血管系统血流量影响最大的因素为 ΔP 和 r^4。动脉半径的轻微改变即能对组织器官的血流灌注量造成极大的影响。事实上，体循环血流阻力（SVR）是指体循环系统中阻力血管（小动脉和微动脉）半径变化引起的血流阻力总和。SVR 的计算方法为：跨外周毛细血管床的压力阶差（平均动脉压－右心房压）除以跨外周毛细血管床的血流量（即 SVR = BP/CO）。SVR 的正常值范围是 800～1500 dynes-s/cm^5。

自主神经系统通过交感神经、副交感神经、代谢产物（局部氧张力、二氧化碳水平、活性氧簇、血液 pH 值）、内皮来源信号分子（NO、内皮素）调节体循环血管张力。机体通过对自主神经传出信号的组成性和反馈性调节，调控心率、心肌收缩力和血管阻力，实现对 BP 的神经调控。

血压神经调控的主要机制是压力反射环的作用。压力感受器是广泛分布于心血管系统的牵张-敏感性神经末梢；其中，分布于颈动脉（如颈动脉窦）和主动脉的感受器称为高压压力感受器（high-pressure baroreceptors），而分布于心肺组织的感受器则称为低压压力感受器（low-pressure baroreceptors）。传入神经信号在中枢神经系统整合，随后经由自主神经系统中交感神经和副交感神经的分支自动传出相应的反射信号。通常情况下，体循环 BP 升高会提高压力感受器的兴奋频率，抑制交感神经的传出信号（减小血管阻力、减慢心率、抑制心肌收缩力），增强副交感神经的传出信号（减慢心率）；但当体循环 BP 下降时则与之正好相反（具体可参考 Goldman-Cecil Medicine 第 26 版第 47 章"心脏与循环功能"）。

肺循环生理机制

与体循环一样，肺循环也是由逐级变小的动脉、微动脉、毛细血管和静脉组成的分支血管网络系统。肺内毛细血管与肺泡被一层薄薄的肺泡-毛细血管膜分隔，此处为肺内气体交换场所。氧分压（pressure of oxygen, P_{O_2}）在肺内血流调控中发挥着重要的作用；它可以促使血液流向通气良好的肺段，远离通气不良的肺段。

推荐阅读

Berne RM, Levy MN: Physiology: part IV. The cardiovascular system, ed 7, St. Louis, 2017, Elsevier.

Guyton AC, Hall JE: Textbook of medical physiology, ed 13, St. Louis, 2015, Elsevier.

2

Evaluation of the Patient With Cardiovascular Disease

James Kleczka, Noura M. Dabbouseh

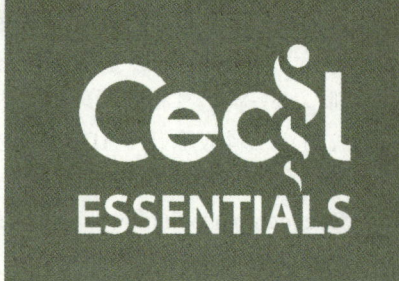

DEFINITION AND EPIDEMIOLOGY

Cardiovascular disease is a major cause of morbidity and mortality around the world, and its spectrum is wide-reaching. Included in this population of patients are people with coronary artery disease (CAD), congestive heart failure, stroke, hypertension, peripheral arterial disease, atrial fibrillation and other arrhythmias, valvular disease, and congenital heart disease. The impact of cardiovascular disease is unmistakable: It is the leading cause of death in both males and females in the United States, with reports estimating that heart disease accounts for between one in three and one in four deaths. It accounted for more inpatient hospital days in the years of 1990-2009 than other disorders such as chronic lung disease and cancer. The high number of inpatient days associated with cardiovascular disease led to a total economic cost of more than $297 billion in the year 2008 alone. In 2011, an estimated $316.6 billion in health care costs and lost productivity was attributable to heart disease and stroke.

Given these facts, the proper evaluation of a patient with cardiovascular disease is imperative in order to potentially decrease an individual's morbidity and mortality and potentially impact health care expenditures. An understanding of the basics of the pathophysiology of heart disease as well as a thorough history and detailed physical examination are required to accurately assess and manage patients with cardiovascular disease.

PATHOLOGY

The term *cardiovascular disease* encompasses a wide array of patient problems. The heart's circulation, myocardium, rhythm, valves, and pericardial structures may be affected, as can the arterial or venous vascular systems. *Coronary artery disease (CAD)*, discussed in depth in Chapter 7, is a leading cause of morbidity and mortality. While many patients do have silent CAD or asymptomatic coronary atherosclerosis, this still impacts patient morbidity. At presentation, patients with symptomatic CAD may have stable angina or an acute coronary syndrome, further stratified into unstable angina (UA), non–ST segment elevation myocardial infarction (NSTEMI), or ST segment elevation myocardial infarction (STEMI). The initial presentation for some patients with CAD is sudden cardiac death, the result of arrhythmia often caused by atherosclerosis of the coronary vasculature.

Congestive heart failure is the end result of many cardiac disorders and has been historically classified as systolic or diastolic in etiology. More recently, the terms heart failure with reduced ejection fraction (HFrEF) and heart failure with preserved ejection fraction (HFpEF), which is often due to diastolic dysfunction, have gained widespread acceptance. In patients with ventricular enlargement or systolic dysfunction, the term cardiomyopathy is appropriate whether or not a patient has clinically demonstrated signs of heart failure. Various forms of cardiomyopathy may lead to systolic dysfunction and a decline in ejection fraction. Without proper management, this will inevitably lead to alterations in hemodynamics that result in development of pulmonary vascular congestion, edema, and a decline in functional capacity, all symptoms of clinical heart failure. Diastolic dysfunction can be present with systolic dysfunction and is often the result of uncontrolled hypertension or infiltrative disorders such as hemochromatosis or amyloidosis. Various forms of heart failure are further discussed in Chapter 4.

Stroke is caused by cerebral hypoperfusion, which can result from such problems as carotid disease, thromboembolism, or emboli of infectious origin. A more detailed discussion can be found in Section "Neurologic Disease" Chapter 13.

Peripheral arterial disease (PAD), addressed in Chapter 11, includes such entities as aneurysms of the ascending, descending, and abdominal aorta and its branches; aortic or peripheral arterial dissection; carotid disease; and atherosclerosis of branch vessels of the aorta and vessels in the limbs. PAD is often present in patients with CAD.

Atrial fibrillation and *hypertension* (see Chapter 8) are not uncommon and increase in prevalence with age. Although they are not typically the primary cause of mortality, these problems often predispose to other causes of cardiovascular disease mortality, such as stroke and heart failure. Arrhythmias other than atrial fibrillation are also common and can lead to significant morbidity and mortality.

Valvular heart disease may lead to cardiomyopathy and is found in all age groups.

Congenital heart disease includes a wide variety of disorders, ranging from valve abnormalities and coronary anomalies to cardiomyopathy and other structural abnormalities including shunts and malformations of the cardiac chambers. With advances in surgical techniques and medical therapy, life expectancy has improved significantly for patients with congenital heart disease. Congenital heart disease is discussed further in Chapter 5.

CLINICAL PRESENTATION

Technologic advancements have allowed for specialized testing to assist in the diagnosis of cardiovascular diseases. We now rely on such tests as angiography, ultrasound scanning, and advanced imaging modalities such as high-resolution computed tomography and magnetic resonance imaging to determine how to manage an individual case. However, these techniques should be used not as a primary method of assessment but rather to supplement the findings from a thorough history and physical examination. Despite the availability of rather costly imaging techniques and laboratory tests, a relatively inexpensive but detailed history and physical examination is a clinician's strongest tool in helping to establish a diagnosis.

心血管疾病患者的评估

王婧莹　戴晨光　魏荧　石静　译　刘嘉慧　刘靖　审校　李悦　通审

定义和流行病学

心血管疾病是全球范围内发病和死亡的主要原因之一，包括冠状动脉疾病（CAD）、充血性心力衰竭、卒中、高血压、周围动脉疾病、心房颤动及其他类型心律失常、心脏瓣膜病和先天性心脏病等。据统计，心血管疾病是美国人群的主要死因，占总死亡人数的1/4～1/3。在1990—2009年，心血管疾病患者的住院天数远超慢性肺部疾病和癌症等其他疾病。仅2008年，因心血管疾病造成的住院花费就超过2970亿美元。2011年，因心脏病和卒中导致的医疗花费和生产力下降造成经济损失达3166亿美元。

因此，对心血管疾病患者进行适当评估可降低个体的发病率和死亡率，并减少医疗支出。掌握心脏病的基础病理生理学知识，结合详尽的病史和详细的体格检查，对于准确评估和管理心血管疾病患者至关重要。

病理学

"心血管疾病"包括心脏循环、心肌、节律、瓣膜、心包结构和动静脉血管系统异常导致的一系列疾病。其中，CAD是导致高发病率和死亡率的主要原因（详见第7章）。部分患者是隐匿型CAD或无症状冠状动脉粥样硬化，这也会影响发病率。目前，有症状CAD分为稳定型心绞痛和急性冠脉综合征，急性冠脉综合征进一步细分为不稳定型心绞痛（UA）、非ST段抬高型心肌梗死（NSTEMI）和ST段抬高型心肌梗死（STEMI）。部分CAD患者首发症状即为心源性猝死，通常由冠状动脉粥样硬化引起的心律失常所导致。

充血性心力衰竭是多种心脏疾病的终末期，按病因分为收缩性心力衰竭和舒张性心力衰竭两种。目前，按射血分数分为射血分数降低的心力衰竭（HFrEF）和射血分数保留的心力衰竭（HFpEF）（通常由舒张功能障碍引起）亦被广泛接受。对于心室扩张或收缩功能障碍的患者，无论其是否存在心力衰竭的临床表现，均可定义为心肌病。各种类型的心肌病均可导致收缩功能障碍和射血分数降低，若未及时治疗，最终将引起血流动力学改变，导致临床心力衰竭症状如肺淤血、水肿和功能储备降低等。舒张功能障碍可与收缩功能障碍同时存在，通常由未控制的高血压或浸润性疾病如血色病、淀粉样变性引起。各种类型的心力衰竭介绍详见第4章。

卒中是由颈动脉疾病、血栓栓塞或感染性栓子导致的脑灌注不足引起的，详见《神经与老年医学分册》第13章。

第11章将介绍周围动脉疾病（PAD），包括升主动脉、降主动脉、腹主动脉及其分支动脉瘤；主动脉或外周动脉夹层；颈动脉疾病以及主动脉分支血管和四肢血管的动脉粥样硬化。CAD的患者通常会伴随PAD。

心房颤动和高血压（详见第8章）较为常见，且发病率随患者年龄增长而增加。它们通常不是患者死亡的直接原因，但常导致其他心血管疾病（如卒中和心力衰竭）死亡风险增加。除心房颤动外，其他心律失常同样具有较高的发病率和死亡率。

心脏瓣膜病可导致心肌病，且在各年龄段均可发病。

先天性心脏病包括瓣膜异常、冠状动脉畸形、心肌病、结构异常如心脏腔室分流和畸形等多种类型。随着外科手术与药物治疗的发展，先天性心脏病患者的预期寿命已显著延长。第5章将进一步讨论先天性心脏病。

临床表现

技术的革新使得多种检查方法如血管造影术、超声扫描、高分辨率计算机断层成像与磁共振成像均可协助诊断与管理心血管疾病患者。然而这些检查手段应作为病史采集和体格检查后的补充内容，而非主要评估方法。相对于较昂贵的影像学技术和实验室检查，详尽的病史采集和体格检查仍是帮助临床医生确定诊断的最有力依据。

TABLE 2.1	Cardiovascular Causes of Chest Pain				
Condition	Location	Quality	Duration	Aggravating or Alleviating Factors	Associated Symptoms or Signs
Angina	Retrosternal region: radiates to or occasionally isolated to neck, jaw, shoulders, arms (usually left), or epigastrium	Pressure, squeezing, tightness, heaviness, burning, indigestion	<2-10 min	Precipitated by exertion, cold weather, or emotional stress; relieved by rest or nitroglycerin; variant (Prinzmetal) angina may be unrelated to exertion, often early in the morning	Dyspnea; S_3, S_4, or murmur of papillary dysfunction during pain
Myocardial infarction	Same as angina	Same as angina, although more severe	Variable; usually >30 min	Unrelieved by rest or nitroglycerin	Dyspnea, nausea, vomiting, weakness, diaphoresis
Pericarditis	Left of the sternum; may radiate to neck or left shoulder, often more localized than pain of myocardial ischemia	Sharp, stabbing, knifelike	Lasts many hours to days; may wax and wane	Aggravated by deep breathing, rotating chest, or supine position; relieved by sitting up and leaning forward	Pericardial friction rub
Aortic dissection	Anterior chest; may radiate to back, interscapular region	Excruciating, tearing, knifelike	Sudden onset, unrelenting	Usually occurs in setting of hypertension or predisposition, such as Marfan syndrome	Murmur of aortic insufficiency; pulse or blood pressure asymmetry; neurologic deficit

A patient who is given the opportunity to outline his or her symptoms in his or her own words can help lead a clinician toward the right diagnosis. For example, many patients who deny chest pain when asked specifically about this symptom will go on to describe the symptom of chest pressure, which patients often feel is distinct from "pain." Gathering further historical details such as provoking factors (e.g., activity, extreme emotional stress, or rest or unprovoked symptoms), location, quality, intensity, and radiation of the symptom is imperative when taking a thorough history. One should delve into aggravating or alleviating factors and whether there are other symptoms that accompany the primary symptom. It is also important to note the pattern of the symptom in terms of stability or progression in intensity or frequency over time. An assessment of functional status should always be a part of the history in a patient with cardiovascular disease; a recent decline in exercise tolerance can help determine severity of disease.

A detailed past medical history and review of systems are necessary in order to understand if the cardiovascular condition is isolated or part of a syndrome. For example, a patient may have arrhythmias in the setting of hyperthyroidism. Rheumatologic disorders often affect the heart. And cancer can increase the risk of thromboembolism, of pericardial effusion and, with some therapies, cardiomyopathy. A comprehensive list of medications must be reviewed, and a social history must be taken detailing alcohol use, smoking, and occupational history. Patients should also be questioned regarding major risk factors such as hypertension, hyperlipidemia, and diabetes mellitus. A thorough family history is needed, not only to identify such entities as early-onset CAD but also to assess for other potentially inherited disorders, such as familial cardiomyopathy or arrhythmic disorders (e.g., long-QT syndrome).

Chest Pain

Chest pain is one of the cardinal symptoms of cardiovascular disease, but it may also be present in many noncardiovascular diseases (Tables 2.1 and 2.2). Chest pain may be caused by cardiac ischemia but also may be related to aortic pathology such as dissection, pulmonary disease such as pneumonia, gastrointestinal pathology such as gastroesophageal reflux, or musculoskeletal pain related to chest wall trauma. Issues with organs in the abdominal cavity such as the gallbladder or pancreas can also cause chest pain. It is therefore very important to characterize the pain in terms of location, quality, quantity, duration, radiation, aggravating and alleviating factors, and associated symptoms. These details will help determine the origin of the pain.

Myocardial ischemia due to obstructive CAD often leads to typical angina pectoris. Angina is often described as tightness, pressure, burning, or squeezing discomfort that patients may not identify as true pain. Patients frequently describe angina as a sensation of "bricks on the center of the chest" or an "elephant standing on the chest." Angina is more common in the morning, and the intensity may be affected by heat or cold, emotional stress, or eating. This discomfort is typically located in the substernal region or left side of the chest. Anginal pain may radiate to other parts of the body, such as the left shoulder and arm (particularly the ulnar aspect), the neck, the jaw, or the epigastrium. Pain that radiates to the back may raise suspicion for aortic dissection. Anginal chest pain is usually brought on with exertion, in particular with more intense activity or walking up inclines, in extremes of weather, or after large meals. It is typically brief in duration, lasting 2 to 10 minutes, and frequently resolves with rest or administration of nitroglycerine within 1 to 5 minutes. Associated symptoms often include nausea, diaphoresis, dyspnea, palpitations, and dizziness. Patients typically report a stable pattern of angina that is relatively predictable and reproducible with a given amount of exertion. When this pain begins to increase in frequency and severity or occurs with lesser amounts of exertion or at rest, one must then consider unstable angina. Anginal pain that occurs at rest with increased intensity and lasts longer than 30 minutes may represent acute myocardial infarction (MI). Some patients endorse a feeling of doom when suffering an MI. Angina-like pain at rest may also occur with coronary vasospasm and noncardiac chest pain.

There are several other potential causes of chest pain that may be confused with angina pectoris (see Table 2.2). Pain associated

表 2.1 胸痛的心血管病因					
分类	位置	性质	持续时间	加重或缓解因素	伴随症状或体征
心绞痛	胸骨后,可放射至(有时只限于)颈部、上颌、肩部、上臂(多为左侧)或上腹部	压迫感,压榨感,紧缩感,沉重感,烧灼感,消化不良	<2～10 min	可由运动、寒冷及情绪激动诱发,休息或含服硝酸甘油后可缓解;变异型心绞痛可与活动无关,常于清晨发作	呼吸困难,疼痛时出现第三心音、第四心音或乳头肌功能异常杂音
心肌梗死	与心绞痛相同	与心绞痛相同,但更为剧烈	多变,通常>30 min	休息及含服硝酸甘油不能缓解	呼吸困难,恶心,呕吐,无力,大汗
心包炎	胸骨左缘,可放射至颈部或左肩,常较心肌缺血局限	锐痛,刺痛,刀割样	持续数小时至数日,可有起伏	深呼吸、转动胸部及仰卧时加剧,前倾坐位可缓解	心包摩擦音
主动脉夹层	前胸,可向背部、肩胛区放射	剧烈,撕裂样,刀割样	突然发作,不缓解	常有高血压、马方综合征等易患因素	主动脉瓣关闭不全杂音,脉搏或血压不对称,神经功能异常

患者自行描述症状可帮助临床医生正确评估心血管疾病,例如部分患者会否认存在胸痛症状,但当其进一步描述不适时会使用"胸部压迫感"等词汇,他们并不认为这种"胸部压迫感"等同于"胸痛"。在进行病史采集时,需重视细节如是否存在诱发因素(如活动、情绪激动、休息或无诱因)、症状的部位、性质、强度和放射痛、加重或缓解因素及伴随症状等。同时,要注意症状的强度和频率是否进行性加重。机体活动能力测评是心血管疾病患者评估的重要组成部分,近期运动耐力下降有助于明确疾病的严重程度。

为了解心血管疾病是单发的抑或是综合征的一种,需详细采集既往史并进行系统回顾。例如,甲状腺功能亢进症患者可能出现心律失常;风湿免疫性疾病通常存在心脏症状;肿瘤会增加血栓栓塞和心包积液的风险,部分抗肿瘤治疗会导致心肌病。同时,需详细采集用药史、吸烟饮酒史、职业史、是否存在危险因素(如高血压、高脂血症、糖尿病)等。最后需关注家族史,以帮助识别早发性 CAD 并评估是否存在潜在遗传性疾病,如家族性心肌病或心律失常等(如长 QT 间期综合征)。

胸痛

胸痛是心血管疾病的主要症状之一,但亦可出现在其他疾病中(表 2.1 和表 2.2)。例如,心肌缺血、主动脉病变(如夹层)、肺部疾病(如肺炎)、胃肠道疾病(如胃食管反流病)、肌肉骨骼疾病(如胸壁创伤)、腹腔脏器(如胆囊、胰腺)相关异常亦可引起胸痛。因此,需从疼痛的部位、性质、程度、持续时间、有无放射痛、加重或缓解因素及伴随症状等多方面进行病史采集,以明确疼痛的病因。

阻塞性 CAD 引起的心肌缺血通常会导致典型心绞痛。心绞痛常被描述为紧缩感、压迫感、灼烧感及压榨样不适感而非疼痛。患者经常描述心绞痛为"胸口压着砖块"或"大象踩在胸前"的感觉。心绞痛好发于清晨,冷热、情绪激动或进食会增加其严重程度,位置多在胸骨下段或左侧胸部,亦可放射至左肩及左臂(尺侧为著)、颈部、下颌或上腹部等部位。放射至背部的疼痛需与主动脉夹层鉴别。心绞痛多在劳累时出现,特别是在剧烈运动、爬坡、处于极端天气或饱餐后。疼痛持续时间通常较短,多为 2～10 min,休息或服用硝酸甘油 1～5 min 后可缓解。伴随症状包括恶心、大汗、呼吸困难、心悸和头晕等。稳定型心绞痛患者症状可被预测并反复出现,常由运动所诱发。当疼痛发作频繁、剧烈或在轻微活动甚至静息时出现,需考虑为不稳定型心绞痛。当静息时出现心绞痛、疼痛剧烈并持续超过 30 min,需考虑为急性心肌梗死(MI)。部分患者在心肌梗死时会有"濒死感"。静息时的"心绞痛样"症状也可能由冠状动脉痉挛和非心源性疾病引起。

临床上存在其他可能与心绞痛混淆的潜在胸痛原因(见表 2.2)。急性心包炎患者多存在病毒前驱症状,

TABLE 2.2 Noncardiac Causes of Chest Pain

Condition	Location	Quality	Duration	Aggravating or Alleviating Factors	Associated Symptoms or Signs
Pulmonary embolism (chest pain often not present)	Substernal or over region of pulmonary infarction	Pleuritic (with pulmonary infarction) or angina-like	Sudden onset (minutes to hours)	Aggravated by deep breathing	Dyspnea, tachypnea, tachycardia; hypotension, signs of acute right ventricular heart failure, and pulmonary hypertension with large emboli; pleural rub; hemoptysis with pulmonary infarction
Pulmonary hypertension	Substernal	Pressure; oppressive	—	Aggravated by effort	Pain usually associated with dyspnea; signs of pulmonary hypertension
Pneumonia with pleurisy	Located over involved area	Pleuritic	—	Aggravated by breathing	Dyspnea, cough, fever, bronchial breath sounds, rhonchi, egophony, dullness to percussion, occasional pleural rub
Spontaneous pneumothorax	Unilateral	Sharp, well localized	Sudden onset; lasts many hours	Aggravated by breathing	Dyspnea; hyperresonance and decreased breath and voice sounds over involved lung
Musculoskeletal disorders	Variable	Aching, well localized	Variable	Aggravated by movement; history of exertion or injury	Tender to palpation or with light pressure
Herpes zoster	Dermatomal distribution	Sharp, burning	Prolonged	None	Vesicular rash appears in area of discomfort
Esophageal reflux	Substernal or epigastric; may radiate to neck	Burning, visceral discomfort	10–60 min	Aggravated by large meal, postprandial recumbency; relief with antacid	Water brash
Peptic ulcer	Epigastric, substernal	Visceral burning, aching	Prolonged	Relief with food, antacid	—
Gallbladder disease	Right upper quadrant; epigastric	Visceral	Prolonged	Spontaneous or after meals	Right upper quadrant tenderness may be present
Anxiety states	Often localized over precordium	Variable; location often moves from place to place	Varies; often fleeting	Situational	Sighing respirations; often chest wall tenderness

with acute pericarditis is typically sharp, is located to the left of the sternum, and radiates to the neck, shoulders, and back. This may be rather severe pain that is present at rest and can last for hours. It typically improves with sitting up and forward and worsens with inspiration. Oftentimes history of causative viral prodrome can be elicited.

Acute aortic dissection usually causes sudden onset of severe tearing chest pain that radiates to the back between the scapulae or to the lumbar region. Typically, there is a history of hypertension, and pulses may be asymmetric between the extremities. A murmur of aortic regurgitation may also be heard. Pain associated with pulmonary embolism is also acute in onset and is usually accompanied by shortness of breath. This pain is typically pleuritic, worsening with inspiration.

Dyspnea

Dyspnea is another hallmark symptom of cardiovascular disease, but it is also a primary symptom of pulmonary disease. It is defined as an uncomfortable heightened awareness of breathing. This can be an entirely normal sensation in individuals performing moderate to extreme exertion, depending on their level of conditioning. When it occurs at rest or with minimal exertion, dyspnea is considered abnormal. Dyspnea may accompany a large number of noncardiac conditions such as anemia due to a lack of oxygen-carrying capacity, pulmonary disorders such as obstructive or restrictive lung disease and asthma, obesity due to an increased work of breathing and restricted filling of the lungs, and deconditioning. In the cardiovascular patient, dyspnea may be caused by ventricular dysfunction, either systolic or diastolic; CAD and resultant ischemia; a large pericardial effusion causing impaired filling and resulting depressed cardiac output (cardiac tamponade); or valvular heart disease that, when severe, can lead to a drop in cardiac output. In cases of left ventricular dysfunction and valvular disease, the mechanism of dyspnea often involves increased intracardiac pressures that lead to pulmonary vascular congestion. Fluid then leaks into the alveolar space, impairing gas exchange and causing dyspnea.

Breathing difficulties can also be secondary to a low-output state without pulmonary vascular congestion. Patients often notice dyspnea with exertion, but it can also occur at rest in patients with severe cardiac disease. Shortness of breath at rest is also a symptom in patients with pulmonary edema, large pleural effusions, anxiety, or pulmonary embolism. A patient with left ventricular systolic or diastolic failure may describe the acute onset of breathing difficulty when sleeping. This problem, called paroxysmal nocturnal dyspnea (PND), is caused by pulmonary edema that is redistributed in a prone position; it is usually secondary to left ventricular failure. These patients often notice the acute onset of dyspnea followed by coughing roughly 2 to 4 hours after going to sleep. This can be a very uncomfortable feeling, and it leads

表 2.2 胸痛的非心血管病因

分类	位置	性质	持续时间	加重或缓解因素	伴随症状或体征
肺栓塞（常无胸痛）	胸骨下或肺梗死区	胸膜炎性（肺梗死时）或心绞痛样	突然发作，数分钟至数小时	深呼吸可加剧	呼吸困难，呼吸急促，心动过速；低血压，急性右心室衰竭体征，大栓子时出现肺动脉高压；胸膜摩擦音；肺梗死时出现咯血
肺动脉高压	胸骨下	受压、压迫感	—	劳力时加剧	疼痛常伴有呼吸困难，肺动脉高压体征
肺炎合并胸膜炎	局限于病变区域	胸膜炎性	—	呼吸时加剧	呼吸困难，咳嗽，发热，支气管呼吸音，干啰音，羊咩音，叩诊浊音，偶有胸膜摩擦音
自发性气胸	单侧	锐痛，高度局限	突然发作，持续数小时	呼吸时加剧	呼吸困难，过清音，肺部呼吸音及语音传导减低
肌肉骨骼疾病	多变	酸痛，高度局限	多变	运动后加剧，有活动史或外伤史	触诊或轻压后疼痛
带状疱疹	沿神经分布	锐痛，烧灼感	持续性	无	不适区域可见水疱性皮疹
胃食管反流	胸骨下或上腹部，可放射至颈部	烧灼感，脏器不适感	10～60 min	大量进食或饭后卧位加重，抑酸药可缓解	胃灼热
消化性溃疡	上腹部，胸骨下	脏器烧灼感，钝痛	持续性	进食、抑酸药可缓解	—
胆囊疾病	右上腹部，上腹部	脏器性	持续性	自发出现或餐后加剧	右上腹部可有压痛
焦虑状态	常局限于心前区	多变，位置常发生变化	可变，通常短暂	情境性	叹息样呼吸，胸壁常有压痛

胸痛常为锐痛，位于胸骨左侧，向颈部、肩部及背部放射。可在休息时出现并持续数小时，疼痛剧烈，在前倾坐位时减轻，在吸气时加重。

主动脉夹层患者多呈突发性剧烈撕裂样胸痛，放射至背部肩胛区或腰部，通常有高血压病史，四肢脉搏不对称，可闻及主动脉瓣反流杂音。肺栓塞引起的胸痛常急性发作，伴有呼吸困难，疼痛常为胸膜炎性，随吸气而加重。

呼吸困难

呼吸困难是心血管疾病的另一种典型症状，也是肺部疾病的主要症状。呼吸困难被定义为一种呼吸不适感，同时也是中高强度运动时的正常生理表现，因个人体能水平而异。当静息或轻微运动时出现呼吸困难，则考虑为病理性的。呼吸困难见于多种非心血管疾病，如贫血导致的携氧能力降低、肺部疾病如阻塞性或限制性肺疾病和哮喘、肥胖导致的呼吸作功增加和肺部充盈受限，以及身体功能减退等。在心血管疾病患者中，呼吸困难可能由心室功能障碍（收缩性或舒张性）、CAD诱发的心肌缺血、大量心包积液导致的充盈障碍和心输出量下降（心脏压塞），或严重心脏瓣膜病造成的心输出量下降等原因引起。左心室功能障碍和心脏瓣膜病患者呼吸困难的机制通常是心腔内压力升高引起的肺血管淤血，液体渗入肺泡间隙影响气体交换，最终导致呼吸困难。

呼吸困难也可继发于无肺血管淤血的低心排血量状态。患者通常在运动时出现呼吸困难，严重心脏病患者在休息时也可出现。静息时气短亦可见于肺水肿、大量胸腔积液、焦虑或肺栓塞。左心室收缩性或舒张性功能衰竭患者在睡眠时突发呼吸困难的症状称为夜间阵发性呼吸困难（PND），是由于卧位时液体重新分布引起的肺水肿造成的，通常继发于左心衰竭。此类患者通常会在入睡后2～4 h突发呼吸困难，随后出现咳嗽。患者会因极度不适而立即坐起或离床，症状多

the patient to sit up immediately or get out of bed. Symptoms typically resolve over 15 to 30 minutes. Patients with left ventricular failure also often complain of orthopnea, which is dyspnea that occurs when one assumes a prone position. This is relieved by sleeping on multiple pillows or remaining seated to sleep. In severe cases of dyspnea due to heart failure, patients may have an immediate feeling of shortness of breath when attempting a supine position.

Patients with sudden onset of dyspnea may be experiencing flash pulmonary edema, which is very rapid and acute accumulation of fluid in the lungs. This can be associated with severe CAD and may also be a cause of dyspnea in patients with coarctation of the aorta and renal artery stenosis. Sudden dyspnea is associated with pulmonary embolism, and this symptom is typically accompanied by pleuritic chest pain and possibly hemoptysis in such patients. Pneumothorax can cause dyspnea accompanied by acute chest pain. Dyspnea due to lung disease is present with exertion, although in severe cases it may be present at rest. This is often accompanied by hypoxia and is relieved by pulmonary bronchodilators or steroids or both. Dyspnea may also be an "angina equivalent." Not all patients with CAD develop typical anginal chest pain. Dyspnea that comes on with exertion or emotional stress, is relieved with rest, and is relatively brief in duration might be a manifestation of significant CAD. This type of dyspnea is also usually improved with the administration of nitroglycerine.

Palpitation

Palpitation is another symptom commonly seen in the cardiovascular patient. This is the subjective sensation of rapid or forceful beating of the heart. Patients are often able to describe in detail the sensation they feel, such as jumping, skipping, racing, fluttering, or an irregularity in the heartbeat. It is important to ask the patient about the onset of the palpitations because they may begin abruptly at rest, only with exertion, with emotional stress, or with ingestion of certain foods such as chocolate. One should also inquire about associated symptoms such as chest pain, dyspnea, dizziness, and syncope. It is important to note other medical issues, such as thyroid disease, and bleeding, which can lead to anemia, because these conditions may be associated with arrhythmias. A social history focusing on drug use and intake of alcohol, caffeine, or medications is important because use of many substances can lead to certain rhythm disturbances. Certain over-the-counter medicines contain pseudoephedrine, which can cause increased heart rate and palpitations. The family history is also important, because there are many inherited disorders (e.g., long-QT syndromes) that might lead to significant arrhythmias.

Potential etiologies of palpitations include premature atrial or ventricular beats, which are typically described as isolated skips and can be uncomfortable. Supraventricular tachycardias such as atrial flutter, AV nodal reentrant tachycardia, and paroxysmal atrial tachycardia often start and stop abruptly and can be rapid. Atrial fibrillation is an irregular heart rhythm originating from the atria. It can lead to rapid heart rates, which can be symptomatic. Even slowly conducted atrial fibrillation can be symptomatic for some patients. Ventricular arrhythmias are more often associated with severe dizziness or syncope. Gradual onset of tachycardia with a gradual decline in HR is more indicative of sinus tachycardia or anxiety.

Syncope

Syncope may be caused by a variety of cardiovascular diseases. It is the transient loss of consciousness due to inadequate cerebral blood flow. In the patient presenting with syncope as a primary complaint, one must try to differentiate true cardiac causes from neurologic issues such as seizure and metabolic causes such as hypoglycemia. Determination of the timing of the syncopal event and associated symptoms is very helpful in determining the etiology. True cardiac syncope is typically very sudden, with no prodromal symptoms. It is typically caused by an abrupt drop in cardiac output that may be due to tachyarrhythmias such as ventricular tachycardia or fibrillation, bradyarrhythmias, such as complete heart block, severe valvular heart disease such as aortic or mitral stenosis, or obstruction of flow due to left ventricular outflow tract (LVOT) obstruction. It can also be caused by cardiac tamponade as well as by hemodynamically significant pulmonary embolism. True cardiac syncope often has no accompanying aura, though palpitations can be experienced in patients with tachyarrhythmia, or with pulmonary embolism or tamponade (due to frequently higher heart rates in these scenarios). In situations such as aortic stenosis or LVOT obstruction, syncope typically occurs with exertion. Patients may regain consciousness rather quickly with true cardiac syncope. It should be noted that some syncope is associated with a generalized shaking (i.e., convulsive syncope), which can mimic epileptic activity. Convulsive activity should not cause the clinician to rule out a cardiac etiology for syncope.

Neurocardiogenic syncope involves an abnormal reflexive response to a change in position. When one rises from a prone or seated position to a standing position, the peripheral vasculature usually constricts, and the HR increases, to maintain cerebral perfusion. With neurocardiogenic syncope, the peripheral vasculature abnormally dilates, the HR slows or doesn't increase normally, or both. This leads to a reduction in cerebral perfusion and syncope. A similar mechanism is responsible for carotid sinus syncope and syncope associated with micturition and cough. The patient usually describes a gradual onset of symptoms such as flushing, dizziness, diaphoresis, and nausea before losing consciousness, which lasts seconds. When these patients wake, they are often pale and have a lower HR.

In the patient with syncope due to seizures, a prodromal aura is typically present before loss of consciousness occurs. Patients regain consciousness much more slowly and at times are incontinent, complain of headache and fatigue, and have a "postictal" confusional state. Syncope due to stroke is rare, because there must be significant bilateral carotid disease or disease of the vertebrobasilar system causing brainstem ischemia. Neurologic deficits accompany the physical examination findings in these patients.

The history is very important in determining the cause of a syncopal episode. This was previously studied by Calkins and colleagues, who found that men older than 54 years of age who had no prodromal symptoms were more likely to have an arrhythmic cause of their episodes. However, those with prodromal symptoms such as nausea, diaphoresis, dizziness, and visual disturbances before passing out were more likely to have neurocardiogenic syncope. Many inherited disorders such as long-QT syndrome and other arrhythmias, hypertrophic cardiomyopathy with LVOT obstruction, and familial dilated cardiomyopathy lead to states conducive to syncope. For this reason, detailed family history is necessary.

Edema

Edema often accompanies cardiovascular disease but may be a manifestation of liver disease (cirrhosis), renal disease (nephrotic syndrome), thyroid disease (myxedema) or local issues such as chronic venous insufficiency or thrombophlebitis. Edema related to cardiac disease is caused by increased venous pressures that alter the balance between hydrostatic and oncotic forces. This leads to extravasation of fluid into the extravascular space. These patients, therefore, are intravascularly "volume up," which has implications for therapeutic approaches. Peripheral edema is common with right-sided heart failure, whereas the same process in left-sided heart failure leads to pulmonary edema. Left- and right-sided heart failure often coexist.

在 15～30 min 后缓解。左心衰竭患者常出现端坐呼吸，即卧位时呼吸困难，高枕或坐位睡眠可缓解。在心力衰竭导致严重呼吸困难的病例中，患者在尝试平卧位时会立即感到呼吸急促。

急性肺水肿可由于肺组织中液体迅速蓄积而突发呼吸困难，见于严重 CAD，也可见于主动脉缩窄和肾动脉狭窄患者。肺栓塞可引起突发呼吸困难，常伴有胸膜炎性疼痛或咯血。气胸导致的呼吸困难常伴急性胸痛。肺部疾病引起的呼吸困难多在劳累时出现，症状严重时在静息时也会出现，常伴有缺氧，应用肺支气管扩张剂、激素或二者合用时可缓解。并非所有 CAD 都会出现典型"心绞痛样"胸痛，部分可表现为劳累或情绪激动后出现、休息可缓解、持续时间较短的呼吸困难，且常可在服用硝酸甘油后缓解。

心悸

心悸是心血管疾病患者的另一种常见症状，是心脏快速而有力搏动的主观感觉。患者通常能够详细描述他们的感受，如心搏增强、心搏脱落、心率加快、扑动或心搏不规则。询问患者心悸的发作时间非常重要，因为心悸可能在休息时突然发作，也可能仅在活动、情绪激动或摄入某些食物（如巧克力）时发作。还应询问伴随症状，如胸痛、呼吸困难、头晕和晕厥等。同样也需要重视其他系统疾病，如甲状腺疾病和出血引起的贫血等都可导致心律失常。既往史如摄入麻醉毒品、酒精、咖啡因或药物等也可导致心律失常；部分非处方药含有伪麻黄碱，可导致心率加快和心悸。家族史也很重要，因为许多遗传性疾病（如长 QT 间期综合征）可能会导致严重心律失常。

心悸的病因包括：房性或室性早搏，通常被描述为引起不适感的单发间歇；室上性心动过速如心房扑动、房室结折返性心动过速、阵发性房性心动过速，通常表现为突发突止且心率较快；心房颤动，起源于心房，节律极不规整，常因心率过快而引起不适，即便是缓慢传导的心房颤动也会出现症状；室性心律失常多与严重头晕或晕厥有关；逐渐开始的心动过速并伴随心率逐渐减慢常提示窦性心动过速或焦虑。

晕厥

晕厥可由多种心血管疾病引起，是由于脑血流不足而引起的短暂意识丧失。对于以晕厥为主诉的患者，需将心源性晕厥与神经系统疾病（如癫痫）、内分泌系统疾病（如低血糖）引起的晕厥鉴别。明确晕厥发作时间和伴随症状有助于确定病因。真正的心源性晕厥通常突然发作，无前驱症状，其原因包括快速性心律失常（如室性心动过速或心室颤动）、缓慢性心律失常（如完全性心脏传导阻滞）、严重心脏瓣膜病（如主动脉瓣或二尖瓣狭窄）、左心室流出道（LVOT）梗阻导致的血流受阻。心脏压塞（亦称心包填塞）和伴随血流动力学改变的肺栓塞也可引起心源性晕厥。心源性晕厥通常无伴随症状，但心动过速、肺栓塞或心脏压塞患者可能伴有心悸（此时心率通常较快）。主动脉瓣狭窄或 LVOT 梗阻引起的晕厥通常在运动时发作。心源性晕厥患者通常很快恢复意识。需要注意的是，部分晕厥会伴有全身抽搐（即抽搐性晕厥），表现与癫痫发作相似，因此临床医生需考虑晕厥是否为心脏疾病引起。

神经心源性晕厥是患者体位改变时的异常反射。生理状态下，从卧位、坐位变为立位时会出现外周血管收缩、心率加快以维持脑灌注。神经心源性晕厥患者外周血管异常扩张、心率减慢或不能正常增快，或二者兼有，导致脑灌注不足从而导致晕厥。类似机制见于颈动脉窦性晕厥和排尿、咳嗽相关性晕厥。此类患者在意识丧失前通常会逐渐出现面部潮红、头晕、大汗、恶心等症状并持续数秒，当恢复意识时多面色苍白、心率较慢。

癫痫发作引起的晕厥在意识丧失前通常会有前驱症状。此类患者意识恢复较为缓慢，有时会出现大小便失禁、头痛、乏力或发作后意识模糊。卒中引起的晕厥较为罕见，当患者存在严重的双侧颈动脉疾病或椎基底系统疾病引起脑干缺血时才会导致晕厥，在体格检查时可发现神经功能缺损体征。

病史采集对于明确晕厥发作的病因非常重要。Calkins 及其同事研究发现 54 岁以上男性出现无前驱症状的晕厥多为心律失常引起。然而，晕厥前有恶心、大汗、头晕、视物模糊等前驱症状的患者，则更可能是神经心源性晕厥。许多遗传性疾病如长 QT 间期综合征和其他类型的心律失常、梗阻性肥厚型心肌病和家族性扩张型心肌病也可导致晕厥。因此，需详细采集家族史。

水肿

水肿常见于心血管疾病患者，也可能是肝脏疾病（肝硬化）、肾脏疾病（肾病综合征）、甲状腺疾病（黏液性水肿）或局部病变（慢性静脉功能不全或血栓性静脉炎）的临床表现。心血管疾病患者出现水肿的机制是静脉压增高引起流体静压与胶体渗透压失衡，导致液体渗出到血管外组织间隙中。这些患者血管内"容量增加"，需采取相应治疗。外周水肿常见于右心衰竭，而左心衰竭通过相同的病理机制导致肺水肿。左心衰竭与右心衰竭经常共存。

Edema due to a cardiac etiology is typically bilateral and begins distally with progression in a proximal fashion. The feet and ankles are affected first, followed by the lower legs, thighs, and, ultimately, the abdomen, sometimes accompanied by ascites. If edema is visible, it is usually preceded by a weight gain of at least 5 to 10 pounds. Edema with heart disease is typically pitting, leaving an indentation in the skin after pressure is applied to the area. The edema is usually worse in the evening, and patients often describe an inability to fit into their shoes. There may also be a feeling of abdominal fullness, depressed appetite, and difficulty fitting into other clothing, such as pants, normally. While these patients are lying prone, the edema can shift to the sacral region after several hours, only to accumulate again the next day when they are on their feet again (dependent edema).

Total body edema, or anasarca, may be caused by heart failure but is also seen in nephrotic syndrome, cirrhosis, and severe hypothyroidism. Unilateral edema is more likely associated with a localized issue such as deep venous thrombosis or thrombophlebitis. Other parts of the history may shed light on the etiology of edema. Patients who report PND and orthopnea are likely to have a cardiac etiology, and in fact, PND is the most specific historical finding in heart failure. If there is a history of alcohol abuse and jaundice is present, liver disease should be a considered cause. Edema of the eyes and face in addition to lower-extremity edema is more likely related to nephrotic syndrome, though this may also occur in heart failure. Edema associated with discoloration or ulcers of the lower extremities is often seen with chronic venous insufficiency. In a patient with insidious onset of edema progressing to anasarca and ascites, one must consider a diagnosis of chronic constrictive pericarditis.

Cyanosis

Cyanosis is defined as an abnormal bluish discoloration of the skin resulting from an increase in the level of reduced hemoglobin or abnormal hemoglobin in the blood. When present, it typically represents an oxygen saturation of less than 85% (normal, >90%). There are several types of cyanosis. Central cyanosis often manifests in discoloration of the lips or trunk and usually represents low oxygen saturations due to right-to-left shunting of blood. This can occur with structural cardiac abnormalities such as large atrial or ventricular septal defects, but it also happens with impaired pulmonary function, as in severe chronic obstructive lung disease. Peripheral cyanosis is typically secondary to vasoconstriction in the setting of low cardiac output. This can also occur with exposure to cold and can represent local arterial or venous thrombosis. When localized to the hands, peripheral cyanosis suggests Raynaud's phenomenon. Cyanosis in childhood often indicates congenital heart disease with right-to-left shunting of blood, causing lower oxygen content in systemically circulated blood.

Other

There are other, nonspecific symptoms that may indicate cardiovascular disease. Although fatigue is present with myriad medical conditions, it is common in patients with cardiac disease and can be a manifestation of coronary disease, volume overload, low cardiac output, hypotension, or hypertension. Iatrogenic causes of fatigue in cardiac patients include aggressive medical treatment of hypertension and overdiuresis in patients with heart failure. Fatigue may also be a direct result of medical therapy for cardiac disease itself, such as with β-blocking agents.

Although cough is commonly associated with pulmonary disease, it may also indicate high intracardiac pressures which can lead to pulmonary edema. Cough may be present in patients with heart failure or significant left-sided valve disease. A patient with congestive heart failure may describe a cough productive of frothy pink sputum, as opposed to frank bloody or blood-tinged sputum, which is more typically seen with primary lung pathology. Nausea and emesis can accompany acute myocardial infarction and are often the only symptoms of MI. These "abdominal" symptoms may also be a reflection of heart failure leading to hepatic or intestinal congestion due to high right heart pressures. Anorexia, abdominal fullness, and cachexia may occur with end-stage heart failure, and the term "cardiac cachexia" has been coined to describe this syndrome. Nocturia is also a symptom described with heart failure; renal perfusion improves when the patient lies in a prone position, leading to an increase in urine output. Hoarseness of voice can occur due to compression of the recurrent laryngeal nerve. This may happen with enlarged pulmonary arteries, enlarged left atrium, or aortic aneurysm (Ortner's syndrome).

Despite the myriad symptoms of cardiovascular disease described here, many patients with significant cardiac disease are asymptomatic. Patients with CAD may have periods of asymptomatic ischemia that can be documented on ambulatory electrocardiographic monitoring. Up to one third of patients who have suffered a myocardial infarction are unaware that they had an event. This is more common in diabetics and in older patients. A patient may have severely depressed ventricular function for some time before presenting with symptoms. In addition, patients with atrial fibrillation can be entirely asymptomatic, with this rhythm discovered only after a physical examination or electrocardiogram is performed.

It is also important to note that cardiovascular disease is a leading cause of morbidity and mortality in women, but women have not classically been included in large longitudinal or epidemiologic studies of cardiac disease. Thus, much of our knowledge has been gathered from the study of men, and women may have atypical symptoms and presentations for cardiovascular disease. A high clinical suspicion for cardiovascular disease, the leading cause of death in both men and women, is imperative during evaluation, especially of the patient with cardiovascular disease risk factors.

At times, patients do not report having symptoms related to usual activities of daily living, yet symptoms are present when functional testing is performed. Therefore, assessing functional capacity is a very important part of the history in a patient with known or suspected cardiovascular disease. The ability or inability to perform various activities plays a substantial role in determining the extent of disability and in assessing response to therapy and overall prognosis, and it can influence decisions regarding the timing and type of therapy or intervention. The New York Heart Association Functional Classification is a commonly used method to assess functional status based on "ordinary activity" (Table 2.3). Patients are classified in one of four functional classes. Functional class I includes patients with known cardiac disease who have no limitations with ordinary activity. Functional classes II and III describe patients who have symptoms with less and less activity, whereas patients in functional class IV have symptoms at rest. The Canadian Cardiovascular Society has provided a similar classification of functional status specifically for patients with angina pectoris. These tools are very useful in classifying a patient's symptoms at a given time, allowing comparison at a future point and determination as to whether the symptoms are stable or progressive.

DIAGNOSIS AND PHYSICAL EXAMINATION

General

Like the detailed history, the physical examination is also vital when assessing a patient with cardiovascular disease. This consists of more than simple cardiac auscultation. Many diseases of the cardiovascular system can affect and be affected by other organ systems. Therefore, a detailed general physical examination is essential. The general

心源性水肿通常为对称性，从肢体远端开始逐渐向近心端发展。首先受累的是足和脚踝，其次是小腿、大腿，最后是腹部（可伴腹水）。若水肿明显，通常患者体重增加至少 5～10 磅（2.25～4.5 kg）。心源性水肿的特点是凹陷性水肿，按压皮肤后可留下明显压痕。水肿通常在夜间加重，很多患者会出现穿鞋困难的情况。部分患者还可能出现腹胀和食欲不振等其他临床表现。虽然患者平卧数小时后水肿可以转移到骶骨区域，但次日站立后会再次出现双足水肿（体位性水肿）。

全身性水肿可见于心力衰竭患者，但也可见于肾病综合征、肝硬化和严重甲状腺功能减退症患者。单侧水肿提示局部疾病如深静脉血栓形成或血栓性静脉炎。仔细询问病史有助于明确水肿的病因。有夜间阵发性呼吸困难和端坐呼吸等症状的患者出现水肿通常由心脏疾病引起。若患者有酒精滥用史或出现黄疸，则提示肝脏疾病可能性大。若除下肢水肿外还有眼睑和颜面部水肿，则可能与肾病综合征有关，心力衰竭也可能发生上述情况。水肿伴有下肢颜色改变或溃疡常见于慢性静脉功能不全患者。起病隐匿并进展为全身水肿和腹水的患者，要考虑慢性缩窄性心包炎的可能。

发绀

发绀的定义是指血液中去氧血红蛋白或异常血红蛋白水平增加，引起皮肤或黏膜呈青紫色的改变。当出现发绀时，说明血氧饱和度低于85%（正常应大于90%）。发绀有多种类型：中心性发绀通常表现为嘴唇和躯干发紫，这是血液自右向左分流引起血氧饱和度降低所致，可见于结构性心脏病如较大的房间隔或室间隔缺损，也可见于重度慢性阻塞性肺疾病等肺功能受损的情况；周围性发绀通常继发于低心输出量引起的血管收缩，也可在暴露于寒冷时发生，可能代表局部动脉或静脉血栓形成。当周围性发绀局限于手部时，则为雷诺现象。儿童期的发绀常提示患有自右向左分流的先天性心脏病。

其他

心血管疾病患者还有许多不典型症状。乏力是心脏疾病（如冠状动脉疾病、心脏容量过载、心输出量低、低血压或高血压）常见的临床表现之一。并且高血压患者过度药物治疗或心力衰竭患者过度利尿也可导致出现乏力。此外，心血管疾病治疗用药也可引起乏力，如应用β受体阻滞剂。

咳嗽也可提示存在心腔内压力增高导致的肺水肿，可见于心力衰竭或严重的左心瓣膜病患者。充血性心力衰竭患者可表现为咳粉红色泡沫痰，而咯血或痰中带血则更常见于原发性肺部疾病。恶心和呕吐是急性心肌梗死的伴随症状，也可能提示心力衰竭时由于右心压力升高引起的肝脏或肠道淤血。心力衰竭终末期患者可能出现厌食、腹部饱胀感和恶病质。夜尿增多也是心力衰竭患者的症状之一，当患者处于卧位时，肾脏灌注得到改善，从而引起尿量增加。声嘶可见于喉返神经受压，可发生于肺动脉扩张、左心房扩大或动脉瘤（Ortner综合征）患者。

尽管在这里介绍了心血管疾病的多种症状，但仍有很多严重的心血管疾病患者是无症状的。冠心病患者处于无症状缺血期，可通过动态心电图检测到异常。多达1/3的心肌梗死患者没有意识到他们发生了心脏事件，尤其在糖尿病和老年患者中更常见。部分患者可能在心功能严重降低后才会出现不适症状。此外，部分心房颤动患者完全没有症状，只有在体检或心电图检查时才发现。

心血管疾病是导致女性发病和死亡的主要原因之一，但女性通常不被纳入心脏病的大型流行病学研究。因此，目前我们的大部分认知都是从针对男性的研究中获得的，而女性可能存在非典型的心血管疾病症状和体征。在临床评估过程中，无论男性或女性，有心血管疾病危险因素者都应怀疑患心血管疾病的可能。

评估心脏功能对于已知或怀疑患有心血管疾病的患者非常重要。是否具有进行各种活动的能力是确定失能程度、评估疗效和整体预后的重要内容，并且可能影响进行治疗或干预的时机和方法。美国纽约心脏协会心功能分级是根据日常活动评估心功能状态的常用方法（表2.3）。患者被分为Ⅰ～Ⅳ级，Ⅰ级患者有心脏疾病但日常活动不受限制；Ⅱ级、Ⅲ级患者的日常活动轻度或明显受限；Ⅳ级患者在休息时即会出现不适症状。加拿大心血管学会也为心绞痛患者提供了类似的功能状态分级。这些工具可在特定时间点对患者的症状进行分级并进行动态评估对比，以确定患者的症状进展情况。

诊断和体格检查

一般情况

体格检查对评估心血管疾病患者也是至关重要的。不仅包括心脏听诊，还需考虑其他器官系统的影响，因此，全面详细的体格检查必不可少。

TABLE 2.3	Classification of Functional Status[a]	
Class I	Uncompromised	Ordinary activity does not cause symptoms; symptoms occur only with strenuous or prolonged activity.
Class II	Slightly compromised	Ordinary physical activity results in symptoms; no symptoms at rest.
Class III	Moderately compromised	Less than ordinary activity results in symptoms; no symptoms at rest.
Class IV	Severely compromised	Any activity results in symptoms; symptoms may be present at rest.

[a]*Symptoms* refers to undue fatigue, dyspnea, palpitations, or angina in the New York Heart Association classification and refers specifically to angina in the Canadian Cardiovascular Society classification.

appearance of a patient is helpful: Examination of skin color, breathing pattern, presence of pain, and overall nutritional status can provide clues regarding the diagnosis. Examination of the head may reveal evidence of hypothyroidism, such as hair loss and periorbital edema, and examination of the eyes may reveal exophthalmos associated with hyperthyroidism. Both conditions can affect the heart. Retinal examination may reveal macular edema or flame hemorrhages that can be associated with uncontrolled hypertension. Findings such as clubbing or edema when examining the extremities, and jaundice or cyanosis when evaluating the skin, may provide clues to undiagnosed cardiovascular disease.

Examination of the Jugular Venous Pulsations

Examination of the neck veins can provide a great deal of insight into right heart hemodynamics. The right internal jugular vein should be used, because the relatively straight course of the right innominate and jugular veins allows for a more accurate reflection of the true right atrial pressure. The longer and more winding course of the left-sided veins does not allow for as accurate a transmission of hemodynamics. For examination of the right internal jugular vein, the patient should be placed at a 45-degree angle—higher in patients with suspected elevated venous pressures and lower in those with lower venous pressures. The head should be turned slightly leftward, and a light shined at an angle over the neck can help the exam. Although the internal jugular vein itself is not visible, the pulsations from that vessel are transmitted to the skin and can be seen in most cases. The carotid artery lies in close proximity to the jugular vein, and its pulsations can sometimes be seen as well. Therefore, one must be certain one is observing the correct vessel.

Several techniques can help the clinician differentiate carotid and venous pulsations. A normal carotid pulsation pattern usually appears as a smooth and rapid upstroke, whereas a venous pulsation tends to have three "waves," the *a* wave of atrial contract, the *c* wave of the tricuspid valve closure, and the *v* wave of ventricular contraction. Variations in the appearance of these waves can help the clinician diagnose arrhythmia, constriction and tamponade, valvular heart disease, and heart failure. These are further discussed in the following text. The carotid and venous pulsations can further be distinguished by response to attempted compression of the pulsations or vessel. An arterial pulse will not be obliterated by this maneuver, whereas a venous pulse likely will become diminished or absent with compression. The arterial pulsations will not change with changes in positioning, whereas venous pulsations, as they are essentially reflections of a column of fluid draining into the right heart, will appear higher in the neck/head when a patient is more supine and lower when a patient is more upright. Finally, compression of the abdomen will cause an elevation or increase in prominence of the appearance of a venous wave and will not affect an arterial waveform in the neck.

Both the level of venous pressure and the morphology of the venous waveforms should be noted. Once the pulsations have been located, the vertical distance from the sternal angle (angle of Louis) to the top of the pulsations is determined. Because the right atrium lies about 5 cm vertically below the sternal angle, this number is added to the previous measurement to arrive at an estimated right atrial pressure in centimeters of water. The right atrial pressure is normally 5 to 9 cm H_2O. It can be higher in patients with decompensated heart failure, disorders of the tricuspid valve (regurgitation or stenosis), restrictive cardiomyopathy, or constrictive pericarditis.

With inspiration, negative intrathoracic pressure develops, venous blood drains into the thorax, and venous pressure in the normal patient falls; the opposite occurs during expiration. In a patient with conditions such as decompensated heart failure, constrictive pericarditis, or restrictive cardiomyopathy, this pattern is reversed (Kussmaul sign), and the venous pressure increases with inspiration. When the neck veins are examined, firm pressure should be applied for 10 to 30 seconds to the right upper quadrant over the liver. In a normal patient, this will cause the venous pressure to increase briefly and then return to normal. In the patient with conditions such as heart failure, constrictive pericarditis, or substantial tricuspid regurgitation, the neck veins will reveal a sustained increase in pressure due to passive congestion of the liver. This finding is called hepatojugular reflux.

The normal waveforms of the jugular venous pulse are depicted in Fig 2.1A. The *a* wave results from atrial contraction. The *x* descent results from atrial relaxation after contraction and the pulling of the floor of the right atrium downward with right ventricular contraction. The *c* wave interrupts the *x* descent and is generated by bulging of the cusps of the tricuspid valve into the right atrium during ventricular systole. This occurs at the same time as the carotid pulse. Atrial pressure then increases as a result of venous return with the tricuspid valve closed during ventricular systole; this generates the *v* wave, which is typically smaller than the *a* wave. The *y* descent follows as the tricuspid valve opens and blood flows from the right atrium to the right ventricle during diastole.

Understanding of the normal jugular venous waveforms is paramount, as these waveforms can be altered in different disease states. Abnormalities of these waveforms reflect underlying structural, functional, and electrical abnormalities of the heart (see Fig. 2.1B to G). Elevation of the right atrial pressure leading to jugular venous distention can be found in heart failure (both systolic and diastolic), hypervolemia, superior vena cava syndrome, and valvular disease. The *a* wave is exaggerated in any condition in which a greater resistance to right atrial emptying occurs. Such conditions include pulmonary hypertension, tricuspid stenosis, and right ventricular hypertrophy or failure. *Cannon a waves* occur when the atrium contracts against a closed tricuspid valve, which can occur with complete heart block or any other situation involving AV dissociation. The *a* wave is absent during atrial fibrillation. With significant tricuspid regurgitation, the *v* wave becomes very prominent and may merge with the *c* wave, diminishing or eliminating the *x* descent. With tricuspid stenosis, there is impaired emptying of the right atrium, which leads to an attenuated *y* descent. In pericardial constriction and restrictive

表 2.3	心功能分级 [a]	
I 级	不受限	日常活动不出现症状，只有当剧烈或持久活动时才会出现症状
II 级	轻度受限	日常活动可出现症状，但休息时无症状
III 级	中度受限	小于日常体力活动即可出现症状，休息时无症状
IV 级	严重受限	任何活动都可引起症状，休息时也可出现症状

[a] 在美国纽约心脏协会心功能分级中，症状指过度劳累、呼吸困难、心悸或心绞痛。而加拿大心血管学会心功能分级中，症状仅包括心绞痛。

患者的一般情况如皮肤颜色、呼吸模式、是否存在疼痛和总体的营养状况可为诊断提供线索。头部检查可发现甲状腺功能减退的证据，如脱发、眼眶周围水肿，眼部检查可发现与甲状腺功能亢进有关的突眼症，这两种疾病都可影响心脏功能。高血压控制不佳者视网膜检查可发现黄斑水肿或出血。杵状指或肢体水肿、黄疸或发绀都可为未确诊的心血管疾病提供有价值的线索。

颈静脉搏动检查

颈部血管检查有利于深入了解右心血流动力学变化。一般选取右侧颈内静脉，因为右侧颈内静脉和无名静脉的走行较直，更能准确反映真实的右心房压力。左侧颈内静脉较长且有多处弯曲，不能准确传递血流动力学信息。在检查右侧颈静脉时，通常采取半卧 45°，怀疑患者有静脉压升高时角度应当更高，而怀疑静脉压较低时角度应更低。患者头转向左侧，使光线以一定的角度照在颈部。虽然颈内静脉本身不可见，但来自血管的搏动可以传递到皮肤，大多数情况下可以观察到。颈动脉靠近颈静脉，其搏动有时也可以看到。因此，必须要确认观察的是正确的血管。

几种方法可以帮助临床医生区分颈动脉搏动和颈静脉搏动。正常的颈动脉搏动模式通常为平稳快速的起伏，而静脉搏动往往有三个"波"：心房收缩的 a 波、三尖瓣关闭的 c 波和心室收缩的 v 波。这些波的变化可以帮助临床医生诊断心律失常、心脏压塞、心脏瓣膜病和心力衰竭。具体内容将在下文进一步讨论。可以通过对搏动部位施加轻微压迫来分辨，动脉搏动不会被这种压迫消除，而静脉搏动会随着压迫逐渐减弱或消失，此外，动脉搏动更加有力。动脉搏动不会随着体位的改变而改变，而静脉搏动，因为它们本质上是一柱液体流入右心的反映，当患者仰卧时，颈部/头部的搏动会更高，而当患者更直立时，颈部/头部的搏动会更低。最后，压迫腹部会引起静脉波的升高或增加，而不会影响颈动脉波形。

检查时要注意静脉压力水平和静脉波形。一旦确定了颈静脉搏动的位置，就测量胸骨角到颈静脉搏动最强处的垂直距离。右心房位于胸骨角垂直向下 5 cm 处，所以将先前的测量值加上 5 cm 即为右心房压力。正常右心房压力为 5～9 cmH_2O。失代偿性心力衰竭、三尖瓣反流或狭窄、限制型心肌病和缩窄性心包炎患者的右心房压力会升高。

正常情况下，吸气时胸膜腔内压为负压，静脉血流入胸腔，静脉压下降，呼气时则相反。在患有失代偿性心力衰竭、缩窄性心包炎或限制型心肌病患者中，反应则相反，吸气时颈静脉压增高，称为 Kussmaul 征。当检查颈静脉时，对肝脏右上象限施加 10～30 s 压力，正常情况下会引起静脉压力短暂增加，然后迅速恢复正常。但在心力衰竭、缩窄性心包炎或有严重三尖瓣反流的患者中，颈静脉压因肝脏被动充血导致持续升高，被称为肝颈静脉回流征。

颈静脉搏动的正常波形如图 2.1A 所示。其中 a 波由心房收缩所致；x 降支波由右心房收缩后舒张、右心室收缩时右心房基底部向下牵拉所致；c 波打断了 x 降支波，由心室收缩期时三尖瓣瓣叶凸向右心房所致，与颈动脉搏动同时出现。心室收缩期时三尖瓣关闭，静脉回流导致心房压力升高，形成 v 波，其波幅通常较 a 波低。随后出现的是 y 降支波，由舒张期三尖瓣开放，血流从右心房流向右心室所致。

颈静脉波在不同的疾病状态下会发生改变，波形的异常反映了心脏的潜在结构、功能和电活动异常（图 2.1B～G）。右心房压力升高引起的颈静脉扩张可见于收缩性或舒张性心力衰竭、血容量过多、上腔静脉综合征和瓣膜病。a 波异常高大主要见于引起右心房排空时阻力增加的疾病，常见于肺动脉高压、三尖瓣狭窄、右心室肥厚或右心衰竭。大炮 a 波见于心房收缩时三尖瓣处于关闭状态导致血液回流，可出现于完全性房室传导阻滞或其他任何导致房室分离的情况。心房颤动时，a 波不存在。三尖瓣严重反流患者的 v 波明显增强，可能与 c 波融合，使 x 降支波变浅或消失。y 降支波变浅见于三尖瓣狭窄、右心房射血受阻的患者。而在心包缩窄和限制型心肌病患者中，y 降支波明显

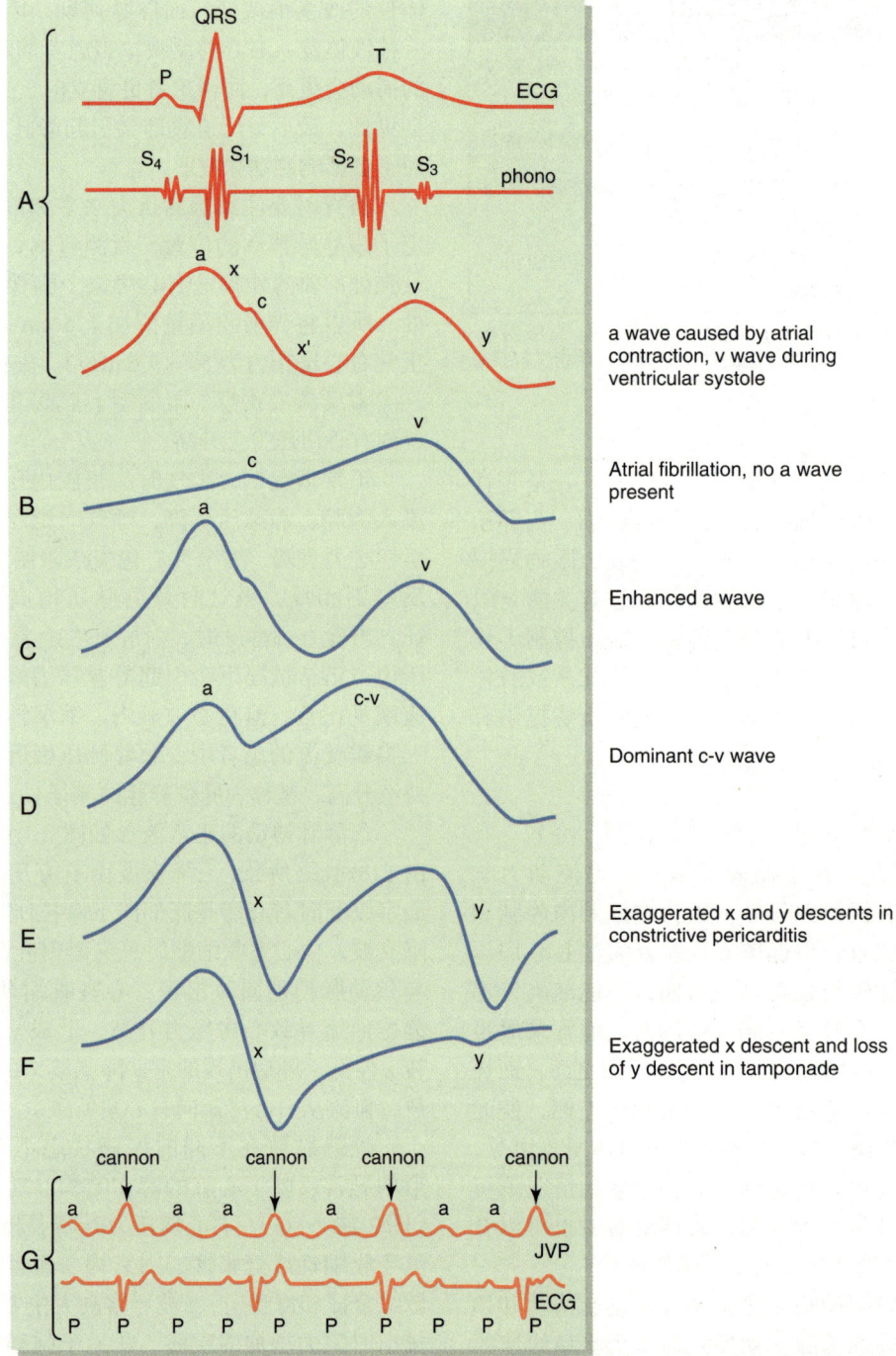

Fig. 2.1 Normal and abnormal jugular venous pulse (JVP) tracings. (A) Normal jugular pulse tracing with simultaneous electrocardiogram (ECG) and phonocardiogram. (B) Loss of the *a* wave in atrial fibrillation. (C) Large *a* wave in tricuspid stenosis. (D) Large *c-v* wave in tricuspid regurgitation. (E) Prominent *x* and *y* descents in constrictive pericarditis. (F) Prominent *x* descent and diminutive *y* descent in pericardial tamponade. (G) JVP tracing and simultaneous ECG during complete heart block demonstrates cannon *a* waves occurring when the atrium contracts against a closed tricuspid valve during ventricular systole. *P*, P waves correlating with atrial contraction; S_1 to S_4, heart sounds.

cardiomyopathy, the *y* descent occurs rapidly and deeply, and the *x* descent may also become more prominent, leading to a waveform with a w-shaped appearance. With pericardial tamponade, the *x* descent becomes very prominent while the *y* descent is diminished or absent.

Examination of Arterial Pressure and Pulse

Arterial blood pressure is measured noninvasively with the use of a sphygmomanometer. Before the blood pressure is taken, the patient ideally should be relaxed, allowed to rest for 5 to 10 minutes in a quiet room, and seated or lying comfortably. The cuff is typically applied

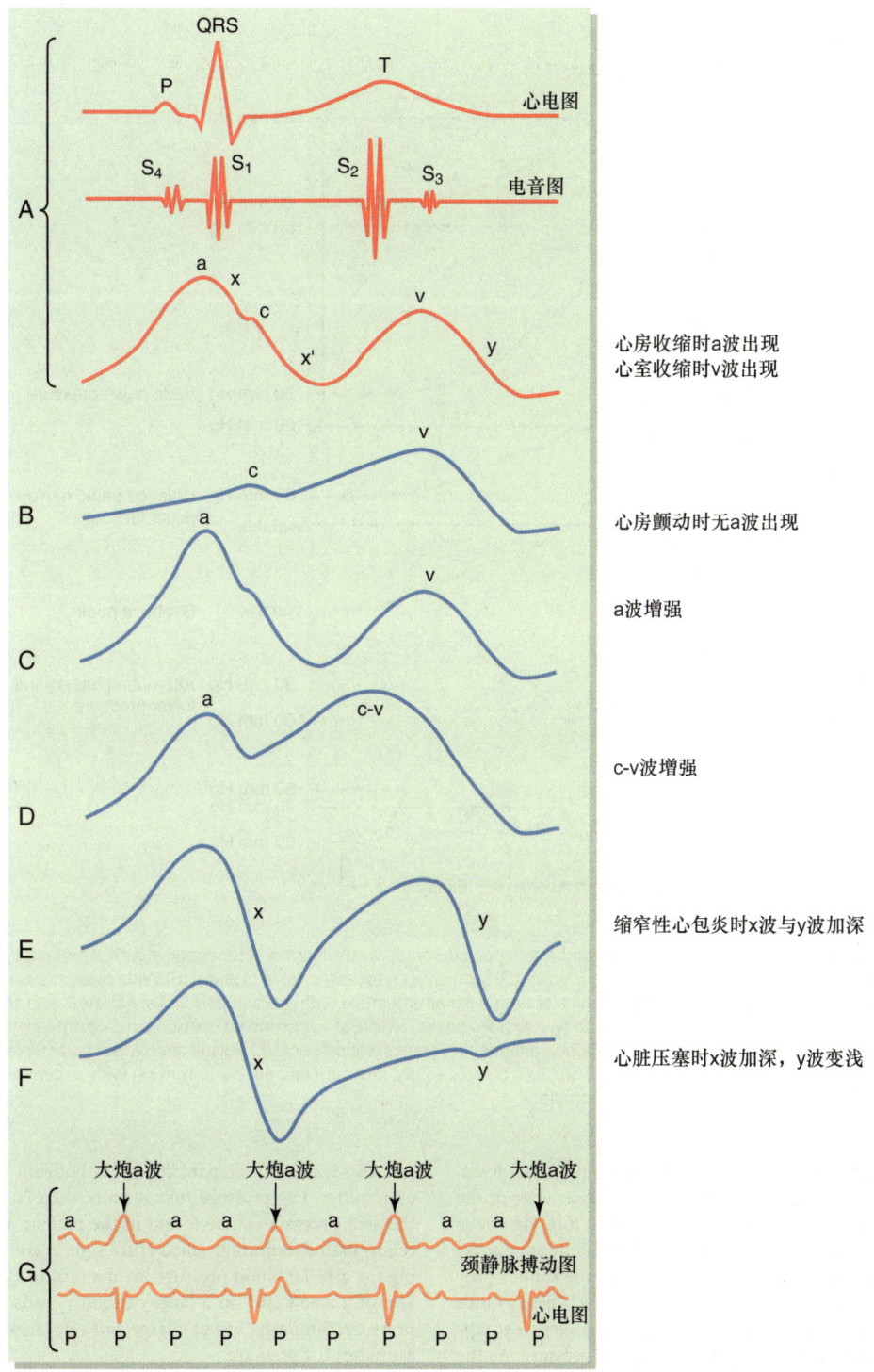

图 2.1 正常和异常的颈静脉搏动图。**A**. 正常颈静脉搏动图与同步的心电图和心音图。**B**. a 波消失见于心房颤动。**C**. a 波增强见于三尖瓣狭窄。**D**. c-v 波增强见于三尖瓣反流。**E**. 缩窄性心包炎时，x 波和 y 波加深。**F**. 心脏压塞时 x 波加深，y 波变浅。**G**. 完全性心脏传导阻滞时的颈静脉搏动图和同步心电图，当心房收缩时心室也处于收缩期，三尖瓣关闭时，显示大炮 a 波。P 波代表心房收缩；$S_1 \sim S_4$ 为心音

加深，并且 x 降支波也可能变得更加突出，出现类似 "w" 形的波形。心脏压塞患者的 x 降支波明显加深，但 y 降支波却变浅甚至消失。

动脉血压和脉搏检查

动脉血压的测量是利用血压计进行无创检查。在测量前，被检查者应在安静环境下放松、休息 5 ～ 10 min。将袖带缠于上臂，使其下缘在肘窝以上约 1 英寸（约

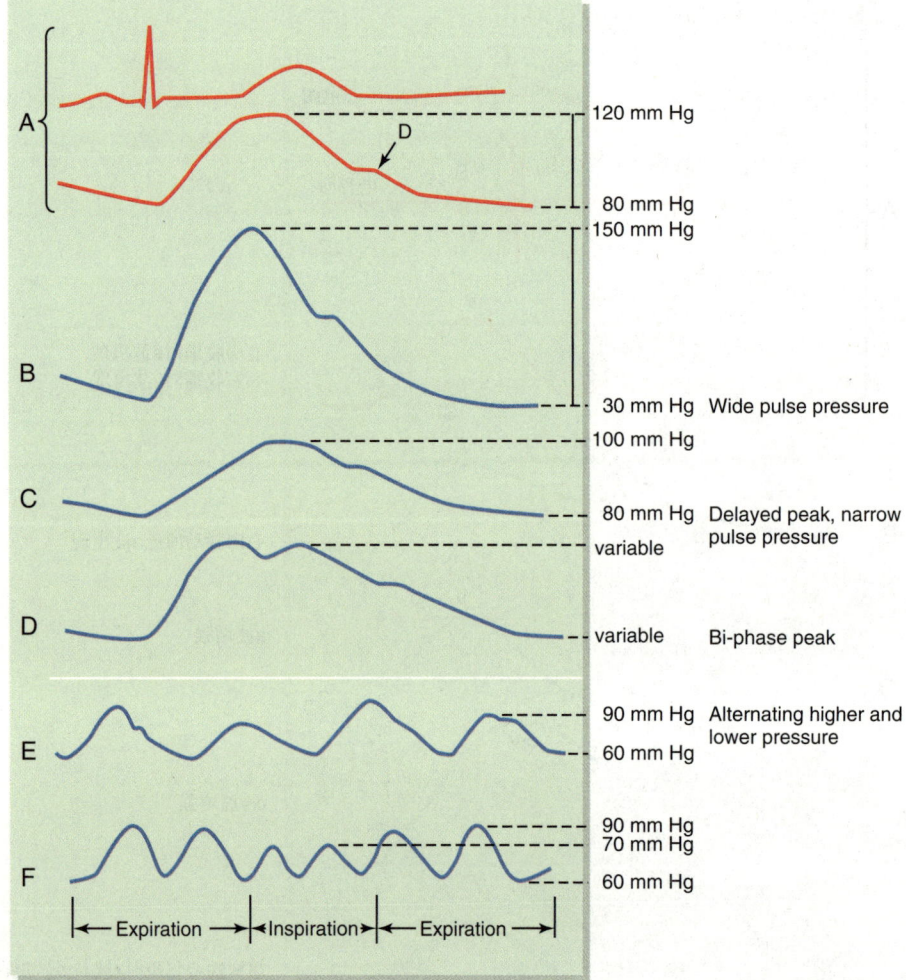

Fig. 2.2 Normal and abnormal carotid arterial pulse contours. (A) Normal arterial pulse with simultaneous electrocardiogram (ECG). The dicrotic wave (D) occurs just after aortic valve closure. (B) Wide pulse pressure in aortic insufficiency. (C) Pulsus parvus et tardus (small amplitude with a slow upstroke) associated with aortic stenosis. (D) Bisferiens pulse with two systolic peaks, typical of hypertrophic obstructive cardiomyopathy or aortic insufficiency, especially if concomitant aortic stenosis is present. (E) Pulsus alternans, characteristic of severe left ventricular failure. (F) Paradoxic pulse (systolic pressure decrease >10 mm Hg with inspiration), most characteristic of cardiac tamponade.

to the upper arm, approximately 1 inch above the antecubital fossa. A stethoscope is then used to auscultate under the lower edge of the cuff. The cuff is rapidly inflated to approximately 30 mm Hg above the anticipated systolic pressure and then slowly deflated (at approximately 3 mm Hg/sec) while the examiner listens for the sounds produced by blood entering the previously occluded artery. These sounds are the Korotkoff sounds. The first sound is typically a very clear tapping sound that, when heard, represents the systolic pressure. As the cuff continues to deflate, the sounds will disappear; this point represents the diastolic pressure.

In normal situations, the pressure in both arms is relatively equal. If the pressure is measured in the lower extremities rather than the arms, the systolic pressure is typically 10 to 20 mm Hg higher. If the pressures in the arms are asymmetric, this may suggest atherosclerotic disease involving the aorta, aortic dissection, or obstruction of flow in the subclavian or innominate arteries. The pressure in the lower extremities can be lower than arm pressures in the setting of abdominal aortic, iliac, or femoral disease. Coarctation of the aorta can also lead to discrepant pressures between the upper and lower extremities. Leg pressure that is more than 20 mm Hg higher than the arm pressure can be found in the patient with significant aortic regurgitation, a finding called Hill's sign. A common mistake in taking the arterial blood pressure involves using a cuff of incorrect size. Use of a small cuff on a large extremity leads to overestimation of pressure. Similarly, use of a large cuff on a smaller extremity underestimates the pressure.

Examination of the arterial pulse in a cardiovascular patient should include palpation of the carotid, radial, brachial, femoral, popliteal, posterior tibial, and dorsalis pedis pulses bilaterally. The carotid pulse most accurately reflects the central aortic pulse. One should note the rhythm, strength, contour, and symmetry of the pulses. A normal arterial pulse (Fig. 2.2A) rises rapidly to a peak in early systole, plateaus, and then falls. The descending limb of the pulse is interrupted by the incisura or dicrotic notch, which is a sharp deflection downward due to closure of the aortic valve. As the pulse moves toward the periphery, the systolic peak is higher and the dicrotic notch is later and less noticeable.

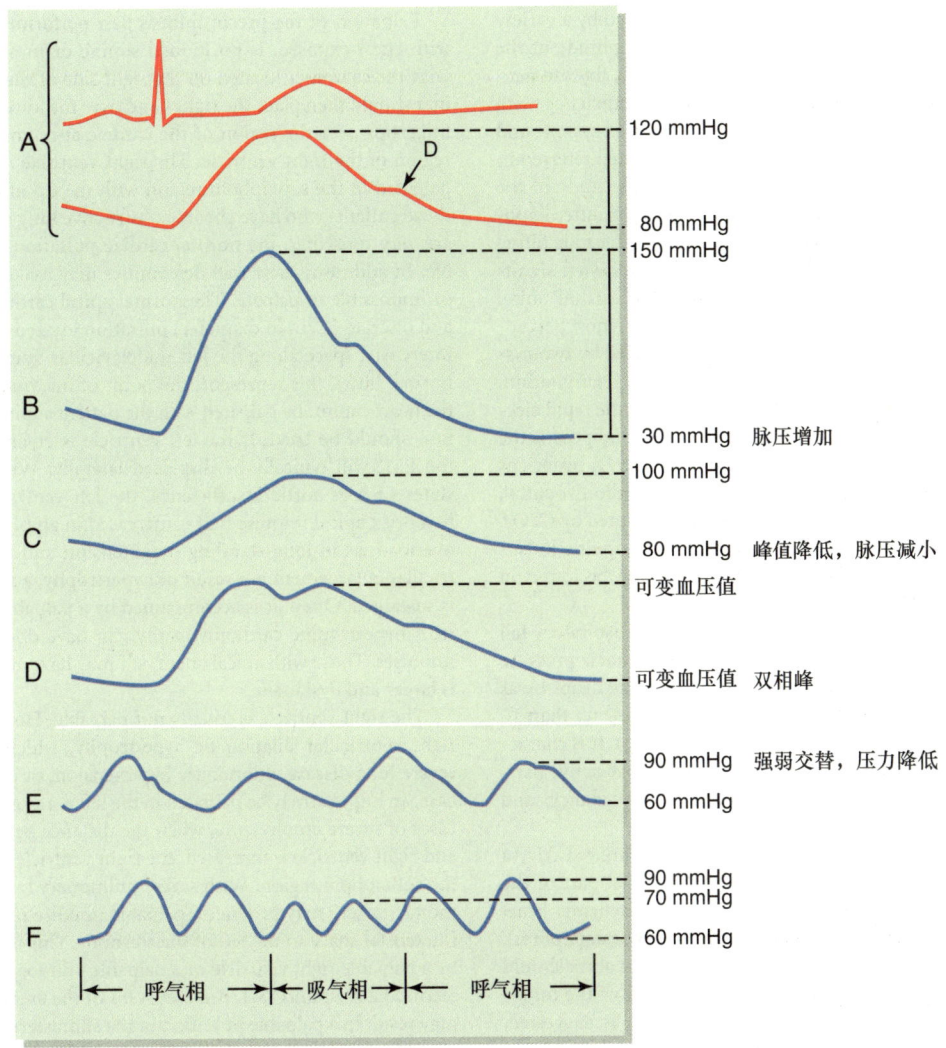

图 2.2　正常和异常的颈动脉脉搏图。**A**.正常动脉脉搏与同步心电图；重搏波（D）发生于主动脉瓣刚刚关闭后。**B**.主动脉瓣关闭不全时脉压增加。**C**.细迟脉（振幅小且缓慢上升）与主动脉瓣狭窄有关。**D**.双峰脉有两个收缩峰，是梗阻性肥厚型心肌病或主动脉瓣关闭不全，尤其是伴主动脉瓣狭窄的特征。**E**.交替脉见于严重的左心衰竭。**F**.奇脉（吸气时收缩压下降大于 10 mmHg）是心脏压塞的特点

2.54 cm）处，然后将听诊器体件置于袖带下缘处准备听诊。向袖带内快速充气，待汞柱升至高出预期收缩压 30 mmHg 时，开始缓慢放气（约 3 mmHg/s），同时注意听诊血液流入之前因受压而闭塞的动脉的声音。这些声音称为 Korotkoff 音。首先听到的响亮拍击声代表收缩压，当袖带继续放气，最终声音消失，此时的血压值为舒张压。

正常情况下，双上肢的血压大致相等。下肢的收缩压比上肢高出 10～20 mmHg。如果双上肢血压不对称，则提示有主动脉的动脉粥样硬化性疾病、主动脉夹层、锁骨下动脉或无名动脉血流受阻。在腹主动脉疾病、髂动脉或股动脉疾病中，会出现下肢血压低于上肢的情况。主动脉缩窄也会出现上肢与下肢血压相差较大。在严重主动脉瓣反流患者中，可以出现下肢血压高出上肢血压超过 20 mmHg，被称为 Hill 征。测量动脉血压的常见错误在于使用了尺寸不合适的袖带。手臂过于粗大时，用标准袖带测量其值会过高，反之，手臂太细时用标准袖带则结果会偏低。

心血管疾病患者的动脉脉搏检查应包括双侧颈动脉、桡动脉、肱动脉、股动脉、腘动脉、胫后动脉和足背动脉的触诊。颈动脉脉搏最能准确地反映中心主动脉脉搏。检查时应注意脉搏的节律、强度、波形及对称性。正常动脉脉搏（图 2.2A）的收缩早期快速达到波峰后进入平台期，随后下降。下降支大幅向下的重搏切迹（波）来源于主动脉瓣关闭。随着脉搏向外周传播，收缩波峰值变得更高，重搏切迹出现得更晚且不明显。

The normal pattern of the arterial pulse can be altered by a variety of cardiovascular diseases (see Fig. 2.2B to F). The amplitude of the pulse increases in conditions such as anemia, pregnancy, thyrotoxicosis, and other states with high cardiac output. Aortic insufficiency, with its resultant increase in pulse pressure (difference between systolic and diastolic pressure), leads to a bounding carotid pulse often referred to as a Corrigan pulse or a water-hammer pulse. The amplitude of the pulse is diminished in low-output states such as heart failure, hypovolemia, and mitral stenosis. Tachycardia, with shorter diastolic filling times, also lowers the pulse amplitude. Aortic stenosis, when significant, leads to a delayed systolic peak and diminished carotid pulse, referred to as *pulsus parvus et tardus*. A bisferiens pulse is most perceptible on palpation of the carotid artery. It is characterized by two systolic peaks and can be found in patients with pure aortic regurgitation. The first peak is the percussion wave, which results from the rapid ejection of a large volume of blood early in systole. The second peak is the tidal wave, which is a reflected wave from the periphery. A bisferiens pulse may also be found in those with hypertrophic cardiomyopathy, in which the initial rapid upstroke of the pulse is interrupted by LVOT obstruction. The reflected wave produces the second impulse. Pulsus alternans is beat-to-beat variation in the pulse and can be found in patients with severe left ventricular systolic dysfunction.

Pulsus paradoxus is an exaggeration of the normal inspiratory fall in systolic pressure. With inspiration, negative intrathoracic pressure is transmitted to the aorta, and systolic pressure typically drops by as much as 10 mm Hg. In pulsus paradoxus, this drop is greater than 10 mm Hg and can be palpable when marked (>20 mm Hg). It is characteristic in cardiac tamponade but can also be seen in constrictive pericarditis, pulmonary embolism, hypovolemic shock, pregnancy, and severe chronic obstructive lung disease.

Because peripheral vascular disease often accompanies CAD, a detailed examination of the peripheral pulses is a crucial part of the physical exam of a patient with known or suspected ischemic heart disease. In addition to the carotid, brachial, radial, femoral, popliteal, dorsalis pedis, and posterior tibial pulses, the abdominal aorta should be palpated. When the abdominal aorta is palpable below the umbilicus, the presence of an abdominal aortic aneurysm is suggested. Impaired blood flow to the lower extremities can cause claudication, a cramping pain located in the buttocks, thigh, calf, or foot, depending on the location of disease. With significant stenosis in the peripheral vasculature, the distal pulses may be significantly reduced or absent. Blood flow in a stenotic artery may be turbulent, creating an audible bruit. With normal aging, the peripheral arteries become less compliant and this change may obscure abnormal findings.

Examination of the Precordium

A complete cardiovascular examination should always include careful inspection and palpation of the chest. Abnormalities of the chest wall including skin findings should be observed. The presence of pectus excavatum is associated with Marfan syndrome and mitral valve prolapse. Pectus carinatum can also be found in patients with Marfan syndrome. Kyphoscoliosis can lead to right-sided heart failure and secondary pulmonary hypertension. One should also assess for visible pulsations, in particular in the regions of the aorta (second right intercostal space and suprasternal notch), pulmonary artery (third left intercostal space), right ventricle (left parasternal region), and left ventricle (fourth to fifth intercostal space at the left midclavicular line). Prominent pulsations in these areas suggest enlargement of these vessels or chambers. Retraction of the left parasternal area can be observed in patients with severe left ventricular hypertrophy, whereas systolic retraction at the apex or in the left axilla (Broadbent sign) is more characteristic of constrictive pericarditis.

Palpation of the precordium is best performed when the patient, with chest exposed, is positioned supine or in a left lateral position with the examiner located on the right side of the patient. The examiner should then place the right hand over the lower left chest wall with fingertips over the region of the cardiac apex and the palm over the region of the right ventricle. The right ventricle itself is typically best palpated in the subxiphoid region with the tip of the index finger. In those patients who have chronic obstructive lung disease, are obese, or are very muscular, the normal cardiac pulsations may not be palpable. In addition, chest wall deformities may make pulsations difficult or impossible to palpate. The normal apical cardiac impulse is a brief and discrete (1 cm in diameter) pulsation located in the fourth to fifth intercostal space along the left midclavicular line. In a patient with a normal heart, this represents the point of maximal impulse (PMI). If the heart cannot be palpated with the patient supine, a left lateral position should be tried. If the left ventricle is enlarged for any reason, the PMI will typically be displaced laterally. With volume overload states such as aortic insufficiency, the left ventricle dilates, resulting in a brisk apical impulse that is increased in amplitude. With pressure overload, as in long-standing hypertension and aortic stenosis, ventricular enlargement is a result of hypertrophy, and the apical impulse is sustained. Often, it is accompanied by a palpable S_4 gallop. Patients with hypertrophic cardiomyopathy can have double or triple apical impulses. Those with apical aneurysm may have an apical impulse that is larger and dyskinetic.

The right ventricle is usually not palpable. However, in those with right ventricular dilation or hypertrophy, which can be related to severe lung disease, pulmonary hypertension, or congenital heart disease, an impulse may be palpated in the left parasternal region. In some cases of severe emphysema, when the distance between the chest wall and right ventricle is increased, the right ventricle is better palpated in the subxiphoid region. With severe pulmonary hypertension, the pulmonary artery may produce a palpable impulse in the second to third intercostal space to the left of the sternum. This may be accompanied by a palpable right ventricle or a palpable pulmonic component of the second heart sound (S_2). An aneurysm of the ascending aorta or arch may result in a palpable pulsation in the suprasternal notch. Thrills are vibratory sensations best palpated with the fingertips; they are manifestations of harsh murmurs caused by such problems as aortic stenosis, hypertrophic cardiomyopathy, and septal defects.

Auscultation

Techniques

Auscultation of the heart is accomplished by use of a stethoscope with dual chest pieces. The diaphragm is ideal for high-frequency sounds, whereas the bell aids in auscultation of low-frequency sounds. When one is listening for low-frequency tones, the bell should be placed gently on the skin with minimal pressure applied. If the bell is applied more firmly, the skin will stretch and higher-frequency sounds will be heard (as when using the diaphragm). Auscultation should ideally be performed in a quiet setting with the patient's chest exposed and the examiner best positioned to the right of the patient. Four major areas of auscultation are evaluated, starting at the apex and moving toward the base of the heart. The mitral valve is best heard at the apex or location of the PMI. Tricuspid valve events are appreciated in or around the left fourth intercostal space adjacent to the sternum. The pulmonary valve is best evaluated in the second left intercostal space. The aortic valve is assessed in the second right intercostal space. These areas should be evaluated from apex to base using the diaphragm and then evaluated again with the bell. Auscultation of the back, the axillae, the right side of the chest, and the supraclavicular areas should also be done. Having the patient perform maneuvers such as leaning forward,

动脉脉搏波形的改变可见于多种心血管疾病（图2.2B～F）。在贫血、妊娠、甲状腺毒症和其他高心排血量状态下，脉搏的幅度增加。主动脉瓣关闭不全引起的脉压（收缩压与舒张压的差值）增大会导致颈动脉搏动起落明显，称为 Corrigan 脉或水冲脉。在心力衰竭、血容量不足和二尖瓣狭窄等低心排血量疾病中，脉搏的幅度减小。心动过速时舒张充盈期缩短，脉搏幅度也会降低。严重的主动脉瓣狭窄会引起收缩期峰值的延迟和颈动脉脉搏减弱，称为细迟脉。双峰脉在触诊颈动脉时最容易察觉。其特征在于具有两个收缩峰，可在单纯主动脉瓣反流患者中发现。第一个峰是冲击波，由收缩早期大量血液快速射出所致；第二个峰为潮汐波，是来自外周的反射波。肥厚型心肌病患者也可出现双峰脉，此情况下脉搏开始快速上升时可被左心室流出道梗阻所中断。交替脉是强弱交替的脉搏，可见于严重左心室收缩功能障碍的患者。

正常人吸气时收缩压下降，而如果下降过度则会出现奇脉。吸气时，胸腔内负压传导到主动脉，收缩压通常可下降多达 10 mmHg。当出现奇脉时，这一下降幅度可大于 10 mmHg，当降幅很大（20 mmHg）时可被触及。这是心脏压塞的特征，也可见于缩窄性心包炎、肺栓塞、低血容量性休克、妊娠和严重的慢性阻塞性肺疾病。

周围血管疾病常伴有 CAD，因此对于已确诊的缺血性心脏病患者，对外周脉搏进行详细检查绝对是有必要的。除了检查颈动脉、桡动脉、肱动脉、股动脉、腘动脉、胫后动脉和足背动脉之外，还应该触诊腹主动脉。当在脐下触及腹主动脉搏动时，提示有腹主动脉瘤。下肢血流不畅可导致跛行，根据病变位置不同可引起臀部、大腿、小腿或足部出现痉挛性疼痛。若外周血管存在严重的狭窄，则远端的脉搏可能明显减弱或消失。狭窄动脉中的血流呈湍流，可闻及杂音。随年龄增长，外周血管的顺应性下降，而这种变化可能会掩盖某些病变。

心前区检查

心血管系统体格检查应包括仔细的胸部视诊和触诊，这可为心脏疾病的诊断提供有价值的线索。胸部视诊时应注意胸廓畸形，包括皮肤的体征。漏斗胸可出现于马方综合征和二尖瓣脱垂患者。脊柱后侧凸可引起右心衰竭和继发性肺动脉高压。此外，还需要评估是否存在肉眼可见的搏动，特别是主动脉区（右侧第 2 肋间隙和胸骨上切迹）、肺动脉区（左侧第 3 肋间隙）、右心室区（左胸骨旁区域）和左心室区（左锁骨中线第 4～5 肋间隙）。这些区域若出现明显的搏动说明这些血管或心腔可能发生了扩张。在严重左心室肥厚患者中可观察到左胸骨旁区域负向搏动；而心脏收缩期出现心尖或左侧腋下负向搏动（Broadbent 征）更多见于缩窄性心包炎患者。

当进行胸部触诊时，患者需要充分暴露胸部，取仰卧位和右侧卧位，检查者位于患者的右侧，将右手置于左侧胸壁下部，指尖放在心尖区，手掌放在右心室区域。右心室的触诊最好用示指指尖在剑突下进行。在慢性阻塞性肺疾病、肥胖或肌肉发达的患者中，正常的心尖搏动可能无法触及。此外，胸壁畸形者也可能难以触及心尖搏动。正常的心尖搏动点位置清晰局限（直径 1 cm），位于左锁骨中线第 4～5 肋间，此处是心尖搏动最强点（PMI）。若患者平卧时心脏搏动无法触及，可采取左侧卧位进行触诊。在容量负荷过重状态，如主动脉瓣关闭不全的患者中，左心室扩大会导致心尖搏动增强。压力负荷过重的情况下，如长期高血压、主动脉瓣缩窄的患者，心室肥厚会导致心室增大，可触及心前区持续搏动（如心尖区抬举样搏动提示左心室肥厚；胸骨左下缘收缩期抬举样搏动提示右心室肥厚）；通常还伴随着可触及的 S_4 奔马律。肥厚型心肌病患者可触及双重或三重心尖搏动。心尖室壁瘤的心尖搏动增强并存在矛盾运动。

右心室搏动通常不易触及。但在严重肺部疾病、肺动脉高压或先天性心脏病引起的右心室扩张或肥厚的患者中，可在左胸骨旁触及搏动。在部分严重的肺气肿患者中，胸壁与右心室之间的距离增加，可在剑突下触及右心室搏动。重度肺动脉高压患者可在胸骨左缘第 2 或第 3 肋间触及明显的肺动脉搏动，可同时伴有右心室搏动或可触及的第二心音（S_2）肺动脉瓣成分。升主动脉或主动脉弓动脉瘤患者可在胸骨上切迹处触及搏动。震颤是一种震动感，在使用指尖触诊时最易触及，是主动脉瓣狭窄、肥厚型心肌病和室间隔缺损等疾病引起的粗糙杂音的表现。

听诊

技巧

心脏听诊是通过双用听诊器来实现的。膜型听诊器适合高频声音，而钟型听诊器对低频声音更敏感。当听诊低频音调时，应将钟型听诊器轻轻放在皮肤上，施加较小压力。如果钟型体件更加紧密地贴于皮肤，会将皮肤拉紧而听到高频声音（如同使用膜型听诊器）。理想状态下，听诊应在安静的环境中进行，充分暴露患者胸部，检查者最好在患者右侧进行听诊。心脏听诊通常从心尖区到心底部依次进行，主要有 4 个听诊区：①二尖瓣区，在心尖或 PMI 听诊最清晰；②三尖瓣区，位于胸骨左缘第 4、5 肋间；③肺动脉瓣区，在胸骨左缘第 2 肋间；④主动脉瓣区，位于胸骨右缘第 2 肋间。这些区域应按照从心尖到心底的顺序，先用膜型再用钟型听诊器进行听诊。此外，也应对背部、腋窝、右侧胸部和锁骨上区域进行听诊。

exhaling, standing, squatting, and performing a Valsalva maneuver may help to accentuate certain heart sounds (Table 2.4).

Normal Heart Sounds

All heart sounds should be described according to their quality, intensity, and frequency. There are two primary heart sounds heard during auscultation: S_1 and S_2. These are high-frequency sounds caused by closure of the valves. S_1 occurs with the onset of ventricular systole and is caused by closure of the mitral and tricuspid valves. S_2 is caused by closure of the aortic and pulmonic valves and marks the beginning of ventricular diastole. All other heart sounds are timed based on these two sounds.

S_1 has two components, the first of which (M_1) is usually louder, heard best at the apex, and caused by closure of the mitral valve. The second component (T_1), which is softer and thought to be related to closure of the tricuspid valve, is heard best at the lower left sternal border. Although there can be two components, S_1 is typically heard as a single sound. S_2 also has two components, which typically can be easily distinguished. A_2, the component caused by closure of the aortic valve, is usually louder and heard earlier and is best heard at the right upper sternal border. P_2, caused by closure of the pulmonic valve, is recognized best over the left second intercostal space. With expiration, a normal S_2 is perceived as a single sound. With inspiration, however, venous return to the right heart is augmented, and the increased capacitance of the pulmonary vascular bed results in a delay in pulmonic valve closure. A slight decline in pulmonary venous return to the left ventricle leads to earlier aortic valve closure. Therefore, physiologic splitting of S_2, with A_2 preceding P_2 during inspiration, is a normal finding.

Additional heart sounds can at times be heard in normal individuals. A third heart sound can sometimes be heard in healthy children and young adults. This is referred to as a physiologic S_3, which is rarely heard after the age of 40 years in a normal individual. A fourth heart sound is caused by forceful atrial contraction into a noncompliant ventricle; it is rarely audible in normal young patients but is relatively common in older individuals.

Murmurs are auditory vibrations generated by high flow across a normal valve or normal flow across an abnormal valve or structure. Murmurs that occur early in systole and are soft and brief in duration are not typically pathologic and are termed *innocent murmurs*. These usually are caused by flow across normal left ventricular or right ventricular outflow tracts and are found in children and young adults. Some systolic murmurs may be associated with high-flow states such as fever, anemia, thyroid disease, and pregnancy and are not innocent, although they are not typically associated with structural heart disease. They are called *physiologic murmurs* because of their association with altered physiologic states. All diastolic murmurs are pathologic.

Abnormal Heart Sounds

Abnormalities in S_1 and S_2 are related to either intensity (Table 2.5) or respiratory splitting (Table 2.6). S_1 is accentuated with tachycardia and with short PR intervals, whereas it is softer in the setting of a long PR interval. S_1 varies in intensity if the relationship between atrial and ventricular systole varies. In those patients with atrial fibrillation, atrial filling and emptying is not consistent because of the variable HR leading to beat-to-beat changes in the intensity of S_1. This also can occur with heart block or AV dissociation. In early mitral stenosis, S_1 is often accentuated, but with severe stenosis, there is decreased leaflet excursion and S_1 is diminished in intensity or altogether absent (Figs. 2.3 and 2.4). As previously mentioned, splitting of S_1 is not frequently heard. However, it is more apparent in conditions that delay closure of the tricuspid valve, including right bundle branch block and Ebstein's anomaly.

TABLE 2.4 Effects of Physiologic Maneuvers on Auscultatory Events

Maneuver	Major Physiologic Effects	Useful Auscultatory Changes
Respiration	↑ Venous return with inspiration	↑ Right heart murmurs and gallops with inspiration; splitting of S_2 (see Fig. 2.3)
Valsalva (initial ↑ BP, phase I; followed by ↓ BP, phase II)	↓ BP, ↓ venous return, ↓ LV size (phase II)	↑ HCM ↓ AS, MR MVP click earlier in systole; murmur prolongs
Standing	↓ Venous return ↓ LV size	↑ HCM ↓ AS, MR MVP click earlier in systole; murmur prolongs
Squatting	↑ Venous return ↑ Systemic vascular resistance ↑ LV size	↑ AS, MR, AI ↓ HCM MVP click delayed; murmur shortens
Isometric exercise (e.g., handgrip)	↑ Arterial pressure ↑ Cardiac output	↑ Gallops ↑ MR, AI, MS ↓ AS, HCM
Post PVC or prolonged R-R interval	↑ Ventricular filling ↑ Contractility	↑ AS Little change in MR
Amyl nitrate	↓ Arterial pressure ↑ Cardiac output ↓ LV size	↑ HCM, AS, MS ↓ AI, MR, Austin Flint murmur MVP click earlier in systole; murmur prolongs
Phenylephrine	↑ Arterial pressure ↑ Cardiac output ↓ LV size	↑ MR, AI ↓ AS, HCM MVP click delayed; murmur shortens

↑, Increased intensity; ↓, decreased intensity; *AI*, aortic insufficiency; *AS*, aortic stenosis; *BP*, blood pressure; *HCM*, hypertrophic cardiomyopathy; *LV*, left ventricle; *MR*, mitral regurgitation; *MS*, mitral stenosis; *MVP*, mitral valve prolapse; *PVC*, premature ventricular contraction; *R-R*, interval between the R waves on an electrocardiogram.

TABLE 2.5 Abnormal Intensity of Heart Sounds

	S_1	A_2	P_2
Loud	Short PR interval Mitral stenosis with pliable valve	Systemic hypertension Aortic dilation Coarctation of the aorta	Pulmonary hypertension Thin chest wall
Soft	Long PR interval Mitral regurgitation Poor left ventricular function Mitral stenosis with rigid valve Thick chest wall	Calcific aortic stenosis Aortic regurgitation	Valvular or subvalvular pulmonic stenosis
Varying	Atrial fibrillation Heart block	—	—

A_2, Component of second heart sound caused by closure of aortic valve; P_2, component of second heart sound caused by closure of pulmonic valve; S_1, first heart sound.

可使患者采取前倾、呼气、站立、蹲位或行 Valsalva 动作增强某些心音（表 2.4）。

正常心音

心音需从性质、强度和频率几方面进行描述。听诊时主要能听到两种心音：第一心音 S_1 和第二心音 S_2，两者均为瓣膜关闭所发出的高频声音。S_1 发生在心室收缩时，由二尖瓣和三尖瓣关闭所产生；S_2 标志着心室舒张期的开始，由主动脉瓣和肺动脉瓣关闭所产生。其他心音听诊的时间均基于这两个心音。

S_1 由两种成分组成：第一种是 M_1，通常较响亮，在心尖部听诊最清楚，由二尖瓣关闭产生；第二种成分是 T_1，较柔和，在胸骨左缘下方最清楚，由三尖瓣关闭产生。虽然 S_1 包括两种成分，但通常听诊仅为一个声音。S_2 也由两种成分组成，通常很容易区分。A_2 由主动脉瓣关闭产生，声音较为响亮且更早，在胸骨右缘第 2 肋间听诊最清楚。由肺动脉瓣关闭产生的 P_2 可于胸骨左缘第 2 肋间闻及。呼气时，S_2 听诊仅为单个声音。然而吸气时，右心回心血量和肺血管床容量增加，导致肺动脉瓣关闭延迟；肺静脉回到左心室的血量也有小幅减少，导致主动脉瓣关闭提前。因此，在吸气时出现 S_2 生理性分裂，A_2 在 P_2 之前出现，是正常现象。

正常个体有时可听到额外心音。健康儿童和年轻人中可听到第三心音，被称为生理性 S_3，但其在 40 岁以上的正常人中很少能听到。第四心音是心房收缩时射血进入顺应性减低的心室所致，在正常年轻人中很少见，但在老年人中相对常见。

杂音是由高速血流通过正常瓣膜或正常血流通过异常瓣膜、异常结构而产生的听觉震动。在收缩早期发生的柔和且持续时间较短的杂音通常不是病理性的，被称为无害性杂音，通常由于血流通过正常的左心室或右心室流出道产生，可见于儿童和年轻人。另外，虽然一些与高血流动力状态如发热、贫血、甲状腺疾病、妊娠相关的收缩期杂音并不一定与结构性心脏病相关，但也并不是无害性杂音。这些杂音与生理状态改变有关，被称为生理性杂音。所有的舒张期杂音都是病理性的。

异常心音

S_1 和 S_2 异常主要表现为强度改变（表 2.5）和呼吸分裂（表 2.6）。S_1 在心动过速和 PR 间期缩短时增强，而在 PR 间期延长时减弱。若心房和心室收缩顺序出现异常，S_1 强度也会发生变化。对心房颤动患者来说，由于心律不规整，心房充盈和排空不一致，导致 S_1 强弱不等。心脏传导阻滞或房室分离时也可能出现上述现象。在轻度二尖瓣狭窄患者中，S_1 通常增强，但当二尖瓣严重狭窄时，瓣叶活动明显受限，S_1 反而减弱甚至完全消失（图 2.3 和图 2.4）。如前所述，S_1 分裂并不常见。但三尖瓣关闭延迟情况可出现，如右束支传导阻滞和埃布斯坦畸形（Ebstein's anomaly）。

表 2.4 生理动作或其他情况对听诊的影响

生理动作或其他情况	主要的生理效应	有意义的听诊变化
呼吸	吸气静脉回心血量↑	↑右心杂音和吸气时奔马律；S_2 分裂（见图 2.3）
Valsalva（初期 BP↑为Ⅰ期；随后 BP↓为Ⅱ期）	↓BP，↓静脉回心血量，↓LV 体积（Ⅱ期）	↑HCM ↓AS，MR 收缩期 MVP 喀喇音提前；杂音延长
站立	↓静脉回心血量 ↓LV 体积	↑HCM ↓AS，MR 收缩期 MVP 喀喇音提前；杂音延长
蹲位	↑静脉回心血量 ↑外周血管阻力 ↑LV 体积	↑AS，MR，AI ↓HCM MVP 喀喇音延迟；杂音缩短
等长运动（如握拳）	↑动脉压 ↑心输出量	↑奔马律 ↑MR，AI，MS ↓AS，HCM
PVC 后或 R-R 间期延长	↑心室充盈 ↑心肌收缩力	↑AS MR 时变化不大
硝酸酯	↓动脉压 ↑心输出量 ↓LV 体积	↑HCM，AS，MS ↓AI，MR，Austin-Flint 杂音 收缩期 MVP 喀喇音提前；杂音延长
去氧肾上腺素	↑动脉压 ↑心输出量 ↓LV 体积	↑MR，AI ↓AS，HCM MVP 喀喇音延迟；杂音缩短

注：↑，强度增加；↓，强度减弱；AI，主动脉瓣关闭不全；AS，主动脉瓣狭窄；BP，血压；HCM，肥厚型心肌病；MR，二尖瓣反流；MS，二尖瓣狭窄；MVP，二尖瓣脱垂；LV，左心室；PVC，室性期前收缩；R-R，心电图上 R 波之间的距离。

表 2.5 异常心音强度

	S_1	A_2	P_2
响亮	PR 间期缩短 二尖瓣狭窄但瓣膜有弹性	高血压 主动脉扩张 主动脉缩窄	肺动脉高压 胸壁薄
柔和	PR 间期延长 二尖瓣反流 左心室功能障碍 二尖瓣狭窄但瓣膜僵硬 胸壁厚	主动脉瓣狭窄钙化 主动脉瓣反流	肺动脉瓣或瓣膜下狭窄
可变化	心房颤动 心脏传导阻滞	—	—

注：A_2，第二心音主动脉瓣成分，由主动脉瓣关闭产生；P_2，第二心音肺动脉瓣成分，由肺动脉瓣关闭产生；S_1，第一心音。

S_2 can be accentuated in the presence of hypertension, when the aortic component will be louder, or in pulmonary hypertension, when the pulmonic component will be enhanced. In the setting of severe aortic or pulmonic stenosis, leaflet excursion of the respective valves is reduced and the intensity of S_2 is significantly diminished. It may become absent altogether if the accompanying murmur obscures what remains of S_2.

There are several patterns of abnormal splitting of S_2. S_2 can remain single throughout respiration if either A_2 or P_2 is not present or if they occur simultaneously. A_2 can be absent, as previously mentioned, with severe aortic stenosis. P_2 can be absent with a number of congenital abnormalities of the pulmonic valve. Splitting may be persistent throughout the respiratory cycle if A_2 occurs early or if P_2 is delayed, as in the presence of right bundle branch block. In that case, splitting is always present but the interval between A_2 and P_2 varies somewhat. In fixed splitting, the interval between A_2 and P_2 is consistently wide and unaffected by respiration. This finding is observed in the presence of an ostium secundum atrial septal defect or right ventricular failure. Paradoxical splitting of S_2 occurs when P_2 precedes A_2. This leads to splitting with expiration and a single S_2 with inspiration. It is commonly found in situations of delayed electrical activation of the left ventricle, as in patients with left bundle branch block or right ventricular pacing. It can also be seen with prolonged mechanical contraction of the left ventricle, as in patients with aortic stenosis or hypertrophic cardiomyopathy.

The third heart sound, S_3, is a low-pitched sound heard best at the apex in mid diastole. Because it is low pitched, it is best recognized with use of the bell on the stethoscope. As stated previously, S_3 can be physiologic in children but is pathologic in older individuals and often associated with underlying cardiac disease. An S_3 occurs during the rapid filling phase of diastole and is thought to indicate a sudden limitation of the expansion of the left ventricle. This can be seen in cases of volume overload or tachycardia. Maneuvers that increase venous return accentuate an S_3, whereas those that reduce venous return diminish the intensity. The fourth heart sound, S_4, is also a low-frequency sound, but in contrast to S_3, it is heard in late diastole, just before S_1. The S_4 gallop occurs as a result of active ejection of blood into a noncompliant left ventricle. Therefore, when atrial contraction is absent, such as in atrial fibrillation, an S_4 cannot be heard. This heart sound is also best recognized with the use of a bell at the apex. It can be heard in patients with left ventricular hypertrophy, acute myocardial infarction, or hyperdynamic left ventricle. At times, an S_3 and an S_4 can be heard in the same patient. In tachycardic states, the two sounds can fuse in mid diastole to form a summation gallop.

S_3 and S_4 gallops are heard in mid diastole and late diastole, respectively. There are other abnormal sounds that can be heard during systole and early diastole. *Ejection sounds* are typically heard in early systole and involve the aortic and pulmonic valves. These are high-frequency sounds that can be heard with a diaphragm shortly after S_1.

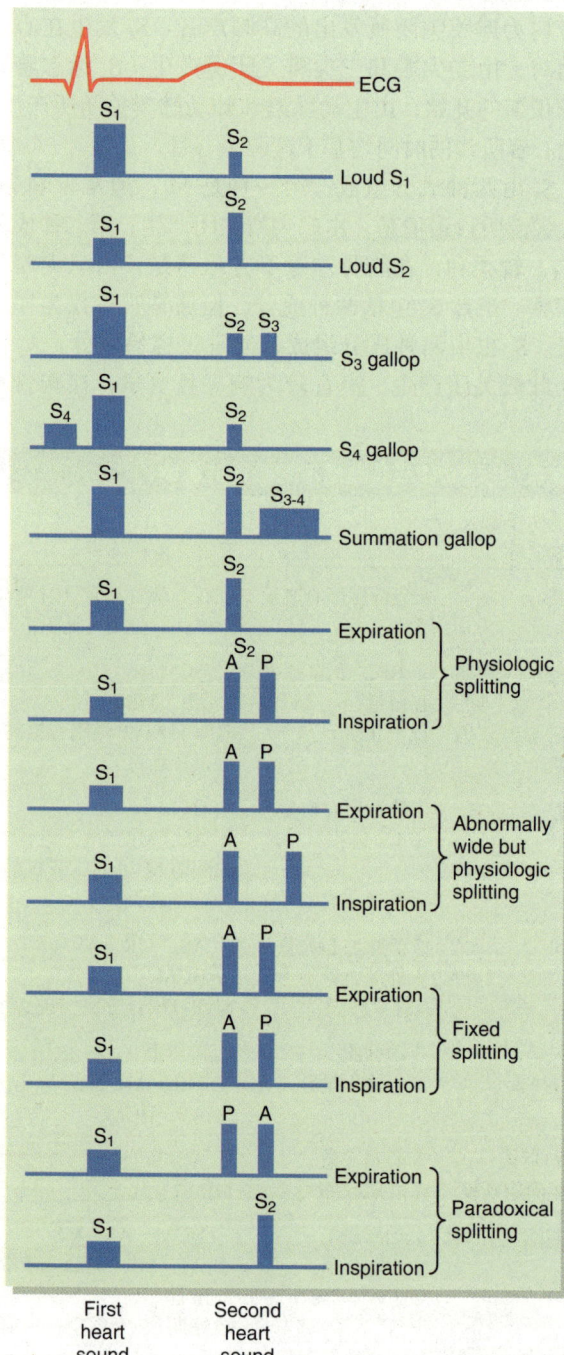

TABLE 2.6 Abnormal Splitting of S_2

Single S_2	Widely Split S_2 With Normal Respiratory Variation	Fixed Split S_2	Paradoxically Split S_2
Pulmonic stenosis	Right bundle branch block	Atrial septal defect	Left bundle branch block
Systemic hypertension	Left ventricular pacing	Severe right ventricular dysfunction	Right ventricular pacing
Coronary artery disease	Pulmonic stenosis		Angina, myocardial infarction
Any condition that can lead to paradoxical splitting of S_2	Pulmonary embolism		Aortic stenosis
	Idiopathic dilation of the pulmonary artery		Hypertrophic cardiomyopathy
	Mitral regurgitation		Aortic regurgitation
	Ventricular septal defect		

S_2, Second heart sound.

Fig. 2.3 Abnormal heart sounds can be related to abnormal intensity, abnormal presence of a gallop rhythm, or abnormal splitting of the second heart sound (S_2) with respiration. A_2, Component of S_2 caused by closure of aortic valve; *ECG*, electrocardiogram; P_2, component of S_2 caused by closure of pulmonic valve.

高血压和肺动脉高压患者的 S_2 可增强，其原因分别为 S_2 的主动脉瓣成分（A_2）和肺动脉瓣成分（P_2）增强。当重度主动脉瓣或肺动脉瓣狭窄时，瓣叶移动受限，S_2 强度明显减弱。若杂音较强，S_2 可能被掩盖而消失。

S_2 异常分裂有几种不同的类型。若 A_2 或 P_2 不存在，或两者同时出现时，S_2 在呼吸周期中均为单音。重度主动脉瓣狭窄患者的 A_2 可消失，几种先天性肺动脉瓣异常患者的 P_2 也可消失。当 A_2 提前出现或 P_2 延迟出现，如右束支传导阻滞时，S_2 在整个呼吸周期中持续分裂。这种情况下，虽然分裂一直存在，但 A_2 和 P_2 之间的时距可发生变化。固定分裂指 A_2 和 P_2 时距固定，不受呼吸影响，见于继发孔型房间隔缺损和右心衰竭。反常分裂指 P_2 早于 A_2 出现，呼气时出现 S_2 分裂，而吸气时 S_2 为单音。反常分裂见于左心室电活动延迟的情况，如左束支传导阻滞或右心室起搏患者，也可见于左心室机械收缩延长，如主动脉瓣狭窄或肥厚型心肌病患者。

第三心音 S_3，在心尖区舒张中期听诊最为明显。其音调低，所以最好应用钟型听诊器进行听诊。如前所述，生理性 S_3 可见于正常儿童，但在成年人中是病理性的，通常与潜在的心脏疾病相关。S_3 发生于舒张期的快速充盈期，被认为与左心室扩张突然受限有关，可见于容量负荷过重或心动过速。增加静脉回流的动作可加重 S_3，而减少静脉回流的动作会减弱 S_3 强度。S_4 也是低频音调，但它与 S_3 不同，S_4 发生在 S_1 之前的舒张晚期。S_4 奔马律是由于血流射入顺应性差的心室所致。因此，当心房收缩不存在，如心房颤动时，则无法闻及 S_4。使用钟型听诊器在心尖部听诊 S_4 最清晰，其可见于左心室肥厚、急性心肌梗死或左心室高动力状态。同一患者中可同时闻及 S_3 和 S_4。心动过速时，这两种心音可在舒张中期融合形成重叠奔马律。

S_3 和 S_4 奔马律分别发生在舒张中期和舒张晚期。另外，在收缩期和舒张早期，还可闻及其他异常心音。喷射音通常出现在舒张早期，与主动脉瓣和肺动脉瓣有关，是高频声音，紧接于 S_1 后出现。

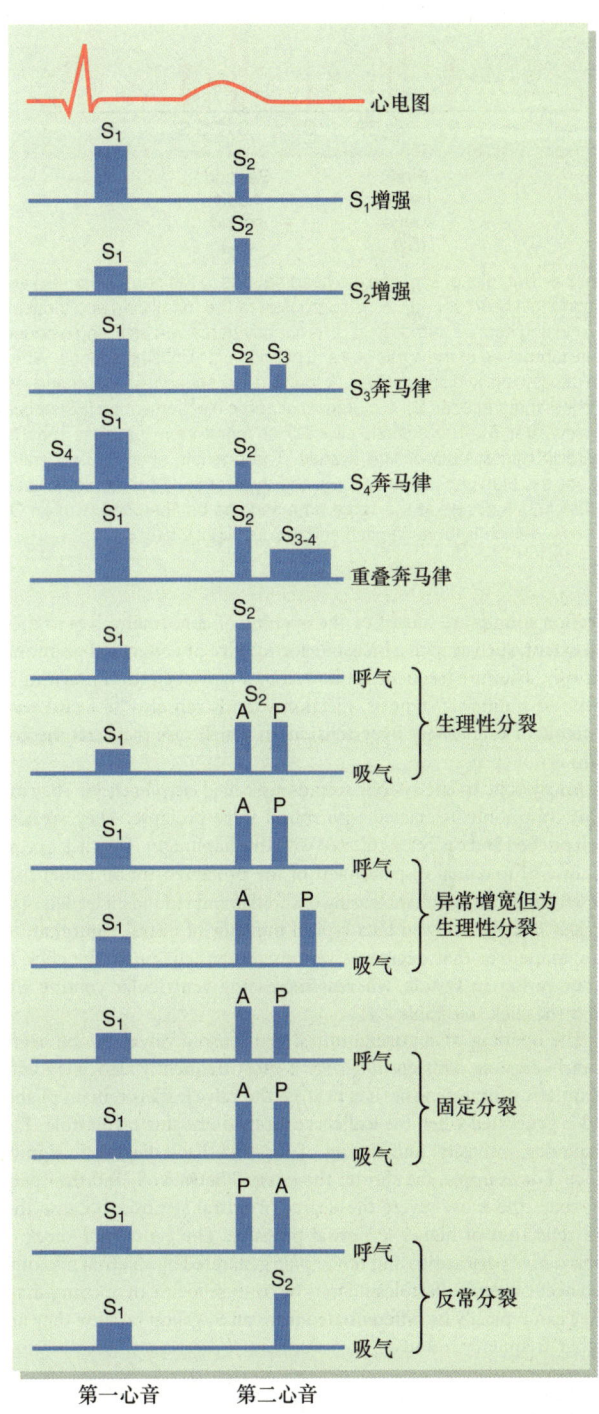

图 2.3　异常心音可能与强度异常、异常奔马律或呼吸时第二心音（S_2）异常分裂有关。A_2，第二心音主动脉瓣成分，由主动脉瓣关闭产生；ECG，心电图；P_2，第二心音肺动脉瓣成分，由肺动脉瓣关闭产生

表 2.6　S_2 的异常分裂

单音 S_2	S_2 分裂增宽伴正常呼吸变异	S_2 固定分裂	S_2 反常分裂
肺动脉瓣狭窄	右束支传导阻滞	房间隔缺损	左束支传导阻滞
高血压	左心室起搏	严重右心室功能障碍	右心室起搏
冠状动脉疾病	肺栓塞		心绞痛，心肌梗死
任何导致 S_2 反常分裂的疾病	肺动脉瓣狭窄		主动脉瓣狭窄
	特发性肺动脉扩张		肥厚型心肌病
	二尖瓣反流		主动脉瓣反流
	室间隔缺损		

注：S_2，第二心音。译者注：高血压和冠状动脉疾病产生单音 S_2 考虑可能由于高血压、动脉粥样硬化时体循环阻力增加，主动脉压力增加，排血时间延长，A_2 关闭延迟与 P_2 同时出现。

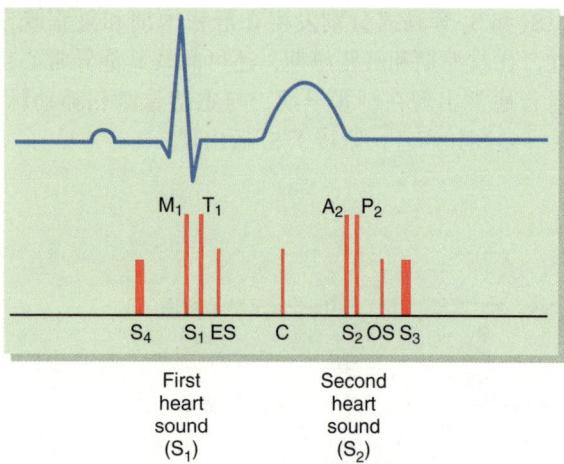

Fig. 2.4 The relationship of extra heart sounds to the normal first (S_1) and second (S_2) heart sounds. S_1 is composed of the mitral (M_1) and tricuspid (T_1) closing sounds, although it is frequently perceived as a single sound. S_2 is composed of the aortic (A_2) and pulmonic (P_2) closing sounds, which are usually easily distinguished. A fourth heart sound (S_4) is soft and low pitched and precedes S_1. A pulmonic or aortic ejection sound (ES) occurs shortly after S_1. The systolic click (C) of mitral valve prolapse may be heard in mid systole or late systole. The opening snap (OS) of mitral stenosis is high pitched and occurs shortly after S_2. A tumor plop or pericardial knock occurs at the same time and can be confused with an OS or an S_3, which is lower in pitch and occurs slightly later.

Ejection sounds are caused by the opening of abnormal valves to their full extent, such as with a bicuspid aortic valve or congenital pulmonic stenosis. They are frequently followed by a typical ejection murmur of aortic or pulmonic stenosis. Ejection sounds can also be heard with systemic or pulmonary hypertension, in which case the exact mechanism is not clear.

Midsystolic to late systolic sounds are called *ejection clicks*. They are most commonly associated with mitral valve prolapse. They are also high pitched and easily auscultated with the diaphragm. The click occurs because of maximal displacement of the prolapsed mitral leaflet into the left atrium and resultant tensing of chordae and redundant leaflets. The click is usually followed by a typical murmur of mitral regurgitation. Any maneuver that decreases venous return will cause the click to occur earlier in systole, whereas increasing ventricular volume will delay the click (see Table 2.4).

The opening of abnormal mitral or tricuspid valves can be heard in early diastole. This *opening snap* is most frequently associated with rheumatic mitral stenosis. It is heard if the valve leaflets remain pliable and is generated when the leaflets abruptly dome during diastole. The frequency, intensity, and timing of the click have diagnostic significance. For example, the shorter the interval between S_2 and the opening snap, the more severe the degree of mitral stenosis, because this is a reflection of higher left atrial pressure. The *pericardial knock* of constrictive pericarditis and *tumor plop* generated by an atrial myxoma also occur in early diastole and may be confused with an opening snap. They can typically be differentiated from an S_3 gallop because they are higher-frequency sounds.

Murmurs

Murmurs are a series of auditory vibrations generated by either abnormal blood flow across a normal cardiac structure or normal flow across an abnormal cardiac structure, both of which result in turbulent flow.

TABLE 2.7 Grading System for Intensity of Murmurs

Grade	Description
1	Barely audible murmur
2	Murmur of medium intensity
3	Loud murmur, no thrill
4	Loud murmur with thrill
5	Very loud murmur; stethoscope must be on the chest to hear it; may be heard posteriorly
6	Murmur audible with stethoscope off the chest

These sounds are longer than individual heart sounds and should be described on the basis of their location, frequency, intensity, quality, duration, shape, and timing in the cardiac cycle. The intensity of a given murmur is typically graded on a scale of 1 to 6 (Table 2.7). Murmurs of grade 4 or higher are associated with palpable thrills. The intensity or loudness of a murmur does not necessarily correlate with the severity of disease. For example, a murmur can be quite harsh when it is associated with a moderate degree of aortic stenosis. If stenosis is critical, however, the flow across the valve is diminished and the murmur becomes rather quiet. In the presence of a large atrial septal defect, flow is almost silent, whereas flow through a small ventricular septal defect is typically associated with a loud murmur.

The frequency of a murmur can be high or low; higher-frequency murmurs are more correlated with high velocity of flow at the site of turbulence. It is also important to notice the configuration or shape of a murmur, such as crescendo, crescendo-decrescendo, decrescendo, or plateau (Fig. 2.5). The quality of a murmur (e.g., harsh, blowing, rumbling) and the pattern of radiation are also helpful in diagnosis. Physical maneuvers can sometimes help clarify the nature of a particular murmur (see Table 2.4).

Murmurs can be divided into three different categories (Table 2.8). Systolic murmurs begin with or after S_1 and end with or before S_2. Diastolic murmurs begin with or after S_2 and end with or before S_1. Continuous murmurs begin in systole and continue through diastole. Murmurs can result from abnormalities on the left or right side of the heart or in the great vessels. Right-sided murmurs become louder with inspiration because of increased venous return. This can help differentiate them from left-sided murmurs, which are unaffected by respiration.

Systolic murmurs should be further differentiated based on timing (i.e., early systolic, midsystolic, late systolic, and holosystolic murmurs). Early systolic murmurs begin with S_1, are decrescendo, and end typically before mid systole. Ventricular septal defects and acute mitral regurgitation may lead to early systolic murmurs. Midsystolic murmurs begin after S_1 and end before S_2, often in a crescendo-decrescendo shape. They are typically caused by obstruction to left ventricular outflow, accelerated flow through the aortic or pulmonic valve, or enlargement of the aortic root or pulmonary trunk. Aortic stenosis, when less than severe in degree, causes a midsystolic murmur that may be harsh and may radiate to the carotids. Pulmonic stenosis leads to a similar murmur that does not radiate to the carotid arteries but may change with inspiration. The murmur of hypertrophic cardiomyopathy may be mistaken for aortic stenosis; however, it does not radiate to the carotids and becomes exaggerated with diminished venous return. Innocent or benign murmurs may also occur as a result of aortic valve sclerosis, vibrations of a left ventricular false tendon, or vibration of normal pulmonary leaflets. They are generally less

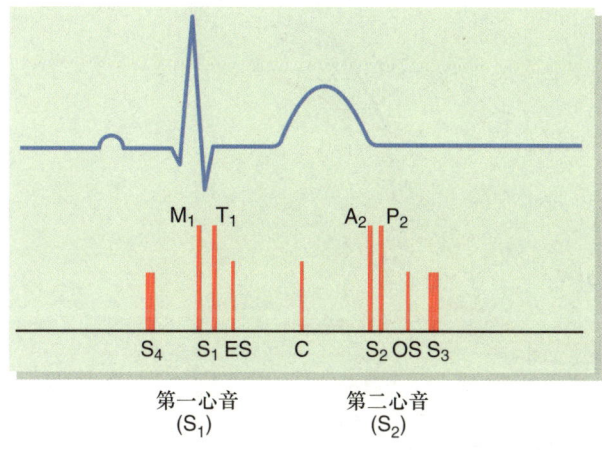

图2.4 额外心音与正常第一音（S_1）和第二心音（S_2）的关系。S_1由二尖瓣成分（M_1）和三尖瓣成分（T_1）组成，通常听诊是单音。S_2由主动脉瓣成分（A_2）和肺动脉瓣成分（P_2）组成，容易出现分裂。第四心音（S_4）柔和，音调低，出现于S_1之前。肺动脉或主动脉喷射音（ES）紧随S_1出现。二尖瓣脱垂的收缩期喀喇音（C）可在收缩中期或收缩晚期闻及。二尖瓣狭窄的开瓣音（OS）为高音调，紧随S_2出现。肿瘤扑落音或心包叩击音可能与OS或S_3同时发生，易混淆，后者为低音调，发生时间稍晚

表 2.7	杂音强度的分级系统
级别	说明
1	几乎听不到杂音
2	中等强度杂音
3	响亮杂音，无震颤
4	响亮杂音伴有震颤
5	非常响亮杂音；听诊器需接触胸壁听诊后方可能闻及
6	听诊器不接触胸壁即可闻及杂音

喷射音是由异常瓣膜完全开放引起，如二叶主动脉瓣或先天性肺动脉瓣狭窄。喷射音后常伴有主动脉瓣或肺动脉瓣狭窄的典型喷射性杂音。喷射音还可见于高血压或肺动脉高压，具体机制尚不清楚。

非喷射性喀喇音（译者注：原文喷射性喀喇音有误）常发生于收缩中晚期，常见于二尖瓣脱垂。喀喇音也是高频音调，应用膜型听诊器进行听诊。喀喇音是由于脱垂的二尖瓣瓣叶在收缩中、晚期发生最大移位时，脱入左心房，使腱索及瓣叶拉紧所致。喀喇音后通常伴有二尖瓣反流的典型杂音。任何减少静脉回流的动作将引起收缩期喀喇音提前出现，而增加左心室血容量的动作则会使其延迟出现（见表2.4）。

异常二尖瓣或三尖瓣的开放可在舒张早期闻及。开瓣音最常见于风湿性二尖瓣狭窄。若瓣叶弹性良好，舒张期瓣叶突然开放可产生开瓣音。开瓣音的频率、强度和出现的时间都具有诊断意义。例如，S_2和开瓣音之间的间隔反映左心房压力，间隔越短说明二尖瓣狭窄程度越严重。缩窄性心包炎产生的心包叩击音和心房黏液瘤产生的肿瘤扑落音也可发生于舒张早期，易与开瓣音混淆。由于它们是高频音调，通常可与S_3奔马律进行区分。

杂音

杂音是由异常血流通过正常心脏组织或正常血流通过异常心脏组织引起的湍流而产生的一种听觉震颤。杂音通常比单个心音持续时间长，应从其部位、频率、强度、性质、持续时间、形态和心动周期的时相等方面对杂音进行描述。杂音按强度分为1～6级（表2.7），4级以上杂音可触及震颤。杂音的强度与疾病的严重程度不一定成正比。例如，中度主动脉瓣狭窄时可闻及粗糙的杂音。但当狭窄非常严重时，通过瓣膜的血流量变少，杂音也就明显变小。当房间隔缺损较大时，几乎听不到杂音，而血液通过较小的室间隔缺损时，杂音却通常非常响亮。

杂音的频率可高可低，高频率的杂音与湍流部位的高流速有关。另外，注意杂音的结构或形态也非常重要，如递增型、递增递减型、递减型、一贯型（图2.5）。杂音的性质（如粗糙样、吹风样、隆隆样）和传导方向也有助于诊断。体位和动作有时也有助于分辨特定杂音的性质（表2.4）。

杂音可分为三种类型（表2.8）：收缩期杂音开始于S_1或S_1之后，结束于S_2或S_2之前；舒张期杂音开始于S_2或S_2之后，结束于S_1或S_1之前；连续性杂音在收缩期和舒张期都持续存在。杂音可由左心、右心或大血管异常引起。深吸气时静脉回心血量增加，右心杂音增强，而左心杂音则不受呼吸影响，可根据该特点进行区分。

收缩期杂音根据时相可进一步分为收缩早期、收缩中期、收缩晚期和全收缩期杂音。收缩早期杂音始于S_1，呈递减型，通常在收缩中期前结束，可见于室间隔缺损和急性二尖瓣反流；收缩中期杂音开始于S_1后，结束于S_2之前，呈递增递减型，通常是由于左心室流出道梗阻、主动脉瓣或肺动脉瓣处流速增加、主动脉根部或肺动脉干扩张引起的。轻中度主动脉瓣狭窄可出现粗糙的收缩中期杂音，并可传导至颈动脉。肺动脉瓣狭窄可出现类似的杂音，但它不向颈动脉传导，且可能随着吸气发生改变。肥厚型心肌病的杂音可能与主动脉瓣狭窄混淆，但前者不向颈动脉传导且随着静脉回心血量的减少而增强。主动脉瓣硬化、左心室假腱索或正常的肺动脉瓣瓣叶发生震动时可引起无害性或良性杂音。此类杂音通常较柔和，持续时间也较短。高动力状态如发热，妊娠或贫血时也可出现

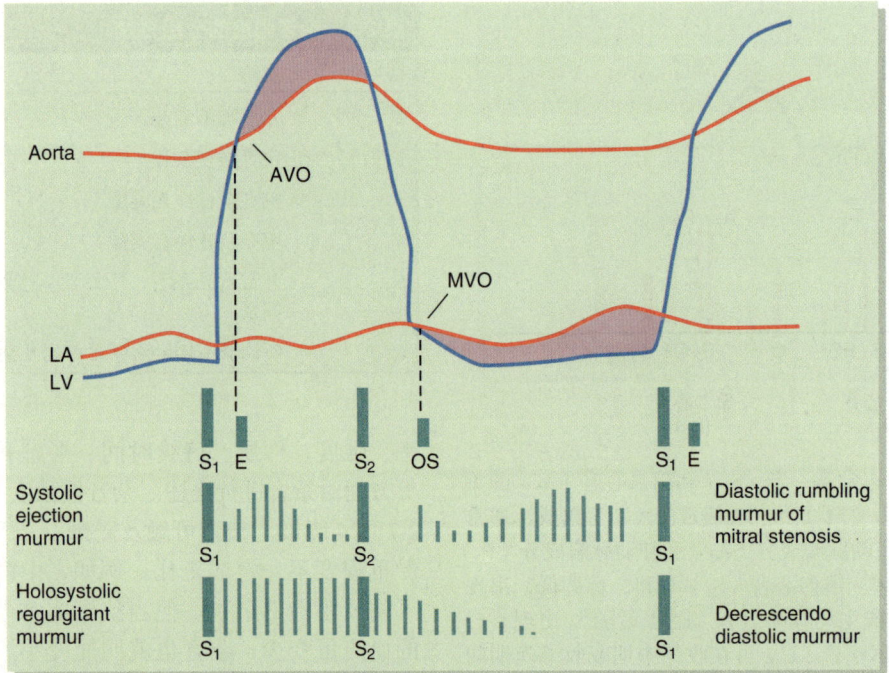

Fig. 2.5 Abnormal sounds and murmurs associated with valvular dysfunction displayed simultaneously with left atrial (LA), left ventricular (LV), and aortic pressure tracings. The *shaded areas* represent pressure gradients across the aortic valve during systole or across mitral valve during diastole; they are characteristic of aortic stenosis and mitral stenosis, respectively. *AVO*, Aortic valve opening; *E*, ejection click of the aortic valve; *MVO*, mitral valve opening; *OS*, opening snap of the mitral valve; S_1, first heart sound; S_2, second heart sound.

TABLE 2.8 Classification of Heart Murmurs

Class	Description	Characteristic Lesions
Systolic		
Ejection	Begins in early systole; may extend to mid or late systole	Valvular, supravalvular, and subvalvular aortic stenoses
	Crescendo-decrescendo pattern	Hypertrophic cardiomyopathy
	Often harsh in quality	Pulmonic stenosis
	Begins after S_1 and ends before S_2	Aortic or pulmonary artery dilation
		Malformed but nonobstructive aortic valve
		↑ Transvalvular flow (e.g., aortic regurgitation, hyperkinetic states, atrial septal defect, physiologic flow murmur)
Holosystolic	Extends throughout systole[a]	Mitral regurgitation
	Relatively uniform in intensity	Tricuspid regurgitation
		Ventricular septal defect
Late	Variable onset and duration, often preceded by a nonejection click	Mitral valve prolapse
Diastolic		
Early	Begins with A_2 or P_2	Aortic regurgitation
	Decrescendo pattern with variable duration	Pulmonic regurgitation
	Often high pitched, blowing	
Mid	Begins after S_2, often after an opening snap	Mitral stenosis
	Low-pitched *rumble* heard best with bell of stethoscope	Tricuspid stenosis
	Louder with exercise and left lateral position	↑ Flow across atrioventricular valves (e.g., mitral regurgitation, tricuspid regurgitation, atrial septal defect)
	Loudest in early diastole	
Late	Presystolic accentuation of mid-diastolic murmur	Mitral stenosis
		Tricuspid stenosis
Continuous		
	Systolic and diastolic components	Patent ductus arteriosus
	"Machinery murmurs"	Coronary atrioventricular fistula
		Ruptured sinus of Valsalva aneurysm into right atrium or ventricle
		Mammary soufflé
		Venous hum

A_2, Component of S_2 caused by closure of aortic valve; P_2, component of S_2 caused by closure of pulmonic valve; S_1, first heart sound; S_2, second heart sound.
[a]Encompasses both S_1 and S_2.

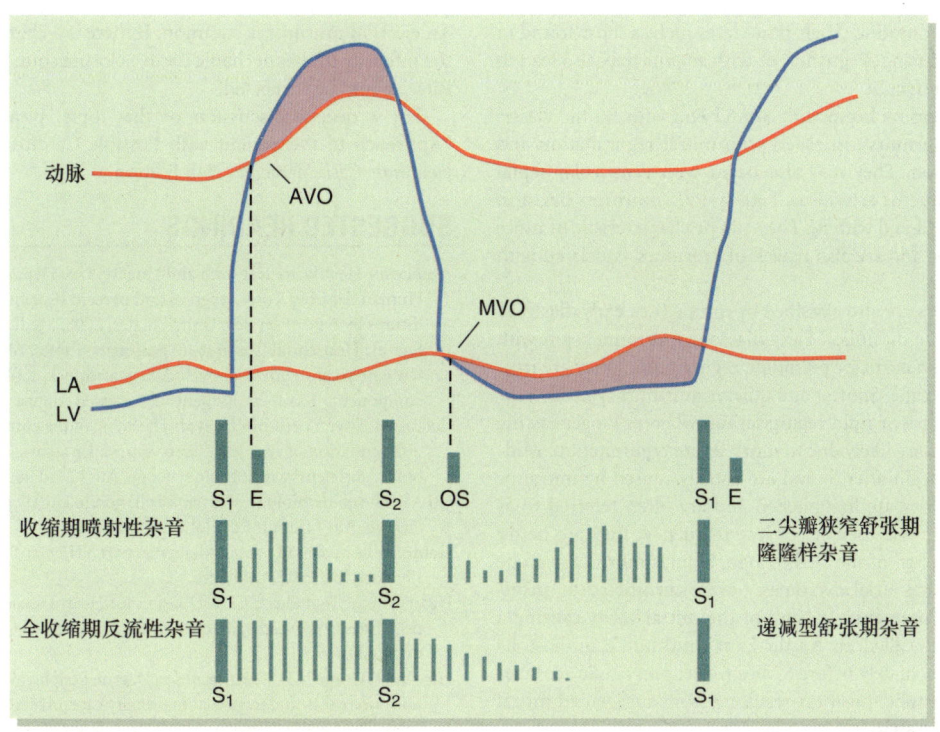

图 2.5 瓣膜功能障碍相关性异常心音和杂音与同步左心房（LA）压、左心室（LV）压和主动脉压图。阴影区域代表收缩期主动脉瓣两侧或舒张期二尖瓣两侧的压力阶差；它们分别为主动脉瓣狭窄和二尖瓣狭窄的特征。AVO，主动脉瓣开放；E，主动脉瓣喷射性咔喇音；MVO，二尖瓣开放；OS，二尖瓣开瓣音；S_1，第一心音；S_2，第二心音

表 2.8 心脏杂音的分类		
分类	描述	特征性病变
收缩期杂音		
喷射性杂音	开始于收缩早期，可持续至收缩中期或晚期；递增-递减型；粗糙；开始于 S_1 之后，结束于 S_2 之前	主动脉瓣、瓣上和瓣下狭窄 肥厚型心肌病 肺动脉狭窄 主动脉或肺动脉扩张 主动脉瓣非阻塞性畸形 经瓣膜血流量增加（如主动脉瓣反流、高动力状态、房间隔缺损、生理性杂音）
全收缩期杂音	持续整个收缩期[a] 强度相对一致	二尖瓣反流 三尖瓣反流 室间隔缺损
收缩晚期杂音	开始时间和持续时间可变，之前常伴有非喷射性咔喇音	二尖瓣脱垂
舒张期杂音		
早期	开始于 A_2 或 P_2 递减型，持续时间可变 通常音调高，吹风样	主动脉瓣反流 肺动脉瓣反流
中期	开始于 S_2 后，通常在开瓣音后出现 低调隆隆样杂音，适用于钟型听诊器 运动或左侧卧位时杂音增强 舒张早期杂音最响亮	二尖瓣狭窄 三尖瓣狭窄 流经房室瓣血流量增加（如二尖瓣反流、三尖瓣反流、房间隔缺损）
晚期	舒张中期杂音持续至收缩前期	二尖瓣狭窄 三尖瓣狭窄
连续性杂音		
	收缩期和舒张期机械性杂音	动脉导管未闭 冠状动脉房室瘘 Valsalva 窦动脉瘤破入右心房或右心室 乳房杂音 静脉营营音

注：A_2，第二心音主动脉瓣成分，由主动脉瓣关闭产生；P_2，第二心音肺动脉瓣成分，由肺动脉关闭产生；S_1，第一心音；S_2，第二心音。
[a] 包括 S_1 和 S_2。

harsh and shorter in duration. High-flow states such as those found in patients with fever, during pregnancy, or with anemia may also lead to midsystolic "flow" murmurs.

Holosystolic murmurs begin with S_1 and end with S_2; the classic examples are the murmurs associated with mitral regurgitation and tricuspid regurgitation. They may also occur with ventricular septal defects and patent ductus arteriosus. Late systolic murmurs begin in mid to late systole and end with S_2. They can be characteristic of more severe aortic stenosis and are also typical of murmurs associated with mitral valve prolapse.

Diastolic murmurs are also classified by timing (i.e., early diastolic, mid diastolic, and late diastolic). Early diastolic murmurs begin with S_2 and can result from aortic or pulmonic regurgitation; they are usually decrescendo in shape. Shorter and quieter murmurs typically represent an acute process or mild regurgitation, whereas longer-lasting and louder murmurs are likely due to more severe regurgitation. Mid-diastolic murmurs begin after S_2 and are usually caused by mitral or tricuspid stenosis. They are low pitched and are often referred to as *diastolic rumbles*. Because they are of low frequency, they are better auscultated with the bell of the stethoscope. Similar murmurs can be heard with obstructing atrial myxomas. Severe chronic aortic insufficiency can lead to premature closure of the mitral valve, causing a mid-diastolic rumble called an Austin-Flint murmur. Late diastolic murmurs occur immediately before S_1 and reflect presystolic accentuation of the mid-diastolic murmurs resulting from augmented mitral or tricuspid flow after atrial contraction.

Continuous murmurs begin with S_1 and last though part or all of diastole. They are generated by continuous flow from a vessel or chamber with high pressure into a vessel or chamber with lower pressure. They are referred to as *machinery murmurs* and are caused by aortopulmonary connections such as a patent ductus arteriosus, AV malformations, or disturbances of flow in arteries or veins.

Other Cardiac Sounds

Pericardial rubs occur in the setting of pericarditis and are coarse, scratching sounds similar to rubbing leather. They are typically heard best at the left sternal border with the patient leaning forward and holding the breath at end-expiration. A classic pericardial rub has three components: atrial systole, ventricular systole, and ventricular diastole. One might also hear a pleural rub caused by localized irritation of surrounding pleura. Continuous venous murmurs, or *venous hums*, are almost always present in children. They can be heard in adults during pregnancy, in the setting of anemia, or with thyrotoxicosis. They are heard best at the base of the neck with the patient's head turned to the opposite direction.

Prosthetic Heart Sounds

Prosthetic heart valves produce characteristic findings on auscultation. Bioprosthetic valves produce sounds that are similar to those of native heart valves, but they are typically smaller than the valves that they replace and therefore have an associated murmur. Mechanical valves have crisp, high-pitched sounds related to valve opening and closure. In most modern valves such as the St. Jude valve, which is a bileaflet mechanical valve, the closure sound is louder than the opening sound.

An ejection murmur is common. If there is a change in murmur or in the intensity of the mechanical valve closure sound, dysfunction of the valve should be suspected.

For a deeper discussion of this topic, please see Chapter 45, "Approach to the Patient with Possible Cardiovascular Disease," in *Goldman-Cecil Medicine*, 26th Edition.

SUGGESTED READINGS

Agency for Healthcare Research and Quality, U.S. Department of Health and Human Services: Total expenses and percent distribution for selected conditions by type of service: United States, 2008. Medical Expenditure Panel Survey: Household Component Summary Tables. Available at: http://www.meps.ahrq.gov/mepsweb/data_stats/quick_tables_search.jsp?component=1&subcomponent=0. Accessed August 5, 2014.

Calkins H, Shyr Y, Frumin H, et al: The value of the clinical history in the differentiation of syncope due to ventricular tachycardia, atrioventricular block, and neurocardiogenic syncope, Am J Med 98:365–373, 1995.

Go AS: The epidemiology of atrial fibrillation in elderly persons: the tip of the iceberg, Am J Geriatr Cardiol 14:56–61, 2005.

Goldman L, Ausiello D: Cecil Medicine: part VIII. Cardiovascular disease, Philadelphia, 2012, Saunders.

Heart Disease Fact Sheet. CDC Division for Heart Disease and Stroke Prevention. https://www.cdc.gov/dhdsp/data_statistics/fact_sheets/fs_heart_disease.htm.

Hirsch AT, Criqui MH, Treat-Jacobson D, et al: Peripheral arterial disease: detection, awareness, and treatment in primary care, JAMA 286:1317–1324, 2001.

Hoffman JI, Kaplan S, Liberthson RR: Prevalence of congenital heart disease, Am Heart J 147:425–439, 2004.

National Heart, Lung and Blood Institute, National Institutes of Health. Unpublished tabulations of National Vital Statistics System mortality data. 2008. Available at: http://www.cdc.gov/nchs/nvss/mortality_public_use_data.htm. Accessed August 5, 2014.

National Heart, Lung and Blood Institute, National Institutes of Health, Unpublished tabulations of National Hospital Discharge Survey, 2009. Available at http://www.cdc.gov/nchs/nhds/nhds_questionnaires.htm. Accessed August 5, 2014.

National Heart, Lung and Blood Institute. Unpublished tabulations of National Health Interview Survey, 1965-2010. Available at: http://www.cdc.gov/nchs/nhis/nhis_questionnaires.htm. Accessed August 5, 2014.

National Heart, Lung and Blood Institute, National Institutes of Health. Morbidity and mortality: 2012 Chart book on cardiovascular, lung, and blood diseases. Available at https://www.nhlbi.nih.gov/research/reports/2012-mortality-chart-book.htm. Accessed September 26, 2014.

National Vital Statistics System, Centers for Disease Control and Prevention: Mortality tables. Available at http://www.cdc.gov/nchs/nvss/mortality_tables.htm. Accessed August 5, 2014.

Pickering TG, Hall JE, Appel LJ, et al: Recommendations for blood pressure measurement in humans and experimental animals: part 1. Blood pressure measurement in humans: a statement for professionals from the Subcommittee of Professional and Public Education of the American Heart Association Council on High Blood Pressure Research, Circulation 111:697–716, 2005.

收缩中期"血流"杂音。

全收缩期杂音开始于 S_1 结束于 S_2。典型杂音见于二尖瓣反流和三尖瓣反流，也可见于室间隔缺损和动脉导管未闭。收缩晚期杂音从收缩中晚期开始，结束于 S_2，是重度主动脉瓣狭窄的特征，也是二尖瓣脱垂的典型杂音。

舒张期杂音也可以根据发生时相进一步分为舒张早期、舒张中期和舒张晚期杂音。舒张早期杂音开始于 S_2，通常呈递减型，可见于主动脉瓣或肺动脉瓣反流。持续时间较短和较柔和的杂音通常代表急性病程或轻度反流，而持续时间长和响亮的杂音代表着更严重的反流。舒张中期杂音开始于 S_2 之后，多由二尖瓣或三尖瓣狭窄引起，为低调的舒张期隆隆样杂音，因此适合用钟型听诊器进行听诊。在阻塞性心房黏液瘤中可闻及类似的杂音。慢性重度主动脉瓣关闭不全可导致二尖瓣关闭过早，出现舒张中期隆隆样杂音，称为 Austin-Flint 杂音。舒张晚期杂音恰好出现在 S_1 之前，反映了心房收缩后二尖瓣或三尖瓣处血流量增加所引起的舒张中期杂音延长至收缩期前。

连续性杂音开始于 S_1，持续至部分或整个舒张期，是因持续性血流由高压血管或心腔流向低压血管或心腔所致，被称为机械性杂音，可见于主肺动脉相通性疾病如动脉导管未闭、动静脉畸形或动静脉血流紊乱等。

其他心音

心包摩擦音见于心包炎，呈粗糙、刮擦样，类似摩擦皮革的声音。通常在胸骨左缘处最响亮，坐位前倾及呼气末屏气时更明显。典型心包摩擦音呈三相：分别对应心房收缩、心室收缩和心室舒张。周围胸膜受到局部刺激时也可闻及胸膜摩擦音。连续静脉杂音又称静脉营营音，基本只见于儿童，也可见于成人妊娠、贫血或甲状腺毒症等情况。当患者头转向对侧时，该杂音在颈根部最响亮。

人工瓣膜音

人工心脏瓣膜的听诊音非常具有特征性。人工生物瓣膜可产生类似于自体心脏瓣膜的声音，但其通常小于被置换的自体瓣膜，因此会伴有杂音。人工机械瓣膜在瓣膜开关时会产生清脆、高调杂音。大多数现代瓣膜如圣犹达（St.Jude）瓣膜为二叶型机械瓣膜，其闭合音大于开放音。喷射性杂音常见。如果人工机械瓣膜的杂音或关闭音强度发生变化，则应当怀疑瓣膜功能障碍。

有关此专题的深入讨论，请参阅 Goldman-Cecil Medicine 第 26 版第 45 章"心血管疾病患者的接诊"。

推荐阅读

Agency for Healthcare Research and Quality, U.S. Department of Health and Human Services: Total expenses and percent distribution for selected conditions by type of service: United States, 2008. Medical Expenditure Panel Survey: Household Component Summary Tables. Available at: http://www.meps.ahrq.gov/mepsweb/data_stats/quick_tables_search.jsp?component=1&subcomponent=0. Accessed August 5, 2014.

Calkins H, Shyr Y, Frumin H, et al: The value of the clinical history in the differentiation of syncope due to ventricular tachycardia, atrioventricular block, and neurocardiogenic syncope, Am J Med 98:365–373, 1995.

Go AS: The epidemiology of atrial fibrillation in elderly persons: the tip of the iceberg, Am J Geriatr Cardiol 14:56–61, 2005.

Goldman L, Ausiello D: Cecil Medicine: part VIII. Cardiovascular disease, Philadelphia, 2012, Saunders.

Heart Disease Fact Sheet. CDC Division for Heart Disease and Stroke Prevention. https://www.cdc.gov/dhdsp/data_statistics/fact_sheets/fs_heart_disease.htm.

Hirsch AT, Criqui MH, Treat-Jacobson D, et al: Peripheral arterial disease: detection, awareness, and treatment in primary care, JAMA 286:1317–1324, 2001.

Hoffman JI, Kaplan S, Liberthson RR: Prevalence of congenital heart disease, Am Heart J 147:425–439, 2004.

National Heart, Lung and Blood Institute, National Institutes of Health. Unpublished tabulations of National Vital Statistics System mortality data. 2008. Available at: http://www.cdc.gov/nchs/nvss/mortality_public_use_data.htm. Accessed August 5, 2014.

National Heart, Lung and Blood Institute, National Institutes of Health, Unpublished tabulations of National Hospital Discharge Survey, 2009. Available at http://www.cdc.gov/nchs/nhds/nhds_questionnaires.htm. Accessed August 5, 2014.

National Heart, Lung and Blood Institute. Unpublished tabulations of National Health Interview Survey, 1965-2010. Available at: http://www.cdc.gov/nchs/nhis/nhis_questionnaires.htm. Accessed August 5, 2014.

National Heart, Lung and Blood Institute, National Institutes of Health. Morbidity and mortality: 2012 Chart book on cardiovascular, lung, and blood diseases. Available at https://www.nhlbi.nih.gov/research/reports/2012-mortality-chart-book.htm. Accessed September 26, 2014.

National Vital Statistics System, Centers for Disease Control and Prevention: Mortality tables. Available at http://www.cdc.gov/nchs/nvss/mortality_tables.htm. Accessed August 5, 2014.

Pickering TG, Hall JE, Appel LJ, et al: Recommendations for blood pressure measurement in humans and experimental animals: part 1. Blood pressure measurement in humans: a statement for professionals from the Subcommittee of Professional and Public Education of the American Heart Association Council on High Blood Pressure Research, Circulation 111:697–716, 2005.

3

Diagnostic Tests and Procedures in the Patient With Cardiovascular Disease

Esseim Sharma, Alan R. Morrison

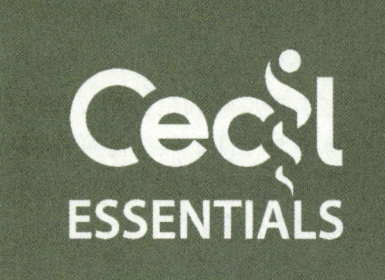

ELECTROCARDIOGRAPHY

The electrocardiogram (ECG) is one of the most basic yet powerful diagnostic tools in cardiovascular medicine. It is critical in the investigation of cardiac arrhythmias, myocardial infarction, and pericardial disease, and may provide additional insight into a variety of other cardiac and noncardiac conditions.

The ECG is a simple and noninvasive procedure that makes use of electrodes placed on the skin of the chest at specific locations in order to measure the electrical activity of the heart. The output is a scroll of wave forms represented as a temporal sequence of deflections on the ECG (Fig. 3.1). The horizontal axis of the graph paper represents time, and at a standard paper speed of 25 mm/second, which is also known as the sweep speed, each small box (1 mm) represents 0.04 seconds, and each large box (5 mm) represents 0.20 seconds. The vertical axis represents voltage or amplitude (1 mm = 0.1 mV). Because the standard ECG demonstrates a 10-second window of time, the heart rate can be calculated by simply counting the number of QRS complexes and multiplying by 6. Alternatively, the heart rate can be estimated by dividing the number of large boxes between complexes (i.e., R-R interval) into 300.

Lead Positioning

The standard ECG consists of 12 leads: six limb leads (I, II, III, aVR, aVL, and aVF) and six chest or precordial leads (V_1 to V_6) (Fig. 3.2). The limb leads view the electrical activity of the heart in the vertical plane, while the precordial leads view the horizontal plane. The electrical activity recorded in each lead represents the direction and magnitude (i.e., vector) of the electrical force as seen from that lead position. Electrical activity directed toward a particular lead is represented as an upward (positive) deflection, and electrical activity directed away from a particular lead is represented as a downward (negative) deflection. Accurate lead placement is essential to reliable interpretation of the ECG.

The limb leads consist of bipolar leads (I, II, and III) and unipolar or augmented leads (leads aVR, aVL, and aVF). The bipolar leads represent electrical forces between the two leads, while augmented leads represent the electrical forces towards the lead. Lead I measures electrical activity between the right and left arms (left arm positive), lead II between the right arm and left leg (left leg positive), and lead III between the left arm and left leg (left leg positive). A vector perpendicular to the limb leads would be isoelectric. In aVR, aVL, and aVF, the vector is positive if electrical forces are directed toward the right arm for aVR, left arm for aVL, and left leg for aVF. Taken together, the six limb leads form a frontal plane of 30-degree arc intervals (Fig. 3.3).

The six standard precordial leads (V_1 to V_6) are attached to the anterior chest wall and are also unipolar leads. Lead placement should be as follows: V_1: fourth intercostal space, right sternal border; V_2: fourth intercostal space, left sternal border; V_3: midway between V_2 and V_4; V_4: fifth intercostal space, left midclavicular line; V_5: level with V_4, left anterior axillary line; V_6: level with V_4, left midaxillary line.

Nonstandard lead configurations can be used in specific clinical scenarios. In patients where there is concern for right ventricular infarction, standard V_1 and V_2 leads are switched, and V_{3R} to V_{6R} are placed at locations on the right chest wall in a mirror image of the standard left-sided chest leads. Posterior leads may be used to increase the sensitivity for diagnosing lateral and posterior wall infarction or ischemia—areas that are often deemed to be *electrically silent* on traditional 12-lead ECGs. To do this, six additional leads are placed in the fifth intercostal space continuing posteriorly from the position of V_6. Shifting the right precordial leads (V_1-V_3) superiorly to the second intercostal space can be used to unmask Brugada syndrome.

Electrocardiographic Intervals

In the normal heart, the electrical impulse originates in the sinoatrial (SA) node, located superiorly in the right atrium, and is conducted through the atria. Given that depolarization of the SA node is too weak to be detected on the surface ECG, the first, low-amplitude deflection on the surface ECG represents a summation atrial vector and is called the *P wave*. The P wave has an electrical axis that moves in sum toward the AV node, generally downward and to the left. The interval between the onset of the P wave and the next rapid deflection (QRS complex) is known as the *PR interval*. It primarily represents the time taken for the impulse to travel through the atrioventricular (AV) node. The normal PR segment ranges from 0.12 to 0.20 seconds. A PR interval greater than 0.20 seconds defines first-degree AV nodal block.

After the wave of depolarization has moved through the AV node, the ventricular myocardium is depolarized in a sequence of four phases. The interventricular septum depolarizes from left to right. This phase is followed by depolarization of the right ventricle and inferior wall of the left ventricle, then the apex and central portions of the left ventricle, and finally the base and the posterior wall of the left ventricle. Ventricular depolarization results in a high-amplitude complex on the surface ECG known as the *QRS complex*. The first downward deflection of this complex is the Q wave, the first upward deflection is the R wave, and the subsequent downward deflection is the S wave. In some individuals, a second upward deflection may occur after the S wave, and it is called *R prime* (R′). Normal duration of the QRS complex is less than 0.10 second. Complexes longer than 0.12 seconds in duration are usually secondary to some form of interventricular conduction delay, including right or left bundle branch block.

心血管疾病的诊断性检查和方法

钟晓丹 杨晓云 李宗哲 王红 译 曾和松 郑金刚 审校 任景怡 通审

心电图

心电图（ECG）是心血管病学中最基本但功能最强大的诊断工具之一，它对心律失常、心肌梗死和心包疾病的诊断至关重要，并可为其他各种心脏和非心脏疾病提供额外的诊断线索。

心电图是一种简便且无创的检查方法，它通过放置在胸部特定位置的电极来测量心脏的电活动。这些电信号输出至体表后就形成一系列随时间变化的波形，并展示在心电图纸上（图3.1）。心电图纸的横轴代表时间，以25 mm/s的标准纸速（也称为扫描速度）计算，每一个小方格（1 mm）代表0.04 s，每一个大方格（5 mm）代表0.20 s。图纸的纵轴表示电压或振幅（1 mm = 0.1 mV）。由于标准心电图显示的时间窗口为10 s，因此只需计算该时间窗口内QRS波群的数量并乘以6即可计算出心率，或者用300除以2个相邻QRS波群之间（即R-R间期）的大方格数量，也可估算出心率。

导联定位

标准心电图由12个导联组成：6个肢体导联（Ⅰ、Ⅱ、Ⅲ、aVR、aVL与aVF）和6个胸部或心前区导联（V_1至V_6）（图3.2）。肢体导联监测心脏垂直平面上的电活动，而心前区导联则监测水平面的电活动。每个导联记录的电活动代表了从该导联位置监测到的电位的方向和大小（即向量）。指向特定导联的电活动表现为除极主波向上（正向波），而远离特定导联的电活动表现为除极主波向下（负向波）。准确放置导联对准确解读心电图至关重要。

肢体导联由标准肢体导联（Ⅰ、Ⅱ、Ⅲ）和加压肢体导联（aVR、aVL与aVF导联）组成。标准肢体导联记录两个导联之间的电位，而加压肢体导联记录朝向导联方向的电位。Ⅰ导联反映左右手臂之间的电活动（左臂为正极），Ⅱ导联反映右臂与左腿之间的电活动（左腿为正极），Ⅲ导联反映左臂与左腿之间的电活动（左腿为正极）。垂直于肢体导联的向量为等电位。在aVR、aVL与aVF中，如果电位指向右臂（aVR）、左臂（aVL）与左腿（aVF），则向量为正。六个肢体导联共同构成了一个间隔为30°的额面系统（图3.3）。

六个标准心前区导联（V_1至V_6）放置在前胸壁上，导联放置位置如下：V_1：胸骨右缘第4肋间；V_2：胸骨左缘第4肋间；V_3：V_2和V_4中间；V_4：左锁骨中线第5肋间；V_5：左腋前线与V_4持平；V_6：左腋中线与V_4持平。

特定临床场景下可以选用非标准导联。对于怀疑右室心肌梗死的患者，可将标准V_1与V_2导联位置对调，并在右侧胸壁上与标准左侧心前区导联镜像对应的位置放置V_{3R}至V_{6R}导联。后壁导联可用于提高诊断侧壁和后壁心肌梗死或缺血的敏感性——相应区域在传统12导联心电图上通常为电位静止区。为此，需要从V_6位置沿着第5肋间向后延伸再放置6个导联。此外，检测Brugada综合征时，可以将右侧心前区导联（$V_1 \sim V_3$）上移至第2肋间。

心电图间期

在正常心脏，心电活动起源于右心房上部的窦房结，并通过心房传导。由于窦房结的除极太弱，无法在体表心电图上被检测到，因此体表心电图上最早出现的是幅度较小的P波，反映整个心房的除极。P波的电轴移动指向房室结方向，通常朝向左下方。从P波开始到其后心室快速除极（QRS波群）之间的时间间期称为PR间期，代表电活动通过房室结所需的时间。正常PR间期为$0.12 \sim 0.20$ s，PR间期大于0.20 s则为一度房室传导阻滞。

除极波通过房室结后，心室肌按四个时相依次除极。首先是室间隔从左到右除极，随后右心室以及左心室下壁除极，接着是左心室的心尖和中间部分，最后是左心室的基底部和后壁。心室除极会在体表心电图上产生一个高振幅的QRS波群。该波群出现的第一个负向波为Q波，第一个正向波为R波，随后的负向波为S波。在部分人群中，S波之后可能会出现第二个正向波，这被称为R'波。正常的QRS波群持续时间小于0.10 s，持续时间超过0.12 s的波群通常继发于某些室内传导延迟，包括右束支或左束支传导阻滞。

The isoelectric segment after the QRS complex is the ST segment, which represents a brief period during which relatively little electrical activity occurs in the heart. The junction between the end of the QRS complex and the beginning of the ST segment is the J point. The upward deflection after the ST segment is the T wave, which represents ventricular repolarization. The QT interval, which reflects the duration and transmural gradient of ventricular depolarization and repolarization, is measured from the onset of the QRS complex to the end of the T wave. The observed QT (QT_{ob}) interval varies with heart rate, but for rates between 60 and 100 beats/minute, the normal QT interval ranges from 0.35 to 0.44 seconds. For heart rates outside this range, the QT interval can be corrected (QT_c) using the following formula (with R-R interval in seconds):

$$QTc = \frac{QTob}{\sqrt{R - R\ interval}}$$

Importantly, patients with interventricular conduction delay due to the presence of bundle branch blocks or pacing will have prolonged QT intervals due to the dispersion of ventricular repolarization, which is not necessarily pathologic. Adjustment of the QT interval in these cases remains controversial.

The TP segment is the isoelectric interval that follows the end of the T wave and lasts till the beginning of the P wave. Because it represents an electrically silent portion of the ECG, the TP segment can be used to measure excursions of other segments, such as the ST or PR segments, to determine the presence of elevation or depression. In some individuals, the T wave may be closely followed by a U wave (0.5 mm deflection, not shown in Fig. 3.1), which can be seen for a variety of reasons, including hypokalemia and central nervous system abnormalities.

Axis

The cardiac axis refers to the overall direction of myocardial depolarization measured in the vertical plane and provides clinically useful information. Though the axis can be calculated for any of the ECG segments mentioned above, the mean QRS axis is the most clinically useful.

Fig. 3.3 illustrates the axial reference system, a reconstruction of the Einthoven triangle, and the polarity of each of the six limb leads of the standard ECG. The normal QRS axis ranges from −30 to +90 degrees. An axis more negative than −30 defines left axis deviation, and an axis greater than +90 defines right axis deviation. Extreme axis deviation is present when the mean QRS axis is between −90 and +180 degrees. A positive QRS complex in leads I and aVF suggests a normal QRS axis between 0 and 90 degrees.

While the precordial leads are not useful in determining cardiac axis, they are helpful in determining the direction of cardiac activation in the horizontal plane. Normally, a small R wave occurs in lead V_1, reflecting septal depolarization, along with a deep S wave, reflecting predominantly left ventricular activation. From V_1 to V_6, the R wave becomes larger (and the S wave smaller) because the predominant forces directed at these leads originate from the left ventricle. The transition from a predominant S wave to a predominant R wave usually occurs between leads V_3 and V_4. A delay in this transition is termed "poor R wave progression" and can be seen in patients with prior anterior myocardial infarctions, among other conditions. In patients with ventricular arrhythmias, the pattern of S and R waves in the precordial leads is essential in localizing the foci of the arrhythmia.

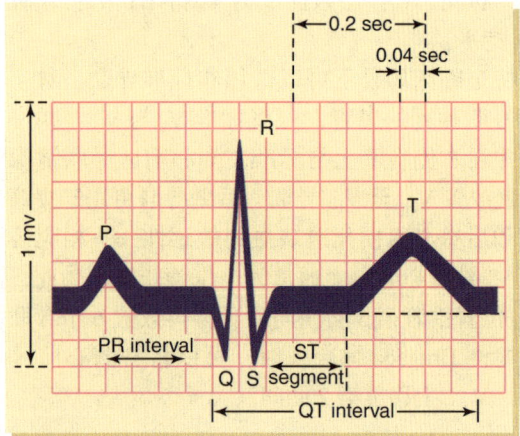

Fig. 3.1 Normal electrocardiographic complex with labeling of waves and intervals.

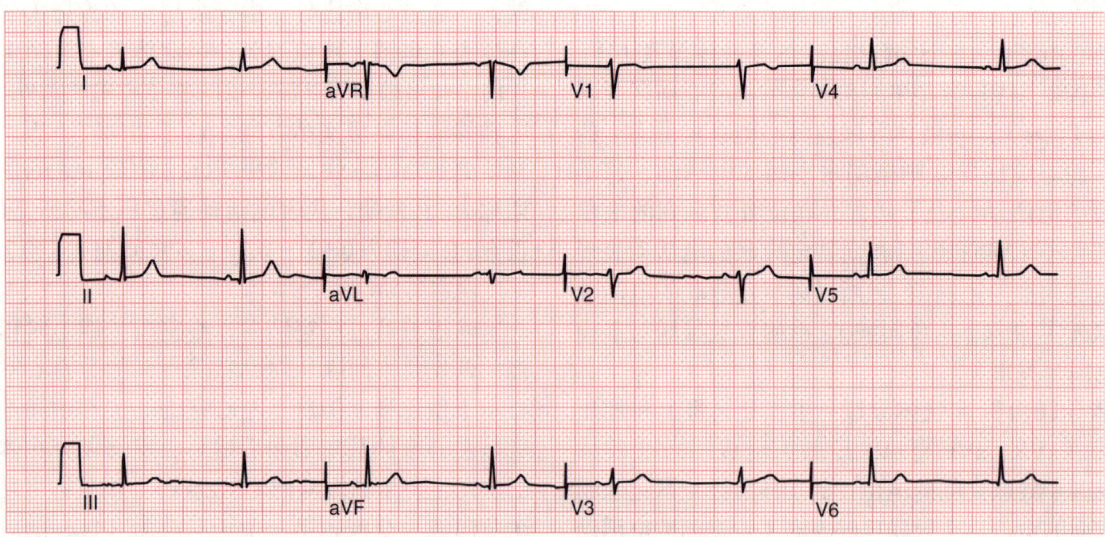

Fig. 3.2 Normal 12-lead electrocardiogram.

QRS 波群之后的等电位段为 ST 段，代表心脏电活动发生相对较少的一个短暂间期。QRS 波群末端与 ST 段起始点交界处为 J 点。ST 段之后的正向波为 T 波，代表心室复极过程。QT 间期是指从 QRS 波起始到 T 波结束的时间，它反映了心室从除极开始至复极结束的持续时间和跨壁梯度。心电图上观察到的 QT 间期（QT_{ob}）随心率而变化，当心率介于 60～100 次/分之间时，正常 QT 间期为 0.35～0.44 s。心率超出此范围时，QT 间期可通过以下公式进行校正（QTc）（R-R 间期以秒为单位）：

$$QTc = \frac{QT_{ob}}{\sqrt{R-R\ 间期}}$$

值得注意的是，由于束支传导阻滞或起搏而导致室内传导延迟的患者会因心室复极离散度增加而出现 QT 间期延长，这种改变不一定是病理性的。在此情况下，是否需要对 QT 间期进行调整仍存在争议。

TP 段是 T 波结束至 P 波开始的等电位间期。由于 TP 段代表了心电图的心电活动静止部分，因此可作为基线用于判断其他波段的偏移情况，如 ST 段或 PR 段是否存在抬高或压低。在部分人群，T 波之后可能紧跟着一个 U 波（振幅 0.5 mm，图 3.1 中未显示）。U 波出现的原因有很多，包括低钾血症和中枢神经系统异常。

电轴

心电轴是指在垂直平面上测量的全部心肌除极的综合向量，可为临床提供有价值的信息。虽然上述任何心电图波段的电轴都可以计算，但平均 QRS 电轴是临床上最有价值的电轴参数。

图 3.3 展示了电轴参考系统、Einthoven 三角的构造以及标准心电图六个肢体导联的极性。正常 QRS 电轴范围为 –30° 至 +90°，电轴位于 –30° 至 –90° 定义为电轴左偏，位于 +90° 至 180° 定义为电轴右偏。当平均 QRS 电轴在 –90° 至 +180° 之间时，为电轴极度偏移。QRS 波群在 I 与 aVF 导联为正向，表明其平均 QRS 电轴在 0 至 90° 之间的正常范围。

虽然心前区导联不能用于确定电轴，但可帮助确定水平面上心脏电活动方向。正常情况下，V_1 导联会出现一个小 r 波，反映室间隔除极，伴随出现的深 S 波则主要反映左心室的激活。指向心前区导联的电位主要来自于左心室，因此自 V_1 至 V_6 导联 R 波逐渐增高，而 S 波逐渐变浅。从 S 波优势过渡到 R 波优势的移行区通常发生在 V_3 与 V_4 两个导联。移行区延迟被称为"R 波递增不良"，见于既往前壁心肌梗死和其他情况。在室性心律失常患者中，心前区导联 S 波与 R 波的波形对心律失常病灶起源定位至关重要。

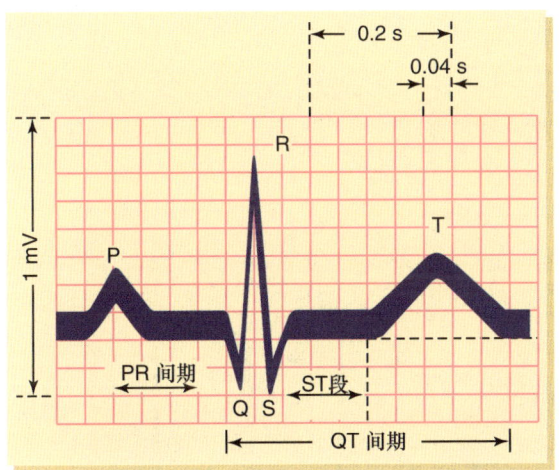

图 3.1　正常心电图，标记各个波和间期

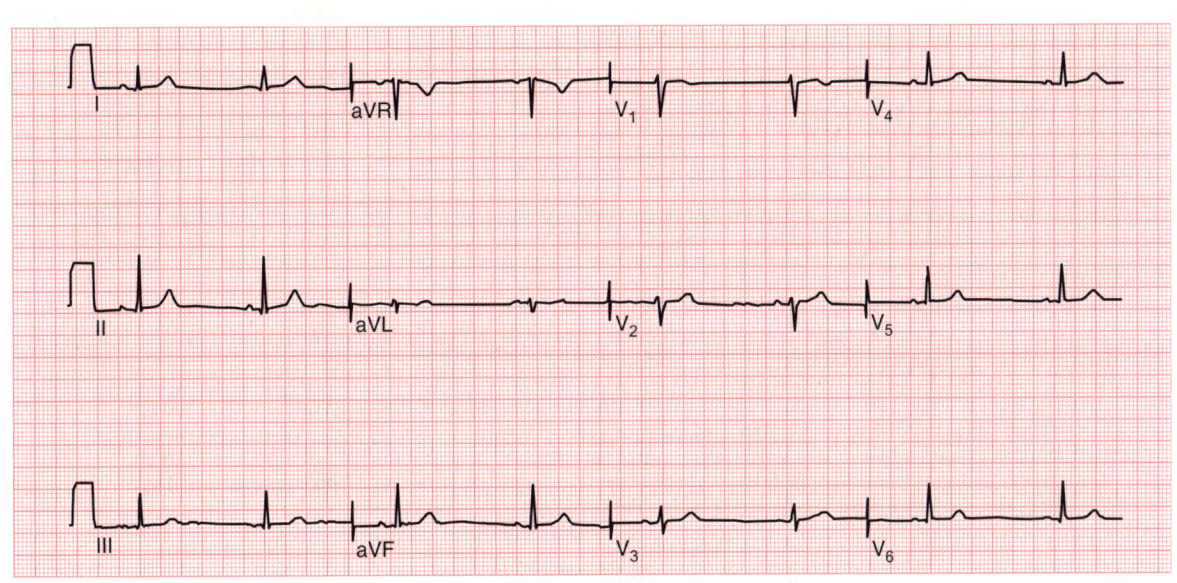

图 3.2　正常 12 导联心电图

ABNORMAL ELECTROCARDIOGRAPHIC PATTERNS

Chamber Abnormalities and Ventricular Hypertrophy

Because of the downward and leftward vector direction, the P wave is normally upright in leads I, II, and aVF, inverted in aVR, and biphasic in V_1. Left atrial abnormality (i.e., enlargement, hypertrophy, or increased wall stress) is characterized by a wide P wave in lead II (0.12 second) and a deeply inverted terminal component in lead V_1 (able to contain one small box or 1 mm^2). Right atrial abnormality is identified when the P waves in the limb leads are tall and peaked and at least 2.5 mm high and (able to contain two stacked small boxes).

Left ventricular hypertrophy may result in increased QRS voltage, slight widening of the QRS complex, late intrinsicoid deflection, left axis deviation, and abnormalities of the ST-T segments (Fig. 3.4A). Multiple criteria with various degrees of sensitivity and specificity for detecting left ventricular hypertrophy are available. The most frequently used criteria are given in Table 3.1.

Right ventricular hypertrophy is characterized by tall R waves in leads V_1 through V_3; deep S waves in leads I, aVL, V_5, and V_6; and right axis deviation (see Fig. 3.4B). The R wave is greater than 7 mm and the R-S ratio is greater than 1 in lead V_1. Other causes of a tall R-wave in V_1 must be excluded, including posterior wall myocardial infarction,

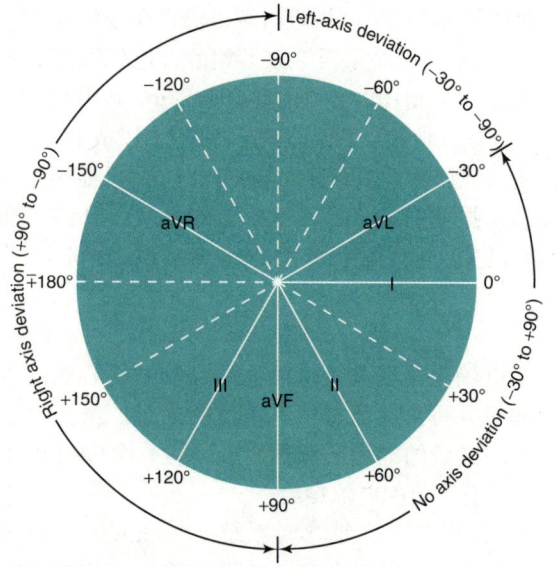

Fig. 3.3 Hexaxial reference figure for frontal plane axis determination, indicating values for abnormal left and right QRS axis deviations.

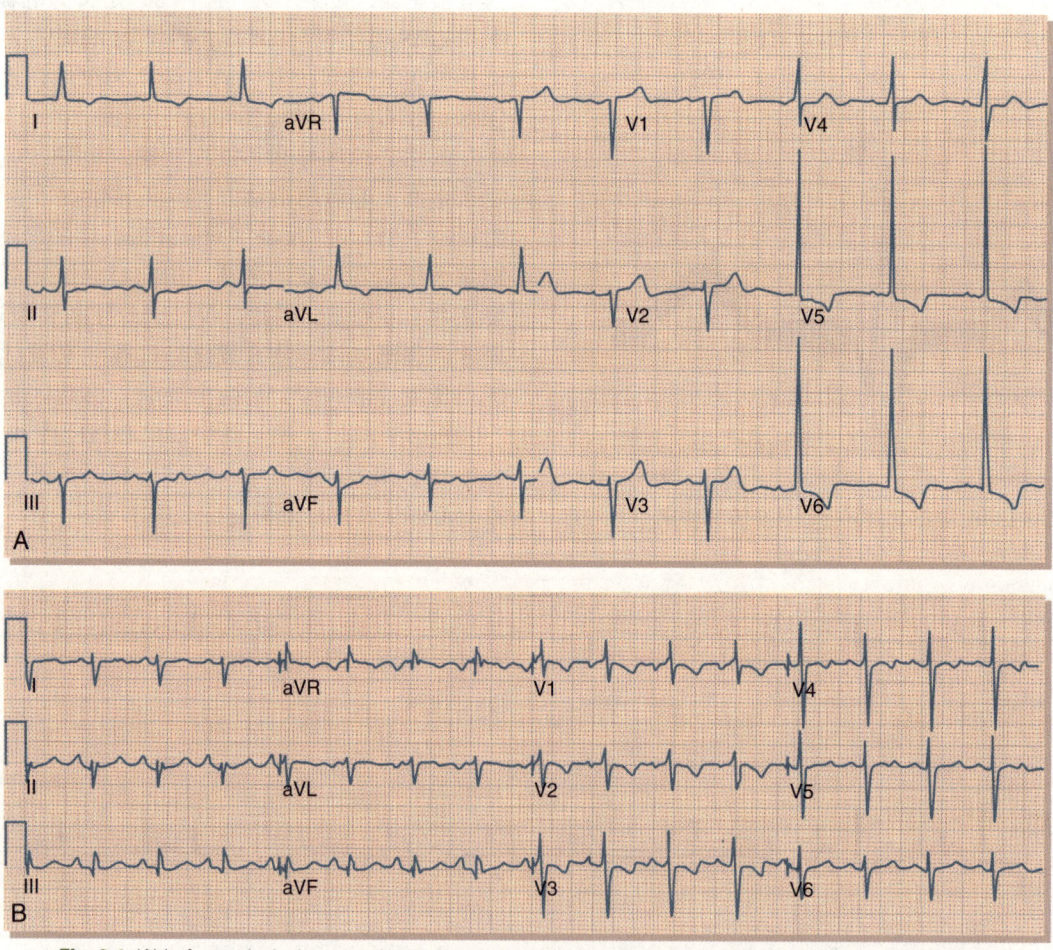

Fig. 3.4 (A) Left ventricular hypertrophy as seen on an electrocardiographic recording. Characteristic findings include increased QRS voltage in precordial leads (i.e., deep S in lead V_2 and tall R in lead V_5) and downsloping ST depression and T-wave inversion in lateral precordial leads (i.e., strain pattern) and leftward axis. (B) Right ventricular hypertrophy with tall R wave in right precordial leads, downsloping ST depression in precordial leads (i.e., RV strain), right axis deviation, and evidence of right atrial enlargement.

异常心电图

腔室异常和心室肥厚

由于心房除极的综合向量向下、向左，P 波在 Ⅰ、Ⅱ 与 aVF 导联通常向上，在 aVR 导联向下，在 V_1 导联呈正负双向。左心房异常（即扩大、肥厚或房壁应力增加）的特征是 P 波在 Ⅱ 导联增宽（≥ 0.12 s）以及在 V_1 导联出现宽而深的负向波（可包含一个小方格或 1 mm^2）。右心房异常则会在肢体导联出现高而尖的 P 波，其高度 ≥ 2.5 mm（可包含两个小方格）。

左心室肥厚可导致 QRS 波群电压增高、QRS 波群轻微增宽、类本位曲折延迟、电轴左偏和 ST-T 异常改变（图 3.4A）。目前有多种检测左心室肥厚的标准，其敏感性和特异性各不相同。表 3.1 列出了最常用的标准。

右心室肥厚的特征是 $V_1 \sim V_3$ 导联 R 波增高，Ⅰ、aVL、V_5 与 V_6 导联出现深 S 波，以及电轴右偏（图 3.4B）。V_1 导联的 R 波通常高于 7 mm 且 R/S 比值大于 1。诊断右心室肥厚时，必须排除可以导致 V_1 导联 R

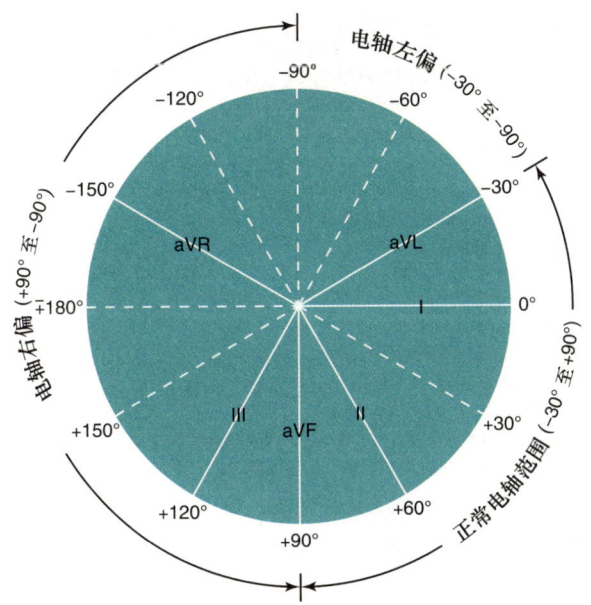

图 3.3　额面六轴参考图，显示电轴左右异常偏移的角度

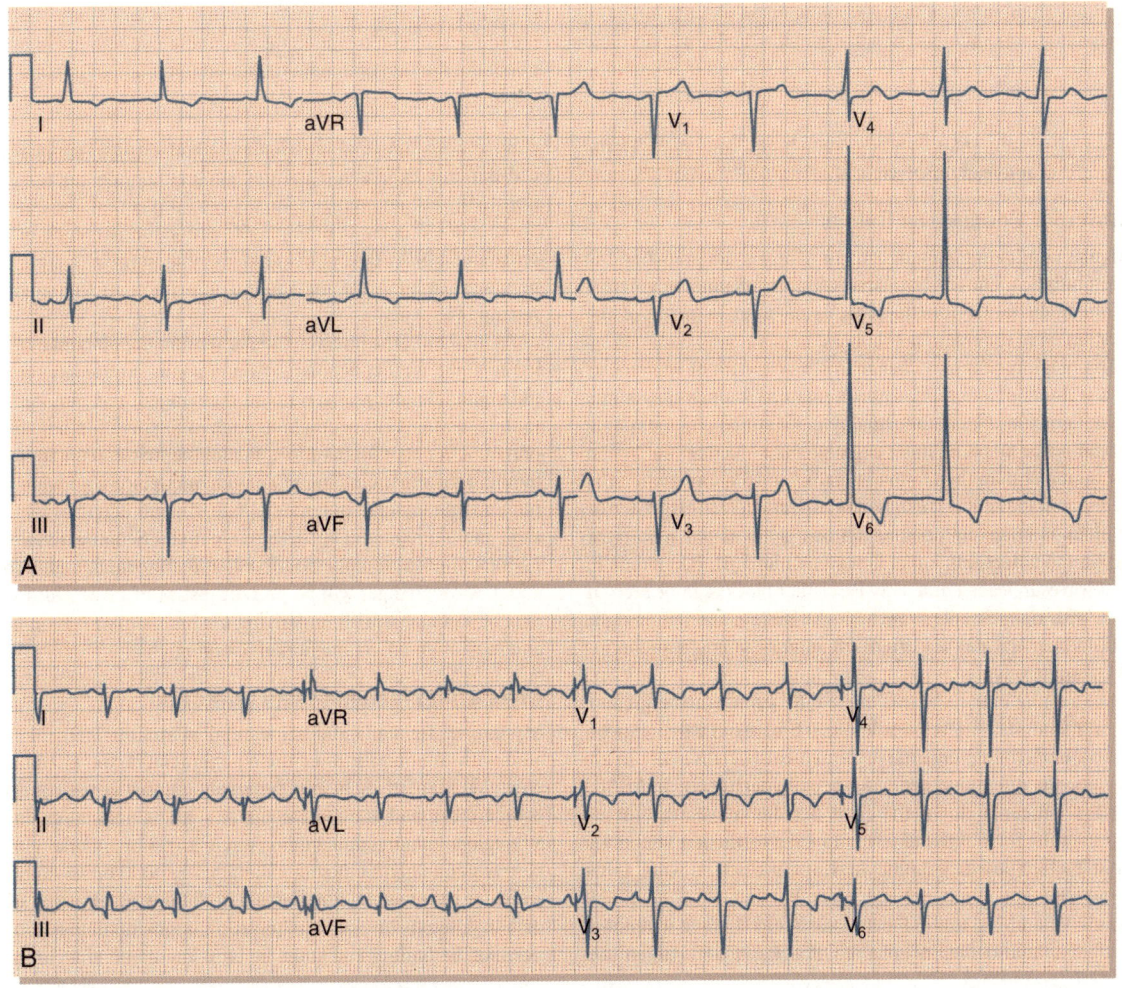

图 3.4　（A）左心室肥厚的心电图表现：特征性变化包括心前区导联的 QRS 波电压增高（即 V_2 导联的深 S 波和 V_5 导联的高 R 波），心前区侧壁导联的 ST 段呈下斜型压低和 T 波倒置（即劳损波形）以及电轴左偏。（B）右心室肥厚的心电图表现：右侧心前区导联出现高 R 波，ST 段下斜型压低（即右心室劳损），电轴右偏和右心房扩大

TABLE 3.1 Electrocardiographic Manifestations of Atrial Abnormalities and Ventricular Hypertrophy

Left Atrial Abnormality
P-wave duration ≥0.12 second
Notched, slurred P wave in leads I and II
Biphasic P wave in lead V_1 with a wide, deep, negative terminal component

Right Atrial Abnormality
P-wave duration ≤0.11 second
Tall, peaked P waves of ≥2.5 mm in leads II, III, and aVF

Left Ventricular Hypertrophy
Voltage criteria
R wave in lead aVL ≥12 mm
R wave in lead I ≥15 mm
S wave in lead V_1 or V_2 + R wave in lead V_5 or V_6 ≥35 mm
Depressed ST segments with inverted T waves in the lateral leads
Left axis deviation
QRS duration ≥0.09 second
Left atrial enlargement

Right Ventricular Hypertrophy
Tall R waves over right precordium (R-to-S ratio in lead V_1 >1.0)
Right axis deviation
Depressed ST segments with inverted T waves in leads V_1 to V_3
Normal QRS duration (if no right bundle branch block)
Right atrial enlargement

TABLE 3.2 Electrocardiographic Manifestations of Fascicular and Bundle Branch Blocks

Left Anterior Fascicular Block
QRS duration ≤0.1 second
Left axis deviation (more negative than −45 degrees)
rS pattern in leads II, III, and aVF
qR pattern in leads I and aVL

Right Posterior Fascicular Block
QRS duration ≤0.1 second
Right axis deviation (+90 degrees or greater)
qR pattern in leads II, III, and aVF
rS pattern in leads I and aVL
Exclusion of other causes of right axis deviation (e.g., chronic obstructive pulmonary disease, right ventricular hypertrophy)

Left Bundle Branch Block
QRS duration ≥0.12 second
Broad, slurred, or notched R waves in lateral leads (I, aVL, V_5, and V_6)
QS or rS pattern in anterior precordium leads (V_1 and V_2)
ST-T-wave vectors opposite to terminal QRS vectors

Right Bundle Branch Block
QRS duration ≥0.12 second
Large R′ wave in lead V_1 (rsR′)
Deep terminal S wave in lead V_6
Normal septal Q waves
Inverted T waves in leads V_1 and V_2

Wolff-Parkinson-White, right bundle branch block, muscular dystrophy, dextrocardia, and lead misplacement.

Interventricular Conduction Delays

The ventricular conduction system consists of two main branches, the right and left bundles. The left bundle further divides into the anterior and posterior fascicles. Conduction block can occur in either of the major branches or in the fascicles (Table 3.2).

Fascicular block results in a change in the sequence of ventricular activation but does not substantially prolong overall conduction time. Left anterior fascicular block abnormality is identified when extreme left axis deviation occurs (i.e., more negative than −45 degrees), when the R wave is greater than the Q wave in leads I and aVL, and when the S wave is greater than the R wave in leads II, III, and aVF. Left posterior fascicular block is relatively uncommon but is associated with right axis deviation (>90 degrees); small Q waves in leads II, III, and aVF; and small R waves in leads I and aVL. Fascicular blocks can be seen in conjunction with right bundle branch block (RBBB), and left or right axis deviations can indicate concurrent left anterior or posterior fascicular blocks, respectively.

Complete bundle branch blocks cause QRS prolongation greater than 120 milliseconds. A left bundle branch block (LBBB) can be indicative of underlying coronary or myocardial disease—most commonly fibrosis due to ischemic injury or hypertrophy. In LBBB, depolarization proceeds down the right bundle, across the interventricular septum from right to left, and then to the left ventricle. Characteristic electrocardiographic findings include a wide QRS complex; a broad R wave in leads I, aVL, V_5, and V_6; a deep QS wave in leads V_1 and V_2; and ST depression and T-wave inversion opposite the terminal deflection of the QRS (Fig. 3.5A). Given the abnormal sequence of ventricular activation and repolarization with LBBB, many ECG abnormalities, such as Q-wave myocardial infarction (MI) and left ventricular hypertrophy, are difficult to evaluate. Sgarbossa's criteria can help to identify the presence of MI in the setting of LBBB, though its sensitivity is limited. A new LBBB may be a sign of an acute myocardial infarction in the correct clinical setting (Fig. 3.6B).

With RBBB, the interventricular septum depolarizes normally from left to right, as this depolarization depends on the left bundle. Thus, the initial QRS deflection remains unchanged, and thus it is important to note that ECG abnormalities such as Q-wave MI can still be interpreted. After septal activation, the left ventricle depolarizes, followed by the right ventricle. The ECG is characterized by a wide QRS complex; a large R′ wave in lead V_1 (R-S-R′); and deep S waves in leads I, aVL, and V_6, representing delayed right ventricular activation (see Fig. 3.5B). Ventricular repolarization is still abnormal, and secondary ST and T wave changes will be present just as in LBBB. Although RBBB may be associated with underlying cardiac disease, it is quite common and may often reflect the fibrosis of aging.

Myocardial Ischemia and Infarction

Myocardial ischemia and myocardial infarction (MI) may be associated with abnormalities of the ST segment, T wave, and QRS complex. Myocardial ischemia primarily affects repolarization of the myocardium and is often associated with horizontal or downsloping ST-segment depression and T-wave inversion. These changes may be transient, such as during an anginal episode or an exercise-related stress, or they may be long-lasting in the setting of progressive angina or MI. T-wave inversion without ST-segment depression can be a nonspecific finding and must be correlated with the clinical findings

表 3.1　心房异常和心室肥厚的心电图表现
左心房异常 P 波时限 ≥ 0.12 s Ⅰ、Ⅱ 导联 P 波顶峰粗钝、有切迹 V_1 导联的 P 波呈双相，出现宽而深的负向波
右心房异常 P 波时限 ≤ 0.11 s Ⅱ、Ⅲ、aVF 导联出现 ≥ 2.5 mm 的高而尖的 P 波
左心室肥厚 电压标准 　　aVL 导联 R 波 ≥ 12 mm 　　Ⅰ 导联 R 波 ≥ 15 mm 　　V_1 或 V_2 导联中 S 波 + V_5 或 V_6 导联中的 R 波 ≥ 35 mm 侧壁导联 ST 段压低，T 波倒置 电轴左偏 QRS 波持续时间 ≥ 0.09 s 左心房扩大
右心室肥厚 右侧心前区出现高 R 波（V_1 导联的 R/S 比值 > 1.0） 电轴右偏 $V_1 \sim V_3$ 导联 ST 段压低，T 波倒置 QRS 波时限正常（如果不伴右束支传导阻滞） 右心房扩大

表 3.2　分支与束支传导阻滞的心电图表现
左前分支阻滞 QRS 波时限 ≤ 0.1 s 电轴左偏（超过 −45°） Ⅱ、Ⅲ、aVF 导联 QRS 波呈 rS 型 Ⅰ、aVL 导联 QRS 波呈 qR 型
左后分支阻滞 QRS 波时限 ≤ 0.1 s 电轴右偏（+90° 或以上） Ⅱ、Ⅲ、aVF 导联 QRS 波呈 qR 型 Ⅰ、aVL 导联 QRS 波呈 rS 型 排除导致电轴右偏的其他原因（如慢性阻塞性肺疾病、右心室肥厚等）
左束支传导阻滞 QRS 波时限 ≥ 0.12 s 侧壁导联（Ⅰ、aVL、V_5 与 V_6）中的 R 波增宽、顶峰粗钝或有切迹 前壁心前区导联（V_1、V_2）呈 QS 或 rS 型 ST-T 方向与 QRS 波群主波方向相反
右束支传导阻滞 QRS 波时限 ≥ 0.12 s V_1 导联出现大 R 波（rsR′ 型） V_6 导联终末 S 波加深 间隔 Q 波正常 V_1 与 V_2 导联 T 波倒置

波增高的其他原因，包括后壁心肌梗死、WPW 综合征、右束支传导阻滞、肌营养不良、右位心和导联放置错误。

室内传导延迟

室内传导系统由两个主要传导束组成，即右束支和左束支。左束支又分为左前分支和左后分支。传导阻滞在主要束支或分支均可发生（表 3.2）。

分支阻滞会导致心室激动顺序的改变，但不会大幅延长总体传导时间。当出现极度电轴左偏（即负值大于 −45°）、Ⅰ 与 aVL 导联的 R 波大于 Q 波、Ⅱ、Ⅲ 与 aVF 导联的 S 波大于 R 波时，即可确定为左前分支阻滞。左后分支阻滞相对少见，但可表现为电轴右偏（>90°）、Ⅱ、Ⅲ 与 aVF 导联出现小 Q 波，以及 Ⅰ 与 aVL 导联出现小 R 波。分支阻滞可与右束支传导阻滞（RBBB）同时出现，电轴左偏或右偏可分别提示右束支传导阻滞伴左前或左后分支阻滞。

完全性束支传导阻滞会导致 QRS 波群增宽时限超过 120 ms。左束支传导阻滞（LBBB）可能是潜在冠状动脉疾病或心肌疾病的征象，最常见于缺血性损伤或肥厚导致的纤维化。左束支传导阻滞时，激动沿右束支下传，从右向左穿过室间隔，然后到达左心室。心电图特征性表现为宽大 QRS 波，Ⅰ、aVL、V_5 与 V_6 导联 R 波增宽，V_1 与 V_2 导联 QS 波加深，以及 ST 段压低和 T 波倒置，方向与 QRS 波群主波方向相反（图 3.5A）。由于左束支传导阻滞时心室激动和复极顺序异常，导致许多心电图异常很难判断，如 Q 波型心肌梗死（MI）和左心室肥厚。Sgarbossa 标准有助于在伴左束支传导阻滞时识别是否存在心肌梗死，但其敏感性不高。在特定的临床场景下，新发的左束支传导阻滞可能提示发生急性心肌梗死（图 3.6B）。

由于室间隔除极依赖于左束支，右束支传导阻滞时，室间隔仍然能从左至右正常除极。因此，QRS 波初始除极保持不变，不会对其他心电图异常（如 Q 波型心肌梗死）的判读产生影响。室间隔激动后，左心室除极，随后是右心室。心电图的特征是 QRS 波群增宽，V_1 导联出现大 R′ 波（R-S-R′），Ⅰ、aVL 与 V_6 导联出现深 S 波，反映右心室激动延迟（见图 3.5B）。心室复极仍然异常，将与左束支传导阻滞一样出现继发性 ST 段和 T 波改变。尽管右束支传导阻滞可能与潜在的心脏疾病有关，但其很常见，常反映衰老引起的心脏纤维化。

心肌缺血和梗死

心肌缺血和心肌梗死（MI）通常表现为 ST 段、T 波和 QRS 波群的异常。心肌缺血主要影响心肌的复极，一般表现为水平或下斜型的 ST 段压低和 T 波倒置。这些变化可能是一过性的，比如在心绞痛发作或劳力负荷时出现，也可能是长期的，比如在进展性心绞痛或心肌梗死时。单纯 T 波倒置不伴有 ST 段压低，可能是非特异性表现，必须结合相关的临床表现来判断是否

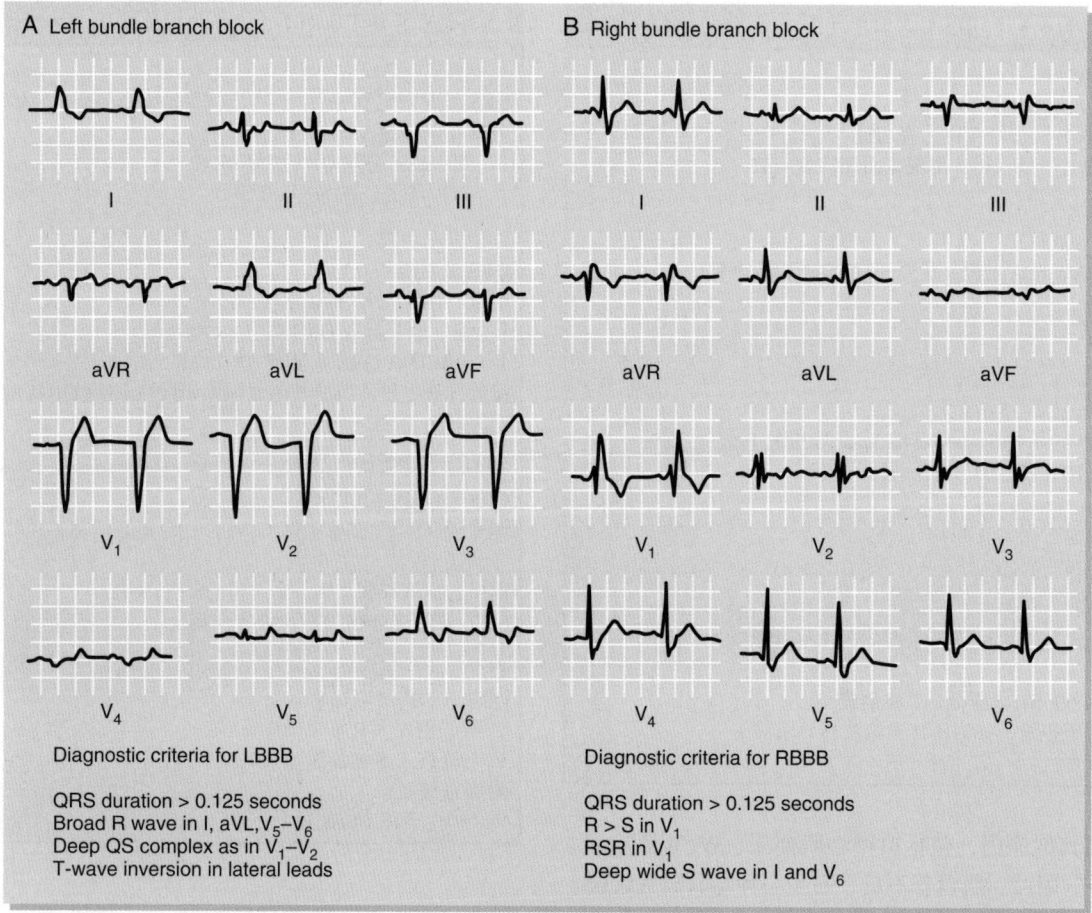

Fig. 3.5 (A) Left bundle branch block (LBBB). (B) Right bundle branch block (RBBB). Criteria for bundle branch blocks are summarized in Table 3.2.

to invoke ischemia or injury. Diffuse T-wave inversions across the precordial leads are often seen in patients with acute cerebral disease, such as stroke or seizures.

ST-segment elevation of 2 mm or more in two or more contiguous leads suggests more extensive myocardial injury, and in the right clinical presentation, is often considered to be an acute MI until proven otherwise (Fig. 3.6A). Vasospastic or Prinzmetal angina may be associated with reversible ST-segment elevation without MI. ST-segment elevation may occur in other settings not related to acute ischemia or infarction. Persistent, localized ST-segment elevation in the same leads as pathologic Q waves is consistent with a ventricular aneurysm. Acute pericarditis is also associated with diffuse ST-segment elevation across multiple contiguous and noncontiguous leads but is also associated with PR depression relative to the TP interval. Diffuse J-point elevation in association with upward-coving ST segments is a normal variant common among young men and is often referred to as *early repolarization*.

A pathologic Q wave is one of the criteria used to diagnose MI. Infarcted myocardium is impaired at conducting normal electrical activity, and electrical forces are directed away from the surface electrode overlying the infarcted region, producing a Q wave on the surface ECG. A thorough understanding of contiguous leads allows for identification of each region of the myocardium relative to the surface lead, enabling the examiner to localize the area of infarction (Table 3.3). Pathologic Q waves are defined as follows: any Q wave 20 ms or greater or QS complex in leads V_2 to V_3, or a Q wave 30 ms or greater and 0.1 mV deep or greater or QS complex in leads I, II, aVL, aVF or V_4 to V_6 in any 2 leads of a contiguous lead grouping (I, aVL, V_6; V_4 to V_6; II, III, and aVF). Not all MIs result in the permanent formation of Q waves. Small R waves can return many weeks to months after an MI. Abnormal Q waves, or *pseudoinfarction* pattern, may be associated with nonischemic cardiac disease, such as ventricular preexcitation, cardiac amyloidosis, sarcoidosis, idiopathic or hypertrophic cardiomyopathy, myocarditis, and chronic lung disease.

Abnormalities of the ST Segment and T Wave

A number of drugs and metabolic abnormalities may affect the ST segment and T wave (Fig. 3.7). Hypokalemia may result in prominent U waves in the precordial leads along with prolongation of the QT interval. Hyperkalemia may result in tall, peaked T waves. Hypocalcemia typically lengthens the QT interval, whereas hypercalcemia shortens it. A commonly used cardiac medication, digoxin, often results in diffuse, scooped ST-segment depression. Cardiac pacing, LBBB, and RBBB affect ventricular repolarization and alter the ST segment and T-wave. Minor or *nonspecific* ST-segment and T-wave abnormalities may occur in many patients and have no definable cause. In these instances, the physician must determine the significance of the abnormalities based on clinical findings.

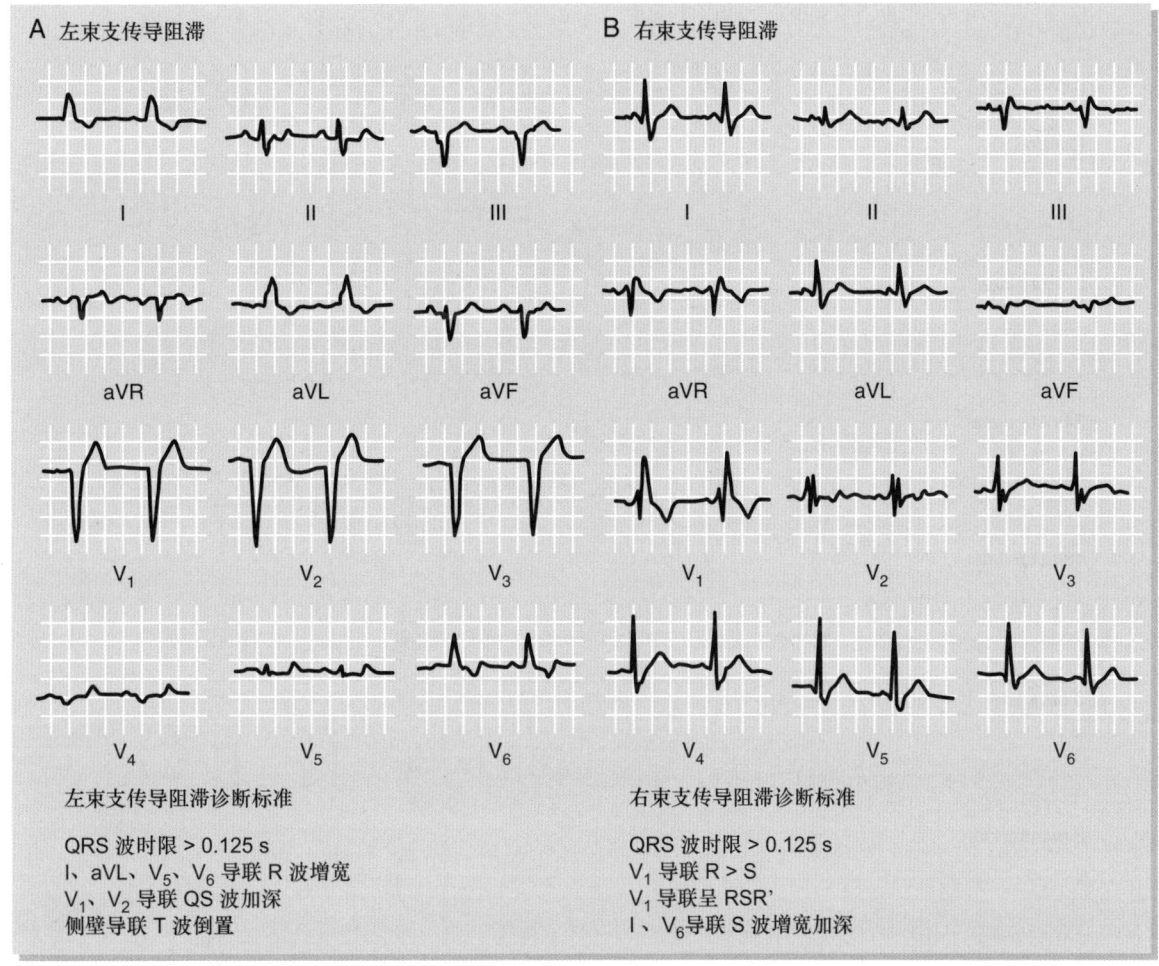

图 3.5 （A）左束支传导阻滞（LBBB）。（B）右束支传导阻滞（RBBB）。束支传导阻滞的诊断标准见表 3.2

存在心肌缺血或损伤。心前区广泛性 T 波倒置常见于急性大脑疾病（如卒中或癫痫）患者。

两个或两个以上相邻导联的 ST 段抬高超过 2 mm 提示更广泛的心肌损伤，在有相应的临床表现时通常考虑为急性心肌梗死（图 3.6A），除非最终证实是与急性心肌梗死无关的其他情况。血管痉挛性或变异型心绞痛可能出现可逆性 ST 段抬高，但无心肌梗死。在有病理性 Q 波的导联出现持续性局部 ST 段抬高提示室壁瘤。急性心包炎时心电图也会出现多个相邻和非相邻导联的广泛性 ST 段抬高，但通常还存在 PR 段压低（以 TP 段为基线）。广泛性 J 点抬高伴 ST 段弓背向下抬高是年轻男性中常见的正常变异，被称为心室早复极。

病理性 Q 波是诊断心肌梗死的标准之一。梗死的心肌无法传导正常的电活动，电位背离梗死区域的体表电极，从而在体表心电图上产生 Q 波。全面考量各连续导联的变化可确定与体表导联相对应的心肌区域，帮助检查者定位心肌梗死部位（表 3.3）。病理性 Q 波的定义为：$V_2 \sim V_3$ 导联出现任何 ≥ 20 ms 的 Q 波或 QS 波群；Ⅰ、Ⅱ、Ⅲ、aVL、aVF（译者注：原文无 Ⅲ 导联，应包括）或 $V_4 \sim V_6$ 导联中任意两个连续导联（Ⅰ、aVL、V_6；$V_4 \sim V_6$；Ⅱ、Ⅲ 与 aVF）出现宽度 ≥ 30 ms 且深度 ≥ 0.1 mV 的 Q 波或 QS 波群。并非所有心肌梗死都会形成永久性 Q 波。心肌梗死后数周至数月，小 R 波可能会恢复。异常 Q 波或假性梗死波可能与非缺血性心脏病有关，如心室预激、心脏淀粉样变性、结节病、特发性或肥厚型心肌病、心肌炎和慢性肺部疾病等。

ST 段和 T 波异常

一些药物和代谢异常可能会影响 ST 段和 T 波（图 3.7）。低钾血症可能导致心前区导联出现明显增高的 U 波伴 QT 间期延长。高钾血症可导致 T 波高尖。低钙血症通常会延长 QT 间期，而高钙血症则会缩短 QT 间期。地高辛是一种常用的心脏病药物，常导致广泛性、鱼钩样 ST 段压低。心脏起搏、左束支传导阻滞和右束支传导阻滞会影响心室复极并导致 ST 段和 T 波改变。许多患者在无明确原因情况下会出现轻微或非特异性 ST-T 异常改变，此时，医生须结合临床来明确这些异常 ST-T 改变的意义。

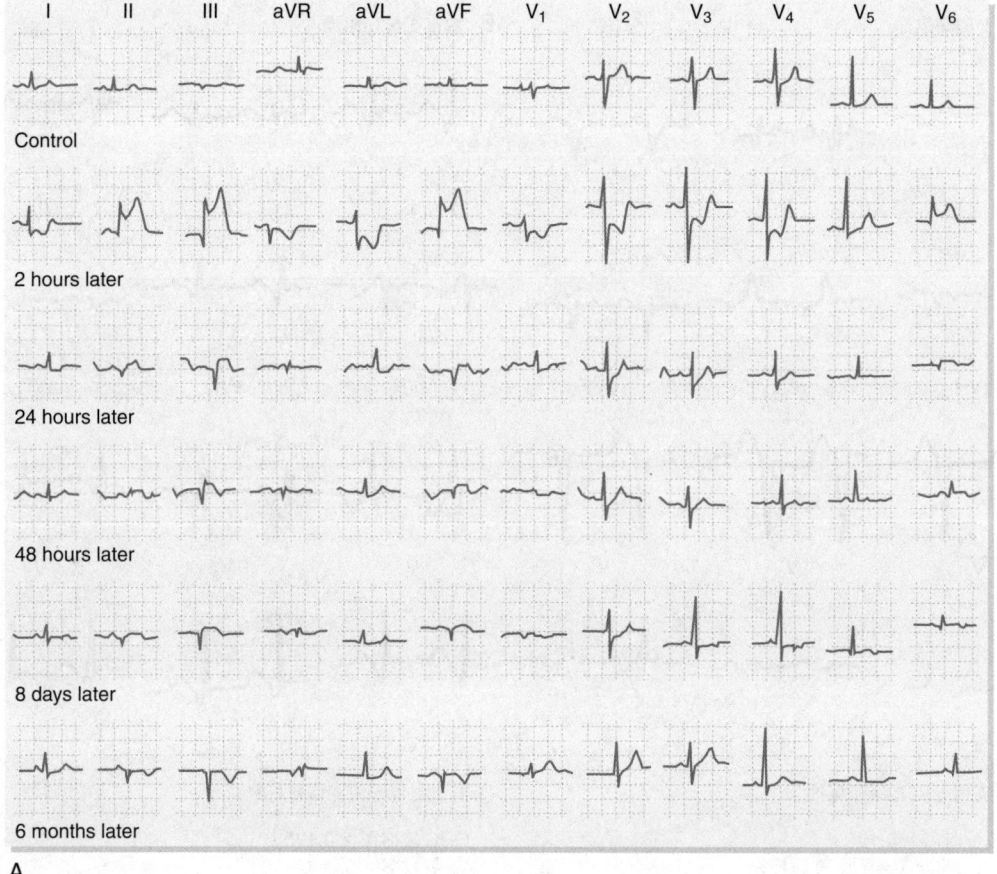

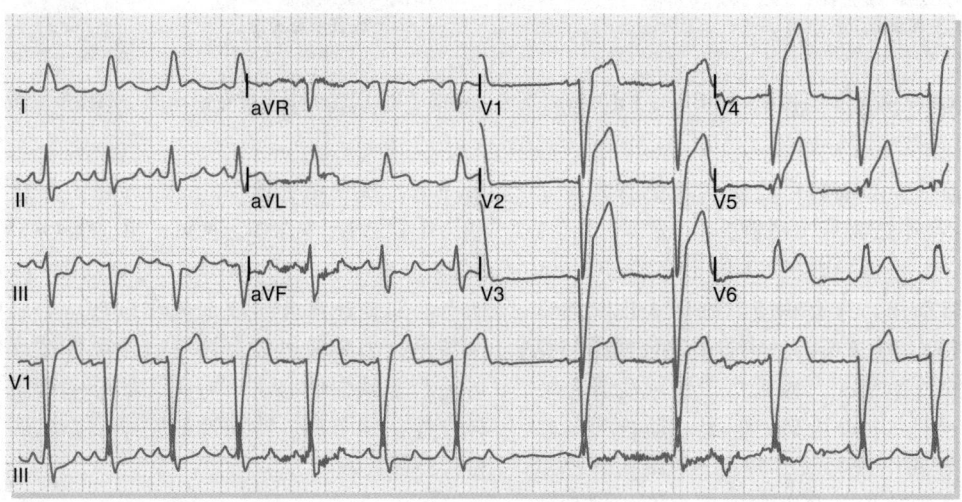

Fig. 3.6 (A) Evolutionary changes in a posteroinferior myocardial infarction (MI). Control tracing is normal. The tracing recorded 2 hours after onset of chest pain demonstrated development of early Q waves, marked ST-segment elevation, and hyperacute T waves in leads II, III, and aVF. A larger R wave, ST-segment depression, and negative T waves have developed in leads V_1 and V_2. These early changes indicate acute posteroinferior MI. The 24-hour tracing demonstrates further evolutionary changes. In leads II, III, and aVF, the Q wave is larger, the ST segments have almost returned to baseline, and the T wave has begun to invert. In leads V_1 to V_2, the duration of the R wave exceeds 0.04 seconds, the ST segment is depressed, and the T wave is upright. (In this example, electrocardiographic changes of true posterior involvement extend past lead V_2; ordinarily, only leads V_1 and V_2 may be involved.) Only minor further changes occur through the 8-day tracing. Six months later, the electrocardiographic pattern shows large Q waves, isoelectric ST segments, and inverted T waves in leads II, III, and aVF and shows large R waves, isoelectric ST segment, and upright T waves in leads V_1 and V_2, indicative of an old posteroinferior MI. (B) Electrocardiogram from a patient with an underlying left bundle branch block (LBBB) who experienced an acute anterior MI. Characteristic ST segment elevation and hyperacute T waves are seen in leads V_1 through V_6 and leads I and aVL despite the presence of the LBBB. This is not always the case, and a patient with typical symptoms, an LBBB, and no definite ischemic ST-segment elevations should be treated as if the individual is having a myocardial infarction or acute coronary syndrome.

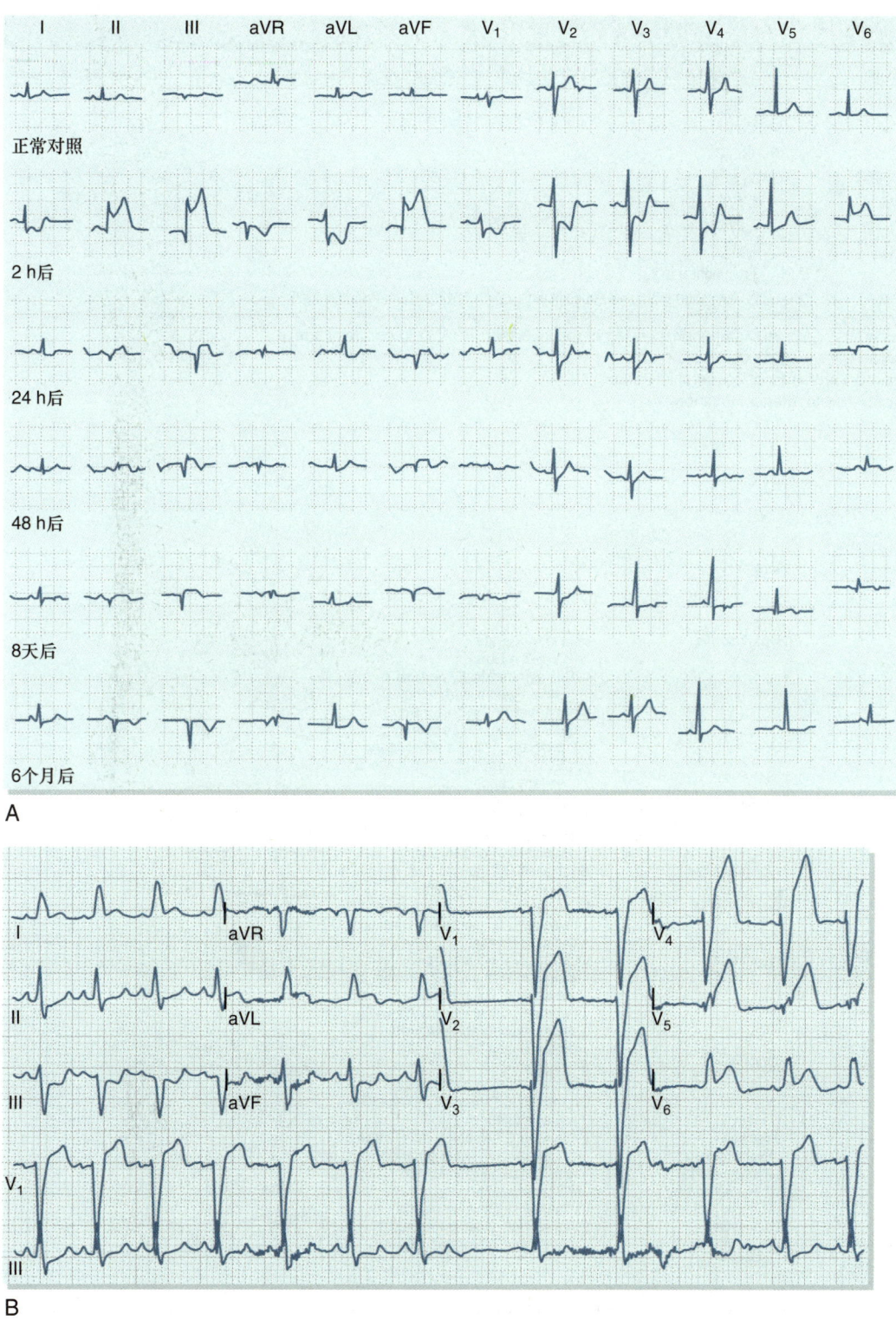

图 3.6 （A）下后壁心肌梗死的心电图演变过程。对照为正常心电图。胸痛发作 2 h 后记录心电图显示 Ⅱ、Ⅲ 与 aVF 导联出现早期 Q 波、ST 段显著抬高和 T 波高耸直立。V_1 与 V_2 导联出现 R 波增高、ST 段压低和 T 波倒置。这些早期变化提示急性下壁及后壁心肌梗死。24 h 后记录的心电图显示了进一步的动态改变。Ⅱ、Ⅲ 与 aVF 导联 Q 波增大，ST 段几乎恢复到基线，T 波开始倒置。V_1~V_2 导联 R 波时限超过 0.04 s，ST 段压低，T 波直立（在本例中，正后壁受累的心电图变化在 V_2 以外导联也见到；而通常情况下，只有 V_1 和 V_2 导联发生变化）。8 天后心电图仅记录到轻微的进一步变化。6 个月后，心电图显示 Ⅱ、Ⅲ 与 aVF 导联出现宽而深的大 Q 波、ST 段恢复正常、T 波倒置，V_1 与 V_2 导联出现大 R 波、ST 段恢复正常、T 波直立，提示陈旧性下壁及后壁心肌梗死。（B）一例左束支传导阻滞患者发生急性前壁心肌梗死的心电图。尽管存在左束支传导阻滞，在 V_1~V_6 导联以及 Ⅰ 与 aVL 导联仍可看到特征性 ST 段抬高和急性期高耸直立的 T 波。但并非所有患者都有这种特征性改变。对于有典型症状但没有确定的缺血性 ST 段抬高心电图表现的左束支传导阻滞患者，应将其视为心肌梗死或急性冠脉综合征进行治疗

TABLE 3.3 Electrocardiographic Localization of Myocardial Infarction

Infarct Location	Leads Depicting Primary Electrocardiographic Changes	Likely Vessel Involved[a]
Inferior	II, III, aVF	RCA
Septal	V_1, V_2	LAD
Anterior	V_3, V_4	LAD
Anteroseptal	V_1 to V_4	LAD
Extensive anterior	I, aVL, V_1 to V_6	LAD
Lateral	I, aVL, V_5 to V_6	CIRC
High lateral	I, aVL	CIRC
Posterior[b]	Prominent R in V_1	RCA or CIRC
Right ventricular[c]	ST elevation in V_1; more specifically, V_4R in setting of inferior infarction	RCA

CIRC, Circumflex artery; *LAD*, left anterior descending coronary artery; *RCA*, right coronary artery.
[a]This is a generalization; variations occur.
[b]Usually in association with inferior or lateral infarction.
[c]Usually in association with inferior infarction.

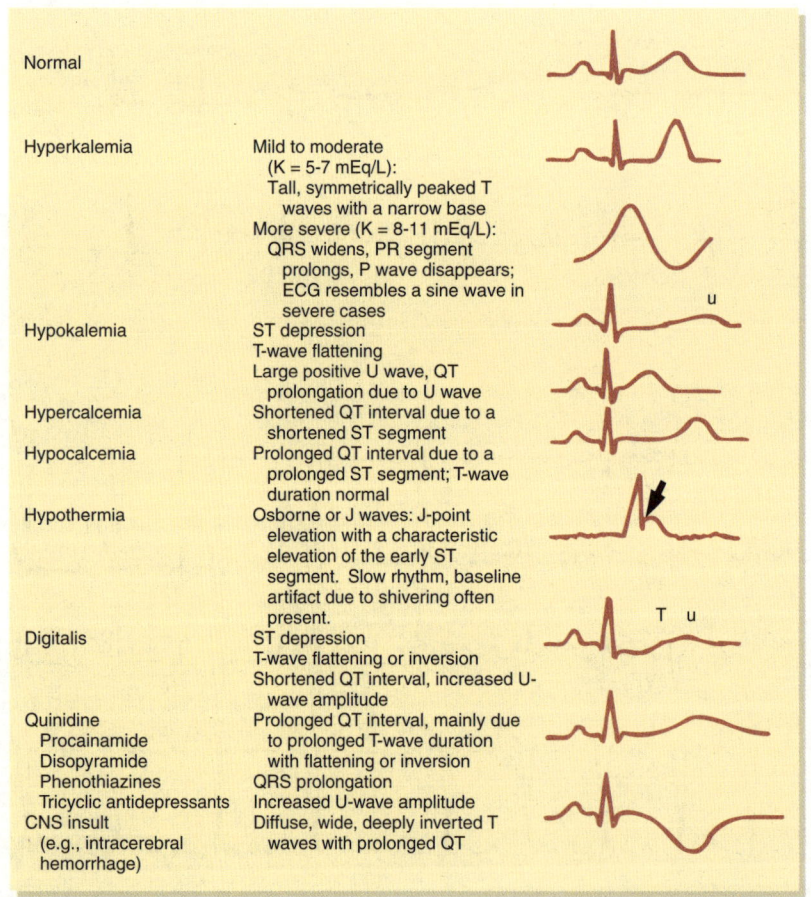

Fig. 3.7 Metabolic and drug influences on the electrocardiographic recording. *CNS*, Central nervous system; *ECG*, electrocardiogram.

AMBULATORY ELECTROCARDIOGRAPHIC RECORDING

Ambulatory ECG monitoring allows clinicians to monitor and capture the presence and frequency of cardiac arrhythmias over a specified period of time. Multiple types of ambulatory recording modalities are available, and the decision to use one or the other largely depends on the duration of surveillance required. Determination of the surveillance duration is influenced by many factors, including the frequency of symptoms (daily, weekly, monthly, or longer), reason for the study

表 3.3 心肌梗死的心电图定位

梗死部位	显示主要心电图变化的导联	可能涉及的血管 [a]
下壁	Ⅱ、Ⅲ、aVF	右冠状动脉
间壁	V_1、V_2	左前降支
前壁	V_3、V_4	左前降支
前间壁	$V_1 \sim V_4$	左前降支
广泛前壁	Ⅰ、aVL、$V_1 \sim V_6$	左前降支
侧壁	Ⅰ、aVL、$V_5 \sim V_6$	左回旋支
高侧壁	Ⅰ、aVL	左回旋支
后壁[b]	V_1 导联 R 波增高	右冠状动脉或左回旋支
右心室[c]	V_1 导联 ST 段抬高；急性下壁心肌梗死时 V_{4R} 导联 ST 段抬高更具特异性	右冠状动脉

[a] 只是常见情况，实际可能存在变异。
[b] 通常伴有下壁或侧壁梗死。
[c] 通常伴有下壁梗死。

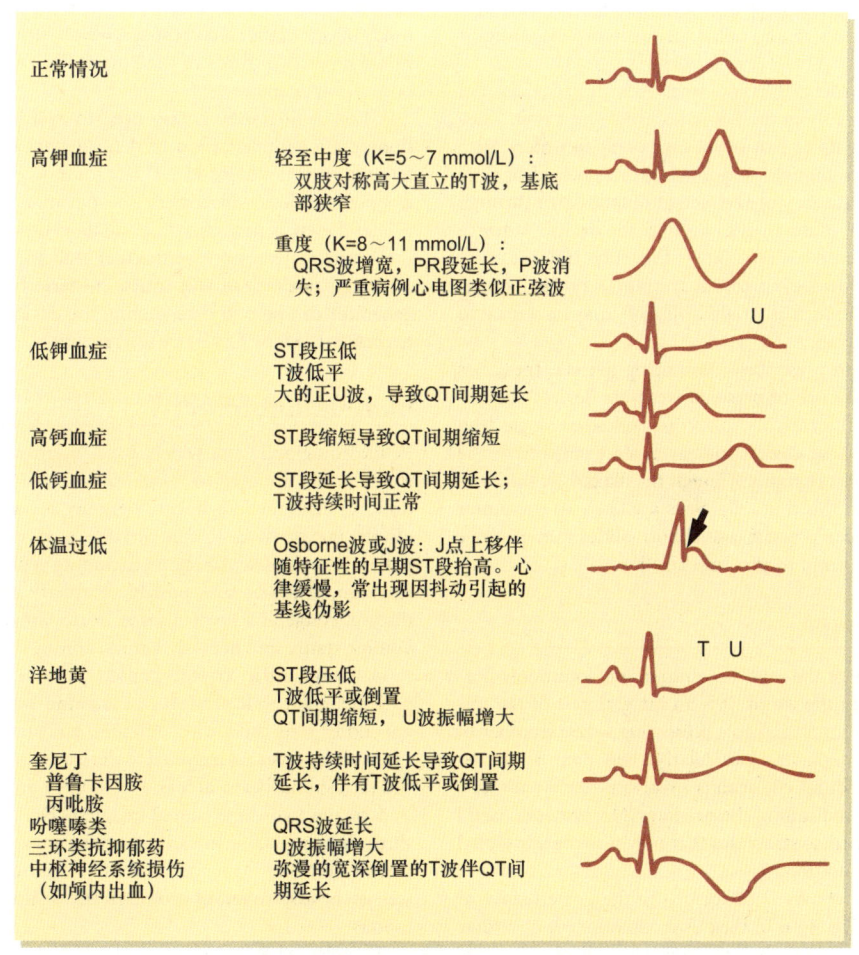

图 3.7 代谢和药物对心电图的影响

动态心电图

动态心电图允许临床医生在指定时间内监测和捕捉心律失常的出现和频率。目前有多种类型的动态心电图记录模式可供选择，使用哪一种主要取决于监测所需的时间。监测持续时间受很多因素的影响，包括症状出现的频率（每天、每周、每月或更长时间）、检查目的（例如对心律失常进行定量分析或捕捉心律失

(i.e., quantifying arrhythmia burden vs. catching an arrhythmic event), and severity of symptoms (lightheadedness vs. stroke).

A Holter monitor collects ECG data from two or three surface leads on a recorder that the patient wears under their clothing, typically for 24 to 72 hours. The device stores all data over this period of time. Patients are asked to write their symptoms in a diary, so that symptoms can be correlated with the rhythm at that time. From these recordings, algorithms analyze and identify abnormal strips for clinician review. Holter monitors are most useful for patients with frequent, daily symptoms, or for quantifying arrhythmic burden such as frequent premature ventricular contractions. Electrocardiographic devices are more recent innovations that also provide continuous ECG recordings through small ECG sensors placed on the chest, usually over a period of two weeks, and can be used instead of Holter monitors.

For patients with more infrequent symptoms, an event recorder can be used to record data for up to a month. Like Holter monitors, surface leads are placed on the chest and connected to a recording device. Unlike Holter monitors, the device only maintains data for 30 to 60 second loops, after which it is erased. Data are only saved when algorithms identify ECG abnormalities, or when patients press a button indicating the presence of symptoms. Therefore, patients must be able to trigger the device. These data are usually uploaded to a monitoring center, where patients can be called for further questioning or counseling.

Implantable loop recorders (ILRs) are small recording devices that are implanted subcutaneously in the left parasternal chest wall. They can record symptoms for up to two years. Like event recorders, data are maintained on a loop, though for a much greater period of time (about thirty minutes). Data are stored either automatically or through a small magnetic activator that patients pass over the device. A device programmer is then used to extract the data in the office. ILRs are especially useful in patients with rare but serious symptoms, or when quantifying arrhythmic burden, such as atrial fibrillation, may be critical to informing the treatment plan.

In addition to clinician prescribed monitoring devices, there has been a recent surge in the use of personal wearable devices such as smartwatches that have the capacity to record and store single lead ECG tracings. Some of these devices may even alert patients to the presence of abnormal heart rhythms. Though the diagnostic utility of these devices is unclear at this time, clinicians are likely to encounter them at an increasing rate in practice, and abnormalities seen on these devices may be used to prompt further investigation.

CHEST RADIOGRAPHY

Chest radiography is one of the most ubiquitous and commonly performed diagnostic tests in the world. It is an integral part of the initial evaluation and work-up for patients presenting with a number of cardiovascular-related complaints, particularly chest pain, shortness of breath, and postprocedural complaints involving cardiac devices. Regardless of the clinical indication, chest radiography provides useful information regarding cardiac structures that may provide additional insight into a patient's condition.

Routinely, chest radiography is performed in the posteroanterior and lateral projections (Fig. 3.8). In the posteroanterior view, cardiac enlargement may be identified when the transverse diameter of the cardiac silhouette is greater than one half of the transverse diameter of the thorax. The heart may appear falsely enlarged when it is displaced horizontally, such as with poor inflation of the lungs or when the image is taken in an anteroposterior projection, which magnifies the heart shadow. The differential diagnosis for cardiac silhouette enlargement on chest radiography includes cardiomegaly, pericardial effusion, prominent epicardial fat pad, or an anterior mediastinal mass.

Left atrial enlargement is suggested when the left-sided heart border is straightened or bulges toward the left. Right atrial enlargement may be confirmed when the right-sided heart border bulges toward the right. Left ventricular enlargement results in downward and lateral displacement of the apex. A rounding of the displaced apex suggests ventricular hypertrophy. Right ventricular enlargement is best assessed on the lateral view and may be diagnosed when the right ventricular border occupies more than one third of the retrosternal space between the diaphragm and thoracic apex.

The aortic arch and thoracic aorta may become dilated and tortuous in patients with severe atherosclerosis, long-standing hypertension, and aortic dissection. A widened mediastinum, which is defined as a width of greater than 8.0 centimeters at the level of the aortic knob, can be seen in acute aortic dissection, although it is not very sensitive or specific for acute dissection.

Pulmonary venous congestion due to elevated left ventricular end-diastolic pressure results in redistribution of blood flow in the lungs and prominence of the apical vessels, which can be seen on chest radiography. Transudation of fluid into the interstitial space may result in fluid in the fissures and along the horizontal periphery of the lower lung fields (i.e., Kerley B lines). As venous pressures further increase, fluid collects in the alveolar space, which early on collects preferentially in the inner two thirds of the lung fields, resulting in a characteristic butterfly appearance.

Chest radiography is also used to evaluate device and lead positioning after implantation of defibrillators or pacemakers. The posteroanterior view helps to evaluate for device and lead integrity as well as potential device placement complications such as pneumothorax. A lateral view is necessary to evaluate ventricular lead positioning. In the lateral view, a right ventricular lead will course anteriorly, while a left ventricular lead will course posteriorly. The shape of the pulse generator can help in determining the device manufacturer, which is necessary to know for device interrogation.

ECHOCARDIOGRAPHY

Echocardiography is a widely used, noninvasive technique in which sound waves are used to image cardiac structures and evaluate blood flow. Transthoracic echocardiography is safe, simple, fast, and relatively inexpensive. It can provide a wealth of information on a patient's cardiovascular status, including ventricular function, valvular function, chamber size, possible coronary artery disease, pericardial disease, congenital heart disease, aortopathy, cardioembolic sources, volume status, and hemodynamics, among many other things.

A piezoelectric crystal housed in a transducer placed on the patient's chest wall produces ultrasound waves. As the sound waves encounter structures with different acoustic properties, some of the ultrasound waves are reflected to the transducer and recorded. Steering the ultrasound beam across a 90-degree arc multiple times per second creates two-dimensional imaging (Fig. 3.9). The development of three-dimensional echocardiographic imaging techniques allows for greater accuracy in measurements of chamber volumes and mass, as well as the assessment of geometrically complex anatomy and valvular lesions.

Doppler echocardiography allows assessment of the direction and velocity of blood flow in the heart and great vessels. When ultrasound waves encounter moving red blood cells, the energy reflected to the transducer is altered. The magnitude of this change (i.e., Doppler shift) is represented as velocity on the echocardiographic display and can be used to determine whether the blood flow is normal or abnormal

常事件）以及症状的严重程度（头昏或卒中）。

Holter 监测器通过患者所佩戴的记录器上连接的 2～3 个体表电极收集心电图数据，通常持续 24～72 h。该设备会存储这段时间内的所有数据。在这一过程中，患者会被要求在日志中写下自己的症状，以便将症状与当时的心律情况联系起来。根据这些记录，算法会分析并识别异常片段，供临床医生查看。Holter 监测器对于日常频繁出现症状的患者，以及在定量分析心律失常负荷（如频发的室性早搏）时最为适用。一些更新的心电图设备也可通过放置在胸部的小型心电图传感器提供连续的心电图记录，通常为两周时间，可用于替代 Holter 监测器。

对于症状不频繁的患者，可使用事件记录器记录长达 1 个月的数据。与 Holter 监测器一样，体表电极被放置在胸部并连接到记录仪。但与 Holter 监测器不同的是，这种设备只循环记录 30～60 s 的数据，之后数据就会被清除。只有当算法识别出异常心电图或患者按下按钮表示出现症状时，数据才会被保存下来。因此，患者必须有能力触发设备。这些数据通常会上传到一家监控中心，由中心联系患者进行进一步的询问或沟通。

植入式循环记录器（ILR）是一种植入在左侧胸骨旁皮下的小型记录装置，记录时间可长达 2 年。与事件记录器一样，数据也是循环保存的，但保存时间更长（约 30 min）。数据可以自动存储或通过患者触发设备上的小型磁性激活器存储，随后在远程中心采用设备编程器进行数据提取。ILR 特别适用于症状发作少但非常严重的患者，以及对心律失常（如心房颤动）负荷情况进行定量分析，这对于制订治疗计划非常关键。

除了临床医生使用的监测设备外，个人可穿戴设备（如能够记录和存储单导联心电图的智能手表）的使用也在迅速增加，其中一些设备甚至可以警示患者异常心律的出现。虽然目前还不清楚这些设备的诊断价值，但医生在临床实践中会越来越多地遇到这些设备，而其提示的心电图异常也可能会被采纳并指引患者进一步的检查。

胸部 X 线检查

胸部 X 线检查即胸片是世界上最常规和最普遍使用的诊断方法之一。对于多数以心血管相关主诉就诊的患者，尤其是胸痛、呼吸困难和心脏装置植入术后患者，胸片是初始评估和系统检查中不可或缺的组成部分。无论临床指征如何，胸片均可提供与心脏结构相关的有价值信息，为明确患者的病情提供进一步的信息。

一般情况下，胸片检查采用后前位和侧位进行投影（图 3.8）。在后前位视图中，当心脏轮廓的横向直径大于胸腔横径的一半时，提示心影增大。当心脏水平移位（如肺部膨胀不良或采用前后位投影）时，心脏阴影会被放大，从而出现假性心影增大。胸片上心脏轮廓增大的鉴别诊断包括心脏肥大、心包积液、心外膜脂肪垫或前纵隔占位。

心脏左缘拉直或向左凸起提示左心房扩大。而右缘向右凸起时，提示右心房增大。左心室增大导致心尖向下和左侧移位。移位的心尖呈圆形表明左心室肥厚。右心室扩大最好在侧位片上进行评估，当右心室边界占据横膈至胸腔顶端之间胸骨后间隙的 1/3 以上时，考虑右心室扩大。

严重动脉粥样硬化、长期高血压和主动脉夹层患者，主动脉弓和胸主动脉可能会扩张和扭曲。纵隔增宽，定义为平动脉结水平纵隔宽度超过 8.0 cm，可见于急性主动脉夹层，尽管其敏感性或特异性都不高。

左心室舒张末压升高引起肺静脉淤血，胸片上可以看到肺部血流重新分布，肺尖血管表现尤为明显。液体向肺间质漏出导致小叶间隔液体潴留，在肺下野外侧形成水平横线（即 Kerley B 线）。随着静脉压力的进一步增加，液体在肺泡间隙潴留，早期主要聚集在肺内中带 2/3 的区域，形成特征性的"蝶翼状"外观。

在植入除颤器或起搏器的患者，胸片也用于评估设备和电极导线位置。后前位视图可帮助评估装置和电极导联的完整性以及潜在的手术并发症，如气胸。判断心室电极导线位置则需要侧位片。在侧位视图上，右心室导线绕行向前，而左心室导线绕行向后。脉冲发生器的形状可以帮助确定设备制造厂家，这在进行植入装置检测时是必须了解的。

超声心动图检查

超声心动图是一种广泛使用的无创技术，使用声波成像评估心脏结构和血流状态。其中，经胸超声心动图使用安全、方便、快速，并且费用相对不高。对于被检患者的心血管情况，超声可以提供非常丰富的信息，包括心室功能、瓣膜功能、心腔大小、可能的冠状动脉疾病、心包疾病、先天性心脏病、主动脉病变、心脏栓子来源、机体容量和血流动力学状态，以及许多其他信息。

放置在患者胸壁表面的超声探头中的压电晶体可以产生超声波。当声波遇到具有不同声学特性的组织结构时，部分超声波被反射并被探头接收和记录下来。超声光束每秒多次与目标结构呈 90°入射时，即可产生二维图像（图 3.9）。三维超声心动图成像技术的发展使得心腔容积和心室质量的测量，以及心脏复杂的几何解剖结构和瓣膜病变的评估都更加准确。

多普勒超声心动图可以评估心脏和大血管中血流的方向和速度。当超声波遇到移动的红细胞时，反射至探头的超声能量会发生变化。在超声心动图上，这种变化的幅度（即多普勒频移）对应血流速度，可用

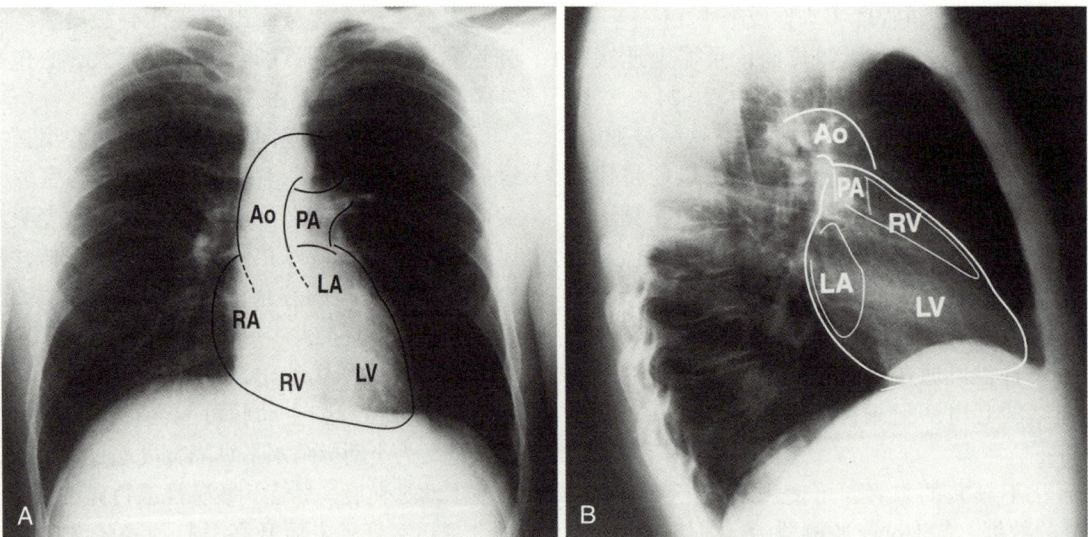

Fig. 3.8 Schematic illustration of the parts of the heart, outlines of which can be identified on a routine chest radiograph. (A) Posteroanterior chest radiograph. (B) Lateral chest radiograph. *Ao,* Aorta; *LA,* left atrium; *LV,* left ventricle; *PA,* pulmonary artery; *RA,* right atrium; *RV,* right ventricle.

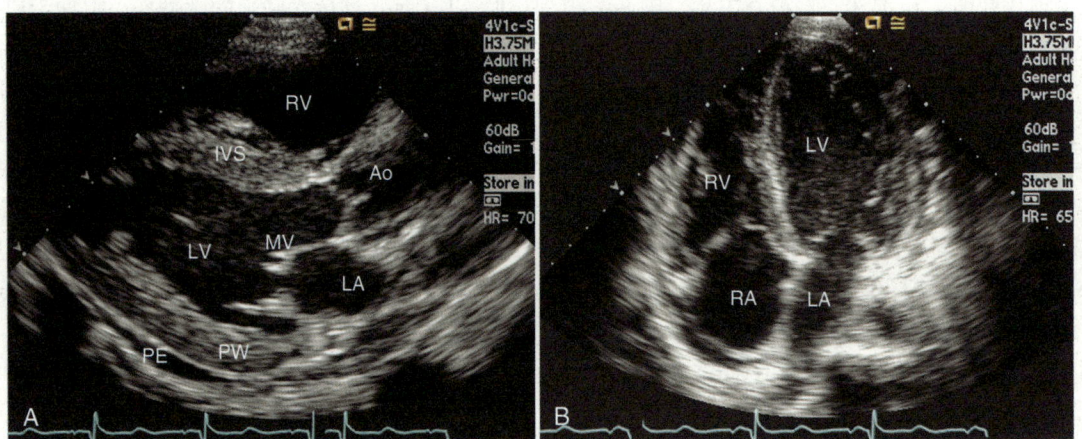

Fig. 3.9 Portions of standard two-dimensional echocardiograms show the major cardiac structures in a parasternal long-axis view (A) and apical four-chamber view (B). *Ao,* Aorta; *IVS,* interventricular septum; *LA,* left atrium; *LV,* left ventricle; *MV,* mitral valve; *PE,* pericardial effusion; *PW,* posterior left ventricular wall; *RV,* right ventricle. (Image courtesy Sheldon E. Litwin, MD, Division of Cardiology, University of Utah, Salt Lake City, Utah.)

(Fig. 3.10). The velocity of a particular jet of blood can be converted to pressure, allowing assessment of pressure gradients across valves or between chambers. Color Doppler imaging allows visualization of blood flow through the heart by assigning a color to the red blood cells based on their velocity and direction (Fig. 3.11). By convention, blood moving away from the transducer is represented in shades of blue, and blood moving toward the transducer is represented in red. Color Doppler imaging is particularly useful in identifying valvular insufficiency and abnormal shunt flow between chambers. The use of Doppler techniques to record myocardial velocities or strain rates can aid in the assessment of myocardial function and hemodynamics.

Ultrasound contrast agents composed of microbubbles can be used in patients who have poorly visualized cardiac structures, such as obese patients or those with chronic lung disease. Ultrasound contrast opacifies the endocardial cavity and aids in assessment of cardiac function (Fig. 3.12). These contrast agents are also necessary in the assessment of potential left ventricular thrombus. Agitated saline, commonly referred to as "bubbles," can be used to assess for intracardiac shunts.

Transesophageal echocardiography (TEE) allows two-dimensional and Doppler imaging of the heart through the esophagus by having the patient swallow a gastroscope mounted with an ultrasound crystal in its tip. Given the proximity of the esophagus to the heart, high-resolution images can be obtained, especially of the left atrium, mitral valve apparatus, and aorta. TEE is particularly useful in diagnosing left atrial appendage thrombi, aortic dissection, endocarditis, prosthetic valve dysfunction, and left atrial masses (Fig. 3.13). TEE has been used for decades intraoperatively during cardiac surgery, and it is now being used with increasing frequency to guide percutaneous cardiac procedures such as transcatheter aortic valve replacement, transcatheter mitral valve repair, and left atrial appendage occlusion.

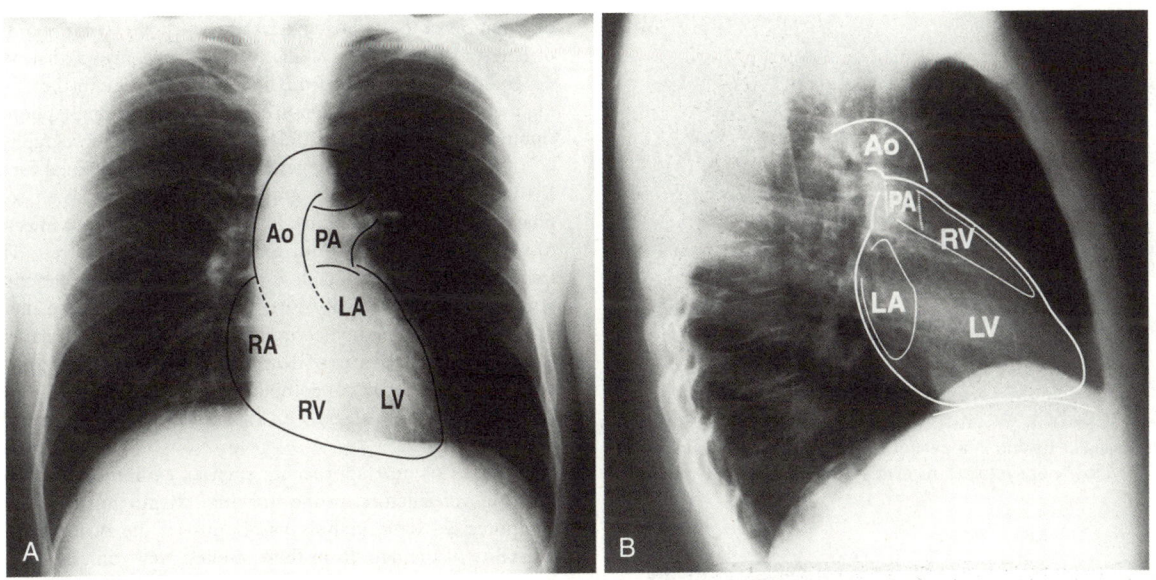

图 3.8 心脏各部分示意图，常规胸部 X 线检查可显示心脏各部分的轮廓。（A）胸部后前位片。（B）胸部侧位片。Ao，主动脉；LA，左心房；LV，左心室；PA：肺动脉；RA，右心房；RV，右心室

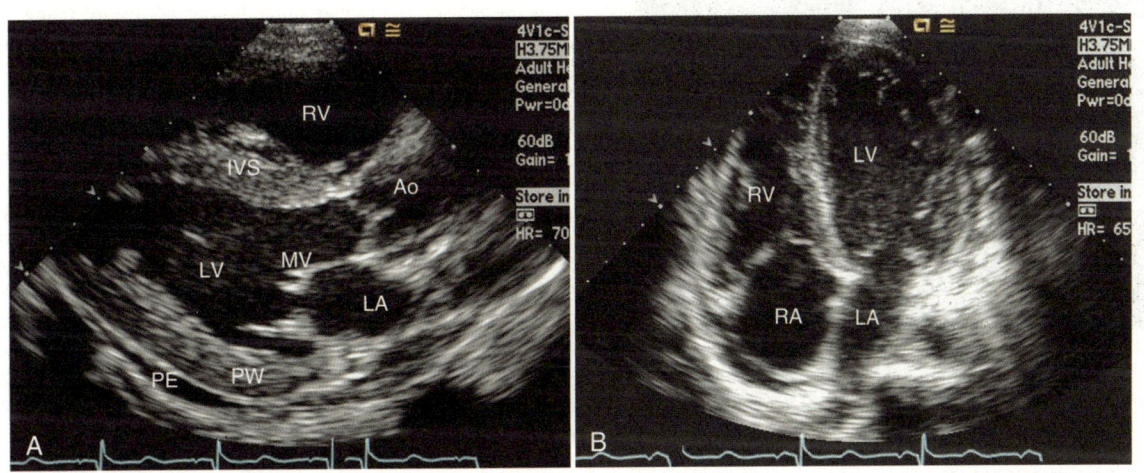

图 3.9 部分标准二维超声心动图显示心脏主要结构，包括胸骨旁左心室长轴视图（A）和心尖四腔心视图（B）。Ao，主动脉；IVS，室间隔；LA，左心房；LV，左心室；MV，二尖瓣；PE，心包积液；PW，左心室后壁；RV，右心室；RA，右心房（图片授权自 Sheldon E. Litwin，MD，Division of Cardiology，University of Utah，Salt Lake City，Utah.）

于确定血流正常与否（图 3.10）。特定的射血流速可转换为压力，从而可以评估跨瓣或 2 个腔室之间的压力阶差。根据体内红细胞流动的速度和方向，彩色多普勒成像用不同的颜色进行表示，即可直观地显示流经心脏的血流（图 3.11）。按惯例，红色表示血流方向指向探头，蓝色则表示血流方向背离探头。彩色多普勒成像在鉴别瓣膜功能不全和心脏腔室间的异常分流方面尤其有价值。使用多普勒技术记录心肌速度或应变率有助于心肌功能和血流动力学的评估。

用含微泡的超声对比剂辅助超声检查，可用于心脏结构显示不佳的患者，比如肥胖或慢性肺病患者。超声对比剂可以填充心腔，帮助评估心脏功能（图 3.12）。在评估可疑的左心室血栓时，超声对比显像也是一个必要检查。盐水混合空气搅动形成的"气泡"对比剂，可用于评估心腔内分流。

经食管超声心动图（TEE）允许通过食管对心脏进行二维和多普勒成像，方法是采用尖端安装有超声晶体类似胃镜的超声探头，经患者口腔插入食管进行显像。由于食管紧邻心脏，此方法可以获得高分辨率的心脏图像，特别是左心房、二尖瓣和主动脉的图像。在诊断左心耳血栓、主动脉夹层、心内膜炎、人工瓣膜功能异常以及左房占位等方面，TEE 的价值尤为明显（图 3.13）。在心脏手术的术中监测方面，TEE 已经使用了几十年，现今则越来越多地用于指导经皮心脏手术，如经导管主动脉瓣置换术、经导管二尖瓣修复术和左心耳封堵术。

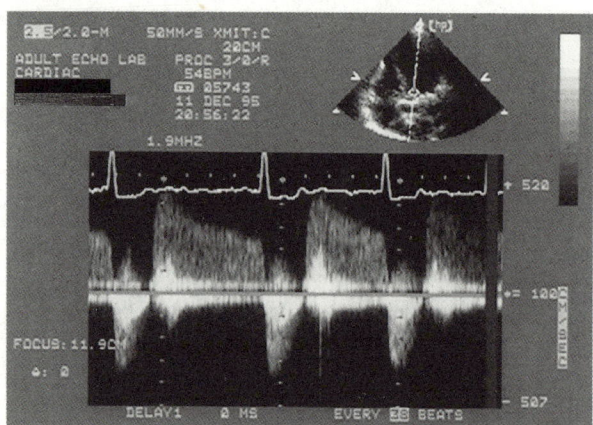

Fig. 3.10 Doppler tracing in a patient with aortic stenosis and regurgitation. The velocity of systolic flow is related to the severity of obstruction.

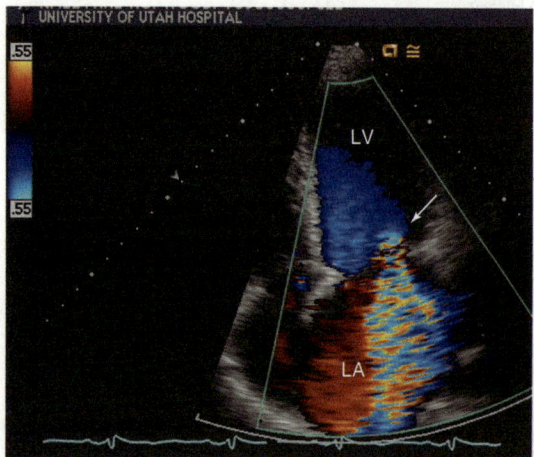

Fig. 3.11 Color Doppler recording demonstrates severe mitral regurgitation. The regurgitant jet seen in the left atrium is represented in *blue* because blood flow is directed away from the transducer. The *yellow* components are the mosaic pattern traditionally assigned to turbulent or high-velocity flow. The *arrow* points to the hemisphere of blood accelerating proximal to the regurgitant orifice (i.e., proximal isovelocity surface area [PISA]). The size of the PISA can be used to help grade the severity of regurgitation. *LA*, Left atrium; *LV*, left ventricle. (Image courtesy Sheldon E. Litwin, MD, Division of Cardiology, University of Utah, Salt Lake City, Utah.)

NUCLEAR CARDIOLOGY

The traditional radiotracer approach to assess ventricular function is equilibrium radionuclide angiocardiography (ERNA), which uses technetium-99m-labeled red blood cells. Serial ERNA can be performed at rest and during various levels of exercise of pharmacologic perturbations to evaluate ventricular function and reserve. ERNA has high reproducibility because there are no geometric assumptions and there is much less operator dependence in the image acquisition. Diastolic parameters can be readily assessed from the ventricular volume curve, which may be very helpful in the assessment of diastolic dysfunction.

In radionuclide imaging of the heart, patients are injected with a radioactive tracer, which distributes throughout the myocardium in proportion to blood flow. Highly specialized cameras then capture the distribution of the radioactive tracer, which allows for quantification of left ventricular size, systolic function, and myocardial perfusion, depending on the tracer used. The two main types of myocardial imaging used in cardiology, often in stress testing, are single-photon emission tomography (SPECT) and positron emission tomography (PET).

In SPECT imaging, images of the heart are obtained for qualitative and quantitative analyses at rest and after stress (i.e., exercise or pharmacologic vasodilation). Radionuclide tracers are injected prior to rest images and just prior to the completion of stress. The most frequently used radionuclide in SPECT imaging is technetium-99m sestamibi. In the normal heart, the radioisotope is equally distributed throughout the myocardium at rest and stress. In patients with ischemia, a localized area of decreased radiotracer uptake occurs after stress but may partially or completely reverse during rest. A persistent defect at peak exercise and rest (i.e., fixed defect) is consistent with MI or scarring.

The use of new approaches such as combined low-level exercise and vasodilators, prone imaging, attenuation correction, and computerized data analysis has improved the quality and reproducibility of the data from these studies. New camera technologies, including those with solid state detector arrays, have demonstrated improved image resolution and allow for reduced radiation exposure. Myocardial perfusion imaging may also be combined with ECG-gated image acquisition (gated SPECT) to allow simultaneous assessment of ventricular function and perfusion. Using this technique, regional wall motion can be evaluated to help assess potential perfusion defects.

PET has been widely used in oncology for many years but has become increasingly popular in cardiology. The commonly used tracers in cardiac PET imaging include rubidium-82 and fluorine-18 fluorodeoxyglucose (FDG). When compared to SPECT, PET has several technical advantages, including higher spatial and temporal resolution, less radiation exposure, and the ability to quantify absolute rather than relative coronary blood flow. These advantages mean that PET is more sensitive and specific compared to SPECT in diagnosing coronary disease, especially in the presence of multivessel disease. Additionally, because PET gives an absolute rather than relative quantification of coronary blood flow, it can be used to assess abnormal microvascular coronary circulation. Despite these clinical advantages of PET over SPECT, the lack of availability of PET cameras and radiotracers, as well as high costs and reimbursement issues, limits the widespread adoption of PET.

In patients with suspected cardiac sarcoidosis, FDG-PET is the imaging modality of choice for diagnosis. FDG-PET can also be used to detect myocardial viability by the use of perfusion and metabolic tracers. In patients with left ventricular dysfunction, metabolic activity in a region of myocardium supplied by a severely stenotic coronary artery suggests viable tissue that may regain more normal function after revascularization (Fig. 3.14).

CARDIAC MAGNETIC RESONANCE IMAGING

Cardiac magnetic resonance imaging (cMRI) is a noninvasive method that is increasingly used for studying the heart and vasculature and has, in fact, become the gold standard for measuring myocardial function, volumes, and scarring. cMRI offers high-resolution dynamic and static images of the heart that can be obtained in any plane, allowing quantification of left ventricular and valvular function. High-quality images can be obtained in a larger proportion of subjects than is typically possible with echocardiography. Obesity, claustrophobia, inability to perform multiple breath-holds of 10 to 20 seconds, and arrhythmias are causes of reduced image quality.

（SPECT）和正电子发射断层成像（PET）。

SPECT 成像时，分别在静息和负荷（即运动负荷或血管舒张药物负荷）后获取心脏图像用于定性和定量分析。放射性核素示踪剂在静息图像采集之前注射，或者在负荷完成后即刻注射。SPECT 成像中最常用的放射性核素示踪剂是锝-99m-甲氧基异丁基异腈（sestamibi，MIBI）。在正常心脏，静息和负荷状态下放射性同位素在整个心肌中是均匀分布的。在缺血心肌，负荷后局部区域放射性示踪剂摄取减少，静息时则可能部分或完全逆转。在运动高峰和静息时都持续存在的摄取缺损（即固定性缺损）则提示心肌梗死或瘢痕心肌。

新方法的使用，如低水平运动负荷和血管扩张剂结合、俯卧位成像、衰减校正和计算机分析，提高了获取数据的质量和可重复性。新的摄像技术，包括那些采用固态探测器阵列的技术，已经证明可以提高图像分辨率，并减少辐射暴露量。心肌灌注成像与心电图门控图像采集（门控 SPECT）相结合，可以同时评估心室功能和心肌灌注。使用该技术可以观察局部室壁运动情况，帮助评估潜在的心肌灌注缺陷。

PET 在肿瘤学领域已经广泛应用多年，在心脏病学领域的应用也日益增多。标记的心脏 PET 成像中常用的示踪剂包括铷-82 和氟-18 脱氧葡萄糖（FDG）。与 SPECT 相比，PET 有几个技术优势，包括更高的空间和时间分辨率，更少的辐射暴露，以及量化绝对而不是相对冠状动脉血流量的能力。这些优势意味着 PET 在诊断冠状动脉疾病时比 SPECT 更为敏感和特异，特别是对于多支血管病变。此外，由于 PET 给出的是绝对而非相对的冠状动脉血流量，因此可用于评估冠状动脉微血管病变。尽管与 SPECT 相比，PET 有上述临床优势，但由于 PET 仪器和所用放射性示踪剂可及性较低，以及费用昂贵和报销问题，PET 的广泛应用受到限制。

在疑似心脏结节病的患者中，FDG-PET 是首选的影像学诊断方法。FDG-PET 还可以通过使用灌注和代谢示踪剂进行心肌灌注/代谢显像检测存活心肌。在左心室功能障碍患者中，严重狭窄的冠状动脉供血区域如存在心肌代谢活动，提示心肌存活，在血运重建后有可能恢复更为正常的心肌功能（图 3.14）。

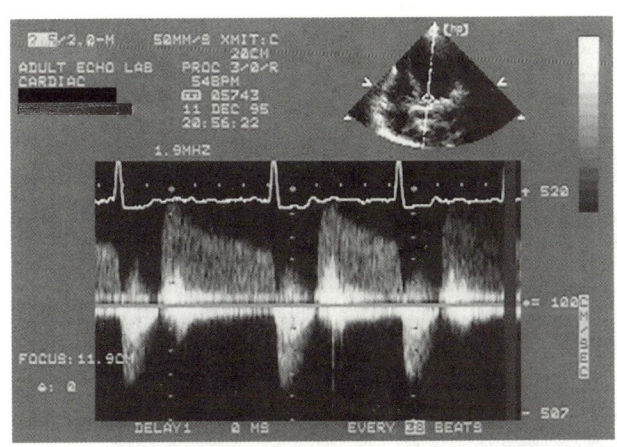

图 3.10　一例主动脉瓣狭窄合并反流患者的多普勒频谱图。收缩期血流速度与瓣膜狭窄的严重程度相关

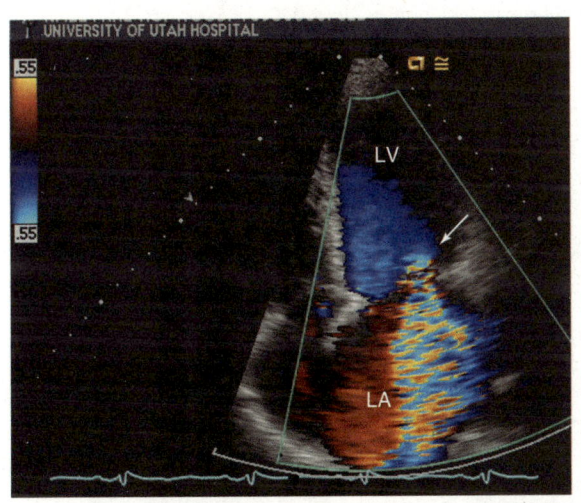

图 3.11　彩色多普勒显示重度二尖瓣反流。左心房看到的反流束显示为蓝色，提示血流方向背离超声探头。黄色的马赛克图案（五彩血流信号）传统上代表湍流或高速血流。箭头指向反流口近端的半圆形血流加速区［即近端等速表面积（PISA）］。PISA 大小可用来帮助评估反流的严重程度。LA，左心房；LV，左心室（图片授权自 Sheldon E. Litwin, MD, Division of Cardiology, University of Utah, Salt Lake City, Utah.）

心脏核素检查

用于评估心室功能的传统核素心脏检查方法是平衡法放射性核素心血管显像（ERNA），使用锝-99m 标记的红细胞作为放射性示踪剂。系列 ERNA 可以在静息状态下和不同水平的运动中或药物干预下进行，用以评估心室功能和心室储备功能。ERNA 不需要对心脏几何形状进行假设，其图像获取对操作者的依赖也少，因此具有很高的可重复性。从心室容积曲线可以很容易地获取舒张参数，这一点在评估心室舒张功能障碍时可能很有帮助。

在心脏的放射性核素成像中，放射性示踪剂被注射入患者体内，在心肌中的分布与血流量成正比。随后高度专业化的摄像机会捕捉到心肌分布的放射性示踪剂，同时依据所使用示踪剂的不同，量化分析左心室大小、收缩功能和心肌灌注情况。心脏病学中主要有两种心肌成像方法，常用于负荷试验，包括单光子发射断层成像

心脏磁共振成像

心脏磁共振成像（cMRI）是一种无创影像学方法，在心血管系统中的应用越来越多，事实上，它已经成为测量和诊断心肌功能、容积和心肌瘢痕组织的金标准。cMRI 可以在任何切面上提供高分辨率的心脏动态和静态图像，允许对左心室和瓣膜功能进行定量评估。与超声心动图通常可获取的图像相比，磁共振可以在更多的受试者中获得高质量的图像。导致磁共振图像质量下降的原因包括肥胖、幽闭恐惧症、患者无法进行多次 10～20 s 的屏气以及存在心律失常。

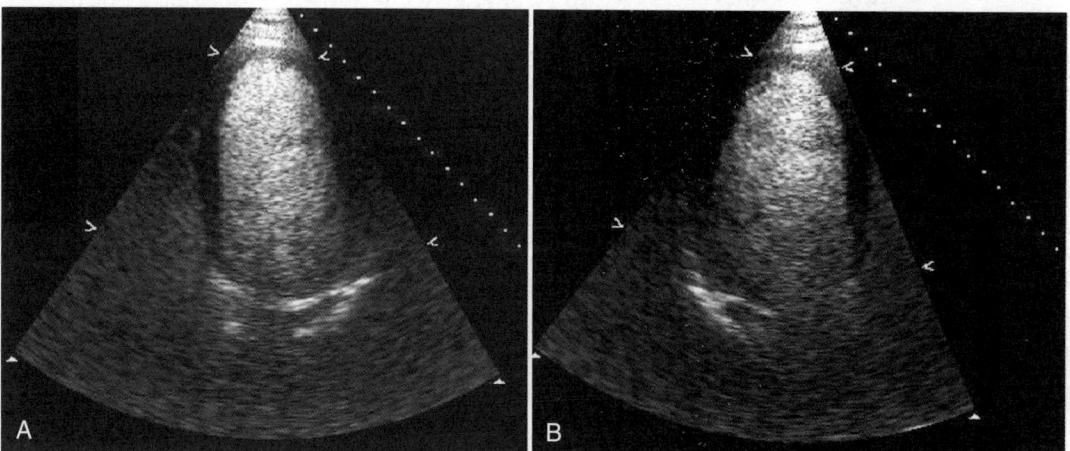

Fig. 3.12 Echocardiogram enhanced with intravenous ultrasound contrast agent: apical four-chamber view (A) and apical long-axis view (B). Highly echo-reflectant microbubbles make the left ventricular cavity appear white, whereas the myocardium appears dark. (Image courtesy Sheldon E. Litwin, MD, Division of Cardiology, University of Utah, Salt Lake City, Utah.)

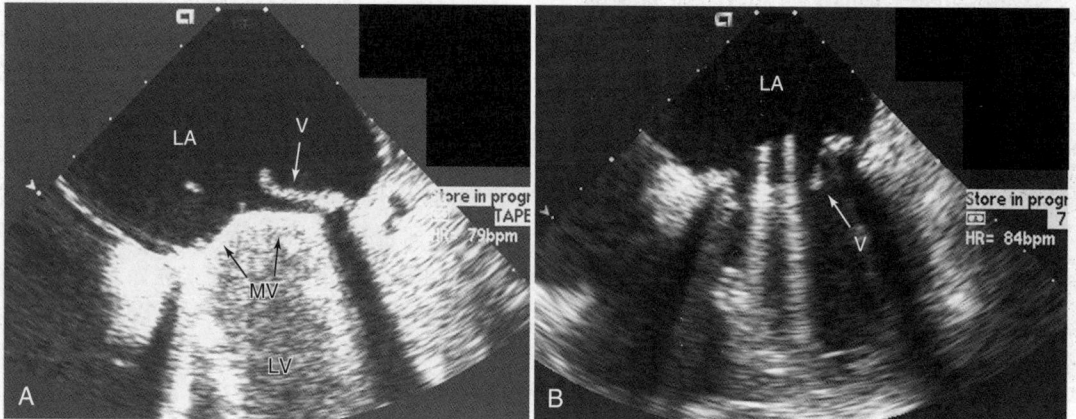

Fig. 3.13 Transesophageal echocardiogram demonstrates a vegetation *(arrow)* adherent to the ring of a bileaflet, tilting-disk mitral valve prostheses. (A) In systole, the leaflets are closed with the vegetation seen in the left atrium. (B) In diastole, the leaflets are open, with the vegetation prolapsing into the left ventricle. Transesophageal echocardiography is the diagnostic test of choice for assessing prosthetic mitral valves because the esophageal window allows unimpeded views of the atrial surface of the valve. *LA*, Left atrium; *LV*, left ventricle; *MV*, prosthetic mitral valve disks; *V*, vegetation. (Courtesy Sheldon E. Litwin, MD, Division of Cardiology, University of Utah, Salt Lake City, Utah.)

cMRI also offers significant advantages over other imaging techniques for the characterization of tissues (e.g., muscle, fat, scar). cMRI is useful in the evaluation of ischemic heart disease because stress-rest myocardial perfusion (Fig. 3.15A) and areas of prior infarction (see Fig. 3.15B to D) can be visualized with excellent spatial resolution. Delayed or late gadolinium enhancement (LGE) in the myocardium is characteristic of scar or permanently damaged tissue. The greater the transmural extent of LGE is in a given segment, the lower the likelihood of improved function in that segment after revascularization. Because of the better spatial resolution, LGE can identify localized or subendocardial scars that are not detectable with nuclear imaging techniques.

MRI is excellent for evaluating a variety of cardiomyopathies (Fig. 3.16). In addition to morphology and function, characteristic patterns of LGE have been reported in myocarditis, cardiac amyloidosis, sarcoidosis, and hypertrophic cardiomyopathy (HCM). In patients with HCM, specific patterns on MRI can help identify those patients at highest risk of sudden cardiac death who would require defibrillators. Similarly, MRI has also been used to help assess right ventricular morphology and function in patients with suspected arrhythmogenic right ventricular cardiomyopathy. The role of MRI in all aspects of cardiac imaging continues to grow.

STRESS TESTING

Stress testing is an important noninvasive tool for evaluating patients with known or suggested coronary artery disease (CAD). During exercise, the increased demand for oxygen by the working skeletal muscles is met by increases in heart rate and cardiac output. In patients with significant CAD, the increase in myocardial oxygen demand cannot be met by a proportional increase in coronary blood flow, and myocardial ischemia may produce chest pain and characteristic ECG

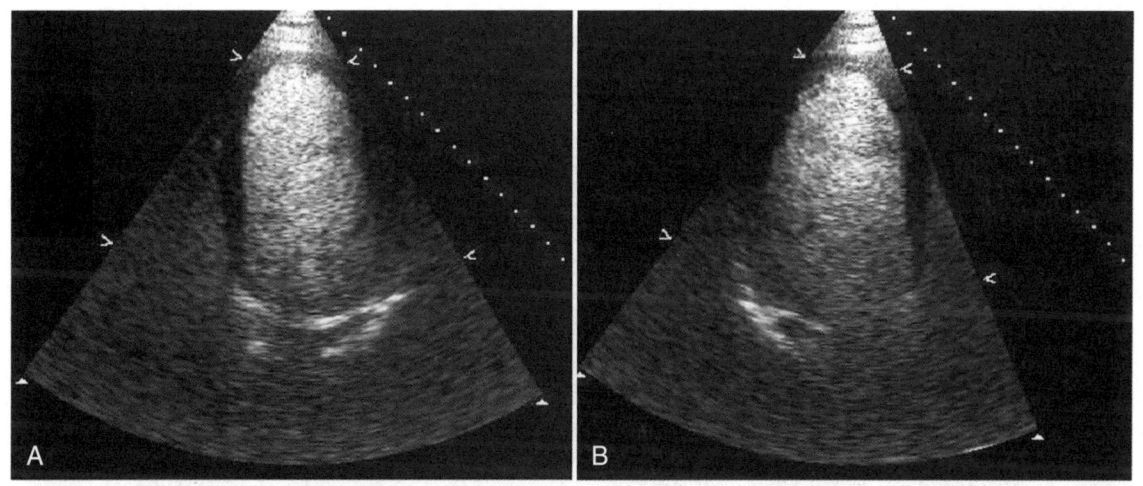

图 3.12 经静脉注射超声造影剂的超声心动图：心尖四腔心视图（**A**）和心尖长轴视图（**B**）。高回声反射的对比剂微泡使左心腔呈白色，而心肌呈黑色。（图片授权自 Sheldon E. Litwin, MD, Division of Cardiology, University of Utah, Salt Lake City, Utah.）

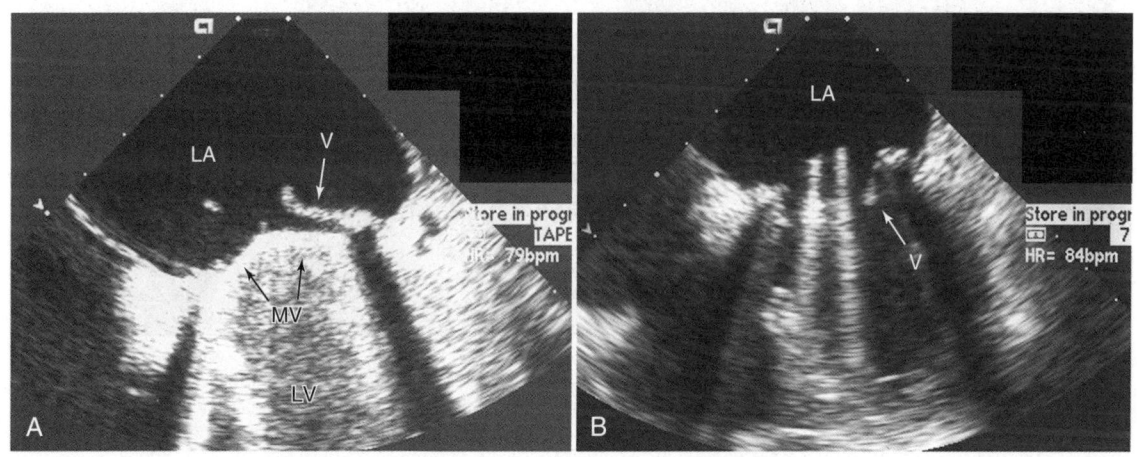

图 3.13 经食管超声心动图显示附着在双叶、倾碟式二尖瓣机械瓣瓣环上的赘生物（箭头）。（**A**）收缩期，二尖瓣闭合，左心房内可见赘生物。（**B**）舒张期，二尖瓣开放，赘生物脱入左心室。经食管超声心动图是评估人工二尖瓣的优选诊断方法，允许无阻碍地观察二尖瓣的左心房面情况。LA，左心房；LV，左心室；MV，人工二尖瓣；V，赘生物（图片授权自 Sheldon E. Litwin, MD, Division of Cardiology, University of Utah, Salt Lake City, Utah.）

与其他成像技术相比，cMRI 在确定组织学特征方面（如肌肉、脂肪、瘢痕）也具有显著优势。采用负荷-静息心肌灌注成像，cMRI 可用于缺血性心脏病的评估（图 3.15A），对既往心肌梗死区域的显示具有极好的空间分辨率（见图 3.15B 至 D）。心肌延迟或晚期钆增强（LGE）显像是心肌瘢痕或永久性损伤的特征表现。特定心肌节段 LGE 的跨壁范围越大，血运重建术后该节段功能改善的可能性越低。由于具有更好的空间分辨率，LGE 可以发现核素成像技术无法检测到的心肌局部或心内膜下瘢痕。

MRI 在评估心肌病方面优势明显（图 3.16）。除形态学和功能评估外，有报道在心肌炎、心脏淀粉样变性、心脏结节病和肥厚型心肌病（HCM）中，LGE 成像具备特征性表现模式。HCM 在 MRI 上的特定征象可以帮助识别需要植入除颤器的心源性猝死高风险患者。同样，MRI 也被用来帮助评估疑似致心律失常型右心室心肌病患者的右心室形态和功能。MRI 于心脏成像各方面的应用还在不断增加中。

负荷试验

负荷试验是评估已知或疑似冠状动脉疾病（CAD）患者的一种重要的无创检查方法。运动时，通过心率和心输出量的提高来满足骨骼肌对氧气需求的增加。在严重冠心病患者，心肌对氧需求量的增加不能通过冠状动脉血流量的相应增加来达到，从而产生心肌缺血并导致胸痛和特征性心电图异常。这些变化，结合

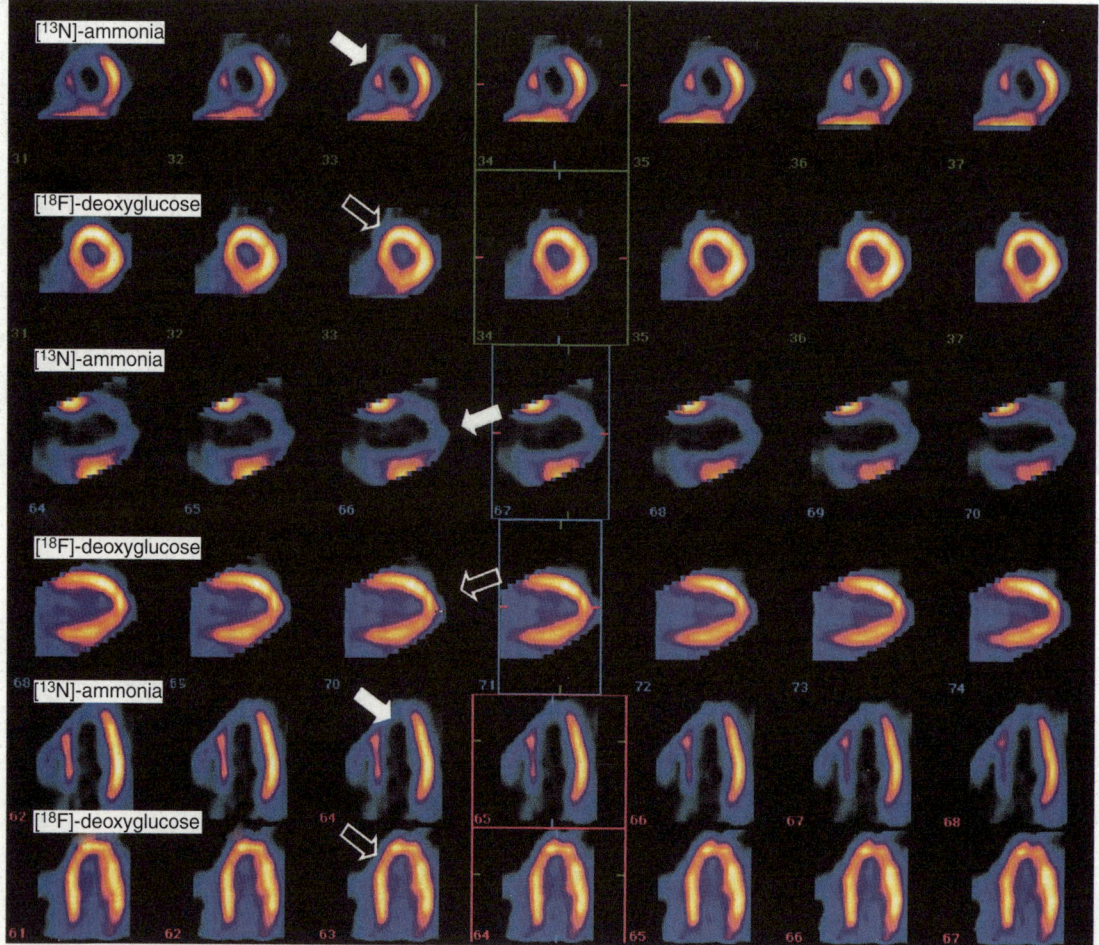

Fig. 3.14 Resting myocardial perfusion (obtained with [^{13}N]-ammonia) and metabolism (obtained with [^{18}F]-deoxyglucose) is seen in positron emission tomography images of a patient with ischemic cardiomyopathy. The study demonstrates a perfusion-metabolic mismatch (reflecting hibernating myocardium) in which large areas of hypoperfused *(solid arrows)* but metabolically viable *(open arrows)* myocardium involve the anterior, septal, and inferior walls and the left ventricular apex. (Courtesy Marcelo F. Di Carli, MD, Brigham and Women's Hospital, Boston, Mass.)

abnormalities. Combined with the hemodynamic response to exercise, these changes can give useful diagnostic and prognostic information for the patient with cardiac abnormalities. The most common indications for stress testing include establishing a diagnosis of CAD in patients with chest pain, assessing prognosis and functional capacity of patients with chronic stable angina or after an MI, evaluating exercise-induced arrhythmias, and assessing for ischemia after a revascularization procedure. Contraindications to stress testing include acute coronary syndromes, poorly controlled hypertension (blood pressure >220/110 mm Hg), severe aortic stenosis (valve area <1.0 cm^2), and decompensated congestive heart failure.

When to Stress Symptomatic Patients

Stress testing is most often used to evaluate symptoms concerning for flow-limiting coronary artery disease and make the diagnosis of CAD. The diagnostic accuracy of the stress test depends on several factors, including the pretest probability of CAD in a given patient, the sensitivity and specificity of the test results in that patient population, the adequacy of stress, and the criteria used to define a positive test. Stress testing, when used to diagnose CAD, is one of the most useful and cost-effective tests in symptomatic patients who have an intermediate pretest probability of CAD, which is defined as a 10% to 90% risk. This is because in patients with a low pretest probability, a positive test does not significantly increase the post-test probability of CAD, and in patients with a high pretest probability, a negative test does not significantly decrease the post-test probability of CAD. The pretest probability of CAD can be calculated through a variety of scores but is most commonly done based on a patient's description of angina (Table 3.4).

Angina has three important components:
1. Substernal chest pain or discomfort
2. The pain or discomfort is provoked by exertion or emotional stress
3. The pain or discomfort is relieved by rest and/or nitroglycerin.

Patients with all three components are said to have *typical angina*. Those with any two of the three components have *atypical angina*, and patients with *nonanginal* chest pain have only one or none of these components.

Other factors that are not solely based on the description of chest discomfort may be present that would increase a patient's pretest

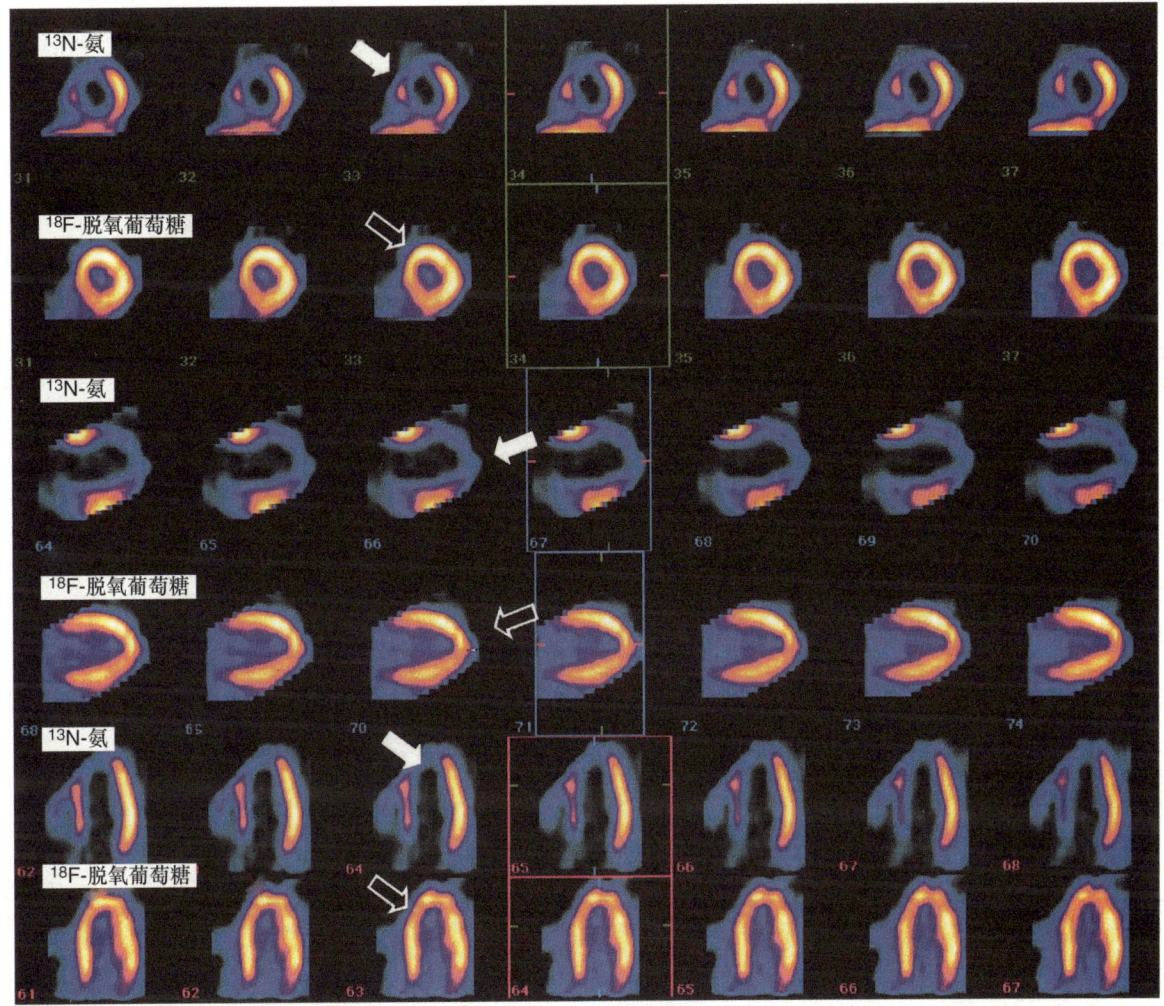

图 3.14 一例缺血性心肌病患者的正电子发射断层成像图像显示静息心肌灌注（^{13}N-氨）和代谢（^{18}F-脱氧葡萄糖）情况。检查结果提示灌注-代谢不匹配（反映冬眠心肌），显示有大面积低灌注心肌（实心箭头）而其代谢仍然活跃（空心箭头），涉及前壁、间隔、下壁和左心室心尖（图像授权自 Marcelo F. Di Carli，MD，Brigham and Women's Hospital，Boston，Mass.）

运动后的血流动力学反应，可以为心脏病患者提供有价值的诊断和预后信息。进行负荷试验最常见的适应证包括：胸痛患者的 CAD 诊断，慢性稳定型心绞痛或心肌梗死后患者预后和功能评估，运动诱发的心律失常的评估，以及血运重建术后心肌缺血的评估。负荷试验的禁忌证包括急性冠脉综合征，高血压控制不佳（血压＞220/110 mmHg），重度主动脉瓣狭窄（瓣膜面积＜1.0 cm²），以及失代偿性充血性心力衰竭。

症状性患者进行负荷试验的时机选择

负荷试验最常用于评估与冠状动脉血流受阻有关的症状以及诊断冠心病。负荷试验诊断的准确性取决于以下几个因素，包括特定患者患 CAD 的验前概率，检测结果在患病群体中的敏感性和特异性，负荷给予是否充分，以及定义阳性结果的标准。在用于诊断 CAD 时，该检查对于有症状且患 CAD 的验前概率为中度（定义为 10%～90% 的患病风险）的患者，是最有价值和成本效益比的检查之一。在验前概率较低的患者，阳性检查结果并不能显著增加 CAD 的诊断可能性，而在验前概率较高的患者，阴性检查结果也并不能显著降低 CAD 的诊断可能性。CAD 的验前概率可以通过各种评分量表来计算，但最常基于患者的心绞痛症状确立（表 3.4）。

心绞痛有以下三个重要特征：
1. 表现为胸骨下疼痛或不适；
2. 疼痛或不适是由于体力活动或情绪紧张引起的；
3. 休息和（或）含服硝酸甘油可减轻疼痛或不适。

胸痛完全符合上述三个特征的患者为典型心绞痛，具有上述三个特征中任意两个的患者为非典型心绞痛，而只符合一个或上述三个均不符合的患者为非心绞痛性胸痛。

其他与胸痛症状不完全相关的因素也可能会增加患者患 CAD 的验前概率。这些因素包括提示冠心病的

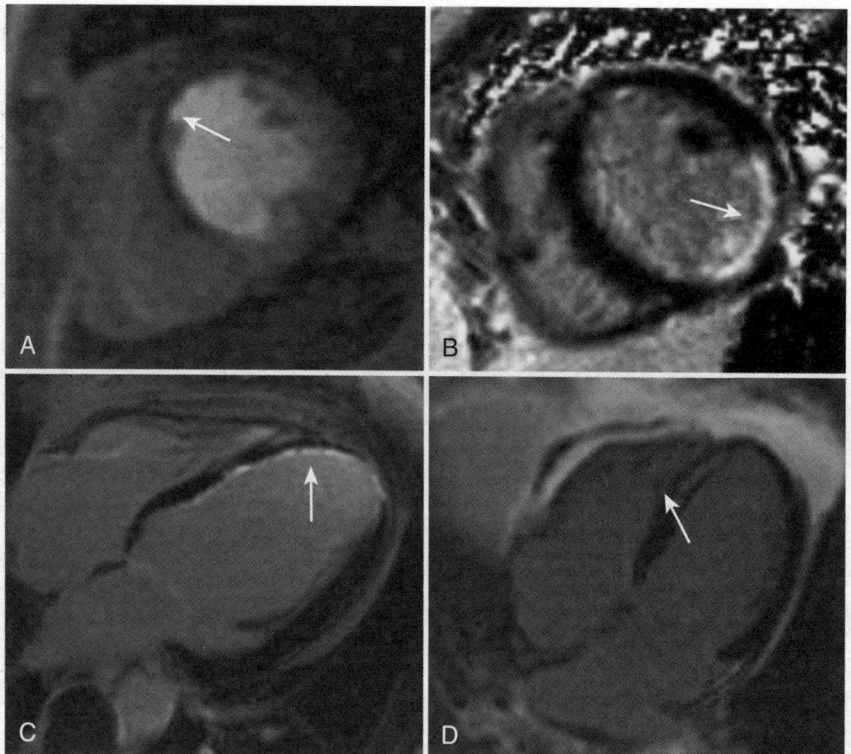

Fig. 3.15 Use of cardiac magnetic resonance imaging in the evaluation of chest pain or ischemic heart disease. (A) First-pass perfusion study during vasodilator stress shows a large septal perfusion defect *(arrow)*. The hypoperfused area appears dark compared with the myocardium with normal perfusion. (B) Example of delayed enhancement imaging of an almost transmural infarction of the mid-inferolateral wall, including the posterior papillary muscle. Infarcted myocardium appears *white*, whereas normal myocardium is *black (arrow)*. (C) Nontransmural (subendocardial) infarction of the septum and apex *(arrow)*. (D) Patient with acute myocarditis mimicking an acute coronary syndrome. Midmyocardial, rather than subendocardial, delayed enhancement is characteristic of myocarditis *(arrow)*.

probability of CAD. These include baseline ECG abnormalities suggestive of CAD and multiple CAD risk factors, such as diabetes, smoking, hypertension, dyslipidemia, or family history of premature CAD. These should be taken into consideration on an individual basis and may require an upward revision of pretest probability.

Stress Modalities

There are two essential components to any stress test: the type of stress and the imaging modality. Stress can either be exercise-induced or pharmacologic. Exercise level is deemed adequate if the patient achieves 85% of his or her maximal predicted heart rate. Submaximal stress tests can still be interpreted but may be limited in the ability to rule out disease due to decreased sensitivity. Indications for terminating a stress test include fatigue, severe hypertension (>220 mm Hg systolic), worsening angina during exercise, developing marked or widespread ischemic ECG changes, significant arrhythmias, or hypotension.

For patients who are able to exercise, the most commonly used exercise protocols are the Bruce and modified Bruce protocols. These protocols require a patient to walk on a treadmill as the speed and incline of the belt increases with each advancing stage. Any patient who can exercise should do so, as duration of exercise and provoked symptoms provide valuable clinical and prognostic information for the physician. The modified Bruce or similar protocols are ideal for older, overweight, unstable, or debilitated patients. Additionally, in patients unable to exercise on a treadmill, bicycle or arm ergometer testing may also be used. In patients who cannot exercise or in those where exercise will interfere with image acquisition, pharmacologic agents may be used.

The most commonly used pharmacologic stress agents are dobutamine, adenosine, and regadenoson, an adenosine derivative and selective adenosine A2A receptor agonist. Dobutamine is a synthetic sympathomimetic that stimulates alpha-1, beta-1, and beta-2 receptors, increasing inotropy and chronotropy, thereby increasing myocardial oxygen demand. It should be used cautiously in patients with a history of atrial or ventricular arrhythmias as it can exacerbate both. Regadenoson is an adenosine receptor agonist that induces coronary vasodilation and is more commonly used in radionuclide myocardial perfusion imaging. Its use is contraindicated in patients with asthma or COPD and active wheezing as well as patients with significant bradyarrhythmias without a pacemaker. It should be used with caution in patients with a history of seizures as it can lower the seizure threshold.

STRESS IMAGING

Exercise or pharmacologic stress testing must be combined with imaging modalities to assess for characteristic changes seen in flow-limiting coronary artery disease. The most basic form of imaging is an ECG, which can be combined with adjunctive echocardiography or radionuclide imaging to increase the diagnostic accuracy of the testing.

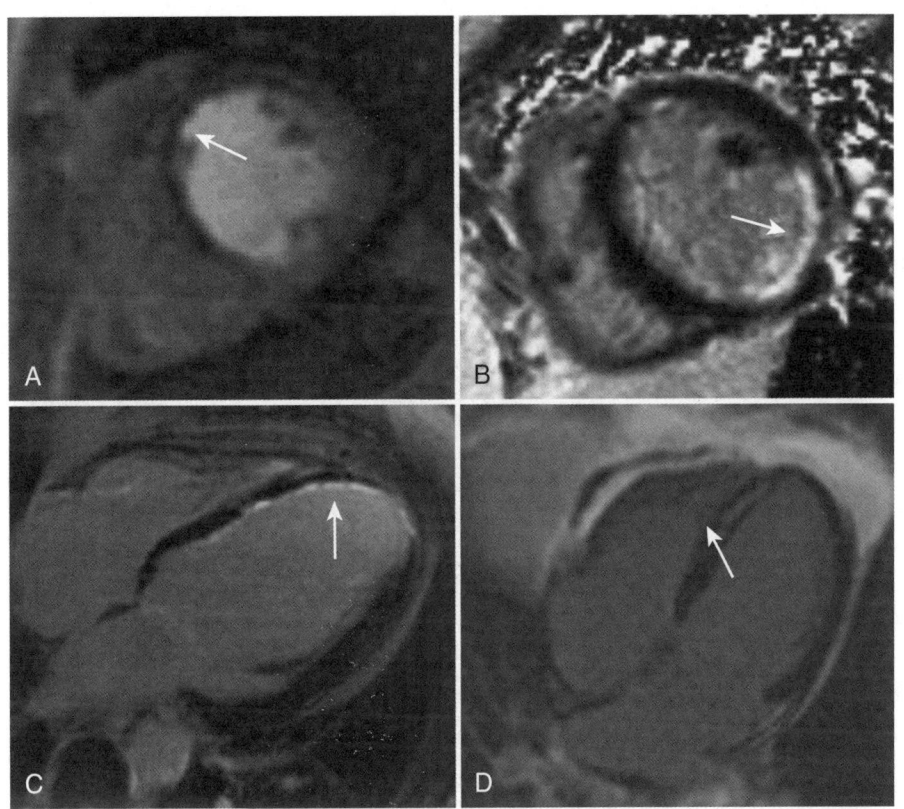

图 3.15 心脏磁共振成像在胸痛评估或缺血性心脏病中的应用。(A) 采用血管扩张剂进行负荷时的首次灌注显像显示较大的室间隔灌注缺损 (箭头)。与灌注正常的心肌相比，灌注不足的心肌区域颜色较黑。(B) 一例延迟增强显像显示下侧壁中段包括后乳头肌在内几乎心肌全层透壁性梗死。梗死心肌呈白色，正常心肌呈黑色 (箭头)。(C) 室间隔和心尖非透壁性 (心内膜下) 心肌梗死 (箭头)。(D) 类似急性冠脉综合征表现的一例急性心肌炎患者。显示心肌中层而非心内膜下的延迟强化，为心肌炎的特征性表现 (箭头)

基线心电图异常，多种冠心病危险因素如糖尿病、吸烟、高血压、血脂异常或早发冠心病家族史。应该在个体化基础上对这些因素加以考虑，必要时需要对验前概率进行相应修正。

负荷试验方法

任何一种负荷试验方法都有两个基本组成要素：负荷方式和成像方式。负荷可以采用运动或药物的方式。当达到患者亚极量即最大预计心率的 85% 时，运动负荷水平认为是足够的。尽管由于其较低的检测敏感性，排除疾病的能力有限，亚极量负荷仍然可以用于疾病解释。不适合进行负荷试验的情况包括疲劳、严重高血压 (收缩压 > 220 mmHg)、典型劳力性心绞痛、显著或广泛的缺血性心电图改变、严重的心律失常或低血压。

对于能够运动的患者，最常用的运动方案是布鲁斯 (Bruce) 和改良的布鲁斯方案。方案要求患者在平板 (跑步机) 上行走，速度和坡度逐级递增。任何能够运动的患者都应该按此方案进行，运动持续的时间和运动诱发的症状可以为医生提供有价值的临床和预后信息。改良的布鲁斯或其类似方案适合于老年人、超重、不稳定或虚弱的患者。此外，对于无法在跑步机上运动的患者，也可以使用踏车或手臂测力仪。对于不能运动的患者或运动会干扰图像采集时，可以使用药物进行负荷。

最常用于负荷试验的药物有多巴酚丁胺、腺苷和瑞加德松 (regadenoson)，后者是一种腺苷衍生物，可以选择性激动腺苷 A2A 受体。多巴酚丁胺是一种合成的拟交感神经介质，刺激 α_1、β_1 和 β_2 受体，增加收缩变力性和心率变时性，从而增加心肌氧耗量。注意有房性或室性心律失常病史的患者慎用，因为有可能导致心律失常加重。瑞加德松是一种腺苷受体激动剂，可以诱发冠状动脉血管扩张，在放射性核素心肌灌注成像时更常使用。对于哮喘或慢性阻塞性肺疾病伴活动性喘息发作的患者，以及缓慢性心律失常没有植入起搏器的患者，禁忌使用。有癫痫发作史的患者也要慎用，因为其会降低癫痫发作阈值。

负荷成像

运动或药物负荷试验需要和成像技术结合起来才能获得冠心病血流受限的特征性变化并进行评估。最基础的方式即 ECG，也可以辅助结合超声心动图或放射性核素显像，用以提高诊断的准确性。

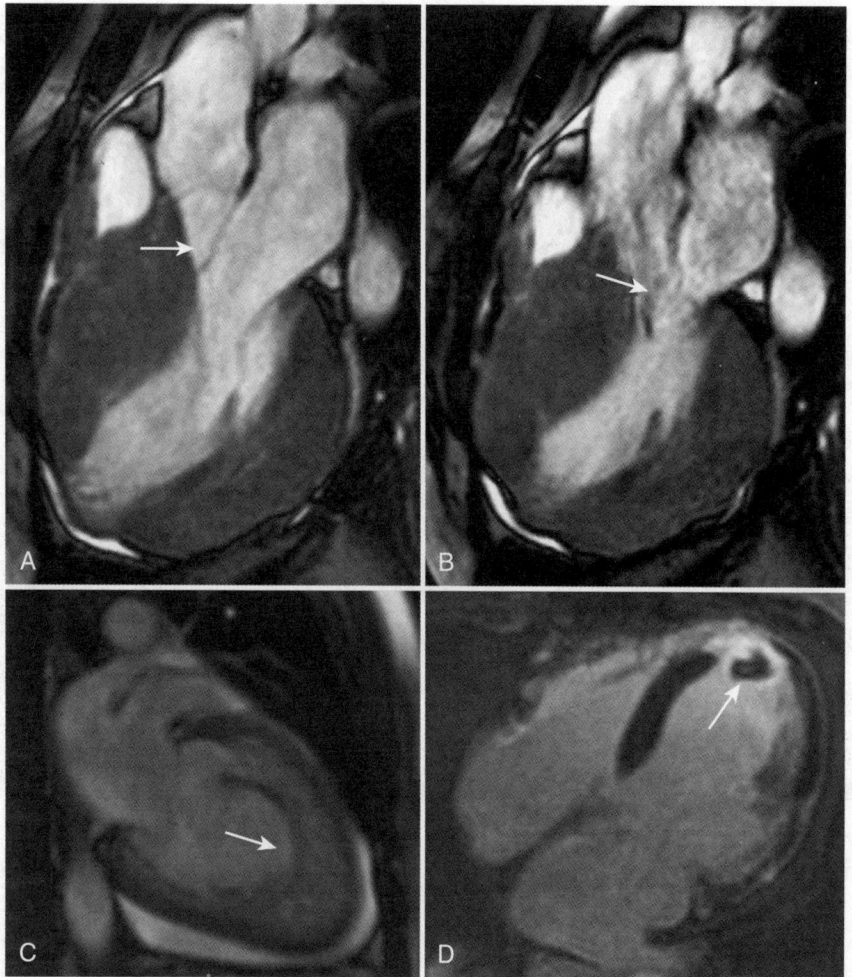

Fig. 3.16 Cardiac magnetic resonance imaging (MRI) is used in the evaluation of cardiomyopathies. (A) Severe left ventricular hypertrophy in a patient with hypertrophic cardiomyopathy. Diastolic frame shows open mitral valve *(arrow)*. (B) Systolic frame shows systolic anterior motion of the mitral valve with flow disturbance in the left ventricular outflow tract *(arrow)*. (C) Patient has left ventricular noncompaction as evidenced by deep trabeculations in the left ventricular apex *(arrow)*. (D) Patient with ischemic cardiomyopathy has transmural apical infarction and adjacent mural thrombus (arrow). (Images courtesy Sheldon E. Litwin, MD, Division of Cardiology, University of Utah, Salt Lake City, Utah.)

TABLE 3.4 Diamond and Forrester Pretest Probability of Coronary Artery Disease by Age, Sex, and Symptoms

Age (Years)	Sex	Typical/Definite Angina Pectoris	Atypical/Probable Angina Pectoris	Nonanginal Chest Pain
≤39	Men	Intermediate	Intermediate	Low
	Women	Intermediate	Very low	Very low
40-49	Men	High	Intermediate	Intermediate
	Women	Intermediate	Low	Very low
50-59	Men	High	Intermediate	Intermediate
	Women	Intermediate	Intermediate	Low
≥60	Men	High	Intermediate	Intermediate
	Women	High	Intermediate	Intermediate

High: >90% pretest probability. Intermediate: between 10% and 90% pretest probability. Low: between 5% and 10% pretest probability. Very low: <5% pretest probability.
From Wolk MJ, Bailey SR, Doherty JU, et al: ACCF/AHA/ASE/ASNC/HFSA/HRS/SCAI/SCCT/SCMR/STS 2013 Multimodality Appropriate Use Criteria for the Detection and Risk Assessment of Stable Ischemic Heart Disease. Journal of the American College of Cardiology 63:380-406, 2014.

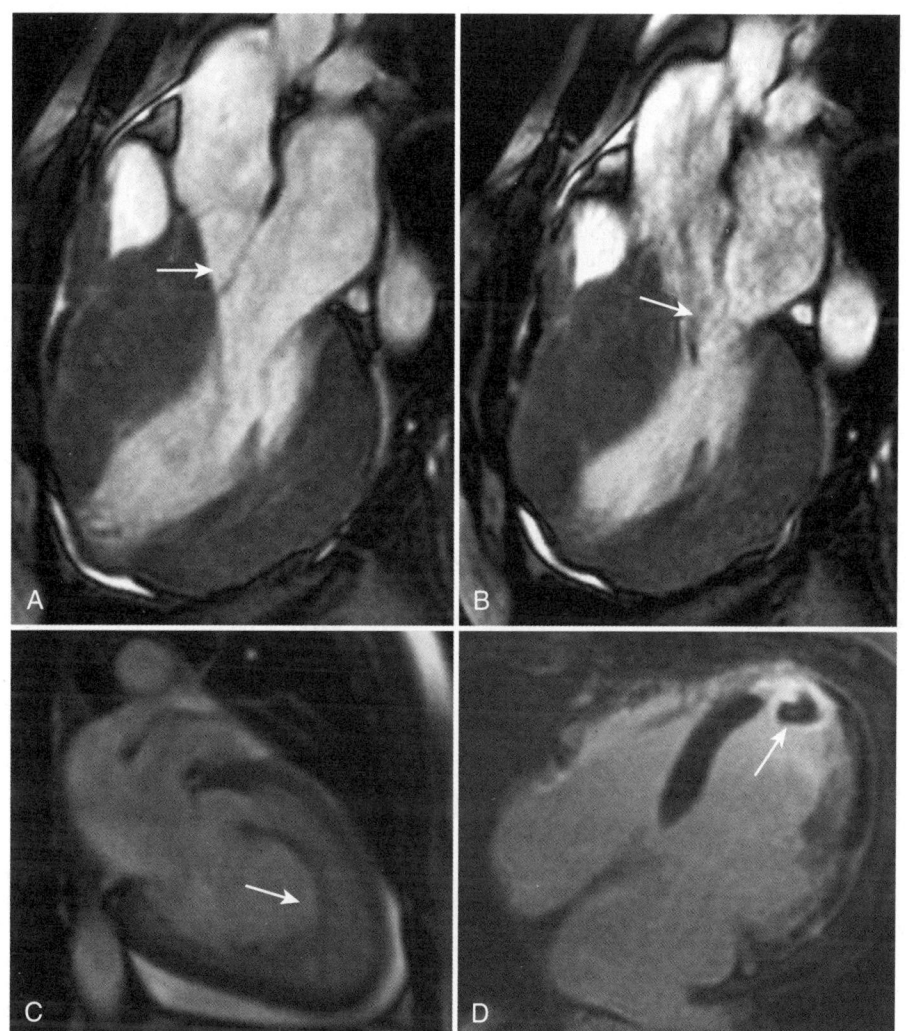

图 3.16 心脏磁共振成像（MRI）用于心肌病的评估。（**A**）一例肥厚型心肌病患者左心室显著肥厚。舒张期显示二尖瓣开放（箭头）。（**B**）收缩期显示二尖瓣收缩期前移，左心室流出道血流紊乱（箭头）。（**C**）一例患者左心室心尖部有较深的肌小梁，提示左心室致密化不全（箭头）。（**D**）一例缺血性心肌病患者心尖透壁性梗死和邻近的附壁血栓（箭头）。（图片授权自 Sheldon E. Litwin，MD，Division of Cardiology，University of Utah，Salt Lake City，Utah.）

表 3.4 · 按年龄、性别和症状评估冠心病验前概率的 Diamond 和 Forrester 测试				
年龄（年）	性别	典型/确定的心绞痛	非典型/可能的心绞痛	非心绞痛性胸痛
≤39	男性	中	中	低
	女性	中	极低	极低
40～49	男性	高	中	中
	女性	中	低	极低
50～59	男性	高	中	中
	女性	中	中	低
≥60	男性	高	中	中
	女性	高	中	中

高：＞90% 验前概率。中：验前概率为 10%～90%。低：验前概率为 5%～10%。极低：验前概率＜5%。
引自 Wolk MJ，Bailey SR，Doherty JU, et al: ACCF/AHA/ASE/ASNC/HFSA/HRS/SCAI/SCCT/SCMR/STS 2013 Multimodality Appropriate Use Criteria for the Detection and Risk Assessment of Stable Ischemic Heart Disease. Journal of the American College of Cardiology 63：380-406，2014.

Stress Electrocardiography

The normal physiologic response to exercise is an increase in heart rate and systolic and diastolic blood pressures. The ECG maintains normal T-wave polarity, and the ST segment remains unchanged or, if depressed, has a rapid upstroke back to baseline. An ischemic ECG response to exercise is defined as 1.5 mm of upsloping ST-segment depression measured 0.08 second past the J point, at least 1 mm of horizontal ST depression, or 1 mm of downsloping ST-segment depression measured at the J point. Given the large amount of artifact on the ECG that may occur with exercise, these changes must be seen in at least three consecutive depolarizations. Other findings that suggest more extensive CAD include early onset of ST depression (6 minutes); marked, downsloping ST depression (>2 mm), especially if present in more than five leads; ST changes persisting into recovery for more than 5 minutes; and failure to increase systolic blood pressure to 120 mm Hg or more or a sustained decrease of 10 mm Hg or more below baseline.

The ECG is not diagnostically useful in the setting of left ventricular hypertrophy, LBBB, Wolff-Parkinson-White syndrome, or chronic digoxin therapy. In these instances, further imaging modalities such as echocardiography, nuclear imaging, or positron-emission tomography (PET) are needed to help diagnose ischemia.

Stress Echocardiography

Two-dimensional echocardiography and Doppler echocardiography are often used in conjunction with exercise or pharmacologic stress testing. The pharmacologic agent typically used is dobutamine. A baseline echocardiogram is performed at rest and during stress. Changes in wall motion are indicative of ischemia and coronary artery disease. In areas of the left ventricle that have wall motion abnormalities at rest, improvement of these wall motion abnormalities with exercise or low-dose dobutamine is indicative of viability.

Relative to myocardial perfusion imaging, the sensitivity of stress echocardiography is slightly lower whereas the specificity is slightly higher. A poor baseline echocardiogram due to limited acoustic windows will limit stress test results. The estimated cost-effectiveness of stress echocardiography is significantly better than nuclear perfusion imaging because of the overall lower cost.

Myocardial Perfusion Imaging (See Also Nuclear Cardiology Section)

Stress testing, using myocardial perfusion imaging with SPECT to compare relative coronary blood flow at stress and at rest, helps to identify areas of perfusion mismatch, indicative of ischemia. Like with other stress modalities, exercise or pharmacologic stress can be used. Commonly used pharmacologic agents include dipyridamole, adenosine, and regadenoson, which are all coronary vasodilators. It is important to note that patients with LBBB have to undergo pharmacologic stress when receiving myocardial perfusion imaging, even if they are able to exercise, as the abnormal septal motion caused by the LBBB can lead to a false perfusion defect during exercise.

Stress Cardiac Magnetic Resonance Imaging

Though either exercise or pharmacologic stress may be combined with cMRI, the contemporary use of stress cMRI usually refers to stress perfusion cMRI with gadolinium contrast that is performed with regadenoson. This technique allows for evaluation of wall motion, perfusion, scar, viability, and microvascular dysfunction, as well as chamber quantification and function, allowing for a comprehensive evaluation of the myocardium and myocardial function. Changes in late gadolinium enhancement between rest and stress has performance characteristics for diagnosing CAD that are at least as good and likely superior to those of conventional stress tests using nuclear myocardial perfusion imaging or echocardiography, and on par with PET imaging.

COMPUTED TOMOGRAPHY OF THE HEART

Newer applications of computed tomography (CT) have greatly advanced our ability to diagnose cardiovascular disease noninvasively. The development of fast gantry rotation speeds and the addition of multiple rows of detectors (i.e., multidetector CT) have allowed unprecedented visualization of the great vessels, heart, and coronary arteries with images acquired during a single breath-hold lasting 10 to 15 seconds. CT is used to diagnose aortic aneurysm, acute aortic dissection, and pulmonary embolism, and it is useful for defining congenital abnormalities and detecting pericardial thickening or calcification associated with constrictive pericarditis. ECG-gated dynamic CT images have been used to quantify ventricular size, function, and regional wall motion, and in contrast to echocardiography, CT is not limited by lung disease or chest wall deformity. However, obesity and implanted prosthetic materials (i.e., mechanical valves or pacing wires) may affect image quality.

The greatest excitement and controversy about cardiac CT relates to the evaluation of coronary atherosclerosis. Electron beam and multidetector CT scans can be used to quickly and reliably visualize and quantitate the extent of coronary artery calcification (Fig. 3.17). The presence of coronary calcium is pathognomonic of atherosclerosis, and the extent of coronary calcium (usually reported as an Agatston score) is a powerful marker of future cardiovascular events. The coronary calcium score adds substantial, independent improvement in risk prediction to the commonly employed clinical risk scores (e.g., Framingham risk score). Moreover, the calcium score is a good marker of the overall atherosclerotic burden. Indications for coronary calcium scoring continue to grow, especially in refining risk predictions in asymptomatic patients at intermediate risk for arteriosclerotic cardiovascular disease.

Contrast-enhanced coronary computed tomography angiography (CCTA) has improved dramatically in recent years. CCTA has a sensitivity of more than 95% in diagnosing significant coronary artery obstruction. Unlike myocardial perfusion imaging, CCTA is an anatomic test, and thus does not give information on perfusion or blood flow across a lesion. Thus, in patients with known coronary disease, CCTA cannot easily differentiate between ischemic and nonischemic chest pain. New technology is being developed to noninvasively determine the hemodynamic significance of a lesion through CCTA, similar to fractional flow reserve in coronary catheterization, though this technology still needs to be rigorously tested and standardized. Evaluation of coronary arteries with CCTA can be significantly limited in patients with extensive coronary calcifications, cardiac devices, or prior stents due to technical limitations.

Concerns that limit the widespread use of cardiac CT most frequently cite the risks of radiation and contrast exposure and the lack of prospective studies showing improvement in outcome with this testing modality. In early studies, the calculated radiation exposure of CCTA was about double that of a diagnostic invasive coronary angiogram, although with prospective ECG-gating, most studies are now equal to or less than a diagnostic angiogram. Contrast use is often higher in a CCTA than in a diagnostic invasive coronary angiogram. The role of CCTA in routine clinical practice continues to evolve.

CARDIAC CATHETERIZATION

Cardiac catheterization is an invasive technique in which fluid-filled catheters are introduced percutaneously into the arterial and/or venous circulation. This method allows direct measurement of intracardiac

负荷心电图

运动的正常生理反应是心率加快，收缩压和舒张压升高；ECG 上 T 波方向正常，ST 段保持不变，或者如果出现压低，会快速回升至基线。运动后出现的缺血性 ECG 定义为：ST 段上斜型压低 1.5 mm 并且压低出现在 J 点后 0.08 s，ST 段水平型压低 1 mm 以上，或者自 J 点起测量 ST 段呈下斜型压低 1 mm 以上。考虑到运动时 ECG 可能会出现大量伪影，上述这些变化必须在至少三次连续波群中出现。其他提示严重 CAD 的指标包括：运动后早期出现 ST 段压低（6 min）；显著的下斜型 ST 段压低（>2 mm），尤其是在 5 个以上导联中出现；ST 段变化在运动恢复期持续 5 min 以上；运动后收缩压未能升高至 120 mmHg 或以上，或持续低于基线水平 10 mmHg 或以上。

在左心室肥厚、LBBB、WPW 综合征或长期服用地高辛的情况下，ECG 对于心肌缺血的诊断价值有限。此时，需要进一步采用超声心动图、心脏核素显像或正电子发射断层成像（PET）等成像方式来帮助诊断。

负荷超声心动图

运动或药物负荷试验常与二维超声心动图和多普勒超声心动图联合应用。常用的激发药物是多巴酚丁胺。在静息和负荷状态下分别进行超声心动图检查。室壁运动改变提示心肌缺血和冠心病。静息时左心室室壁运动异常减弱的区域，如果通过运动或小剂量多巴酚丁胺可以改善，则提示心肌存活。

与心肌灌注成像相比，负荷超声心动图的敏感性稍低，而特异性稍高。如果声窗不佳影响超声心动图成像质量，则负荷试验的结果会受限。负荷超声心动图总体成本较低，因此性价比明显优于核素灌注成像。

负荷心肌灌注成像（参见心脏核素检查部分）

使用 SPECT 心肌灌注成像技术进行负荷试验，比较负荷和静息时的相对冠状动脉血流，可以帮助确定灌注不匹配的心肌缺血区域。同其他成像技术一样，可使用运动或药物进行负荷激发。常用的药物包括：双嘧达莫、腺苷和瑞加德松，都属于冠状动脉血管扩张剂。值得注意的是，LBBB 患者在接受心肌灌注成像时，即使患者能够进行运动，也建议进行药物负荷试验，因为 LBBB 会引起室间隔运动异常而导致运动负荷时出现假性灌注缺损。

负荷心脏磁共振成像

虽然运动或药物负荷试验均可与 cMRI 结合应用，但目前的负荷 cMRI 通常是指同时使用钆造影剂和瑞加德松的负荷灌注 cMRI。这种技术可评估室壁运动、灌注、瘢痕、存活心肌、微血管功能障碍，以及心腔的大小和功能，从而对心肌和心肌功能进行全面评估。在诊断 CAD 方面，静息与负荷钆延迟强化显像的价值不劣于甚至优于传统的负荷试验，包括负荷心肌核素灌注成像或负荷超声心动图，并且与 PET 成像相当。

心脏计算机断层成像

近年来，计算机断层成像（CT）的应用极大地提高了心血管疾病无创诊断的能力。随着机器旋转速度的加快和多排探测器（即多探头 CT）的增加，单次持续 10～15 s 的屏气过程中就能获得大血管、心脏和冠状动脉的图像，实现了前所未有的成像水平。CT 可用于诊断主动脉瘤、急性主动脉夹层和肺栓塞，还可用于诊断先天性畸形，发现与缩窄性心包炎相关的心包增厚或钙化。与超声心动图相比，CT 不受肺部疾病或胸壁畸形的限制。但是，肥胖和植入的人工材料（如机械瓣膜或起搏器导线）可能会影响图像质量。

心脏 CT 的最大亮点和争议在于对冠状动脉粥样硬化的评估。电子束和多探头 CT 扫描可以快速、可靠地观察和量化冠状动脉钙化的程度（图 3.17）。冠状动脉钙化是冠状动脉硬化的病理标志，钙化程度[通常以阿加斯顿评分（Agatston score）表示]是预测未来心血管事件的重要指标。与常用的临床风险模型[如弗雷明汉（Framingham）风险评分]相比，冠状动脉钙化评分在风险预测方面有额外和独立的预测价值。此外，冠状动脉钙化评分还是评价动脉粥样硬化总体负担的良好指标。冠状动脉钙化评分的适应证仍在不断增加，尤其适合于对无症状、动脉粥样硬化性心血管疾病风险中危患者的进一步评估。

近年来，造影剂增强冠状动脉 CT 血管成像（CCTA）有了长足进步。在诊断严重的冠状动脉狭窄时，CCTA 的敏感性超过 95%。与心肌灌注成像不同，CCTA 是一种解剖学检查，不能提供关于病变部位的灌注或血流信息。因此，对于已知有冠状动脉疾病的患者，CCTA 难以区分缺血性和非缺血性胸痛。目前正在开发新的技术，尝试通过 CCTA 无创确定病变的血流动力学意义，类似于冠状动脉导管检查中的血流储备分数，但这项技术仍需进一步进行严格的试验并标准化。由于技术限制，对于冠状动脉广泛钙化、具有心脏植入设备或曾植入过支架的患者，CCTA 评估冠状动脉的价值受到较大限制。

心脏 CT 广泛应用受限的顾虑主要是辐射和造影剂暴露的风险，以及缺乏前瞻性研究证实采用这种检查方式能改善临床结局。在早期研究中，计算出的 CCTA 辐射暴露大约是进行有创冠状动脉造影的 2 倍，不过随着前瞻性心电图门控技术的发展，现在多数情况下辐射暴露相当于或低于诊断性血管造影。CCTA 的造影剂用量通常高于有创的诊断性冠状动脉造影。CCTA 在日常临床实践中的作用仍在不断拓展。

心导管检查

心导管检查是一种侵入性检查技术，经皮将充液导管引入动脉和（或）静脉。这种方法可直接测量

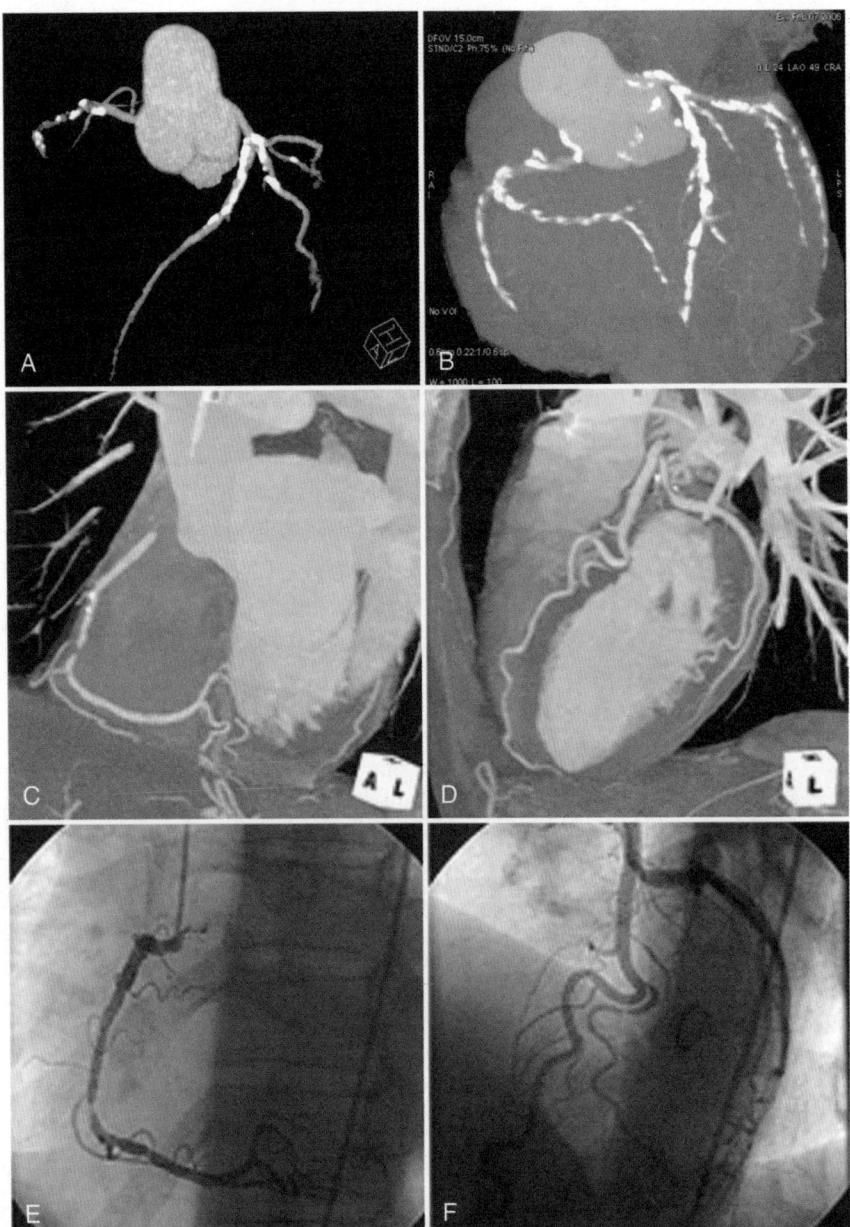

Fig. 3.17 Computed tomography coronary angiography compared with conventional radiographic contrast angiography. (A and B) Volume-rendering technique demonstrates stenosis of the right coronary artery and normal left coronary artery. (C and D) Maximal intensity projection of the same arteries demonstrates severe noncalcified plaque in the right coronary artery with superficial calcified plaque. (E and F) Invasive angiography of the same arteries. (From Raff GL, Gallagher MJ, O'Neill WW, et al: Diagnostic accuracy of noninvasive coronary angiography using 64-slice spiral computed tomography, J Am Coll Cardiol 46:552-557, 2005.)

pressures and oxygen saturation and, with the injection of a contrast agent, visualization of the coronary arteries, cardiac chambers, and great vessels. Cardiac catheterization is indicated when a clinically suggested cardiac abnormality requires confirmation and its anatomic and physiologic importance needs to be quantified. Coronary angiography for the diagnosis of CAD is the most common indication for this test.

Compared with catheterization, noninvasive testing with echocardiography is safer, often cheaper, and equally effective in the evaluation of most valvular and hemodynamic conditions. Most often, catheterization precedes some type of beneficial intervention, such as coronary artery angioplasty, coronary bypass surgery, or valvular surgery. Although cardiac catheterization is usually safe (0.1% to 0.2% overall mortality rate), procedure-related complications such as vascular injury, renal failure, stroke, and MI can occur.

Left Heart Catheterization and Coronary Angiography

Left heart catheterization and coronary angiography first requires the introduction of wires and fluid-filled catheters into the arterial system of the body. In the past, femoral arterial access was the default route, but now, radial arterial access has become increasingly more common.

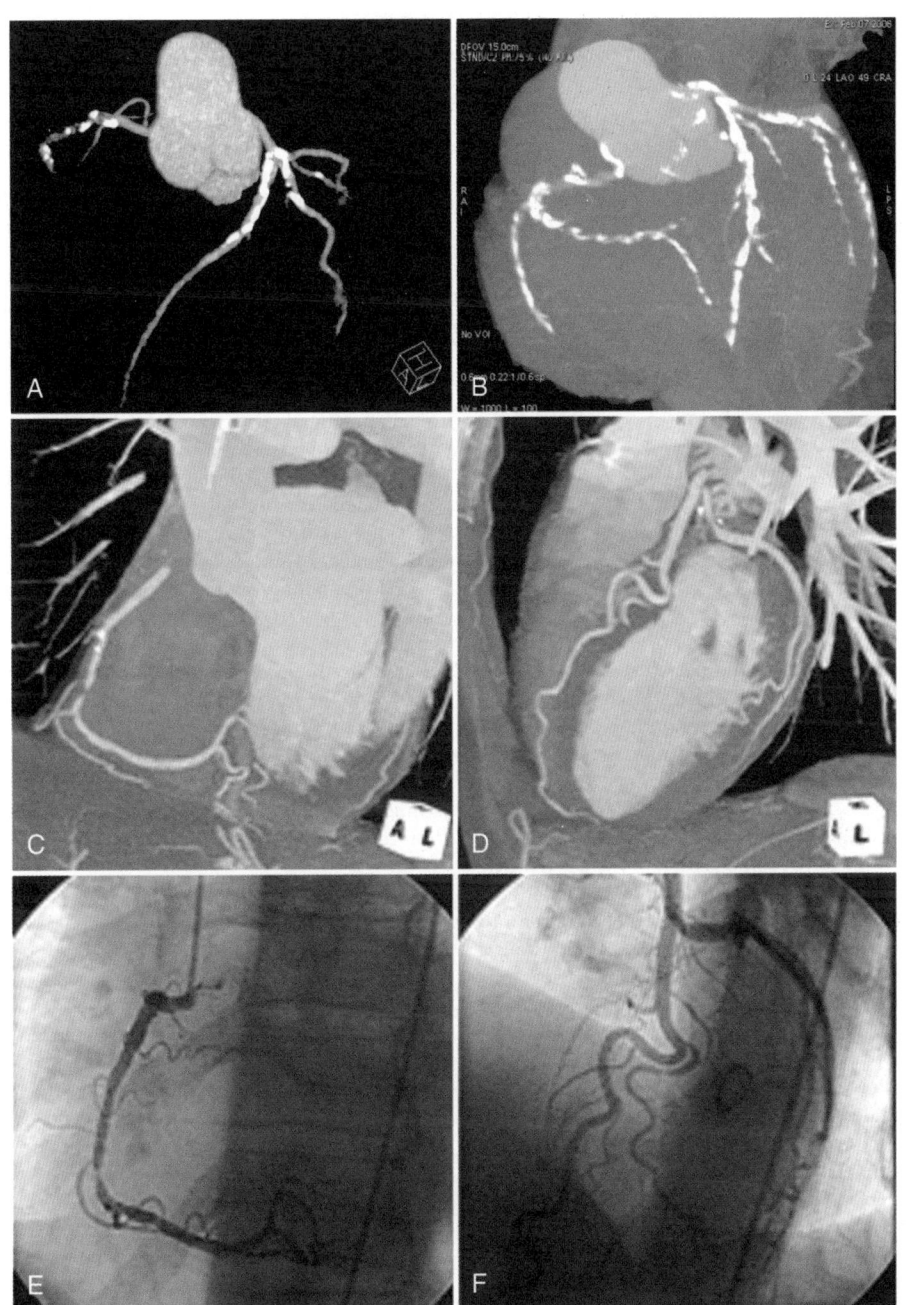

图 3.17 计算机断层成像冠状动脉造影与传统放射造影对比。（A 和 B）容积渲染技术显示右冠状动脉狭窄，左冠状动脉正常。（C 和 D）动脉最大强度投影显示右冠状动脉存在严重的非钙化斑块和钙化斑块。（E 和 F）相同动脉的有创血管造影（引自 Raff GL，Gallagher MJ，O'Neill WW, et al: Diagnostic accuracy of noninvasive coronary angiography using 64-slice spiral computed tomography, J Am Coll Cardiol 46：552-557，2005.）

心腔内压力和血氧饱和度，并通过注射造影剂来观察冠状动脉、心腔和大血管。当临床怀疑心脏异常需要确认，其解剖和生理指标需要进行量化时，就需要进行心导管检查。冠状动脉造影术的主要适应证是诊断 CAD。

与心导管检查相比，无创超声心动图检查更安全、便宜，而且对大多数瓣膜疾病和血流动力学的评估效果一致。通常在进行冠状动脉血管成形术、冠状动脉旁路移植术或瓣膜手术等介入治疗前先进行心导管检查。虽然心导管检查通常是安全的（总死亡率为 0.1%～0.2%），但也会出现手术相关并发症，如血管损伤、肾功能衰竭、卒中和 MI。

左心导管检查和冠状动脉造影

左心导管检查和冠状动脉造影首先需要将导丝和充液导管引入人体动脉系统。以往，股动脉入路是默认的手术入路，而现在则越来越普遍地选择桡动脉入路。在大多数中心，桡动脉入路已取代股动脉入路成

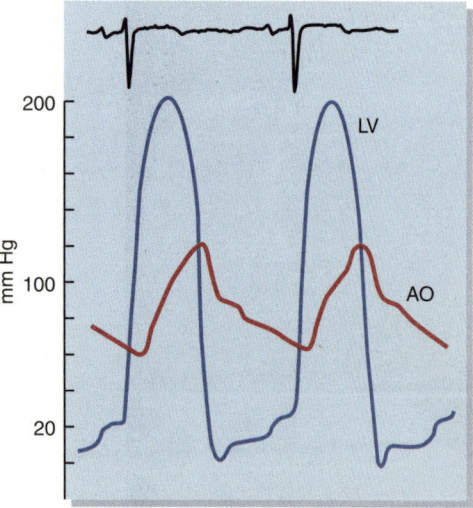

Fig. 3.18 Electrocardiographic tracing and left ventricular (LV) and aortic (AO) pressure curves in a patient with aortic stenosis. A pressure gradient occurs across the aortic valve during systole.

It has replaced femoral arterial access as the default access site in most centers. Radial arterial access is associated with less bleeding, fewer vascular complications, and increased patient comfort and early mobility after the procedure when compared with femoral arterial access. However, it is also associated with higher radiation exposure and increased procedural time.

After access is obtained, wires and fluid-filled catheters are advanced to the aortic root and through the aortic valve into the left ventricle under fluoroscopic guidance. Here, left ventricular size, wall motion, and ejection fraction can be accurately assessed by injecting contrast into the left ventricle (i.e., left ventriculography). Aortic and mitral valve insufficiency can be qualitatively assessed during angiography by observing the reflux of contrast medium into the left ventricle and left atrium, respectively. Left ventricular pressures can be directly measured and recorded, and the catheter can slowly be pulled back across the left ventricular outflow tract (LVOT) and aortic valve to directly assess for any pressure differential that would be consistent with aortic stenosis or LVOT obstruction (Fig. 3.18).

The coronary anatomy can be defined by injecting contrast medium into the coronary tree. Atherosclerotic lesions appear as narrowing of the internal diameter (lumen) of the vessel. A hemodynamically important stenosis is defined as 70% or more narrowing of the luminal diameter. However, the hemodynamic significance of a lesion can be underestimated by coronary angiography, particularly when the atherosclerotic plaque is eccentric or elongated. Intravascular ultrasound, optical coherence tomography, or miniaturized pressure sensors can be used during invasive procedures to help evaluate the severity or estimate the physiologic significance of intermediate lesions.

Right Heart Catheterization

Right heart catheterization is a useful invasive technique that can be performed at bedside or with fluoroscopic guidance. The pulmonary artery (Swan-Ganz) catheter, which is a balloon-tipped catheter used for right heart catheterization, can be left in a patient for a prolonged period of time in a critical care setting to provide continuous information on cardiovascular hemodynamics and filling pressures. Right heart catheterization can be helpful when used in appropriate situations, such as when differentiating noncardiogenic from cardiogenic pulmonary edema, managing mixed shock, managing cardiogenic shock, and classifying and treating pulmonary hypertension.

Right heart catheterization is performed by first accessing the venous system. Common sites of entry for right heart catheterization include the internal jugular vein (usually the right), the right brachial vein, or the femoral veins. The procedure can be performed at the bedside or under fluoroscopic guidance with a balloon-tipped (Swan-Ganz) catheter. The catheter is advanced from the vein to the right atrium, right ventricle, and pulmonary artery, where pressures are measured and recorded. The catheter can then be advanced further until it *wedges* in the distal pulmonary artery. The transmitted pressure measured in this location originates from the pulmonary venous system and is known as the *pulmonary capillary wedge pressure*. In the absence of pulmonary venous disease, the pulmonary capillary wedge pressure reflects left atrial pressure, and if no significant mitral valve pathologic condition exists, it reflects left ventricular diastolic pressure. A more direct method of obtaining left ventricular filling pressures is through left heart catheterization, as described in the previous section. With these two methods of obtaining intracardiac pressures, each chamber of the heart can be directly assessed and the gradients across any of the valves determined (Fig. 3.19).

Cardiac output can be determined by one of two widely accepted methods: the Fick oxygen method and the indicator dilution technique. The basis of the Fick method is that total uptake or release of a substance by an organ is equal to the product of blood flow to that organ and the concentration difference of that substance between the arterial and venous circulation of that organ. If this method is applied to the lungs, the substance released into the blood is oxygen; if no intrapulmonary shunts exist, pulmonary blood flow is equal to systemic blood flow or cardiac output. The cardiac output can be determined by the following equation:

$$\text{Cardiac output} = \frac{\text{Oxygen consumption}}{(\text{Arterial oxygen content} - \text{Venous oxygen content})}$$

Oxygen consumption is measured in milliliters per minute by collecting the patient's expired air over a known period while simultaneously measuring oxygen saturation in a sample of arterial and mixed venous blood (i.e., arterial and venous oxygen content, respectively, measured in milliliters per liter). The cardiac output is expressed in liters per minute and then corrected for body surface area (i.e., cardiac index). The normal range of cardiac index is 2.6 to 4.2 L/min/m^2. Cardiac output can also be determined by the indicator dilution technique, which most commonly uses cold saline as the indicator. With this method, cold saline is injected into the blood, and the resulting temperature change *downstream* is monitored. This action generates a curve in which temperature change is plotted over time, and the area under the curve represents cardiac output.

Detection and localization of intracardiac shunts can be performed by sequential measurement of oxygen saturation in the venous system, right side of the heart, and two main pulmonary arteries. In patients with left-to-right shunt flow, an increase in oxygen *step-up* (i.e., saturation increase from one chamber to the successive chamber) occurs as arterial blood mixes with venous blood. By using the Fick method for calculating blood flow in the pulmonary and systemic systems, the shunt ratio can be calculated. Noninvasive approaches have largely supplanted catheterization laboratory assessment of shunts.

In the past, the Swan-Ganz catheter was routinely used in most patients with shock; however, randomized trials have since been published suggesting no improvement in outcomes in critically ill patients in whom pulmonary artery catheterization was performed.

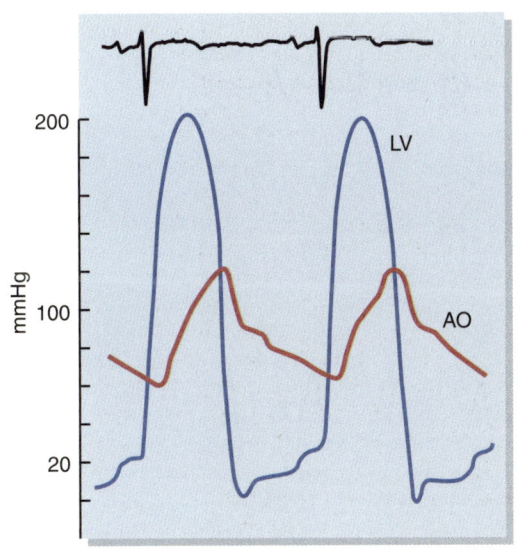

图 3.18 一名主动脉瓣狭窄患者的心电图以及左心室（LV）和主动脉（AO）压力曲线。主动脉瓣在收缩期出现跨瓣压力阶差

为默认的手术入路。与股动脉入路相比，桡动脉入路出血更少，血管并发症更少，患者更舒适，术后早期活动能力更强。不过桡动脉入路也会增加辐射暴露量和手术时间。

建立通道后，在射线透视引导下，将导丝和充液导管推进到主动脉根部，并通过主动脉瓣进入左心室。通过向左心室注入造影剂（即左心室造影），可以准确评估左心室大小、室壁运动和射血分数。在血管造影过程中，通过观察造影剂进入左心室和左心房的流量，可以对主动脉瓣和二尖瓣关闭不全进行定性评估。对左心室压力可直接进行测量和记录，将导管缓慢回撤到左心室流出道（LVOT）和主动脉瓣，可以直接评估主动脉瓣狭窄或 LVOT 梗阻导致的压力阶差（图 3.18）。

向冠状动脉注入造影剂可确定冠状动脉的解剖结构。动脉粥样硬化病变表现为血管内径（管腔）变窄。血流动力学意义上的狭窄是指管腔直径缩小 70% 或以上。然而，冠状动脉造影可能会低估病变的血流动力学意义，尤其是当动脉粥样硬化斑块呈偏心或为长节段病变时。在有创手术中可使用血管内超声、光学相干断层成像或微型压力传感器来帮助评估病变的严重程度或估算其生理意义。

右心导管检查

右心导管检查是一种侵入性检查技术，可在床旁或放射线引导下进行。肺动脉（Swan-Ganz）导管是一种用于右心导管检查、顶端有球囊的导管，在重症监护环境中可长期留置在患者体内，以提供关于心血管血流动力学和充盈压力的连贯信息。在适宜情况下使用右心导管检查非常有价值，如在区分非心源性肺水肿和心源性肺水肿、处理多因素所致的休克、处理心源性休克以及对肺动脉高压进行分类和治疗时。

右心导管检查首先要进入静脉系统。插入的常见部位包括颈内静脉（通常是右侧）、右肱静脉或股静脉。手术可以在床边进行，也可以在射线引导下使用顶端有球囊的（Swan-Ganz）导管进行。导管从静脉进入并推进到右心房、右心室和肺动脉，分别测量和记录压力。然后将导管进一步推进，直至楔入远端肺动脉。在此位置测量到的传输压力来自肺静脉系统，称为肺毛细血管楔压。在没有肺静脉疾病的情况下，肺毛细血管楔压反映的是左心房压；如果没有明显的二尖瓣病变，它同时反映左心室舒张压。获取左心室舒张压的更直接方法是左心导管检查，如上一节所述。有这两种获取心内压力的方法，就可以直接评估心脏的每个腔室，并评估跨任何瓣膜的压力阶差（图 3.19）。

心输出量可通过两种广为接受的方法之一来确定：菲克（Fick）氧气法和指示剂稀释技术。菲克氧气法的基本原理是，器官对某种物质的总摄入量或释放量等于该器官的血流量与该器官动脉和静脉循环中该物质浓度差的乘积。如果将此方法应用于肺部，则释放到血液中的物质为氧气；如果不存在肺内分流，则肺血流量等于全身血流量或心输出量。则心输出量可通过以下公式确定：

$$\text{心输出量} = \frac{\text{耗氧量}}{（\text{动脉氧含量} - \text{静脉氧含量}）}$$

耗氧量可通过收集患者在已知时间内的呼出气体，以 ml/min 为单位测量；同时测量动脉血和混合静脉血样本中的氧饱和度（即动脉和静脉血中的氧含量，以 ml/L 为单位）。心输出量以血流体积（L）/分钟表示，然后根据体表面积进行校正（即心脏指数）。心脏指数的正常范围为 $2.6 \sim 4.2$ L/（min·m^2）。心输出量也可通过指示剂稀释技术来测定，该技术最常用冷盐水作为指示剂。使用这种方法时，将冷盐水注入血液，并监测下游温度的变化。这一过程会产生一条温度随时间变化的曲线，曲线下的面积代表心输出量。

可通过连续测量静脉系统、右心和两条肺动脉主干的血氧饱和度来检测和确定心内分流部位。在左向右分流的患者中，当动脉血与静脉血混合时，氧含量变化出现增加（即下一个心腔较相连上一个心腔的氧饱和度增加）。通过使用菲克氧气法计算肺部和全身系统的血流，可以计算出分流比值。无创方法目前在很大程度上取代了有创导管检查对分流的评估。

以往大多数休克患者都会常规使用 Swan-Ganz 导管；但后来发表的随机临床试验表明，对危重患者进

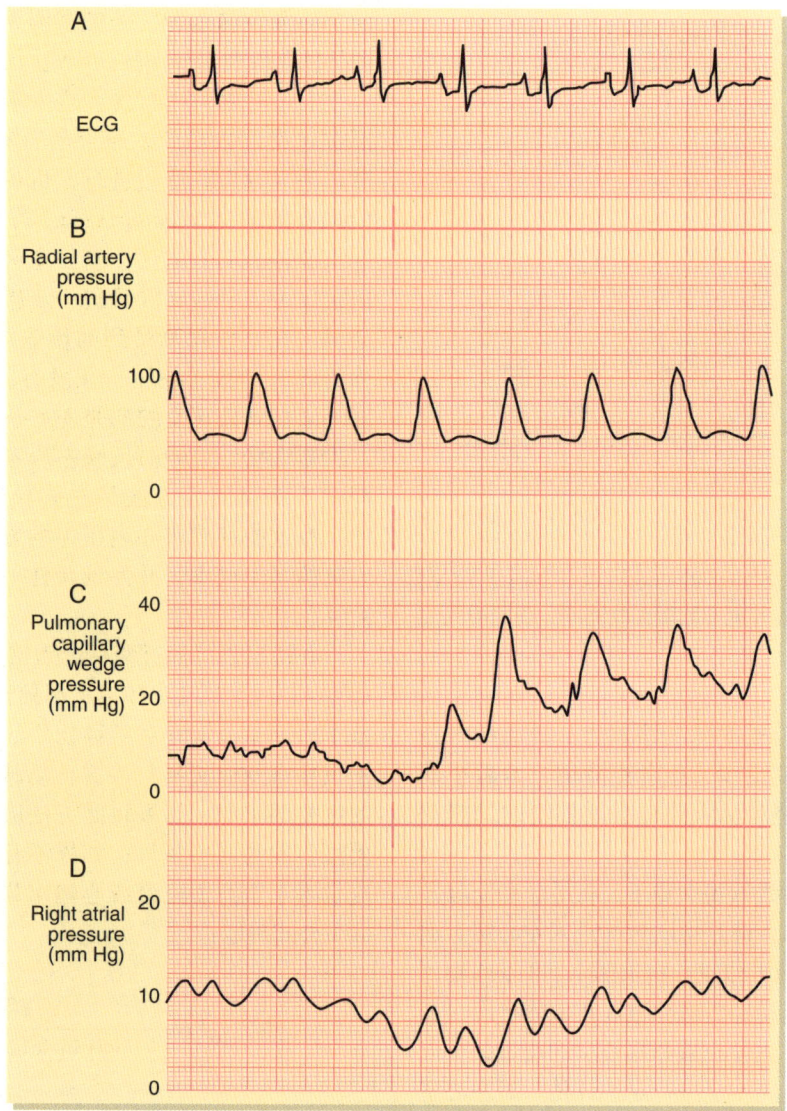

Fig. 3.19 Electrocardiographic (ECG) (A) and Swan-Ganz flotation catheter (C) recordings are shown. The recordings of a catheter in the radial artery and Swan-Ganz floating catheter in the right atrium are shown in B and D, respectively. The left portion of tracing C was obtained with the balloon inflated, yielding the pulmonary arterial wedge pressure. The right portion of tracing C was recorded with the balloon deflated, depicting the pulmonary arterial pressure. In this patient, the pulmonary arterial wedge pressure (i.e., left ventricular filling pressure) is normal, and the pulmonary artery pressure is elevated because of lung disease.

Certainly, improvements in noninvasive imaging techniques have made the Swan-Ganz catheter much less important in diagnosing cardiac conditions such as cardiac tamponade, constrictive pericarditis, right ventricular infarction, and ventricular septal defect. This led to a decline in the routine use of Swan-Ganz catheters in intensive care units. However, the use of these catheters has resurged, likely due to the increased use of advanced heart failure therapies and mechanical support, where continuous hemodynamic monitoring is essential for optimal therapy titration (Table 3.5).

ENDOMYOCARDIAL BIOPSY

Biopsy of the right ventricular endomyocardium can be performed. With this technique, a bioptome is introduced into the venous system through the right internal jugular vein and guided into the right ventricle by fluoroscopy. Small samples of the endocardium are taken for histologic evaluation. The primary indication for endomyocardial biopsy is the diagnosis of rejection after cardiac transplantation and documentation of cardiac amyloidosis; however, endomyocardial biopsy may have some use in diagnosing specific etiologic agents responsible for myocarditis.

NONINVASIVE VASCULAR TESTING

Assessment for the presence and severity of peripheral vascular disease is an important component of the cardiovascular evaluation. Comparison of the systolic blood pressure in the upper and lower extremities is one of the simplest tests to detect hemodynamically important arterial disease. Normally, the systolic pressure in the thigh is similar to that in the brachial artery. An ankle-to-brachial pressure

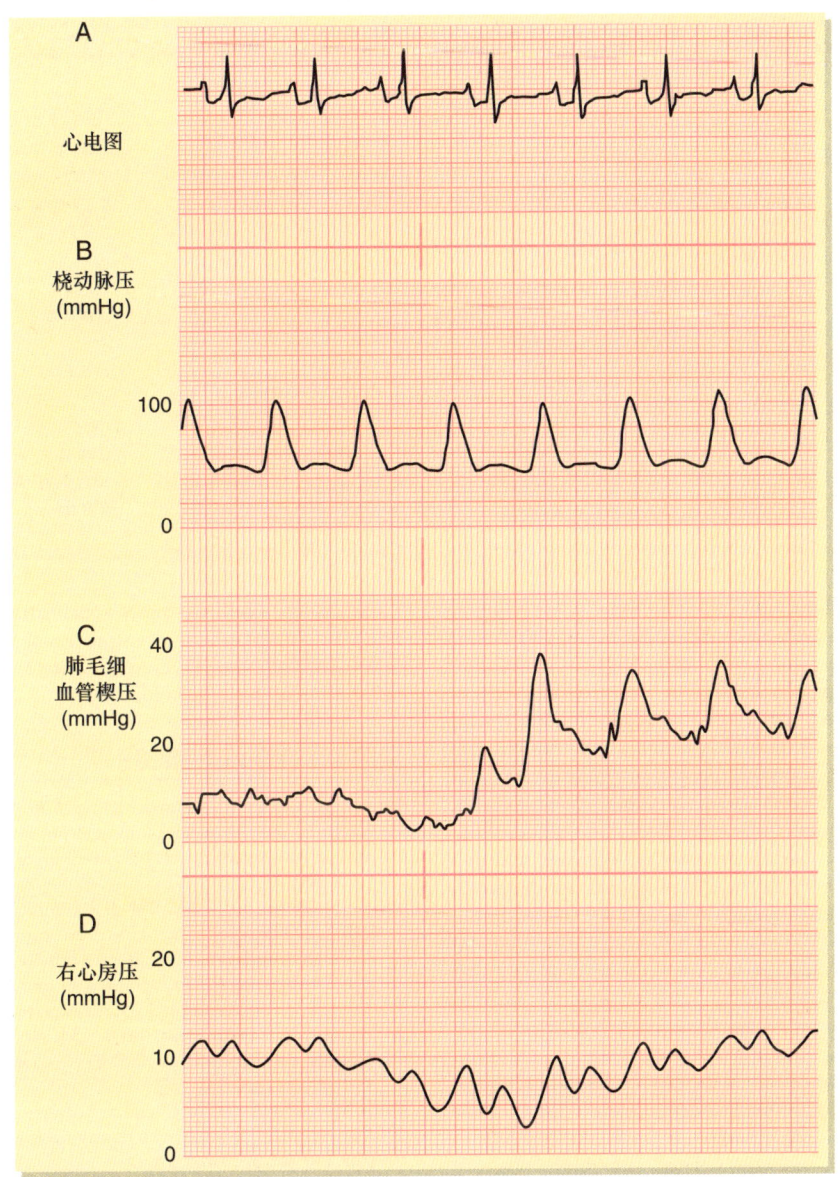

图 3.19 图示为心电图（ECG）（A）和 Swan-Ganz 漂浮导管（C）记录。B 和 D 分别显示桡动脉导管和右心房 Swan-Ganz 漂浮导管的记录。C 曲线的左侧部分是在球囊充盈的情况下获得的，从而得出肺毛细血管楔压。C 曲线的右侧部分是在球囊排气的情况下记录的，显示的是肺动脉压。该患者的肺毛细血管楔压（即左心室充盈压）正常，肺动脉压因肺部疾病而升高

行肺动脉导管置入术后，预后并无改善。当然，无创成像技术的改进使得 Swan-Ganz 导管在诊断心脏疾病（如心脏压塞、缩窄性心包炎、右心室心肌梗死和室间隔缺损）方面的重要性大大降低。因此重症监护病房常规使用 Swan-Ganz 导管的情况有所减少。但是近来这些导管的使用又重新兴起，可能是由于先进的心衰疗法和机械支持治疗的使用增加，而持续的血流动力学监测对于优化治疗至关重要（表 3.5）。

心内膜心肌活检

可对右心室心内膜进行活检。采用这种技术时，通过右颈内静脉将活检钳引入静脉系统，在射线的引导下进入右心室。抓取少量心内膜样本进行组织学评估。心内膜心肌活检的主要适应证是诊断心脏移植后的排斥反应和确诊心肌淀粉样变性；然而，心内膜心肌活检也可用于心肌炎时的特定病原体的诊断。

无创血管检查

评估是否存在周围血管疾病及其严重程度是心血管评估的重要组成部分。比较上下肢的收缩压是检测大动脉疾病血流动力学改变最简单的测试方法之一。正常情况下，踝动脉的收缩压与肱动脉的收缩压相似。

TABLE 3.5 Differential Diagnosis Using a Bedside Balloon Flow-Directed (Swan-Ganz) Catheter

Disease State	Thermodilution Cardiac Output	PCW Pressure	RA Pressure	Comments
Cardiogenic shock	↓	↑	nl or ↓	↑ Systemic vascular resistance
Septic shock (early)	↑	↓	↓	↑ Systemic vascular resistance; myocardial dysfunction can occur late
Volume overload	nl or ↑	↑	↑	
Volume depletion	↓	↓	↓	
Noncardiac pulmonary edema	nl	nl	nl	
Pulmonary heart disease	nl or ↑	nl	↑	↑ PA pressure
RV infarction	↓	↓ or nl	↑	
Pericardial tamponade	↓	nl or ↑	↑	Equalization of diastolic RA, RV, PA, and PCW pressure
Papillary muscle rupture	↓	↑	nl or ↑	Large v waves in PCW tracing
Ventricular septal rupture	↑	↑	nl or ↑	Artifact caused by RA → PA sampling higher in PA than RA; may have large v waves in PCW tracing

nl, Normal; *PA*, pulmonary artery; *PCW*, pulmonary capillary wedge; *RA*, right atrium; *RV*, right ventricle; ↑, increased; ↓, decreased.

ratio (i.e., ankle-brachial index) of less than or equal to 0.9 is abnormal. Patients with claudication usually have an index ranging from 0.5 to 0.8, and patients with rest pain have an index less than 0.5. In some patients, measuring the ankle-brachial index after treadmill exercise may help to determine the importance of borderline lesions. During normal exercise, blood flow increases to the upper and lower extremities with corresponding decreases in peripheral vascular resistance, whereas the overall ankle-brachial index remains unchanged. In the presence of a hemodynamically significant lesion, the reduced flow across the lesions causes a consequent pressure decrease, and as a result, the ankle-brachial index decreases in proportion to the severity of the stenosis. Some patients, especially those with diabetes or chronic kidney disease, may have falsely elevated ankle-brachial indices due to vascular stiffness (>1.3). In these patients, a toe-brachial index can be measured. In general, a toe-brachial index less than 0.6 indicates abnormal perfusion in the foot, though the site of the occlusive disease would have to be identified with further studies.

After significant vascular disease in the extremities has been identified, plethysmography can be used to determine the location and severity of the disease. With this method, a pneumatic cuff is positioned on the leg or thigh, and when inflated, temporarily obstructs venous return. Volume changes in the limb segment below the cuff are converted to a pressure waveform, which can be analyzed. The degree of amplitude reduction in the pressure waveform corresponds to the severity of arterial disease at that level.

Doppler ultrasound uses reflected sound waves to identify and localize stenotic lesions in the peripheral arteries. This test is particularly useful for patients with severely calcified arteries, for whom pneumatic compression is not possible and ankle-brachial indices are inaccurate. In combination with real-time imaging (i.e., duplex imaging), this technique is useful in assessing specific arterial segments and bypass grafts for stenotic or occlusive lesions.

Magnetic resonance angiography and CTA allow high-quality and comprehensive imaging of the entire peripheral arterial circulation in a single study. The three-dimensional nature of these studies and the ability to perform extensive postprocessing views, including cross-sectional views, of all vessels, even those that are very tortuous, are attractive features of these modalities.

SUGGESTED READINGS

Fihn SD, Blakenship JC, Alexander KP, et al: 2014 ACC/AHA/AATS/PCNA/SCAI/STS Focused update of the guideline for the diagnosis and management of patients with stable ischemic heart disease, Circulation 130:1749-1767, 2014.

Kligfield P, Gettes LS, Bailey JJ, et al: Recommendations for the standardization and interpretation of the electrocardiogram: part I: the electrocardiogram and its technology a scientific statement from the American Heart Association Electrocardiography and Arrhythmias Committee, Council on Clinical Cardiology; the American College of Cardiology Foundation; and the Heart Rhythm Society endorsed by the International Society for Computerized Electrocardiology, J Am Coll Cardiol 49:1109-1127, 2007.

Otto CM: Textbook of clinical echocardiography, ed 6, Chapter 2, Normal anatomy and flow patterns on transthoracic echocardiography, Philadelphia, Elsevier, pp. 33-65, 578p.

Rybicki FJ, Udelson JE, Peacock, WF, et al: 2015 ACR/ACC/AHA/AATS/ACEP/ASNC/NASCI/SAEM/SCCT/SCMR/SCPC/SNMMI/STR/STS Appropriate utilization of cardiovascular imaging in emergency department patients with chest pain: a joint document of the American College of Radiology Appropriateness Criteria Committee and the American College of Cardiology Appropriate Use Criteria Task Force, J Am Coll Cardiol 13:e1-e29, 2016.

St. John Sutton M, Morrison AR, Sinusas AJ, Ferrari VA: Heart failure: a companion to braunwald's heart disease, ed 4, Mann DL, Felker GM, editors: Philadelphia, Elsevier Inc, 2019, Chapter 32, Cardiac imaging in heart failure, p.418-448. 739p.

Wolk MJ, Bailey SR, Doherty JU, et al: ACCF/AHA/ASE/ASNC/HFSA/HRS/SCAI/SCCT/SCMR/STS 2013 Multimodality appropriate use criteria for the detection and risk assessment of stable ischemic heart disease, J Am Coll Cardiol 63:380-406, 2014.

表 3.5　使用床旁球囊漂浮（Swan-Ganz）导管进行鉴别诊断

疾病状态	热稀释法心输出量	PCW 压力	RA 压力	注释
心源性休克	↓	↑	nl 或 ↓	↑全身血管阻力
感染中毒性休克（早期）	↑	↓	↓	↑全身血管阻力；晚期可发生心肌功能障碍
容量负荷过度	nl 或 ↑	↑	↑	
容量不足	↓	↓	↓	
非心源性肺水肿	nl	nl	nl	
肺源性心脏病	nl 或 ↑	nl	↑	↑PA 压力
右室心肌梗死	↓	↓ 或 nl	↑	
心脏压塞	↓	nl 或 ↑	↑	均衡的舒张期 RA、RV、PA 和 PCW 压力
乳头肌断裂	↓	↑	nl 或 ↑	PCW 描记曲线出现大 v 波
室间隔穿孔	↑	↑	nl 或 ↑	由于肺动脉压力高于右心房，导管自右心房至肺动脉的压力测量过程中可出现误差；PCW 描记曲线可能出现大 v 波

nl，正常；PA，肺动脉；PCW，肺毛细血管楔（压）；RA，右心房；RV，右心室；↑，上升；↓，下降。

踝臂压比值（即踝臂指数）小于或等于 0.9 即为异常。跛行患者的指数通常在 0.5 至 0.8 之间，而静息性下肢痛患者的指数则小于 0.5。对于某些患者，在跑步机运动后测量踝臂指数可能有助于确定边缘病变的严重程度。正常运动时，上肢和下肢的血流量增加，外周血管阻力相应降低，而总体踝臂指数保持不变。如果存在明显的血流动力学改变，病变处的血流减少会导致压力下降，因此踝臂指数会随狭窄的严重程度成比例地下降。有些患者，尤其是糖尿病或慢性肾病患者，可能会因血管僵硬而导致踝臂指数假性升高（＞1.3）。对于这些患者，可以测量趾臂指数。一般来说，趾臂指数小于 0.6 表示足部灌注异常，但闭塞性病变的部位必须通过进一步检查才能确定。

在确定下肢有明确的血管疾病后，可以使用体积描记法来确定病变的位置和严重程度。这种方法将充气袖带放置在小腿或大腿上，当袖带充气时，静脉回流会暂时受阻。袖带下方肢体的血容量变化会转换成压力波形，并对其进行分析。压力波形的振幅降低程度与该处动脉疾病的严重程度相对应。

多普勒超声利用反射声波来识别和定位外周动脉的狭窄病变。这项检查对动脉严重钙化的患者尤其实用，因为对这些患者无法进行气压检测，且踝臂指数也不准确。结合实时成像（即双相成像），该技术可用于评估特定动脉段和移植旁路的狭窄或闭塞性病变。

通过磁共振血管成像和 CTA，可以在一次检查中对整个外周动脉循环进行高质量的全面成像。这些检查的三维属性以及具备对所有血管（即使是非常迂曲的血管）进行广泛后处理（包括横截面视图）的能力，是其优势。

推荐阅读

Fihn SD, Blakenship JC, Alexander KP, et al: 2014 ACC/AHA/AATS/PCNA/SCAI/STS Focused update of the guideline for the diagnosis and management of patients with stable ischemic heart disease, Circulation 130:1749-1767, 2014.

Kligfield P, Gettes LS, Bailey JJ, et al: Recommendations for the standardization and interpretation of the electrocardiogram: part I: the electrocardiogram and its technology a scientific statement from the American Heart Association Electrocardiography and Arrhythmias Committee, Council on Clinical Cardiology; the American College of Cardiology Foundation; and the Heart Rhythm Society endorsed by the International Society for Computerized Electrocardiology, J Am Coll Cardiol 49:1109-1127, 2007.

Otto CM: Textbook of clinical echocardiography, ed 6, Chapter 2, Normal anatomy and flow patterns on transthoracic echocardiography, Philadelphia, Elsevier, pp. 33-65, 578p.

Rybicki FJ, Udelson JE, Peacock, WF, et al: 2015 ACR/ACC/AHA/AATS/ACEP/ASNC/NASCI/SAEM/SCCT/SCMR/SCPC/SNMMI/STR/STS Appropriate utilization of cardiovascular imaging in emergency department patients with chest pain: a joint document of the American College of Radiology Appropriateness Criteria Committee and the American College of Cardiology Appropriate Use Criteria Task Force, J Am Coll Cardiol 13:e1-e29, 2016.

St. John Sutton M, Morrison AR, Sinusas AJ, Ferrari VA: Heart failure: a companion to braunwald's heart disease, ed 4, Mann DL, Felker GM, editors: Philadelphia, Elsevier Inc, 2019, Chapter 32, Cardiac imaging in heart failure, p.418-448. 739p.

Wolk MJ, Bailey SR, Doherty JU, et al: ACCF/AHA/ASE/ASNC/HFSA/HRS/SCAI/SCCT/SCMR/STS 2013 Multimodality appropriate use criteria for the detection and risk assessment of stable ischemic heart disease, J Am Coll Cardiol 63:380-406, 2014.

Heart Failure and Cardiomyopathy

Daniel J. Levine, Hyeon-Ju Ryoo Ali, Rayan Yousefzai

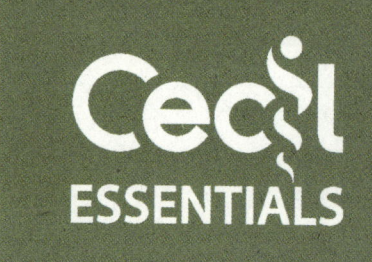

DEFINITION AND CLASSIFICATION

Heart failure (HF) is a clinical syndrome defined by inability of the heart to maintain output under normal filling pressures and/or impairment in relaxation of ventricles causing an increase in filling pressures. Patients experience fatigue and exercise intolerance if cardiac output is low and dyspnea and peripheral edema if the ventricular filling pressure is elevated. There are numerous ways to classify HF—by the type of cardiac impairment, causes of cardiomyopathy, patient's symptoms, or hemodynamic profiles.

Ejection Fraction

Most patients with HF have disorders in both systolic and diastolic function. However, ejection fraction (EF) is an important distinguishing characteristic in most clinical trials and, therefore, in guidelines for therapy. By imaging, cardiac function can be categorized as reduced EF (<40%) or preserved EF (≥50%). Patients with midrange EF (40% to 50%) are treated similarly to patients with reduced EF. HF with reduced EF (HFrEF) is associated with significant morbidity and mortality, especially in the elderly and those with severely low EF (<30%). HF with preserved EF (HFpEF) is less well studied with fewer effective targeted therapies. Increasing awareness of HFpEF has led to recognition of its prevalence with associated morbidity and mortality and the need for more research into optimal management.

Causes

Table 4.1 lists the common causes of cardiomyopathy leading to HF. Ischemic cardiomyopathy is the most common cause of HF and is estimated to account for about 60% of all HF admissions in the United States. This serves as a basis for clinical practice. Patients who present with new cardiomyopathy may undergo cardiac catheterization to exclude underlying coronary artery disease (CAD). Common causes of nonischemic cardiomyopathy include hypertension, chemotherapy, substance use, familial cardiomyopathy, and systemic disorders affecting the heart, such as amyloidosis and hemochromatosis. Worldwide, infections are a common cause of nonischemic cardiomyopathy including Chagas disease (endemic in South America), tuberculosis, and HIV.

Additional nonmyocardial processes that lead to HF include primary pericardial disorders. Pericardial tamponade limits the compliance of the heart, resulting in elevated filling pressures. Other causes include radiation-induced pericarditis, viral pericarditis, postsurgical pericardial thickening, and idiopathic fibrosis of the pericardium.

Valvular pathology including regurgitant and stenotic lesions can also lead to signs and symptoms of HF. Undetected, they can lead to morphologic changes in ventricular size and function. Most studies of HF exclude patients with uncorrected valvular diseases. Diagnosis and treatment of valvular heart disease is reviewed separately (see Chapter 6, "Valvular Heart Disease").

Types of Cardiomyopathy

Historically, cardiomyopathy has been classified morphologically as "dilated," "hypertrophic," and "restrictive." Dilated cardiomyopathy commonly leads to impairment in systolic function, or HFrEF. Common causes of dilated cardiomyopathy include myocardial infarction or infectious myocarditis.

Ventricular hypertrophy causes impairment in relaxation of ventricles, elevated filling pressures, and HFpEF. The most common cause of hypertrophy of ventricles is long-standing hypertension. Older women are at higher risk, as well as patients with diabetes, atrial fibrillation, obesity, hyperlipidemia, and CAD. Hypertrophic cardiomyopathy (HCM) is a genetic disorder in which a mutation in the sarcomeric proteins leads to thickening of ventricles and impaired filling. Patients with known family history of HCM should be tested by genetic analysis; current tests achieve a diagnostic yield of 30% to 60%. More than 130 genes associated with cardiomyopathy and arrhythmias have been identified. Genetic testing should be performed in centers with experienced geneticists and genetic counselors.

Restrictive cardiomyopathy also impairs ventricular relaxation and leads to HFpEF. This type of cardiomyopathy can be due to fibrosis as in radiation heart disease, or deposition of insoluble proteins as in amyloidosis. Restrictive cardiomyopathy is much less common than the other two types.

High-output HF is an under-recognized entity. It is characterized by an increased cardiac output that still fails to meet the metabolic and perfusion demands. Possible causes include obesity, anemia, hyperthyroidism, vitamin B1 deficiency, arteriovenous shunts and liver disease.

Functional Impairment

HF is a clinical syndrome with management strategies targeted to patients' symptoms and function status. Thus, it is paramount to have a unified language to stratify patients' degree of symptoms. Table 4.2 displays two classification methods: the "stages" as defined by the American College of Cardiology Foundation and the American Heart Association (ACCF/AHA) and the "classes" as defined by the New York Heart Association (NYHA).

ACCF/AHA Stages of HF

Patients in ACCF/AHA stage A have risk factors—such as hypertension, diabetes, metabolic syndrome, history of cardiac toxins, and family history of cardiomyopathy—without the diagnosis of CAD or cardiac remodeling. In stage B, patients may have prior history of MI or evidence of cardiomyopathy, but do not have symptoms. Stage C

心力衰竭与心肌病

任景怡 译 石静 审校 郑金刚 通审

定义和分类

心力衰竭（HF，简称心衰）是指心脏在正常充盈压下不能维持射血和（或）心室舒张功能受损导致充盈压升高的临床综合征。心输出量降低时，表现为疲劳和运动不耐受；心室充盈压升高时，表现为呼吸困难和外周水肿。可以根据心脏功能损害类型、心肌病病因、临床症状或血流动力学特征等，对心衰进行分类。

射血分数

大部分心力衰竭患者都存在收缩和舒张功能障碍。在大多数临床试验和治疗指南中，将射血分数（EF）作为一个重要的分类标准。通过影像学检查，心功能可分为射血分数降低（＜40%）和射血分数保留（≥50%）两种类型。射血分数降低的心力衰竭（HFrEF）多伴有高发病率和高死亡率，尤其是在老年人和 EF 严重降低（＜30%）的患者中。对射血分数保留的心力衰竭（HFpEF）研究较少，有效的针对性治疗也较少。随着对 HFpEF 的认识不断加深，有必要对其患病率、发病率、死亡率以及最佳治疗方案进行深入研究。

病因

表 4.1 列出了导致 HF 的常见心肌病病因。缺血性心肌病是 HF 的最常见原因，约占美国所有因 HF 入院人数的 60%，为临床实践的主体。新发心肌病患者可接受心导管检查以排除潜在的冠状动脉疾病（CAD）。非缺血性心肌病的常见原因包括高血压、化疗、药物滥用、家族性心肌病和影响心脏的全身性疾病（如淀粉样变性和血色素沉着病）。在世界范围内，感染是非缺血性心肌病的常见原因，包括恰加斯病（Chagas disease，南美洲流行）、结核病和 HIV 感染。

其他非心肌疾病如原发性心包疾病亦会导致 HF；心脏压塞会限制心脏顺应性，导致充盈压升高；其他原因包括放射性心包炎、病毒性心包炎、术后心包增厚和特发性心包纤维化。

瓣膜病变（包括反流和狭窄病变）也会导致 HF 的体征和症状。如果一直未被检查发现，最终会导致患者心室形态学和功能变化。大多数 HF 研究排除了患有未纠正瓣膜病变患者。心脏瓣膜病的诊断和治疗将单独讨论（见第 6 章"心脏瓣膜病"）。

心肌病的类型

既往心肌病根据形态学分为"扩张型""肥厚型"和"限制型"。扩张型心肌病通常导致收缩功能异常或 HFrEF，其常见原因包括心肌梗死和感染性心肌炎。

心室肥厚会导致心室舒张障碍、充盈压升高和 HFpEF。心室肥厚的最常见原因是长期高血压状态。老年女性、糖尿病、心房颤动、肥胖、高脂血症和 CAD 患者心室肥厚风险更高。肥厚型心肌病（HCM）是一种遗传性疾病，其肌节蛋白突变会导致心室增厚和充盈受损。有 HCM 家族史的患者应接受基因检测分析，基因检测诊断率可达 30%～60%。目前已发现 130 多个与心肌病和心律失常相关的基因，基因检测应在拥有经验丰富的遗传学家和遗传咨询师的中心进行。

限制型心肌病引起心室舒张功能异常并导致 HFpEF。这种类型的心肌病可能是由于纤维化（如放射性心脏病）或不溶性蛋白质沉积（如淀粉样变性）引起。限制型心肌病较其他两种类型少见得多。

高心输出量性心力衰竭是一种尚未被充分认识的疾病，其特征是心输出量增加，但仍不能满足代谢和灌注需求，其可能的原因包括肥胖、贫血、甲状腺功能亢进、维生素 B_1 缺乏、动静脉分流和肝脏疾病。

功能障碍

HF 是一种临床综合征，需要根据患者的不同症状和功能采取相应的治疗策略。因此，最重要的是确定一种统一的标准对患者的症状程度进行分层。表 4.2 列出了两种分类方法：美国心脏病学会基金会和美国心脏协会（ACCF/AHA）定义的"分期"和纽约心脏协会（NYHA）定义的"分级"。

心力衰竭的 ACCF/AHA 分期

ACCF/AHA A 期患者有高血压、糖尿病、代谢综合征、心脏毒性物质使用病史和心肌病家族史等危险因素，但未确诊为 CAD 或心脏重塑。B 期患者可能有心肌梗死病史或心肌病证据，但无症状。C 期患者

TABLE 4.1	Causes of Cardiomyopathy
Myocardial infarction
Infection
HIV
Lyme
Chagas
Viral myocarditis
Tuberculosis
Iatrogenic
Chemotherapy: bleomycin, doxorubicin (Adriamycin)
Antiretroviral medications
Radiation
Phenothiazines
Chloroquine
Clozapine
Toxins
Alcohol
Cocaine
Methamphetamines
Cobalt, lead, lithium, mercury, carbon monoxide, beryllium
Endocrine and metabolic
Thyroid dysfunction
Thiamine deficiency
Pellagra
Hypophosphatemia, hypocalcemia, uremia
Inflammatory
Systemic lupus erythematosus
Scleroderma
Rheumatoid arthritis
Giant cell arteritis
Kawasaki disease
Infiltrative cardiomyopathy
Amyloidosis
Sarcoidosis
Hemochromatosis
Other structural
Valvular disease: progressive stenosis or regurgitation, acute chordae tendineae rupture, thrombosis of replaced valve
Infective endocarditis
Takotsubo cardiomyopathy
Idiopathic dilated cardiomyopathy
Idiopathic restrictive cardiomyopathy
Peripartum cardiomyopathy
Arrhythmogenic right ventricular dysplasia
Congenital heart disease
Fabry disease
Danon disease
Friedreich's ataxia
Myotonic dystrophy
Duchenne-Becker muscular dystrophy
Rhythm
Tachy-mediated cardiomyopathy
Pacing-mediated cardiomyopathy

constitutes clinical signs and symptoms of HF, while stage D encompasses patients whose HF is refractory to appropriate therapy.

NYHA Functional Classification of HF

The NYHA classification characterizes functional impairment of patients in symptomatic HF (ACCF/AHA stages C and D). Class I patients are asymptomatic with ordinary activity and may also fall under stage B. Patients in class II have *some* limitation at *moderate* levels of physical activity while patients in class III have *any* limitations at *mild* levels of activity. Patients with symptoms at rest are categorized as class IV.

Hemodynamic Profiles

The impact of HF on circulatory physiology can be broadly categorized into four groups based on the degree of impairment of cardiac output and elevation of filling pressures (Fig. 4.1). Reduced cardiac output (cardiac index, CI ≤2.2 L/min/m^2) leads to impairment in end-organ perfusion. Patients may complain of fatigue, dizziness, or diminished urine output. On physical exam, extremities are cool due to low cardiac output and the compensatory vasoconstriction of the capillary beds to maintain perfusion. This finding helps identify the "cold" patients in the low-output state.

Elevated filling pressures can cause hydrostatic pressure to increase beyond the oncotic pressure, leading to extravasation of fluid into the interstitial space. Fluid may be retained in the lungs causing dyspnea, in the gut causing loss of appetite or nausea, and in the extremities causing peripheral edema.

Most patients who present in acute HF exacerbation are "warm and wet." Despite elevated filling pressures and congestion, they are still adequately perfused and can be treated with diuresis without hemodynamic support. "Cold and wet" patients are further decompensated. They require inotropic support to maintain adequate blood pressures and to perfuse the kidneys and permit effective diuresis. Some patients, despite diuresis, may remain in a poor perfusion state due to underlying cardiac disease. These patients are "cold and dry" and may require advanced therapies that will be described later.

PATHOPHYSIOLOGY

Frank-Starling Law

Under normal conditions, an increase in preload, or left ventricular end-diastolic pressure (LVEDP), increases stroke volume, as described by the Frank-Starling law (Fig. 4.2). In HF, the low cardiac output triggers an adaptive neurohormonal response that is designed to increase preload and stroke volume. However, due to the depressed myocardial contractility, the same increase in preload does not lead to increase in stroke volume or cardiac output. The consequence is dysregulation of an adaptive mechanism that leads to excessive filling pressures and fluid retention. Treatment consists of augmenting stroke volume by reducing afterload and increasing myocardial contractility with an inotrope. Diuresis can also reduce LVEDP, filling pressures, and congestive symptoms. Treatment of decompensated HF is discussed further in the section titled "Diagnosis and Management of Acute Decompensation."

Adaptive Neurohormonal Response

Our understanding of HF has changed over the years. It is no longer sufficient to consider morphologic characteristics or hemodynamic profiles of this clinical syndrome. HF is a clinical syndrome marked by sympathetic activation and neurohormonal dysregulation. The neurohormonal dysregulation and adaptive response are important targets for HF management strategies.

In response to low cardiac output, the sympathetic nervous system is triggered, releasing epinephrine and norepinephrine. The adrenalins increase heart rate and cause ventricular relaxation. They also trigger the G-coupled receptor pathways, increasing cyclic adenosine monophosphate (cAMP) production. Increased cAMP concentration leads to calcium influx and augments myocardial contractility.

In the kidneys, the juxtaglomerular cells in afferent arterioles sense decreased blood flow and in turn release renin. The consequent activation of the renin-angiotensin-aldosterone system (RAAS) is a cascade

表 4.1 心肌病病因
心肌梗死
感染
艾滋病
莱姆病
恰加斯病
病毒性心肌炎
结核病
医源性
化疗：博来霉素、多柔比星（阿霉素）
抗逆转录病毒药物
放射
吩噻嗪类
氯喹
氯氮平
毒性物质
酒精
可卡因
甲基苯丙胺
钴、铅、锂、汞、一氧化碳、铍
内分泌和代谢
甲状腺功能障碍
硫胺素缺乏症
糙皮病
低磷血症、低钙血症、尿毒症
炎症性疾病
系统性红斑狼疮
硬皮病
类风湿关节炎
巨细胞动脉炎
川崎病
浸润性心肌病
淀粉样变性
结节病
血色素沉着病
其他结构性
瓣膜疾病：进行性狭窄或关闭不全、急性腱索断裂、置换瓣膜血栓形成
感染性心内膜炎
应激性心肌病
特发性扩张型心肌病
特发性限制型心肌病
围产期心肌病
致心律失常性右心室发育不良
先天性心脏病
法布里病
达农（Danon）病
弗里德赖希（Friedreich）共济失调
肌强直性营养不良
进行性假肥大性肌营养不良症
心律失常性心肌病
心动过速介导性心肌病
起搏介导性心肌病

伴 HF 的临床体征和症状，而 D 期 HF 患者对适当治疗无效。

心力衰竭的 NYHA 心功能分级

NYHA 心功能分级描述了有症状 HF 患者的功能障碍（ACCF/AHA C 和 D 期）。Ⅰ级患者在日常活动时无症状，也可能属于 B 期。Ⅱ级患者在中等程度体力活动中会受限，而Ⅲ级患者在轻度活动时即受限。静息时有症状的患者被归类为Ⅳ级。

血流动力学特征

根据心输出量受损程度和充盈压升高程度，HF 对循环生理的影响大致可分为四类（图 4.1）。心输出量减少 [心脏指数，$CI \leq 2.2 \, L/(min \cdot m^2)$] 会导致终末器官灌注受损。患者可能会出现疲劳、头晕或尿量减少等症状。体格检查时，由于心输出量减少，毛细血管床代偿性血管收缩以维持灌注，患者可出现四肢发凉的症状。这一表现有助于识别低心输出量状态下的"冷"患者。

充盈压升高可引起静水压超过胶体渗透压，从而导致液体渗出到组织间隙。液体滞留在患者肺部引起呼吸困难，滞留在消化道会引起食欲不振或恶心，滞留在四肢则引起外周水肿。

大多数心力衰竭急性加重的患者都处于"湿暖"状态。尽管循环生理上表现为充盈压升高、充血，但血流灌注仍然充足，可以利尿治疗而无需血流动力学支持。"湿冷型"患者会进一步失代偿，需要正性肌力支持来维持足够的血压和肾脏灌注，同时进行有效的利尿治疗。有些患者尽管进行了利尿治疗，但由于潜在的心脏疾病，仍可能处于灌注不良状态。这些患者"干冷"，可能需要采用稍后介绍的高阶治疗。

病理生理学

Frank-Starling 定律

正常情况下，前负荷或左心室舒张末期压力（LVEDP）增加可增加每搏输出量，如 Frank-Starling 定律所述（图 4.2）。HF 患者心输出量降低会触发适应性神经激素反应，从而增加前负荷和每搏输出量。然而，由于心肌收缩力减弱，前负荷增加不会导致每搏输出量或心输出量相应增加，引起适应性机制失调，最终导致充盈压过高和液体潴留。其治疗包括降低后负荷以增加每搏输出量和使用强心剂增加心肌收缩力。利尿也可以降低 LVEDP、充盈压以及缓解充血症状。失代偿性 HF 的治疗将在"急性失代偿心衰的诊断和治疗"一节中进一步讨论。

适应性神经激素反应

多年来，我们对 HF 的理解发生了变化。仅仅考虑这种临床综合征的形态学特征或血流动力学特征已远远不够。HF 是一种以交感神经激活和神经激素失调为特征的临床综合征。神经激素失调和适应性反应是 HF 管理策略的重要目标。

当心输出量减少时，交感神经系统会被触发，释放肾上腺素和去甲肾上腺素。肾上腺素会增加心率，引起心室松弛。同时会触发 G 偶联受体通路，增加环磷酸腺苷（cAMP）的产生。cAMP 浓度增加会导致钙内流，增强心肌收缩力。

在肾脏中，入球小动脉中的肾小球旁细胞感知到血流减少，进而释放肾素。随后，肾素-血管紧张素-醛固酮系统（RAAS）被激活，这是一系列酶级联反

TABLE 4.2 ACCF/AHA Stages and NYHA Functional Classification of HF

ACCF/AHA Stages		NYHA Functional Classification	
A	Risk factors for HF without cardiomyopathy or HF symptoms	None	
B	Cardiomyopathy without HF symptoms	I	No HF symptoms
C	Cardiomyopathy with HF symptoms	I	No HF symptoms
		II	Some HF symptoms with moderate activity
		III	Any HF symptoms with mild activity
		IV	HF symptoms at rest
D	HF refractory to medical therapy	IV	HF symptoms at rest

ACCF, American College of Cardiology Foundation; *AHA*, American Heart Association; *HF*, heart failure; *NYHA*, New York Heart Association. Data from Yancy CW, Jessup M, Bozkurt B, et al: 2013 ACCF/AHA guidelines for the management of heart failure: a report of the American College of Cardiology Foundation/American Heart Association Task Force on Practice Guidelines, *J Am Coll Cardiol* 62:e147-e239, 2013.

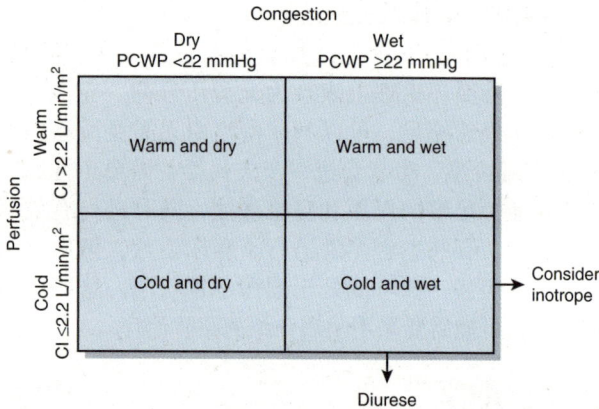

Fig. 4.1 Assessment of hemodynamic profiles in patients with heart failure. *CI*, Cardiac index; *PCWP*, pulmonary capillary wedge pressure. (Modified from Thibodeau JT, Drazner MH. The role of the clinical examination in patients with heart failure. JACC Hear Fail. 2019;6(7):544-551. https://doi.org/10.1016/j.jchf.2018.04.005.)

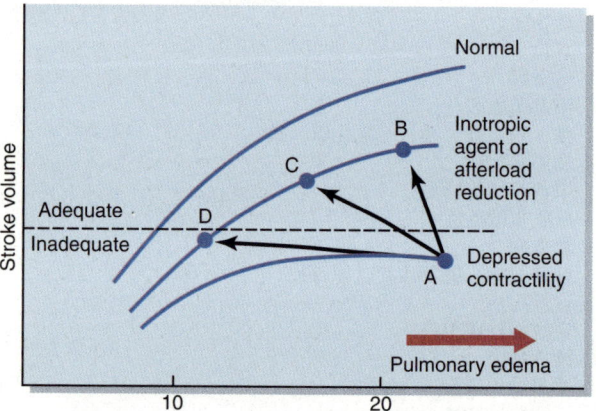

Fig. 4.2 Frank-Starling curve. Pulmonary edema occurs when the left ventricular end-diastolic pressure (LVEDP) is elevated such that hydrostatic pressures in pulmonary vasculature exceed oncotic pressures. For most patients, this threshold is approximately LVEDP = 20 mm Hg. Diuresis or venodilation reduces the filling pressures and can shift patients along the same curve correlating with lower LVEDP. Inotropic agents or afterload reduction can improve the cardiac output and improve stroke volume, shifting the pressure-volume curve upwards and to the left, moving patients from point A to point B. Adding diuresis or venodilation can shift patients from point A to point C. Excessive diuresis or venodilation shifting from point A to point D may cause excessive decline in LVEDP. While these patients may be at lower risk of pulmonary edema, their stroke volume may be impaired and result in inadequate cardiac output.

of enzyme activity that promotes end-organ perfusion by vasoconstriction, fluid retention at the level of the kidneys, and increased fluid intake by stimulating thirst.

Over time, these mechanisms become dysregulated. The adrenalins augment chronotropy and inotropy, which increase wall stress and myocardial oxygen consumption. Angiotensin II causes vasoconstriction that places the myocardium under higher afterload. Initially, cardiac muscles become hypertrophied to compensate for the workload; however, ventricles eventually dilate and lose contractility. Aldosterone also exacerbates ventricular remodeling, leading to progressive decline in cardiac function and loss of myocytes with subsequent fibrosis in a process known as apoptosis.

Atrial natriuretic peptide and brain natriuretic peptide (BNP) are counterregulatory hormones that are released in response to myocardial stress. They promote natriuresis and arterial vasodilation. Neprilysin degrades BNP and thereby inhibits the counterregulatory mechanism and inhibits natriuresis. This pathway is the target of novel drug therapies described in the section titled "Guideline-directed Medical Therapy."

DIAGNOSIS AND MANAGEMENT OF ACUTE DECOMPENSATION

Patients with HF frequently experience acute decompensation. Careful history and exam, as well as laboratory and imaging findings can help distinguish HF from other causes of dyspnea, such as chronic obstructive pulmonary disease (COPD) exacerbation or pneumonia.

History
Symptoms
HF is a clinical diagnosis. Thus, presenting symptoms, exam findings, and patients' response to HF treatments help establish the diagnosis.

Most patients with HF exacerbation present with dyspnea. Patients may also experience orthopnea (shortness of breath while lying flat) or paroxysmal nocturnal dyspnea or PND (waking up with shortness of breath) due to redistribution of fluid from the periphery to the lungs. Orthopnea and PND are specific for HF (specificity = 74% to 77% for orthopnea and 80% to 84% for PND) and can help discriminate among different etiologies for dyspnea.

Elevation of venous pressures (preload to the right ventricle) cause symptoms of systemic venous congestion. Patients may complain of

表 4.2　心力衰竭的 ACCF/AHA 分期及 NYHA 功能分级

ACCF/AHA 分期		NYHA 功能分级	
A	有心衰危险因素，但无心肌病或心衰症状	无	
B	无心衰症状的心肌病	I	无心衰症状
C	伴心衰症状的心肌病	II	活动轻度受限。中等程度活动可引起心衰症状
		III	活动明显受限。轻度活动即引起心衰症状
		IV	静息时即有心衰症状
D	药物难治性心衰	IV	静息时即有心衰症状

ACCF，美国心脏病学会基金会；AHA，美国心脏协会；HF，心力衰竭；NYHA，纽约心脏协会
数据来自 Yancy CW, Jessup M, Bozkurt B, et al: 2013 ACCF/AHA guidelines for the management of heart failure: a report of the American College of Cardiology Foundation/American Heart Association Task Force on Practice Guidelines, J Am Coll Cardiol 62: e147-e239, 2013.
译者注：原表右列 C 期对应 NYHA 功能分级有误。

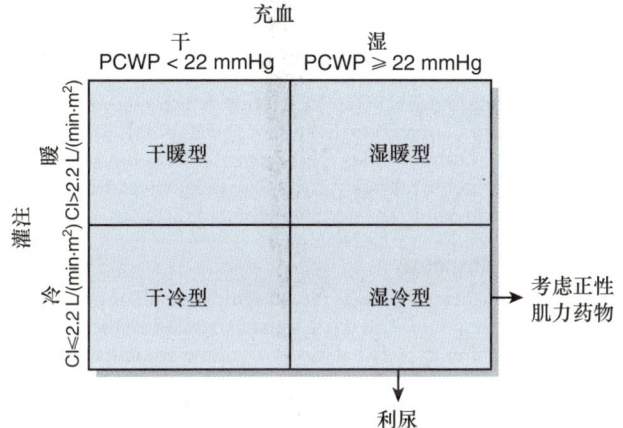

图 4.1　心力衰竭患者血流动力学特征评估。CI，心脏指数；PCWP，肺毛细血管楔压［修改自 Thibodeau JT, Drazner MH. The role of the clinical examination in patients with heart failure. JACC Hear Fail. 2019；6（7）：544-551. https://doi.org/10.1016/j.jchf.2018.04.005.］

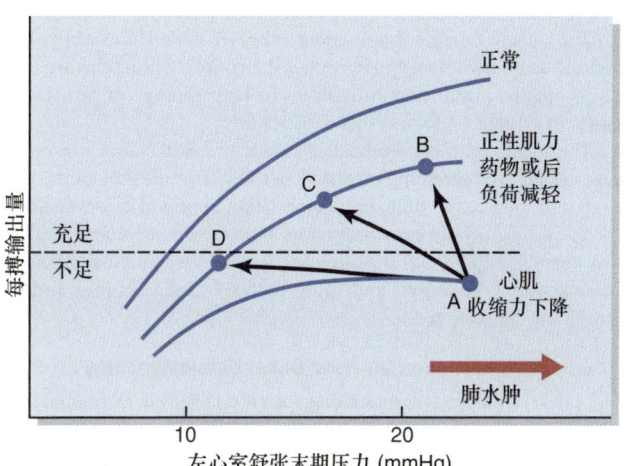

图 4.2　Frank-Starling 曲线。当左心室舒张末期压力（LVEDP）升高，导致肺血管的静水压超过充盈压时，即会发生肺水肿。对于大多数患者，该阈值约为 LVEDP = 20 mmHg。使用利尿剂或扩张静脉可降低充盈压，并可使患者沿着与 LVEDP 降低相关的同一曲线移动。正性肌力药物或减轻后负荷可改善心输出量并增加每搏输出量，使压力-容积曲线向上向左移动，从 A 点移动至 B 点。增加利尿或扩张静脉可从 A 点转移至 C 点。过度利尿或扩张静脉将从 A 点转移到 D 点，可能导致 LVEDP 过度下降。虽然这些患者发生肺水肿的风险较低，但他们的每搏输出量可能受损并导致心输出量不足

应，通过血管收缩促进终末内脏器官灌注，在肾脏水平形成液体潴留，并通过刺激口渴症状来增加液体摄入量。

随着时间的推移，这些机制会失调。肾上腺素通过增强心肌变时性和变力性，从而增加壁张力和心肌氧耗量；血管紧张素 II 导致血管收缩，使心肌承受更高的后负荷；最初，心肌肥大以代偿工作负荷的增加，然而，心室最终扩张且收缩力下降；醛固酮加剧心室重塑，导致心脏功能逐步下降，心肌细胞逐渐丢失，随后在细胞凋亡的过程中发生纤维化。

心房利钠肽和脑利钠肽（BNP）是响应心肌应激而释放的反调节激素。它们促进排钠和动脉血管舒张。脑啡肽酶降解 BNP，从而抑制反调节机制并抑制排钠。该途径是"指南指导的药物治疗"部分中描述的新型药物治疗的靶标。

急性失代偿心衰的诊断和治疗

心衰患者经常出现急性失代偿。详细的病史和体格检查，以及实验室和影像学检查结果有助于鉴别心衰与其他原因导致的呼吸困难（如慢性阻塞性肺疾病加重或肺炎）。

病史

症状

心衰是一种临床诊断。因此，症状体征、检查结果和患者对心衰治疗的反应有助于确定诊断。

大多数心衰加重患者表现为呼吸困难。由于液体从外周重新分布到肺部，患者也可能出现端坐呼吸（平躺时呼吸困难）、阵发性夜间呼吸困难（PND，因呼吸困难而憋醒）。端坐呼吸和 PND 对心衰诊断是特异性的（端坐呼吸特异性为 74%～77%；PND 特异性为 80%～84%），可以帮助鉴别不同病因的呼吸困难。

静脉压（右心室前负荷）升高会导致全身静脉充血症状。患者可能出现由于肠道水肿引起的食欲减退、

decreased appetite, nausea, and abdominal fullness from intestinal edema of the gut. Transudation of fluid into the abdominal compartment may cause ascites and increased abdominal girth. Many patients complain of leg swelling or inability to fit into their shoes. Asking patients about sudden weight gain (e.g., 2-3 lb in a few days or 5 lb in a week) can also help assess the degree of fluid accumulation and identify targets for therapy.

Patients with inadequate cardiac output due to HF experience fatigue, exercise intolerance, or presyncope. Reduced end-organ perfusion can lead to altered mental status and diminished urine output. These symptoms are important clues to the hemodynamic profile of the patient and are critical for determining their need for inotropic support.

Precipitating Factors for Acute HF Exacerbation

Acute HF exacerbation may result from a new-onset primary cardiac dysfunction or decompensation of known chronic HF due to noncardiac causes. Cardiac dysfunction causes of acute HF exacerbation include acute myocardial infarction, other primary nonischemic cardiomyopathy, conduction disorders, valvular pathology, or pericardial issues (see Table 4.1 for a comprehensive list).

The most common noncardiac causes of heart failure exacerbation are diet indiscretion (increased salt intake or alcohol consumption) and medication noncompliance. Other common causes include infections (e.g., viral upper respiratory tract infection) or acute blood loss anemia. High blood pressure can also increase afterload acutely, increase filling pressures, and cause reduced cardiac output and/or worsening congestion.

Additional Information for New-Onset Cardiomyopathy

Once heart failure exacerbation diagnosis is established, additional history elements can help determine cause of cardiomyopathy. Questions should be focused on symptoms and risk factors of coronary artery disease, given that myocardial infarction is the most common cause of cardiomyopathy in the United States. Other helpful information includes past medical history including valvular disease, arrhythmias, autoimmune diseases, congenital heart disease, cancer, radiation, or cardiotoxic therapy, such as anthracycline derivatives. Social history should include duration and quantity of alcohol intake and cocaine use. Symptoms suggestive of other systemic disorders affecting the heart, such as neuropathy in amyloidosis, may be helpful and relevant for treatment options. Family history may be important in cases such as early-onset coronary artery disease, autoimmune disorders, congenital heart disease, and familial cardiomyopathies.

Exam Findings

Exam findings should be focused on signs of elevated filling pressures and reduced cardiac output to establish the diagnosis of heart failure. Other exam maneuvers not reviewed here include those relevant to myocardial ischemia, valvular disease, and arrhythmias that are reviewed in Chapters 6, 7, and 8.

Edema, JVD, and HJR

Elevated filling pressures in the heart are detected by several physical exam cues. Pulmonary auscultation may demonstrate rales, rhonchi, or even wheezing. Edema may be found in the lower extremities, but also in the abdomen in the form of ascites.

Jugular venous distension (JVD) is assessed with the patient situated at 30 to 45 degrees and breathing quietly. The vertical distance between the sternal notch and top of the JVD meniscus is the jugular venous height to which 5 cm should be added for true central venous pressure (normal range = 5-9 cm H_2O). Hepatojugular reflux (HJR) is elevation of filling pressures by more than 3 cm H_2O while compressing the right upper quadrant for at least 10 seconds. Valvular disease, specifically tricuspid regurgitation, may falsely elevate the JVD meniscus and make these exam findings less reliable.

Cardiac Examination: S_3 and S_4

The point of maximal impulse (PMI) may be displaced (below the fifth intercostal space and lateral to the midclavicular line) suggestive of cardiomegaly. On auscultation of the heart, a third heart sound (S_3) may be heard in early diastole. The sound is the result of blood passively traveling from the atrium into an already filled ventricle. This is typically associated with left ventricular systolic dysfunction and incomplete ejection of blood during systole. S_4 is heard in late diastole and results from the atrial kick pushing the remaining fluid into a stiffened ventricle. S_4 suggests diastolic dysfunction.

Bendopnea

Bendopnea is a recently described simple stress maneuver that can be used if the aforementioned exams are not helpful in discriminating among the many causes of dyspnea. Patients are asked to bend forward while sitting in a chair for 30 seconds, which increases filling pressures. Patients may develop dyspnea or "bendopnea," particularly if they have a low cardiac index. This maneuver has been associated with increased 6-month mortality, composite end point of death, heart failure–related admission, and need for advanced therapies.

Square Wave Response

Another stress maneuver to assess the left ventricular filling pressure is the square wave response. This is particularly useful when the JVD and HJR are limited due to body habitus or tricuspid regurgitation. The blood pressure cuff is inflated to the point of hearing the first Korotkoff sound. Then the patient is asked to Valsalva (i.e., bear down) in order to reduce the preload and decrease pulmonary venous return to the left ventricle. In normal patients, the Korotkoff sound disappears due to a drop in blood pressure. In patients with pulmonary congestion, the pulmonary intravascular volume maintains forward flow during Valsalva, and the Korotkoff sound remains the same. The persistence of Korotkoff sound, therefore, is a positive test and is suggestive of elevated left ventricular pressures and pulmonary congestion.

Laboratory Data and Imaging

Patients who have symptoms and signs concerning for acute heart failure exacerbation should all receive an electrocardiogram (ECG) and a chest radiograph. An ECG may show evidence of new ischemia or old infarct suggesting MI as the potential cause for cardiomyopathy. A chest radiograph may demonstrate signs of pulmonary edema, such as Kerley B lines and pleural effusions (Fig. 4.3). The BNP is often elevated, although it is neither sensitive nor specific. In fact, BNP is most useful for its negative predictive value. A low BNP (or NT-pro-BNP) can exclude HF in patients with combined cardiopulmonary disease who present acutely with dyspnea. The troponin may be elevated in acute myocardial infarction or demand ischemia. Laboratory testing should include a basic metabolic panel to establish baseline electrolytes and kidney function. The liver function test results help assess the degree of congestion and cardiohepatic syndrome. The complete blood count can give clues to the etiology, such as leukocytosis in the setting of acute infection or anemia.

All patients with new-onset heart failure should have an echocardiogram. It may reveal wall motion abnormalities consistent with CAD, valvular stenosis or regurgitation, or pericardial effusion. Ventricular wall thickness and chamber sizes can also be assessed. Thickened ventricles may raise concerns for genetic hypertrophic cardiomyopathy,

恶心和腹胀等症状；液体漏入腹腔可引起腹水和腹围增大；许多患者出现腿部水肿或无法穿鞋等症状。询问患者近期体重突然增加的情况［如几天内增重 2～3 磅（0.91～1.36 kg）或 1 周内增重 5 磅（2.27 kg）］也有助于评估液体潴留的程度并确定治疗目标。

心衰引起心输出量不足的患者会出现疲劳、运动不耐受或晕厥前期等症状。终末内脏器官灌注减少可导致精神状态改变和尿量减少。这些症状是了解患者血流动力学特征的重要线索，也是确定患者是否需要正性肌力药物支持的关键。

急性心衰加重的诱发因素

急性心衰加重可由新发的原发性心功能障碍或非心脏原因引起已知慢性心衰失代偿诱发。心功能障碍导致急性心衰加重的原因包括急性心肌梗死、其他原发性非缺血性心肌病、传导障碍、瓣膜病和心包疾病（见表 4.1）。

心衰加重最常见的非心脏原因是饮食不当（盐摄入量或酒精摄入量增加）和不遵医嘱服药。其他常见原因包括感染（如病毒性上呼吸道感染）或急性失血性贫血。高血压还可急性增加后负荷，增加充盈压力，导致心输出量减少和（或）使充血加重。

新发心肌病的其他信息

一旦心衰加重的诊断确定，其他病史因素可以帮助确定心肌病的病因。鉴于心肌梗死是美国最常见的心肌病原因，应重点关注冠状动脉疾病的症状和危险因素。其他有用的信息包括既往史，如心脏瓣膜病、心律失常、自身免疫性疾病、先天性心脏病、癌症、放疗或有心脏毒性药物（如蒽环类药物衍生物）的治疗史。社会史应包括酒精摄入以及可卡因的使用及持续时间和剂量。其他影响心脏的全身性疾病的症状（如淀粉样变性的神经病变）有助于治疗方案的选择。家族史在早发性冠状动脉疾病、自身免疫性疾病、先天性心脏病和家族性心肌病等病例中很重要。

体格检查结果

体格检查应侧重于充盈压升高和心输出量减少的体征上，以确定心衰的诊断。其他未在此概述的检查技巧（包括与心肌缺血、心脏瓣膜病和心律失常相关的检查技巧）在第 6、7 和 8 章概述。

水肿、颈静脉怒张和肝颈静脉回流征

心脏充盈压升高的体征可通过几种体格检查检测到。如肺听诊可表现为湿啰音、干啰音，甚至哮鸣音。水肿可出现在下肢，也可出现在腹部，表现为腹水。

评估颈静脉怒张（JVD）时患者应取 30°～45° 半卧位，保持平静呼吸。胸骨切迹与 JVD 液柱的弯月面之间的垂直距离为颈静脉高度，再加上 5 cm 即为真正的中心静脉压（正常范围 = 5～9 cmH$_2$O）。肝颈静脉回流征（HJR）是指在压迫腹部右上象限至少 10 s 的同时，颈静脉压力升高 3 cmH$_2$O 以上。心脏瓣膜病，特别是三尖瓣反流，可能会假性升高 JVD 液柱的弯月面，从而使检查结果的可靠性降低。

心脏体格检查：S_3 和 S_4

心尖搏动点（PMI）的移位（位于第 5 肋间隙下方和锁骨中线外侧）提示心脏肥大。心脏听诊可在舒张早期闻及第三心音（S_3），这种声音由血液被动地从心房进入已经充盈的心室产生。这通常与左心室收缩功能障碍和收缩期不完全射血有关。在舒张后期可闻及 S_4 心音，这是由于心房将剩余的血液推入僵硬的心室所致，S_4 提示舒张功能不全。

俯身呼吸困难

如果前面提到的检查不能帮助鉴别呼吸困难的原因，俯身呼吸困难是新近描述的一种简单且易于使用的压力操作。患者需坐在椅子上且身体保持前倾 30 s，该动作增加了充盈压。患者可能出现呼吸困难或"俯身呼吸困难"，特别是当他们的心脏指数较低时。该操作与 6 个月死亡率、复合死亡终点、心力衰竭相关入院以及对高阶治疗的需求增加有关。

方波响应

另一种评估左心室充盈压的应力操作是方波响应，尤其是当 JVD 和 HJR 由于体型或三尖瓣反流的存在而影响评估时尤为有用。将血压袖带充气至能听到第一个 Korotkoff 音，然后要求患者进行 Valsalva 动作（如蹲下），以减少前负荷，减少肺静脉血液回流至左心室。在正常患者中，Korotkoff 音会因血压下降而消失。在肺淤血患者中，肺血管内容积在 Valsalva 期间保持向前流动，Korotkoff 音保持不变。因此，持续的 Korotkoff 音是一个阳性的测试结果，提示左心室压力升高和肺淤血。

实验室和影像学检查

有急性心衰加重症状和体征的患者都应接受心电图和胸片检查。如果心电图发现新发的缺血或陈旧的心肌梗死，提示心肌梗死是心肌病的潜在病因。胸片可显示肺水肿征象，如 Kerley B 线和胸腔积液（图 4.3）。BNP 指标常升高，尽管它既不敏感也不具有特异性。事实上，BNP 最有价值的是其阴性预测值。低 BNP（或 NT-proBNP）可排除表现为急性呼吸困难的合并心肺疾病患者的心衰。肌钙蛋白可在急性心肌梗死或心肌缺血时升高。实验室检查应包括基本代谢检查，以确定基线电解质和肾功能情况。肝功能检查结果有助于评估充血程度和肝心综合征。全血细胞计数可以提示病因，如急性感染时的白细胞增多或贫血。

所有新发心衰患者都应做超声心动图检查。它可能显示 CAD 时的室壁运动异常、瓣膜狭窄、反流或心包积液，心室壁厚度和腔室大小也具有评估价值。心室增厚应引起对遗传性肥厚型心肌病、长期高血压性

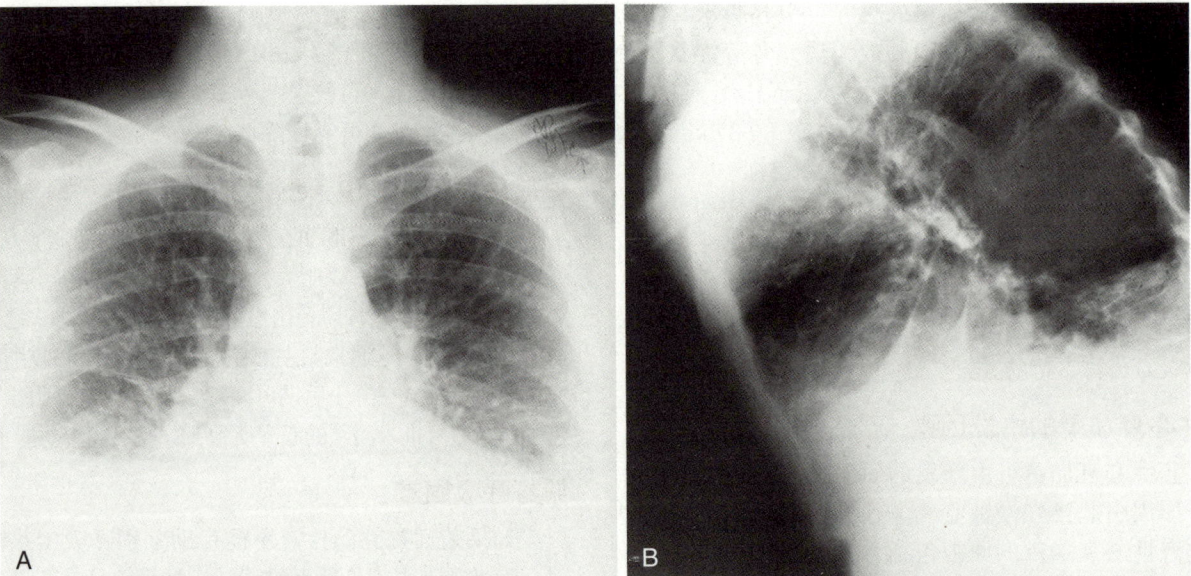

Fig. 4.3 (A) Posteroanterior chest radiograph demonstrating pulmonary edema. Notice the increased interstitial markings, more prominent in central zones, and Kerley B lines, which are horizontal markings at the lung periphery. There is also a prominent horizontal line in left lung, suggestive of fluid layering in the major fissure. Both costovertebral angles are obscured, suggesting bilateral pulmonary effusion. (B) Lateral chest radiograph demonstrating pulmonary edema. Fluid is layering in the lower lung zones suggestive of pulmonary effusion.

long-standing hypertension hypertrophic heart, or infiltrative disease such as amyloidosis (Fig. 4.4). Newer techniques including strain imaging can be used to evaluate for infiltrative disease as well as early changes due to toxic chemotherapeutic agents.

Additional Testing to Determine Etiology

Appropriate patients with symptoms, signs, ECG, and/or troponin results concerning for myocardial infarction causing heart failure exacerbation should undergo coronary angiography and revascularization. Some patients presenting with new heart failure diagnosis have a history of coronary artery disease but do not have typical anginal symptoms. For these patients, the Surgical Treatment for Ischemic Heart Failure (STITCH) trials demonstrated that myocardial viability assessment with nuclear stress testing does not, in fact, improve mortality. However, the ACCF/AHA 2013 guidelines make weak recommendations to obtain noninvasive imaging such as nuclear stress test or stress echocardiogram prior to proceeding with revascularization. Evidence of ischemia and significant myocardial viability may be one of the factors to be considered for catheterization.

If the above work-up is negative, additional testing for nonischemic cardiomyopathy can be pursued. A cardiac MRI can reveal specific patterns of enhancement that are indicative of infiltrative disorders (e.g., cardiac amyloidosis and sarcoidosis). Additional laboratory testing may include thyroid function test, human immunodeficiency virus (HIV) test, iron studies, and hepatitis C virus antibodies.

Prompt recognition and work-up for cardiac amyloidosis has become more important as novel therapies have become available that are important to initiate early in the disease progression. Features concerning for amyloidosis include low voltage on ECG, left ventricular hypertrophy, and evidence of other organ manifestation such as gastrointestinal symptoms (diarrhea, nausea), neuropathy, and chronic kidney disease. Laboratory testing should include levels of serum and urine protein electrophoresis (SPEP and UPEP) along with serum and/or urine immunofixation. Imaging techniques include echocardiography, specifically strain imaging that tends to spare the apex, and nuclear imaging called pyrophosphate (PYP) scan. The latter is sensitive and specific for transthyretin, or wild-type amyloidosis. Definitive diagnosis is achieved with direct visualization of the amyloid deposits in tissue samples. Biopsy can be done on the abdominal fat pad, cardiac muscle, rectal mucosa, salivary gland, and liver.

Right heart catheterization is another diagnostic tool for assessment of acute HF exacerbation. The routine use of pulmonary artery catheters (PACs) for patients with HF exacerbation has not been shown to improve mortality, length of stay, or rehospitalization rates (the Evaluation Study of Congestive Heart Failure and Pulmonary Artery Catheterization Effectiveness, ESCAPE). The ACCF/AHA 2013 guidelines still recommend use of PACs with patients who do not respond to standard therapies and when there is a degree of uncertainty regarding the patient's volume status despite routine clinical assessment. Right heart catheterization is also used to estimate cardiac output, assess candidacy for advanced therapy, and perform cardiac biopsy.

Acute Management
Diuresis

The mainstay treatment for acute HF exacerbation is intravenous (IV) loop diuretics. Intravenous administration of diuretics should be equal to or exceed the dose of home oral medications. Oral diuretics may be less effective in this setting due to bowel edema which can impair absorption via the gut. Diuresis should be targeted toward symptom management, improvement in vital signs, resolution of acute kidney injury (AKI), change in weight, and net output of urine. Some patients with prolonged diuretic use can develop resistance to loop diuretics. These patients may benefit from thiazide administration to block fluid reabsorption in the distal convoluted tubules. Patients who do not respond to maximal diuretic regimen can be considered for ultrafiltration.

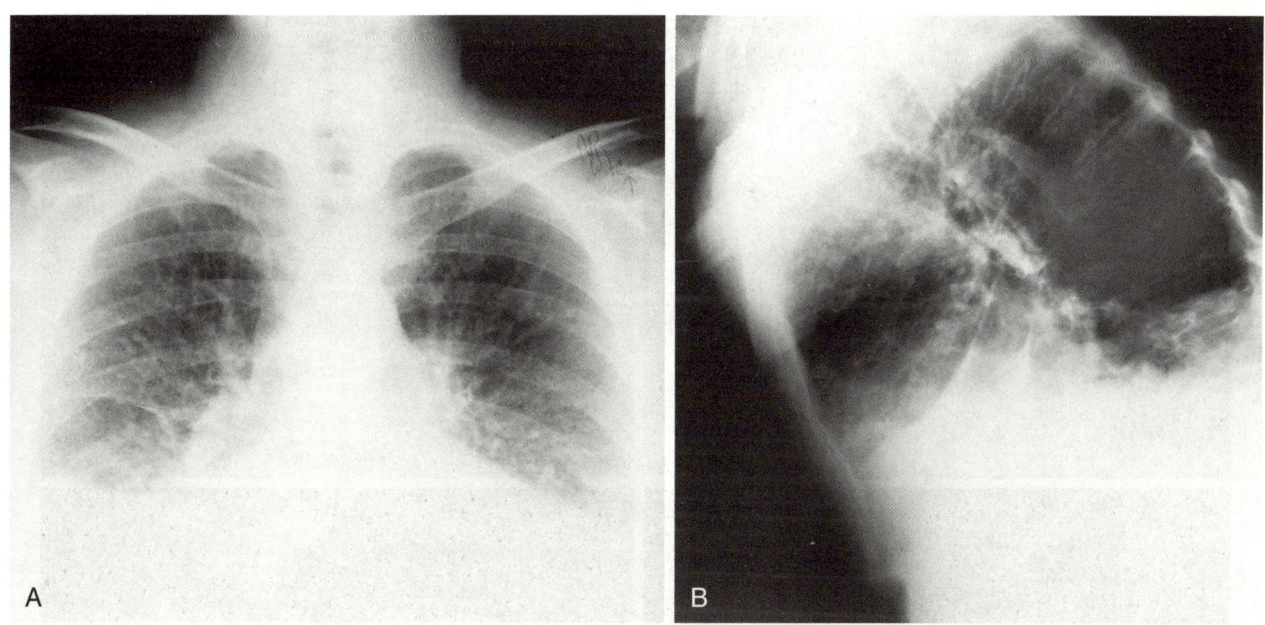

图4.3 （A）后前位胸片显示肺水肿。可见肺间质纹理增多，在中央区域更为明显，以及 Kerley B 线，它们是肺边缘的水平纹理。左肺也有一条明显的水平线，提示肺大裂中有液体分层。两侧肋脊角均不清晰，提示双侧肺积液。（B）侧位胸片显示肺水肿。下肺区域有液体分层，提示有胸腔积液

心脏肥厚或浸润性疾病（如淀粉样变性）的关注（图4.4）。包括应变成像在内的新技术可用于评估浸润性疾病以及由毒性化疗药物引起的早期心脏变化。

确定病因的补充检查

症状、体征、心电图和（或）肌钙蛋白结果提示心肌梗死为心衰加重病因的患者应接受冠状动脉造影和血运重建术。一些新诊断为心衰的患者有冠状动脉疾病史，但没有典型的心绞痛症状。对于这些患者，缺血性心力衰竭的外科治疗（Surgical Treatment for Ischemic Heart Failure, STITCH）试验表明，通过核素负荷试验评估存活心肌来指导治疗，实际上并不能改善死亡率。然而，ACCF/AHA 2013 指南仍推荐在进行血运重建术之前进行无创成像检查，如负荷核素试验或负荷超声心动图，但推荐级别较低。如发现心肌缺血和心肌明显存活的证据，可能是需要考虑行心脏导管检查的因素之一。

如果上述检查为阴性，可以进行非缺血性心肌病的其他检查。心脏 MRI 可以显示浸润性疾病的特定强化模式（如心脏淀粉样变性和结节病）。其他的实验室检查可能包括甲状腺功能检查、人类免疫缺陷病毒（HIV）检测、铁检测和丙型肝炎病毒抗体检测。

随着新的治疗方法的出现，及时对心脏淀粉样变性识别和检查变得越来越重要，因为早期启动新型疗法对控制疾病进展至关重要。淀粉样变性的特征包括心电图低电压、左心室肥厚和其他器官表现，如胃肠道症状（腹泻、恶心）、神经病变和慢性肾病。实验室检测应包括血清和尿蛋白电泳（SPEP 和 UPEP）水平以及血清和（或）尿液免疫固定电泳。成像技术包括超声心动图，特别是倾向于保留心尖的应变成像，以及称为焦磷酸盐（PYP）扫描的核成像。后者对转甲状腺素蛋白或野生型淀粉样变性具有敏感性和特异性，组织样本中观察到淀粉样蛋白沉积可明确诊断。可在腹部脂肪垫、心肌、直肠黏膜、唾液腺和肝脏进行活检。

右心导管检查是评估急性心衰加重的另一种诊断工具。对于心衰加重患者常规使用肺动脉导管（PAC）并未被证明可以改善死亡率、住院时间或再住院率（充血性心力衰竭和肺动脉导管有效性评估研究：ESCAPE）。ACCF/AHA 2013 指南仍然推荐对标准治疗无反应的患者以及尽管进行了常规临床评估，但患者的容量状况仍存在一定程度的不确定性时使用 PAC。右心导管检查也用于评估心输出量，评估患者是否应进行高阶治疗以及心脏活检。

急性期管理

利尿

急性心衰加重的主要治疗是静注（IV）袢利尿剂。静脉给予利尿剂应等于或超过家庭口服药物的剂量。口服利尿剂在这种情况下可能效果较差，因为肠道水肿会影响肠道内药物的吸收。利尿剂应针对症状管理、改善生命体征、缓解急性肾损伤（AKI）、改变体重和净排尿量来给予。一些长期使用利尿剂的患者会对其产生耐药性，这些患者可能从处方噻嗪类药物中获益，以阻断远曲小管的液体重吸收。对最大化利尿方案无反应的患者可考虑超滤治疗。

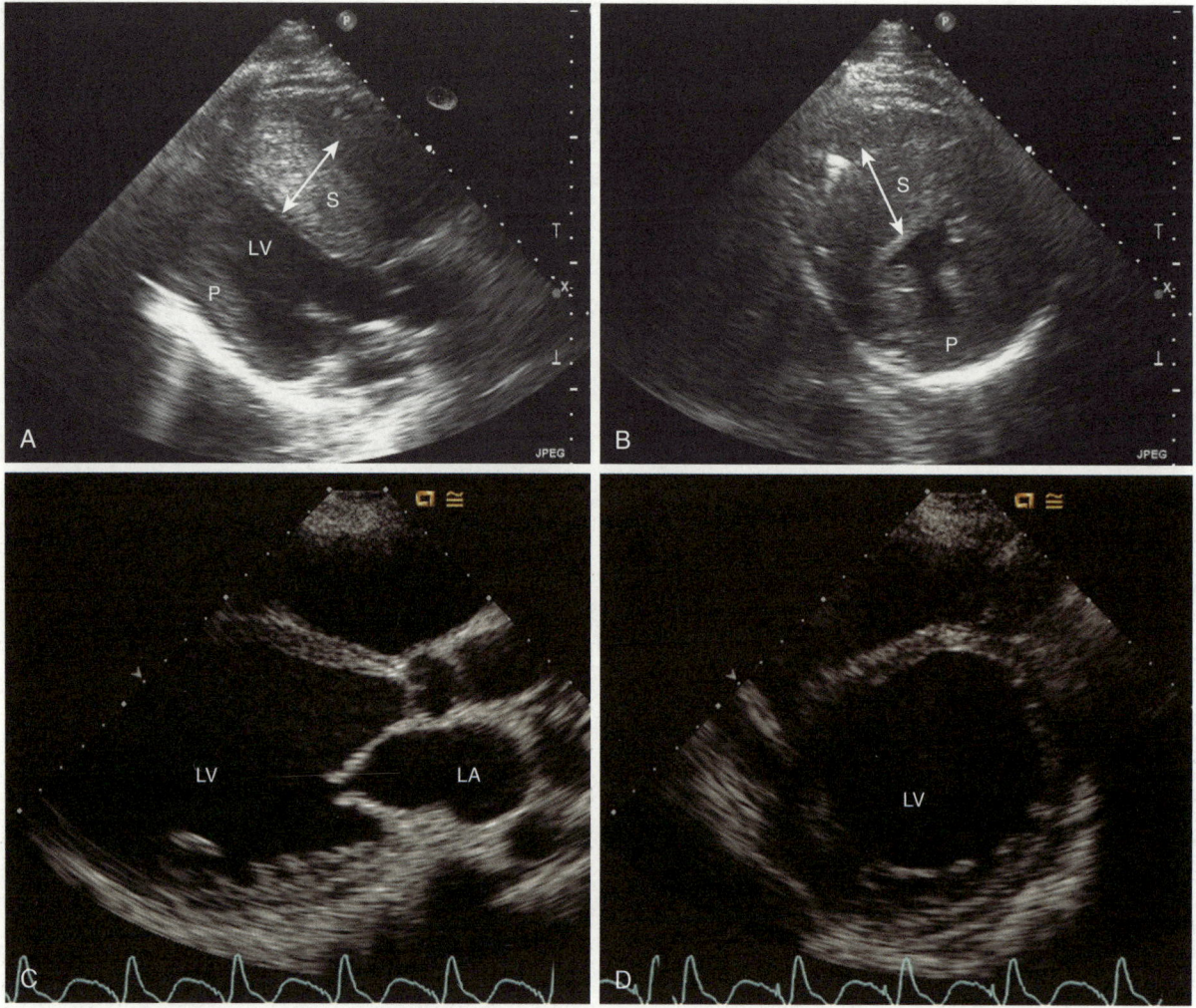

Fig. 4.4 Examples of hypertrophic cardiomyopathy on (A) long axis view and (B) short axis view. The posterior wall "P" and interventricular septum, "S" are markedly thickened. Examples of dilated cardiomyopathy on (C) long axis view and (D) short axis view. The left ventricular cavity "LV" and left atrium "LA" are enlarged.

Afterload Reduction

Patients may be hypertensive in the setting of HF exacerbation. Acutely lowering the blood pressure can quickly reduce the afterload, lower ventricular filling pressures, and reduce the degree of pulmonary vascular congestion. Patients in respiratory distress may experience prompt relief of their symptoms with afterload reduction. Intravenous therapy options for acute afterload reduction include nitroglycerin, nitroprusside, and nesiritide.

Cardiogenic Shock Management

Some patients in acute HF exacerbation present in "cold" hemodynamic profiles and have significantly reduced cardiac output. These patients may require inotropic support for end-organ perfusion. The use of inotropes can improve perfusion of kidneys and patients' response to diuresis. More information regarding the different types of inotropes and their use is detailed in the section titled "Inotropic Support."

Guideline-Directed Medical Therapy

In the current age, the goal in heart failure therapy is to not only control symptoms and slow progression of disease, but also to recover some cardiac function. New pharmacotherapies have become available that not only improve functional status but lower mortality and reduce hospitalizations. Thus, it is imperative to understand and follow guideline-directed medical therapy (GDMT) for all patients with HF (Fig. 4.5).

All patients with HF should be advised to make lifestyle modifications to reduce the risk of development or progression or cardiac disease. Blood pressure control, weight loss, and management of diabetes can significantly reduce the risk of CAD and ventricular remodeling. Patients with any stage of heart failure, regardless of whether they have symptoms, should be treated with ACE inhibitors or aldosterone receptor II blockers (ARBs), as well as statins if there is evidence of coronary artery disease or the atherosclerotic cardiovascular disease (ASCVD) risk score is greater than 7.5%.

For patients with HFrEF stage C (i.e., patients with any symptoms), several medications have been shown to reduce mortality and improve quality of life. All patients should be treated with specific β-blockers known to improve mortality in HFrEF patients, as well as a medication for afterload reduction (ACE inhibitors, ARBs, or angiotensin receptor blocker–neprilysin inhibitors, i.e., ARNIs). The other therapies described in the following sections have been proven effective for only certain subpopulations.

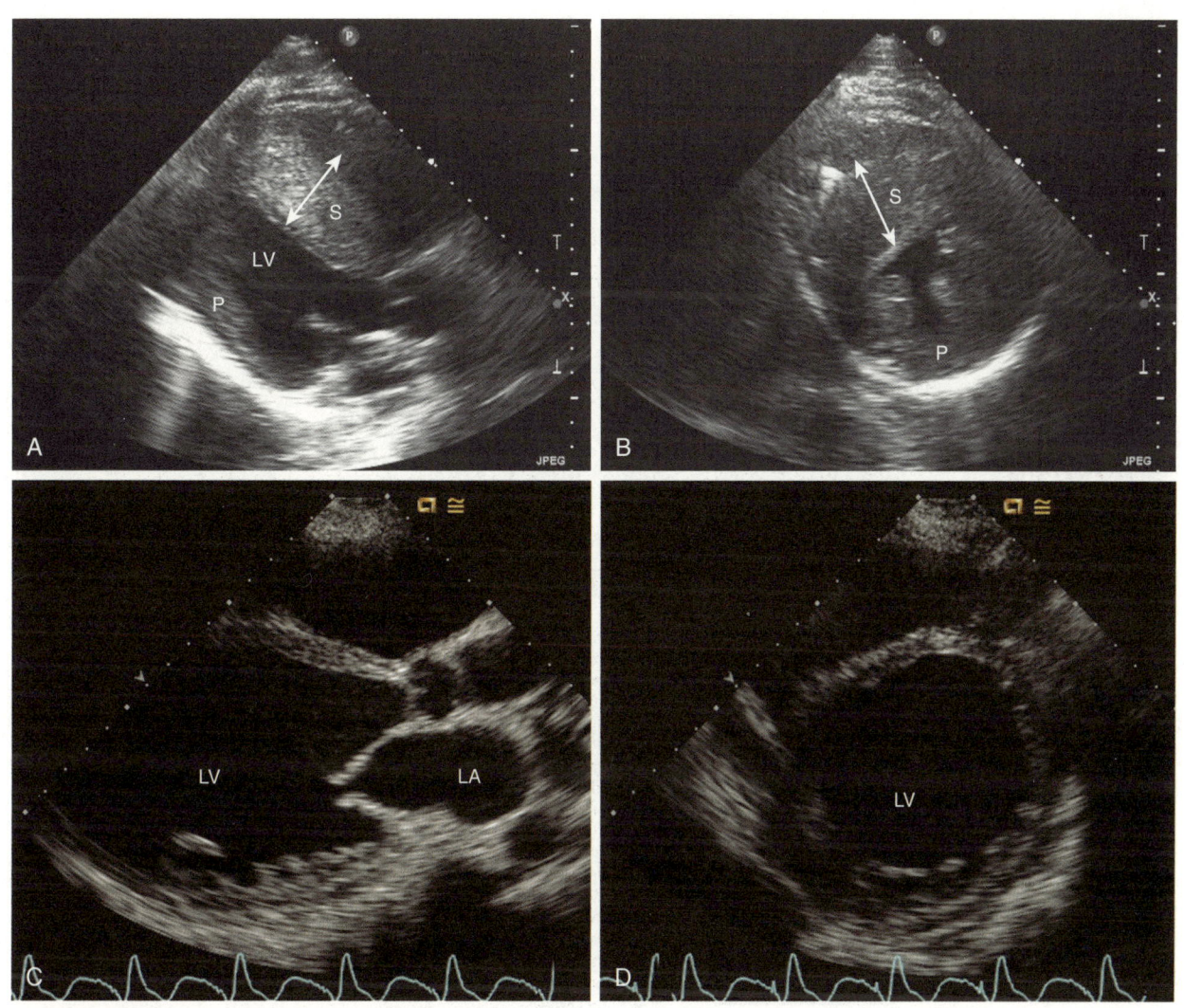

图 4.4　肥厚型心肌病的示例。（A）长轴视图和（B）短轴视图。后壁"P"和室间隔"S"明显增厚。扩张型心肌病的示例：（C）长轴视图和（D）短轴视图。左室腔"LV"和左心房"LA"增大

降低后负荷

在心衰加重的情况下，患者可能处于高血压状态。急性降压治疗可迅速减小后负荷，降低心室充盈压力，减轻肺血管充血程度。呼吸窘迫患者可因后负荷降低而迅速缓解症状，急性降低后负荷的静脉治疗包括硝酸甘油、硝普钠和奈西立肽等选择。

心源性休克的处理

一些心衰急性加重的患者表现为"冷型"血流动力学特征，心输出量明显减少。这些患者可能需要正性肌力支持来维持终末内脏器官灌注。使用正性肌力药物可以改善肾脏灌注和患者对利尿的反应。更多关于不同类型的正性肌力药物及其使用的详细信息，请参阅"正性肌力药物支持"部分。

指南指导的药物治疗

如今，心衰治疗的目标不仅是控制症状和延缓疾病的进展，而且还需恢复一定的心脏功能。新的药物疗法不仅改善了心脏功能，而且降低了死亡率和住院率。因此，了解并遵循指南指导的药物治疗（GDMT）对所有心衰患者至关重要（图 4.5）。

应建议所有心衰患者改变生活方式，以降低心脏病发生或进展的风险。控制血压、减轻体重和控制糖尿病可以显著降低冠心病和心室重构的风险。任何阶段的心衰患者，无论是否有症状，都应接受 ACE 抑制剂（ACEI）或血管紧张素Ⅱ受体阻滞剂（ARB）（译者注：原文醛固酮受体有误）治疗，如果有证据表明冠状动脉疾病或动脉粥样硬化性心血管疾病（ASCVD）风险评分大于 7.5%，也应接受他汀类药物治疗。

对于 HFrEF C 期患者（即有症状的患者），已证明某几种药物可降低死亡率并改善生活质量。所有患者应接受可改善 HFrEF 患者死亡率的特定 β 受体阻滞剂治疗，以及降低后负荷药物（ACEI、ARB 或血管紧张素受体阻滞剂-脑啡肽酶抑制剂，即 ARNI）。以下章节中描述的其他治疗方法已被证明仅对某些心衰人群有效。

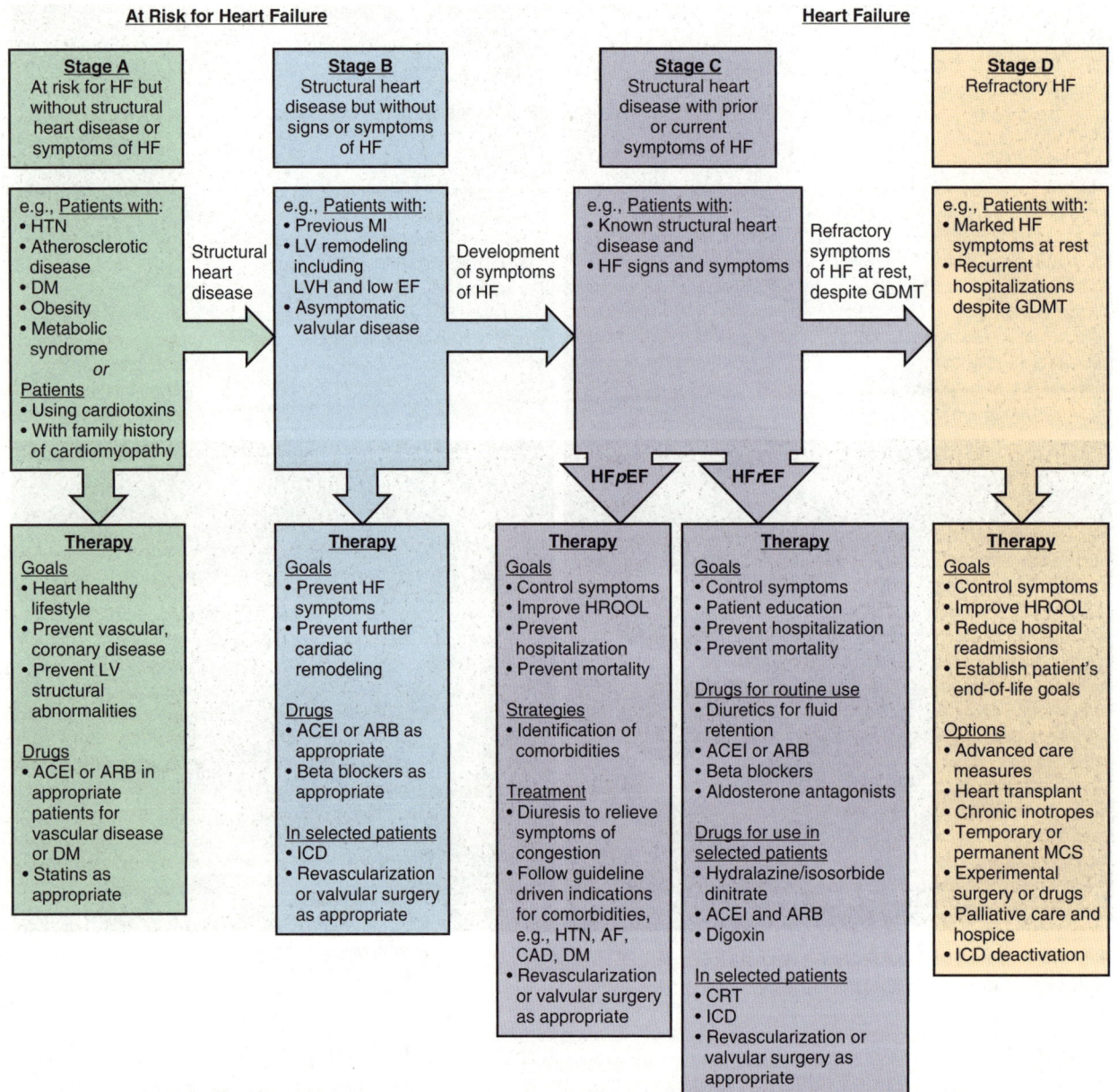

Fig. 4.5 Clinical overview by HF stage A-D. *ACEI*, Angiotensin-converting enzyme inhibitor; *AF*, atrial fibrillation; *ARB*, angiotensin receptor blocker; *CAD*, coronary artery disease; *CRT*, cardiac resynchronization therapy; *DM*, diabetes mellitus; *EF*, ejection fraction; *GDMT*, guideline-directed medical therapy; *HF*, heart failure; *HRQOL*, health-related quality of life; *HTN*, hypertension; *ICD*, implantable cardiac defibrillator; *LV*, left ventricular; *LVH*, left ventricular hypertrophy; *MCS*, mechanical circulatory support. (Adapted from ACCF/AHA 2013 Guidelines.)

ACE Inhibitor, ARB, and ARNI

All patients with stage C HFrEF, regardless of symptom burden, should be on an ACE inhibitor, an ARB, or an ARNI. By inhibiting RAAS, ACE inhibitors and ARBs reduce afterload and inhibit fibrosis. Multiple trials from the 1980s to the early 2000s including CONSENSUS, SOLVD, Val-HeFT, and CHARM demonstrated an improvement in mortality (by 16% to 40%) and reduced hospitalizations for HF exacerbations in patients treated with ACE inhibitors or ARBs.

The ARNI is a novel medication that combines the ARB, valsartan, with a neprilysin inhibitor called sacubitril. Neprilysin is an endopeptidase that breaks down vasoactive peptides such as BNP and bradykinin. By inhibiting neprilysin, the sacubitril promotes the action of the BNP, which increases diuresis. In the PARADIGM randomized controlled trial (RCT) ARNIs were found to be superior to ACE inhibitors (number needed to treat, NNT = 21 for composite end point of HF admissions or mortality). The PIONEER study also demonstrated ARNIs could be safely started during hospitalization and readmission due to HF exacerbations. The 2017 American College of Cardiology and American Heart Association (ACC/AHA) updates to the guidelines recommend patients on ACE inhibitors or ARBs should be

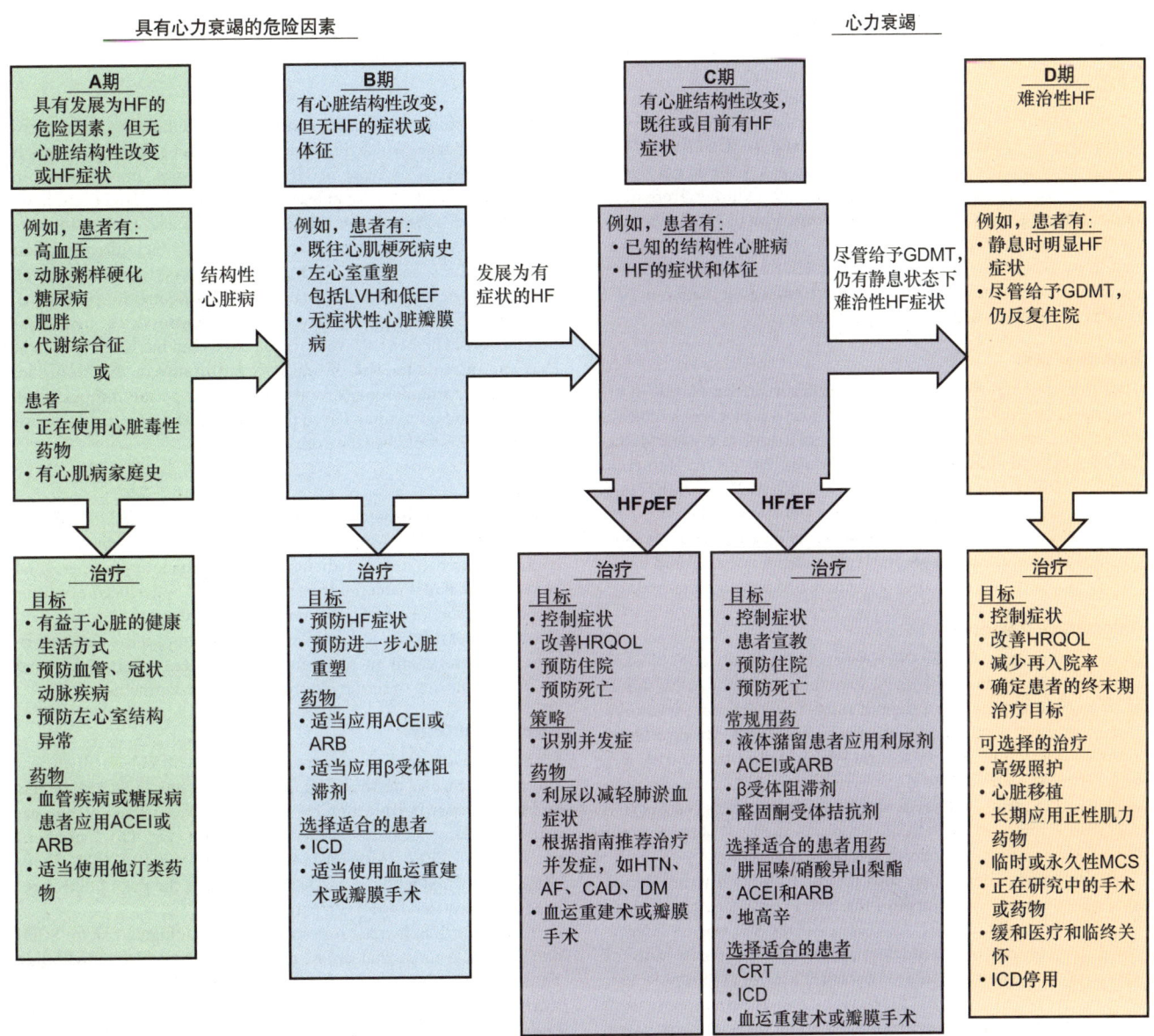

图 4.5 心衰 A～D 期临床概况。ACEI, 血管紧张素转换酶抑制剂; AF, 心房颤动; ARB, 血管紧张素受体阻滞剂; CAD, 冠状动脉疾病; CRT, 心脏再同步化治疗; DM, 糖尿病; EF, 射血分数; GDMT, 指南指导的药物治疗; HF, 心力衰竭; HRQOL, 健康相关生活质量; HTN, 高血压; ICD, 植入式心脏复律除颤器; LVH, 左心室肥厚; MCS, 机械循环支持（改编自 ACCF/AHA 2013 Guidelines.）

ACEI、ARB 和 ARNI

所有 C 期 HFrEF 患者，无论症状负担如何，都应服用 ACEI、ARB 或 ARNI。通过抑制 RAAS，ACEI 和 ARB 能够减小后负荷，抑制纤维化。从 20 世纪 80 年代到 21 世纪初，包括 CONSENSUS、SOLVD、Val-HeFT 和 CHARM 在内的多项试验表明，在接受 ACEI 或 ARB 治疗的患者中，死亡率得到改善（16%～40%），因心衰加重的住院率降低。

ARNI 是一种新型药物，结合了 ARB（缬沙坦）和一种名为沙库巴曲的脑啡肽酶抑制剂。脑啡肽酶是一种内肽酶，可分解血管活性肽，如 BNP 和缓激肽。通过抑制脑啡肽酶，沙库巴曲促进 BNP 的作用（沙库巴曲增加 BNP 活性），从而增加利尿。在随机对照试验（RCT）PARADIGM 研究中发现，ARNI 优于 ACEI（HF 入院或死亡的复合终点，需治人数 NNT = 21）。PIONEER 研究还表明，ARNI 可在住院期间和因心衰加重而再次入院时安全地开始使用。2017 年美国心脏病学会和美国心脏协会（ACC/AHA）更新了指南，建议服用 ACEI 或 ARB 的患者应改用 ARNI。服用 ACEI 的患者在停用 ACEI 后应有 36 h 的洗脱期，以避免缓激肽蓄积引起的血管性水肿。

包括 PEP-CHF、CHARM-preserved 和 I-PRESERVE 在内的几项随机对照试验研究了 ACEI 和 ARB 对 HFpEF

switched to ARNIs. Patients on ACE inhibitors should have a washout period of 36 hours after ACE inhibitors are discontinued to avoid angioedema secondary to bradykinin accumulation.

The therapeutic potential of ACE inhibitors and ARBs for the HFpEF patient population has been investigated by several RCTs, including PEP-CHF, CHARM-preserved, and I-PRESERVE. These studies unfortunately showed ACE inhibitors and ARBs do not significantly reduce cardiovascular mortality or heart failure exacerbations in this patient group. The Prospective Comparison of ARNI with ARB Global Outcomes in HFpEF (PARAGON-HF) also demonstrated no significant risk reduction of mortality or HF-related hospitalizations for ARNIs. Guidelines currently do not recommend initiation of ACE inhibitors, ARBs, or ARNIs for HFpEF patients.

Beta-Blockers

The three types of β-blockers found to be effective in Stage C HFrEF are bisoprolol, carvedilol, and metoprolol succinate. β-Blockers inhibit the sympathetic nervous system, reduce myocardial work, improve endothelial integrity, and ultimately reduce ventricular remodeling. Numerous studies—MERIT-HF, CAPRICORN, COPERNICUS, COMET, and CIBIS-II—have demonstrated a significant reduction in mortality (31% to 40%) and the composite end point of mortality and heart failure exacerbation admissions. The trials on HFpEF patients are small and inadequately powered, but many show a trend toward improving mortality.

Aldosterone Antagonist

Patients with stage C HFrEF, NYHA class II-IV already on β-blockers and afterload reduction with an ACE inhibitor, ARB, or ARNI should be started on aldosterone receptor antagonists assuming creatinine clearance greater than 30 and normal potassium levels. The direct inhibition of aldosterone further reduces ventricular fibrosis and remodeling. The RALES trial showed a 30% reduction in all-cause mortality, sudden cardiac death, and HF hospitalizations for patients with NYHA class II-IV symptoms. EMPHASIS-HF also showed a 37% reduction in the composite end point of death and HF readmissions.

Patients with HFpEF may also benefit from aldosterone receptor antagonists. The Treatment of Preserved Cardiac Function Heart Failure with an Aldosterone Antagonist (TOPCAT) was an international, placebo-controlled, randomized study for patients with EF 45% or greater. The study showed a small effect size of spironolactone reducing HF hospitalizations (12.0% vs. 14.2%). However, subsequent analyses showed a significant regional variation, suggesting that North American participants may have been more compliant with the medications and likely may have derived greater benefit.

Ivabradine

Patients with symptomatic HFrEF (stage C, NYHA class II-IV) with high resting heart rate (≥70 beats per minute) despite treatment with a high dose of β-blocker may benefit from the addition of ivabradine. Ivabradine works by inhibiting I_f—the "funny channel"—at the sinus node. The SHIFT trial demonstrated that patients in NYHA II-IV class with EF 35% or less already on GDMT treated with ivabradine experienced a 5% absolute risk reduction in heart failure exacerbations and 2% absolute reduction in cardiovascular mortality.

Hydralazine and Nitrates

Vasodilators such as hydralazine and nitrates reduce afterload, myocardial work, and in theory, reduce ventricular remodeling. Their efficacy, however, has only been shown among African Americans with HFrEF stage C and NYHA III-IV symptoms already on GDMT. For patients with HFpEF, nitrates have been shown to improve exercise tolerance but do not improve mortality (NEAT-HFpEF, 2015). The ACC/AHA 2017 updates to the guidelines do not yet recommend vasodilators for HFpEF patients.

Digoxin

Digoxin increases myocardial contractility by inhibiting sodium-potassium exchange, which increases intracellular calcium. Digoxin is associated with a decrease in HF hospitalizations, improvement in quality of life, and increase in exercise tolerance. The DIG trials, however, showed no impact on mortality. Digoxin also has an unfavorable side effect profile. It can cause arrhythmias (ectopic, re-entrant cardiac rhythms, and heart block), GI side effects (nausea, anorexia), and neurologic side effects (visual effects, disorientation, confusion). Patients who are elderly and have low body mass index or renal dysfunction are at higher risk. Many medications can increase the digoxin level and increase the risk of toxicity (clarithromycin, erythromycin, itraconazole, amiodarone, dronedarone, cyclosporine, propafenone, verapamil, and quinidine). Given these risks and benefits, patients with stage C HFrEF could benefit from digoxin.

Diuretics

For patients with chronic heart failure, diuretics are used to maintain euvolemia and target symptom management. Loop diuretics are most commonly used, but some patients develop resistance over time. Distal convoluted tubules become hypertrophied and water becomes reabsorbed past the loop of Henle, reversing the effect of loop diuretics. Small doses of thiazide and metolazone, which impact the distal nephrons, can significantly increase diuresis. Their use requires close and careful monitoring of serum electrolytes and renal function.

Device Therapy

Cardiomyopathy confers an increased risk of ventricular arrhythmias and sudden cardiac death (SCD). Patients with low EF of 35% or less and NYHA class II-III symptoms should receive an implantable cardiac defibrillator (ICD) for primary prevention (Fig. 4.6). Numerous trials—SCD-HeFT, CARE-HF, MADIT-CRT, and REVERSE—have demonstrated reduction in SCDs that outweigh the risk of device-related complications for HFrEF patients.

Patients with ischemic cardiomyopathy are at higher risk for SCDs due to the scar tissue that can be a nidus for ventricular arrhythmias. Thus, patients with ischemic cardiomyopathy (EF ≤30%) should also receive an ICD even if they do not have symptoms (NYHA class I). The evidence behind device therapy for HFpEF patients, however, is less clear. The DANISH trials demonstrated 3% mortality benefit but 1.5% device-related complications.

Device therapy in the form of cardiac resynchronization therapy (CRT), also termed "biventricular pacing," has also been shown to improve functional capacity, reduce HF rehospitalizations, and improve all-cause mortality. Patients derive their benefit from improved contractility and increased forward flow due to ventricular synchrony. Additional benefits include improvement in blood pressure, making it possible to intensify therapy with ACE inhibitors, ARBs, and ARNIs. Patients with HFrEF and a widened QRS of 150 ms or greater with a left bundle branch block pattern should be considered for CRT implantation.

Management of Atrial Fibrillation

HF patients with atrial fibrillation (AF) are at higher risk of stroke, HF exacerbations, and mortality. The AFFIRM trial demonstrated similar outcomes between rate and rhythm control strategies; however, patients with HFrEF were underrepresented. Theoretically, restoring sinus rhythm allows preservation of the atrial kick and improvement in A-V synchrony, which could reduce filling pressures and improve cardiac output. Recently, CASTLE-AF demonstrated that patients with HFrEF

患者群体的治疗潜力。然而，这些研究表明，ACEI 和 ARB 并不能显著减少该患者人群的心血管死亡率或心衰恶化。PARAGON-HF（HFpEF 患者中 ARNI 与 ARB 全球结局的前瞻性比较）研究也显示 ARNI 的死亡率或 HF 相关住院率没有显著降低。指南目前不建议 HFpEF 患者开始使用 ACEI、ARB 或 ARNI。

β 受体阻滞剂

在 C 期 HFrEF 患者中有效的三种 β 受体阻滞剂是比索洛尔、卡维地洛和琥珀酸美托洛尔。β 受体阻滞剂抑制交感神经系统，减少心肌作功，改善血管内皮完整性，最终减少心室重构。许多研究——MERIT-HF、CAPRICORN、COPERNICUS、COMET 和 CIBIS-II——已经证明 β 受体阻滞剂显著降低死亡率（31%～40%）以及死亡率和因心衰加重入院的复合终点。针对 HFpEF 患者的试验规模较小且证据力度不足，但许多试验显示出降低死亡率的趋势。

醛固酮受体拮抗剂

C 期 HFrEF、NYHA II～IV 级患者在已经使用 β 受体阻滞剂、ACEI、ARB 或 ARNI 类药物降低后负荷后，如果肌酐清除率大于 30 ml/min 且血钾水平正常，则应开始使用醛固酮受体拮抗剂，直接抑制醛固酮，进一步减少心室纤维化和重构。RALES 试验显示，该类药物的使用可使 NYHA II～IV 级患者的全因死亡率、心源性猝死和心衰住院率降低 30%。EMPHASIS-HF 试验也显示死亡和 HF 再入院的复合终点降低了 37%。

HFpEF 患者也可能受益于醛固酮受体拮抗剂。TOPCAT（醛固酮受体拮抗剂治疗射血分数保留的心力衰竭）研究是一项针对 EF ≥ 45% 患者的国际、安慰剂对照、随机临床试验，研究显示螺内酯降低心衰住院率的效果较小（12.0% vs. 14.2%）。然而，随后的分析显示了显著的地区差异，表明北美参与者对药物依从性更高，并可能获得更大的益处。

伊伐布雷定

尽管接受了高剂量 β 受体阻滞剂治疗，但有症状的 HFrEF（C 期，NYHA II～IV 级）患者如果静息心率仍较高（≥ 70 次 / 分），加用伊伐布雷定可能会使患者受益。伊伐布雷定通过抑制窦房结的 I_f 通道起作用。SHIFT 试验表明，在 NYHA II～IV 级患者中，接受了包含伊伐布雷定在内的指南指导的药物治疗（GDMT）的 EF ≤ 35% 患者，心衰加重的绝对风险降低了 5%，心血管死亡率绝对降低了 2%。

肼屈嗪和硝酸盐

血管扩张剂如肼屈嗪和硝酸盐可减轻后负荷和心肌作功，理论上可减少心室重构。然而，它们的疗效仅在已经使用 GDMT 的 HFrEF C 期和 NYHA III～IV 级症状的非裔美国人中显示出来。对于 HFpEF 患者，硝酸盐已被证明可以提高运动耐量，但不会降低死亡率（NEAT-HFpEF，2015）。ACC/AHA 2017 指南的更新尚未推荐 HFpEF 患者使用血管扩张剂。

地高辛

地高辛通过抑制钠钾交换来增加细胞内钙，从而提高心肌收缩力。地高辛与 HF 住院率降低、生活质量改善和运动耐量增加有关。然而，DIG 试验显示其对死亡率没有影响。地高辛也有不利的副作用。它可引起心律失常（异位性、折返性心律失常和心脏传导阻滞）、胃肠道副作用（恶心、厌食）和神经系统副作用（视觉影响、定向障碍、意识混乱）。老年人、低体重指数或肾功能不全的患者风险更高。许多药物（克拉霉素、红霉素、伊曲康唑、胺碘酮、决奈达隆、环孢素、普罗帕酮、维拉帕米和奎尼丁）可增加血浆地高辛水平并增加毒性风险。综合考虑这些风险和益处，C 期 HFrEF 患者可以从地高辛中获益。

利尿剂

对于慢性心衰患者，利尿剂用于维持血容量和目标症状管理。袢利尿剂是最常用的，但随着时间的推移，一些患者会产生耐药性，远曲小管变得肥大，水通过髓袢被重吸收，逆转袢利尿剂的作用。小剂量噻嗪和美托拉宗影响远端肾单位，可显著增强利尿作用。使用这些药物需要密切和仔细地监测血清电解质和肾功能。

器械治疗

心肌病会增加室性心律失常和心源性猝死（SCD）的风险。EF 低于 35% 且 NYHA II～III 级症状的患者应接受植入式心脏复律除颤器（ICD）进行一级预防（图 4.6）。许多试验——SCD-HeFT、CARE-HF、MADIT-CRT 和 REVERSE——已经证明，对于这些 HFrEF 患者，降低 SCD 所获的益处超过出现器械相关并发症的风险。

由于瘢痕组织可能是室性心律失常的病灶，缺血性心肌病患者发生 SCD 的风险较高。因此，缺血性心肌病（EF ≤ 30%）患者即使没有症状（NYHA I 级）也应接受 ICD。然而，HFpEF 患者使用器械治疗的证据尚不清楚。DANISH 试验显示患者的死亡率降低了 3%，但 1.5% 的患者出现了器械相关并发症。

心脏再同步化治疗（CRT）这种形式的器械治疗，也被称为"双心室起搏"，也被证明可以改善运动功能，减少 HF 再住院，并改善全因死亡率。由于心室同步，患者心脏收缩力改善，且前向血流增加。其他益处包括血压的改善，这可能强化 ACEI、ARB 和 ARNI 的药物治疗效果。HFrEF 和 QRS 波宽度 ≥ 150 ms 且伴有左束支传导阻滞的患者应考虑植入 CRT。

心房颤动的处理

合并心房颤动（AF）的心衰患者卒中、心衰加重和死亡的风险更高。AFFIRM 试验表明，心率和节律控制策略之间的结果相似；然而，HFrEF 患者的代表性不足。从理论上讲，恢复窦性心律可以保留心房搏动并改善心房-心室同步，从而降低充盈压并提高心

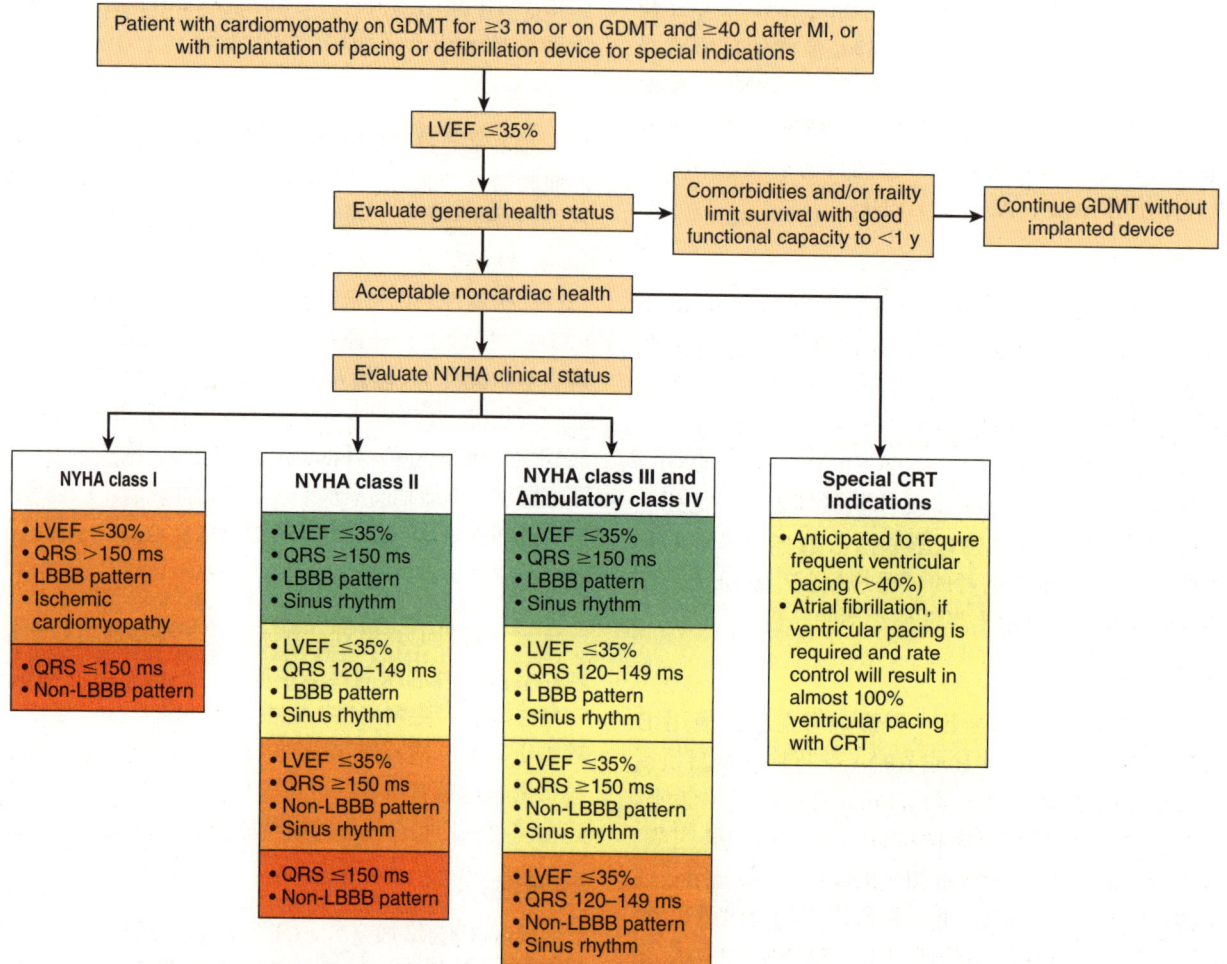

Fig. 4.6 Recommendations for implanted cardiac defibrillator (ICDs) and cardiac resynchronization therapy (CRT) depend on the ejection fraction (EF) and New York Heart Association (NYHA) functional class. *Green* indicates class I recommendations (evidence or agreement that treatment is useful and effective), *yellow* indicates class IIa recommendations (weight of evidence or opinion in favor of treatment), *orange* indicates IIb recommendations (usefulness/efficacy is less well established), and *red* indicates class III recommendations (evidence or general agreement that treatment is not useful/effect and in some cases may be harmful). *GDMT*, Guideline-directed medical therapy; *LBBB*, left bundle branch block; *MI*, myocardial infarction. (Adapted from ACCF/AHA 2013 guidelines.)

NYHA class II-IV experienced significant reduction in death (11.6%) and heart failure exacerbation (15.2%) after catheter ablation to restore sinus rhythm. Although not yet reflected in the guidelines, patients with HFrEF who are symptomatic should be considered for AF ablation.

Invasive Hemodynamic Monitoring of Ambulatory Patients

For patients with recurrent heart failure exacerbations, ambulatory monitoring devices can allow for early detection of increase in filling pressures and timely interventions. CardioMEMS is an implantable device placed in the pulmonary artery that communicates real-time hemodynamics measurements remotely to trained health care professionals. Multiple RCTs have demonstrated their effectiveness. In COMPASS-HF patients with NYHA class III monitored with CardioMEMS experienced a 36% reduction of HF hospitalizations. Similarly, CHAMPION-HF demonstrated CardioMEMS could achieve up to 37% relative risk reduction in HF exacerbations in the first 17 months. Device-related or systems-related complications were found to be exceedingly rare (freedom from complications estimated to be 98.6%). Currently, the device is FDA-approved for patients with heart failure with NYHA class III symptoms who have been hospitalized in the past year. The GUIDE-HF trial is an ongoing investigation to determine the impact of CardioMEMS in the NYHA class II and IV patient population and patients with elevated BNP. Many ICDs now have the capacity to monitor physiologic parameters including heart rate variability and intrathoracic impedance, which may be helpful for patient assessment and management.

Advanced Therapy

Patients with HFrEF stage D, who are refractory to medical therapy, are challenging to manage. Appropriate patients with stage D symptoms despite optimal medical therapy should be referred to centers that provide advanced circulatory support. Recent advances in mechanical support technology have made possible implantation of durable pumps as destination therapy in patients ineligible for other therapy.

INTERMACS Profiles

Patients in HFrEF stage D can be further characterized with profiles developed by the Interagency Registry of Mechanically Assisted Circulatory Support (INTERMACS). The INTERMACS profiles

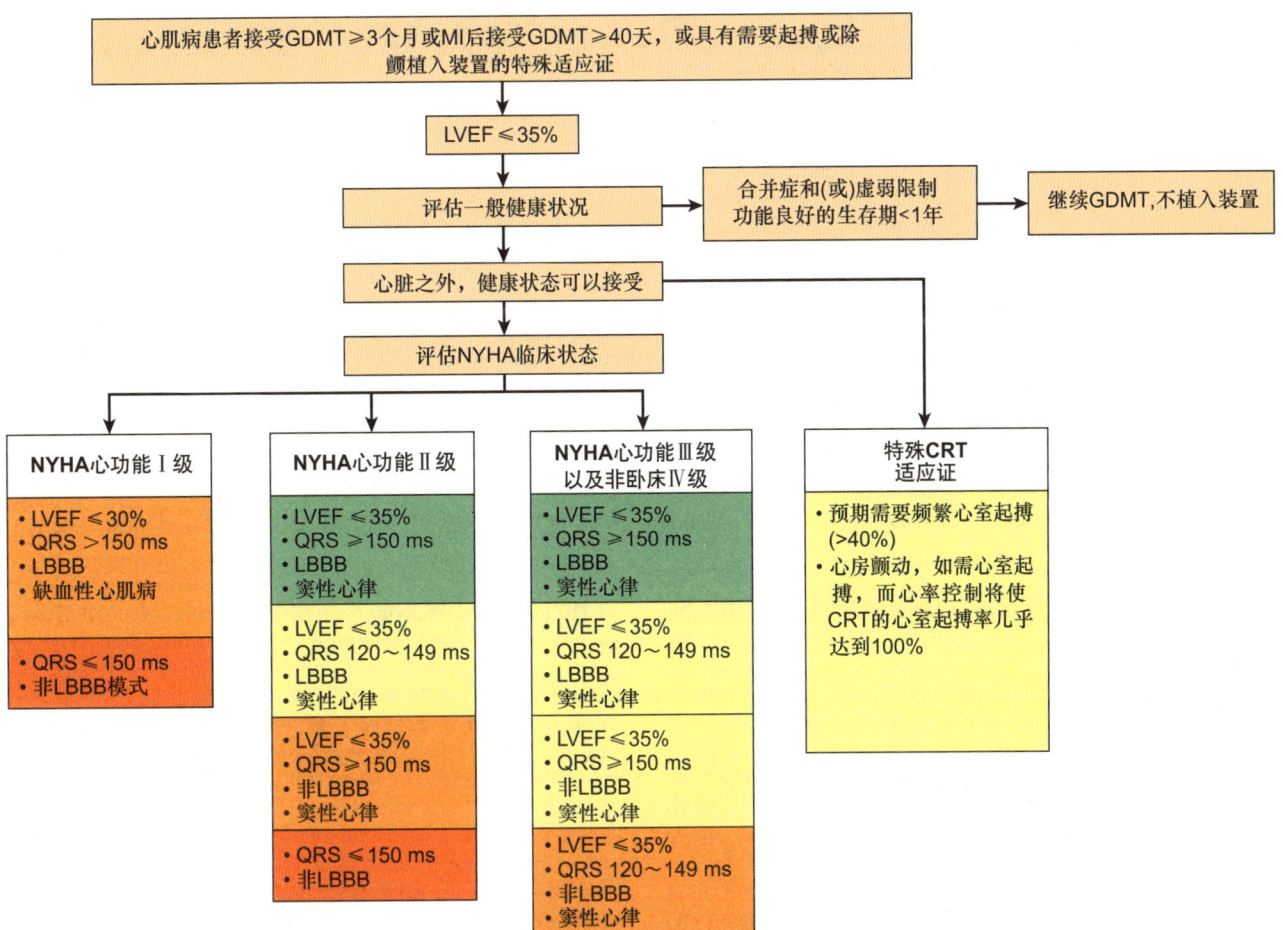

图 4.6 植入式心脏复律除颤器（ICD）和心脏再同步化治疗（CRT）的推荐取决于射血分数（EF）和纽约心脏协会（NYHA）功能分级。绿色表示 I 类建议（证据显示或一致认为治疗是有用和有效的），黄色表示 IIa 类建议（证据的权重或意见支持治疗），橙色表示 IIb 建议（用处/疗效不太确定），红色表示 III 类建议（证据或普遍认为治疗无用/无效，在某些情况下可能有害）。GDMT，指南指导的药物治疗；LBBB，左束支传导阻滞；MI，心肌梗死（改编自 ACCF/AHA 2013 guidelines.）

输出量。最近，CASTLE-AF 试验证明 HFrEF NYHA II～IV 级患者在行导管消融恢复窦性心律后，死亡率（11.6%）和心力衰竭加重率（15.2%）显著降低。尽管指南中尚未明确指出，但有症状的 HFrEF 患者应考虑心房颤动消融术。

门诊患者有创血流动力学监测

复发性心衰患者症状加重时，门诊的监测设备可帮助早期识别充盈压升高并及时干预。CardioMEMS 是一种植入式装置，放置在肺动脉中，远程向训练有素的医疗专业人员传达实时血流动力学测量结果。多个随机对照试验证明了其有效性。在 COMPASS-HF 研究的患者中，CardioMEMS 监测的 NYHA III 级患者心衰住院率降低了 36%。同样，CHAMPION-HF 研究表明，CardioMEMS 在前 17 个月内可将 HF 恶化的相对风险降低 37%。与器械或系统相关的并发症极为罕见（无并发症率估计为 98.6%）。目前，该设备已被 FDA 批准用于过去 1 年中住院治疗的有 NYHA III 级症状的心衰患者。GUIDE-HF 试验是一项正在进行的研究，旨在确定 CardioMEMS 对 NYHA II 级和 IV 级患者人群以及 BNP 升高患者的影响。许多 ICD 现在都具备监测生理参数的功能，包括心率变异性和胸内阻抗，这可能有助于患者的评估和管理。

高阶治疗

对药物治疗无效的 D 期 HFrEF 患者治疗起来具有挑战性。尽管接受了最佳药物治疗，但出现 D 期症状且情况允许的患者仍应转诊至提供高级循环支持的中心。对于不适合其他治疗的患者，机械支持技术的最新进展使长期植入辅助装置成为可能，并以此作为目标治疗。

INTERMACS 分级

HFrEF D 期患者可以通过机械辅助循环支持跨机构登记处（INTERMACS）分级进一步分类。INTERMACS 分级描述了从晚期 NYHA III 级（等级 7）到严重心源性休克（等级 1）的症状范围，并有助

TABLE 4.3 INTERMACS Profiles

INTERMACS Profile	Description	Urgency of Interventions
1: Cardiogenic shock	"Crash and burn": critical cardiogenic shock despite increasing doses of inotropes confirmed with rising lactate or acidosis	Within hours
2: Progressive decline	"Sliding on inotropes": end-organ hypoperfusion evidenced by worsening renal failure and inability to maintain euvolemia despite inotropic support	Within days
3: Stable but inotrope dependent	"Dependent stability": adequate end-organ perfusion and symptom control while on inotropic support or temporary circulatory support device, but unable to wean from inotropes	Within weeks to months
4: Resting symptoms	Symptoms of congestion occur at rest	Within weeks to months
5: Exertion intolerant	"Housebound": comfortable at rest and basic activities of daily living but any other activity causes limiting symptoms	Depends upon nutrition, organ function, activity
6: Exertion limited	"Walking wounded": fatigues after a few minutes of activity. Could confirm cardiac impairment with hemodynamic measures or cardiopulmonary stress test	Depends upon nutrition, organ function, activity
7: Advanced NYHA III	Mild physical exertion is tolerable, but moderate activity causes symptoms	Not yet indicated

INTERMACS, Interagency Registry of Mechanically Assisted Circulatory Support; *NYHA,* New York Heart Association.
Data from Stevenson LW, Pagani FD, Young JB, et al. INTERMACS profiles of advanced heart failure: the current picture. *J Heart Lung Transplant.* 2009;28(6):535-541.

describe the range of symptoms from advanced NYHA class III (profile 7) to critical cardiogenic shock (profile 1) and can help assess the urgency to evaluate for mechanical circulatory support or transplants (Table 4.3). Patients in INTERMACS profiles 5 through 7 can be monitored without immediate plan for advanced heart failure therapy. Patients with resting symptoms (profile 4) or receiving inotropic support (profile 3) may need circulatory support sooner. Patients who are "sliding on inotropes" (profile 2)—demonstrating poor end-organ perfusion despite inotropic support—should be considered for immediate support within days and potentially transferred to a left ventricular assist device (LVAD) and transplant center. Patients in critical cardiogenic shock (profile 1) take precedence in mechanical circulatory support or heart transplant, which may be needed within hours.

Inotropic Support

Patients who have persistent symptoms despite GDMT and volume optimization, found to have elevated filling pressures and/or low cardiac output, may be appropriate candidates for ambulatory inotropic support. Ambulatory inotropes can be used for either bridge to durable mechanical support or palliation of symptoms. The current evidence suggests that ambulatory inotropes compared to GDMT do not improve mortality but may improve heart failure symptoms (improvement in NYHA class by 0.6 more than GDMT).

Inotropes commonly used include milrinone and dobutamine. Milrinone inhibits phosphodiesterase and thereby causes vasodilation. Hemodynamics improve due to reduction in afterload, decrease in pulmonary vascular resistance, and increase in cardiac contractility. Dobutamine is a sympathomimetic agent; it is an agonist for α-1, β-1, and β-2 receptor. This leads to an increase in myocardial contractility and stroke volume as well as decrease in total peripheral resistance, or afterload. Adverse effects include arrhythmias and significant hypotension due to vasodilation. If patients are hypotensive, norepinephrine (α-1 and β-1 receptor agonists) and dopamine (β-1 receptor agonist at medium doses and α-adrenergic receptor agonists at high doses) are preferred agents because they can vasoconstrict and increase blood pressure in addition to increasing myocardial contractility.

Mechanical Circulatory Support

In the setting of acute cardiogenic shock, several options are available for short-term mechanical support.

The intra-aortic balloon pump (IABP) is a counterpulsation pump placed in the aorta and synchronized to native cardiac beats. It reduces the afterload by deflating during systole and improves coronary perfusion pressure by inflating during diastole. The IABP-SHOCK II trials demonstrated no difference in 30-day mortality between patients treated with inotropes alone and those with IABP. Compared to other short-term mechanical supports, IABP provides only a small augmentation in cardiac output (500-600 mL/min/m^2). Potential complications include limb ischemia, thrombosis, and vascular complications.

The Impella ventricular support system is an axial-flow pump that pulls blood from the left ventricle through an inlet area near the tip and expels blood from the catheter into the ascending aorta. There are different sizes of Impella including 2.5 or CP, which are designed for percutaneous peripheral insertion, as well as Impella 5.0 or LD, which are designed for surgical insertion. Depending on the type of Impella, it can provide 2.5 to 5 L/min/m^2 of augmentation. The ISAR-SHOCK and IMPRESS trials, however, have demonstrated no improvement in mortality. In addition to limb ischemia and vascular complications, the rotor in the pump can lyse red blood cells, causing significant hemolytic anemia.

Venous arterial extracorporeal membrane oxygenation (VA-ECMO) is a heart-lung bypass via venous and arterial cannulas that pump the blood from the body through an external oxygenator. Venous blood is drained from the right atrium and returned to the distal arterial system providing near complete temporary circulation support.

In addition to concerns of limb ischemia, hemolysis, and vascular injury due to the cannulas, the north-south syndrome is a feared complication. In this syndrome, only the lower body receives oxygenated blood through the arterial cannula, and the "north"—or the brain and upper body—receives perfusion with the deoxygenated blood. This may occur due to the position of the cannulas or the recovery of native heart function. VA-ECMO is considered as a last resort and is available at only select centers with the surgeons and infrastructure capabilities.

The advancement in durable mechanical circulatory support devices has now made it possible for HF patients in cardiogenic shock to be discharged and managed in ambulatory settings. Since the first heart lung machine in 1953, the durable circulatory supports have undergone significant transformation to reduce their size, noise, and device-related complications (Table 4.4). In order to reduce pump thrombosis, devices have evolved from axial-flow to centrifugal-flow.

表4.3 INTERMACS 分级

INTERMACS 分级	描述	干预措施的紧急程度
1. 严重心源性休克	"治疗失败": 尽管正性肌力药物剂量增加, 但仍有乳酸升高或酸中毒的重症心源性休克	在数小时内
2.（应用正性肌力药物的同时）心力衰竭进展性恶化	"正性肌力药物支持下恶化": 肾功能不全进展, 以及正性肌力药物支持下仍无法维持正常血容量的终末器官灌注不足	在数天内
3. 病情稳定但依赖正性肌力药物	"依赖正性肌力药物下的稳定": 在使用正性肌力药物支持或临时循环辅助装置时, 终末器官灌注充足且症状得到控制, 但无法脱离正性肌力药物支持	在数周至数月内
4. 有静息症状	静息状态下出现充血相关症状	在数周至数月内
5. 不能耐受体力活动	"不能外出活动": 静息和基本日常生活活动下感到舒适, 但任何其他体力活动都会引起症状	取决于营养状态、器官功能、活动能力
6. 体力活动受限	"尚能行走": 体力活动数分钟后感到疲乏。血流动力学监测或心肺运动负荷试验能证实心功能受损	取决于营养状态、器官功能、活动能力
7. 进展型 NYHA 分级Ⅲ级	轻度的体力活动可耐受, 但中度体力活动下出现症状	尚不明确

INTERMACS, 机械辅助循环支持跨机构登记处; NYHA, 纽约心脏协会。
数据引自 Stevenson LW, Pagani FD, Young JB, et al. INTERMACS profiles of advanced heart failure: the current picture. J Heart Lung Transplant. 2009; 28 (6): 535-541.

于评估机械循环支持或心脏移植的紧迫性（表4.3）。在 INTERMACS 分级表中, 等级 5 至 7 的患者可以进行监测且暂不立即计划行高阶心衰治疗。有静息症状（等级 4）或接受正性肌力药物支持（等级 3）的患者可能尽早需要循环支持。"正性肌力药物支持下恶化"的患者（等级 2）——尽管有正性肌力药物支持, 但仍然出现终末内脏器官灌注不良——应考虑在几天内立即接受支持治疗, 并可能转移到能行左心室辅助装置（LVAD）和移植的中心。危重心源性休克患者（等级 1）优先考虑机械循环支持或心脏移植, 这可能需要在数小时内完成。

正性肌力药物支持

尽管有 GDMT 和容量优化, 但对于持续有症状的患者, 发现其充盈压升高和心输出量低, 可能是门诊正性肌力药物支持治疗的合适人选。门诊正性肌力药物可作为过渡到持久的机械辅助装置的桥接治疗, 或用于缓解症状。目前的证据表明, 与 GDMT 相比, 正性肌力药物不能降低死亡率, 但可能改善心衰症状（与 GDMT 相比, NYHA 心功能分级可改善 0.6 级）。

常用的正性肌力药物包括米力农和多巴酚丁胺。米力农抑制磷酸二酯酶, 从而引起血管舒张。血流动力学的改善是由后负荷减小、肺血管阻力降低和心脏收缩力增加导致的。多巴酚丁胺是一种拟交感神经药物, 它是 α_1、β_1 和 β_2 受体的激动剂。这导致心肌收缩力和每搏输出量的增加, 以及总外周阻力或后负荷的减小。副作用包括心律失常和因血管舒张引起的严重低血压。若患者发生低血压, 去甲肾上腺素（α_1 和 β_1 受体激动剂）和多巴胺（中剂量时为 β_1 受体激动剂, 高剂量时为 α 受体激动剂）是首选药物, 因为它们除了能增加心肌收缩力外, 还能收缩血管, 升高血压。

机械循环支持

在急性心源性休克的情况下, 短期机械支持有以下几种选择。

主动脉内球囊反搏（IABP）是放置在主动脉内的反搏泵, 与自然心跳同步。它通过心脏收缩期的球囊放气来减小后负荷, 并通过心脏舒张期的球囊充气来改善冠状动脉灌注压力。IABP-SHOCK Ⅱ 试验表明, 单独使用正性肌力药物治疗的患者和 IABP 患者的 30 天死亡率没有差异。与其他短期机械循环支持相比, IABP 只能少量增加心输出量 [$500 \sim 600$ ml/(min·m^2)]。潜在的并发症包括肢体缺血、血栓和血管并发症。

Impella 心室支持系统是一个轴流泵, 它将血液从左心室通过尖端附近的导管入口抽出, 并将血液通过导管排出到升主动脉。Impella 有不同的尺寸, 包括 2.5 或 CP（用于经皮外周插入）, 以及 Impella 5.0 或 LD（为手术插入而设计）。根据 Impella 的类型, 它可以使心输出量增加 $2.5 \sim 5$ L/(min·m^2)。然而, ISAR-SHOCK 和 IMPRESS 试验没有显示死亡率的改善。除了肢体缺血和血管并发症外, 泵中的转子还会破坏红细胞, 引起明显的溶血性贫血。

静脉动脉体外膜肺氧合（VA-ECMO）是一种通过静脉和动脉插管将血液从人体泵出经过体外氧合器的心肺旁路手术。静脉血从右心房引出并经膜肺氧合后回流到远端动脉系统, 提供近乎完全的临时循环支持。

除了担心肢体缺血、溶血和插管引起的血管损伤外, 南北综合征是一种令人恐惧的并发症。在这种综合征中, 只有下半身通过动脉插管接受含氧血液, 而"北方"——即大脑和上半身接受缺氧血液的灌注。出现这种情况的原因可能是由于插管的位置或原有心脏功能的恢复。VA-ECMO 被认为是终极的治疗手段, 仅可在具有外科医生和相关条件的特定中心使用。

随着长期机械循环支持装置的进步, 心源性休克的 HF 患者已经可以出院并在门诊进行管理了。自 1953 年第一台心肺机诞生以来, 长期机械循环支持经历了重大变革, 以减小其尺寸、噪声和设备相关并发症（表 4.4）。为了减少泵血栓形成, 设备已经从轴流发展到离心流。在后一种配置中, 叶轮垂直于血流,

TABLE 4.4 Parameters of Left Ventricular Assist Device

	HeartMate II	HeartMate III	HVAD
Flow configuration	Axial	Centrifugal	Centrifugal
Impeller bearings	Mechanical	Magnetic levitation	Hybrid
Weight	250 grams	220 grams	160 grams
Variation in speed	No	Yes	No
Implantation site	Chest and abdomen	Pericardial	Pericardial

In the latter configuration, impellers are perpendicular to the flow of the blood to reduce the risk of clot formation. Although older devices required mechanical bearings for the pumps, the latest designs employ magnetic levitation, further reducing thrombotic risks and improving durability. The newest FDA-approved device, HeartMate III, combines continuous flow with frequent variation in the speed, which can further reduce hemostasis and clot formation.

The prospective, multicenter RCT with the HeartMate III demonstrated up to 78% stroke-free 2-year survival rate. With these superior outcomes for the latest LVADs, advanced heart failure patients who are otherwise not candidates for heart transplants can now receive durable circulatory support as destination therapy. In fact, LVADs are now FDA-approved for patients with INTERMACS profiles 1 through 6. Patients who demonstrate signs of cardiorenal syndrome, intolerance to GDMT due to hypotension, and are persistently in NYHA functional classes III to IV despite GDMT should be referred to an advanced heart failure specialist for further evaluation.

Heart Transplant

Heart transplant remains an option for select patients with refractory HF. In recent years, the list of candidates for heart transplantation continues to grow without concurrent increase in available heart donors. Due to the scarcity of organs and high waitlist mortality, particularly in certain geographic areas, the United Network for Organ Sharing (UNOS) released a new set of allocation criteria in order to prioritize the sickest patients (Fig. 4.7). Those in status 1 or 2 will have access to organs that become available in a larger geographic area of up to 500 miles from the donor site.

Patients' survival after heart transplantation has improved but gains are mostly limited to the first year, with 1-year survival estimated to be 85%. The median survival is estimated to be 11 years; those who survive the first year have a longer median survival of 13 years. Survival may be improved by preoperative care including LVAD implantation as bridge to transplant, reducing allograft ischemic time intraoperatively, and optimization of postoperative immunosuppressants and cardiac rehabilitation. Patients are on multiple immunosuppressants, which places them at increased risk of developing opportunistic infections and malignancy. Inadequate immunosuppression can increase the risk of graft failure. These patients undergo close surveillance for the first year and continued monitoring for the rest of their lives.

Palliative Care

Despite advances in HF treatment and prevention, rates of hospitalization for acute decompensation, 30-day readmission, and mortality rates remain high. Only 50% of patients survive after 5 years and 29% die within the first year. Indicators of poor prognosis include functional status, low EF, pulmonary vascular and right ventricular remodeling due to left ventricular failure, cardiorenal and hepatic syndromes, and presence of arrhythmias.

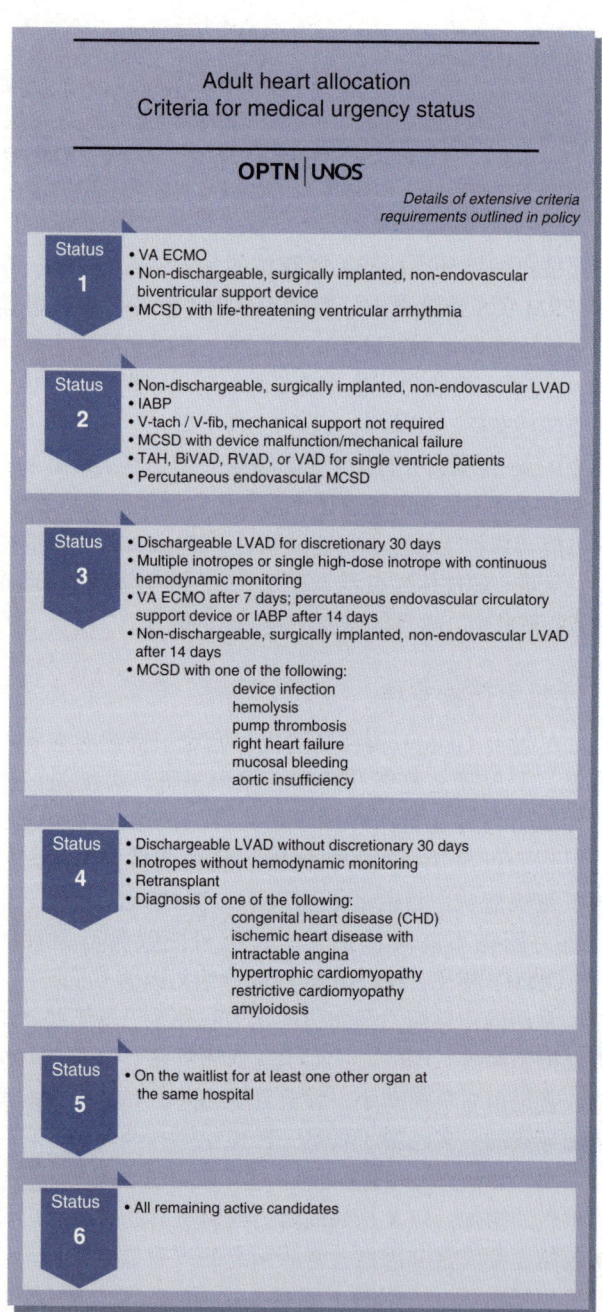

Fig. 4.7 Adult heart allocation criteria. (Adapted from UNOS, https://optn.transplant.hrsa.gov/learn/professional-education/adult-heart-allocation/.)

第4章 心力衰竭与心肌病

表 4.4 左心室辅助装置参数

	HeartMate Ⅱ	HeartMate Ⅲ	HVAD
血流模式	轴流泵	离心泵	离心泵
叶轮轴承	机械的	磁悬浮	混合的
重量	250 g	220 g	160 g
速度变化	无	有	无
植入位置	胸部和腹部	心包	心包

以减少血凝块形成的风险。虽然旧的设备需要机械轴承泵，但最新的设计已采用磁悬浮技术，进一步降低血栓形成的风险，并提高耐用性。最新的 FDA 批准设备 HeartMate Ⅲ 结合了连续流动和频繁变化的速度，可以进一步减轻止血效应和血凝块形成。

使用 HeartMate Ⅲ 的前瞻性多中心随机对照试验显示，无卒中 2 年生存率高达 78%。有了这些最新 LVAD 的卓越疗效，原本不适合心脏移植的晚期心衰患者现在可将接受长期循环支持作为最终治疗手段。事实上，LVAD 现在已被 FDA 批准用于 INTERMACS 等级 1～6 的患者。如果患者表现出心肾综合征的症状、因患低血压而不耐受 GDMT，并且在接受 GDMT 后仍持续处于 NYHA 功能Ⅲ～Ⅳ级，则应转至拥有晚期心衰专家的医疗中心进行进一步评估。

心脏移植手术

心脏移植仍然是难治性心衰患者的一个选择。近年来，心脏移植候选者人数持续增长，但可用的心脏供体量却没有同时增加。针对器官稀缺和较高的移植等待者死亡率，特别是在某些地理区域，器官共享联合网络（UNOS）发布了一套新的分配标准，以便优先考虑病情最严重的患者（图 4.7）。那些处于图 4.7 中状态 1 或 2 的人将有机会在距离捐赠地点 500 英里（805 km）的更大地理区域范围内获得器官。

心脏移植后患者的生存率有所提高，但主要局限于第一年，1 年生存率估计为 85%。中位生存期估计为 11 年；存活超过第一年的患者平均存活时间更长，为 13 年。通过术前照护，包括 LVAD 植入作为移植的桥接，术中减少同种异体移植物缺血时间，优化术后免疫抑制剂治疗和心脏康复，可提高生存率。患者服用多种免疫抑制剂，将使他们发生机会性感染和恶性肿瘤的风险增加。免疫抑制不足会增加移植物失败的风险。这些患者在第一年需接受密切监测，并在余生中继续进行监测。

缓和医疗

尽管在心衰治疗和预防方面取得了进展，但因心衰的急性失代偿住院率、30 天再入院率和死亡率仍然很高。只有 50% 的患者在 5 年后存活，29% 的患者在 1 年内死亡。预后不良的指标包括功能状态、低射血分数、左心衰引起的肺血管和右心室重构、心肾和肝综合征、心律失常等。

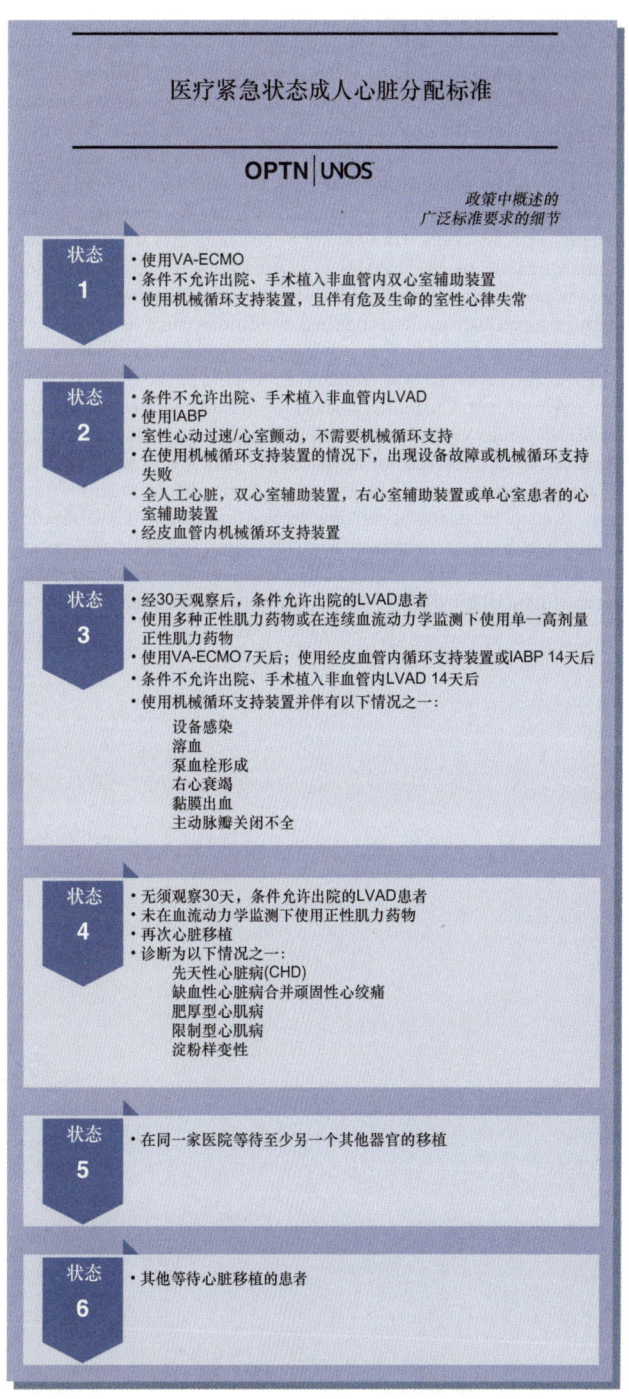

图 4.7 成人心脏分配标准（改编自 UNOS，https://optn.transplant.hrsa.gov/learn/professional-education/adult-heart-allocation/.）

Toward the end of life, patients with HF have significant symptom burden that leads to loss of function and independence. Palliative care provides an interdisciplinary approach to meet the physical and emotional needs of the patient. Patients experience significant improvement in symptom burden, rates of anxiety and depression, as well as reduced hospitalization readmission rates. Palliative care can also assist with end-of-life transition and introduction of hospice care to patients and their families. Palliative care is a class I recommendation for stage D HFrEF patients. The optimization of HF symptom management and increasing access to palliative care are critical for improving care for advanced HF patients.

FUTURE DIRECTIONS

Prevention is still the key to success in treating HF. Treating hypertension and diabetes remain major public health objectives. Recent advances in pharmacologic and device therapies have improved HF-associated mortality and morbidity. Replacement of ACE inhibitors and ARBs with ARNIs has been shown to reduce mortality. CardioMEMs reduce 30-day readmission rates by more than 50%. Patients with advanced HF who are poor candidates for heart transplants can now receive LVADs as destination therapy. In addition, there is promising research and development in diagnosis and treatment of previously underrecognized conditions, such as HFpEF and amyloidosis.

However, access to care remains challenging in the modern health care environment. Currently, costs of novel therapies like ARNIs, cardioMEMs, and LVADs can be prohibitive. There is still limited access to palliative care services for advanced HF patients, even though this "low tech" intervention improves symptom management and reduces costs due to excessive acute care service utilization. Collaboration among health care providers, patient advocates, and policymakers can lead to improvement not only in survival and quality of life but reducing the financial burden to the society and the individual.

SUGGESTED READINGS

Abrahao Hajjar L, Teboul J-L: Mechanical Circulatory Support Devices for Cardiogenic Shock: State of the Art, 1–150, 2019, https://doi.org/10.1186/s13054-019-2368-y.

Gersh BJ, Maron BJ, Bonow RO, et al: 2011 ACCF/AHA Guideline for the diagnosis and treatment of hypertrophic cardiomyopathy: a report of the American College of Cardiology Foundation/American Heart Association Task Force on Practice guidelines developed in collaboration with the American Association for Thoracic Surgery, American Society of Echocardiography, American Society of Nuclear Cardiology, Heart Failure Society of America, J Am Coll Cardiol 58(25):e212–e260, 2011, https://doi.org/10.1016/j.jacc.2011.06.011.

Hershberger RE, Givertz MM, Ho CY, et al: Genetic evaluation of cardiomyopathy—a Heart Failure Society of America Practice Guideline, J Card Fail 24(5):281–302, 2018, https://doi.org/10.1016/j.cardfail.2018.03.004.

Kavalieratos D, Gelfman LP, Tycon LE, et al: Palliative care in heart failure: rationale, evidence, and future priorities, J Am Coll Cardiol 70(15):1919–1930, 2017, https://doi.org/10.1016/j.jacc.2017.08.036.

Martin N, Manoharan K, Thomas J, Davies C, Lumbers RT: Beta-blockers and inhibitors of the renin-angiotensin aldosterone system for chronic heart failure with preserved ejection fraction, Cochrane Database Syst Rev 2018(6), 2018, https://doi.org/10.1002/14651858.CD012721.pub2.

Thibodeau JT, Drazner MH: The role of the clinical examination in patients with heart failure, JACC Hear Fail 6(7):544–551, 2019, https://doi.org/10.1016/j.jchf.2018.04.005.

Yancy CW, Jessup M, Bozkurt B, et al: 2013 ACCF/AHA Guideline for the management of heart failure: a report of the American College of Cardiology Foundation/American Heart Association Task Force on practice guidelines, Circulation 128(16):e240–e327, 2013, https://doi.org/10.1161/CIR.0b013e31829e8776.

Yancy CW, Jessup M, Bozkurt B, et al: 2017 ACC/AHA/HFSA focused update of the 2013 ACCF/AHA guideline for the management of heart failure: a report of the American College of Cardiology/American Heart Association Task Force on Clinical Practice Guidelines and the Heart Failure Society of America, Circulation 136:e137–e161, 2017, https://doi.org/10.1161/CIR.0000000000000509.

在心衰患者的生命终末期会有明显的症状负担，进而导致身体功能衰退和生活无法自理。缓和医疗采用跨学科的方法，旨在满足患者身心两方面的需求。经此治疗，患者的症状负担、焦虑及抑郁状况显著改善，同时再入院率也有所降低。此外，缓和医疗还能帮助患者及其家属更好地面对生命终末期的过渡，并顺利进入临终关怀。对于 D 期 HFrEF 患者而言，缓和医疗是 I 级推荐治疗方案。优化心衰症状的管理、提高缓和医疗的可及性，对于改善心衰晚期患者的照护工作至关重要。

未来方向

预防仍是心衰治疗成功的关键所在。治疗高血压和糖尿病仍是主要的公共卫生目标。近期，药物及器械疗法的进步已降低了心衰相关的死亡率和发病率。以 ARNI 取代 ACEI 和 ARB 的疗法，已证实可以降低死亡率。CardioMEMS 可使 30 天内再入院率降低 50% 以上。对于心脏移植条件不佳的晚期心衰患者，如今的左心室辅助装置可作为最终治疗手段。此外，针对先前未得到充分重视的病症（如射血分数保留型心衰和心肌淀粉样变性）的诊断与治疗，也展现出了良好的研发前景。

然而，在现代医疗环境中，获取医疗服务仍然面临着挑战。目前，诸如 ARNI、CardioMEMS 和左心室辅助装置等新型疗法的费用可能令人望而却步。尽管缓和医疗这种"低技术型"干预能改善病症管理，并减少因过度使用急诊照护服务而产生的费用，但晚期心衰患者获得缓和医疗服务的机会仍然有限。医疗服务提供者、患者权益倡导者和政策制定者之间的合作，不仅可以提高患者的生存率和生活质量，还可以减轻社会和个人的经济负担。

推荐阅读

Abrahao Hajjar L, Teboul J-L: Mechanical Circulatory Support Devices for Cardiogenic Shock: State of the Art, 1–150, 2019, https://doi.org/10.1186/s13054-019-2368-y.

Gersh BJ, Maron BJ, Bonow RO, et al: 2011 ACCF/AHA Guideline for the diagnosis and treatment of hypertrophic cardiomyopathy: a report of the American College of Cardiology Foundation/American Heart Association Task Force on Practice guidelines developed in collaboration with the American Association for Thoracic Surgery, American Society of Echocardiography, American Society of Nuclear Cardiology, Heart Failure Society of America, J Am Coll Cardiol 58(25):e212–e260, 2011, https://doi.org/10.1016/j.jacc.2011.06.011.

Hershberger RE, Givertz MM, Ho CY, et al: Genetic evaluation of cardiomyopathy—a Heart Failure Society of America Practice Guideline, J Card Fail 24(5):281–302, 2018, https://doi.org/10.1016/j.cardfail.2018.03.004.

Kavalieratos D, Gelfman LP, Tycon LE, et al: Palliative care in heart failure: rationale, evidence, and future priorities, J Am Coll Cardiol 70(15):1919–1930, 2017, https://doi.org/10.1016/j.jacc.2017.08.036.

Martin N, Manoharan K, Thomas J, Davies C, Lumbers RT: Beta-blockers and inhibitors of the renin-angiotensin aldosterone system for chronic heart failure with preserved ejection fraction, Cochrane Database Syst Rev 2018(6), 2018, https://doi.org/10.1002/14651858.CD012721.pub2.

Thibodeau JT, Drazner MH: The role of the clinical examination in patients with heart failure, JACC Hear Fail 6(7):544–551, 2019, https://doi.org/10.1016/j.jchf.2018.04.005.

Yancy CW, Jessup M, Bozkurt B, et al: 2013 ACCF/AHA Guideline for the management of heart failure: a report of the American College of Cardiology Foundation/American Heart Association Task Force on practice guidelines, Circulation 128(16):e240–e327, 2013, https://doi.org/10.1161/CIR.0b013e31829e8776.

Yancy CW, Jessup M, Bozkurt B, et al: 2017 ACC/AHA/HFSA focused update of the 2013 ACCF/AHA guideline for the management of heart failure: a report of the American College of Cardiology/American Heart Association Task Force on Clinical Practice Guidelines and the Heart Failure Society of America, Circulation 136:e137–e161, 2017, https://doi.org/10.1161/CIR.0000000000000509.

5
Congenital Heart Disease

Scott Cohen, Michael G. Earing

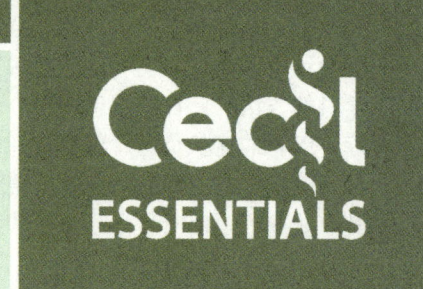

INTRODUCTION

Congenital heart defects are the most common group of birth defects, occurring in approximately 9 of 1000 live births. Without treatment, most patients die in infancy or childhood, with only 5% to 15% surviving into adulthood. Advancements in surgical and medical practices have resulted in survival of approximately 90% of these children to adulthood. Estimates suggest that more adults than children are living with congenital heart disease in the United States and that there is a 5% increase in the size of the adult congenital heart disease population every year.

Most adults living with congenital heart disease have had interventions performed (Table 5.1). Although most children who undergo surgical intervention survive to adulthood, total correction usually is not the rule. Adult patients with congenital heart disease are surviving longer than ever before, and it is becoming apparent that even the simplest lesions can be associated with long-term cardiac complications (i.e., arrhythmias and conduction abnormalities, ventricular dysfunction, residual shunts, valvular lesions, hypertension, and aneurysms) and noncardiac complications (i.e., renal dysfunction, restrictive lung disease, neurocognitive deficits, anxiety, depression, and liver dysfunction). Most adults with congenital heart disease need lifelong follow-up.

ACYANOTIC HEART DISEASE

Atrial Septal Defects

Definition and Epidemiology

Atrial septal defects (ASDs) are communications between the atria that allow shunting of blood from one atrium to the other. They are among the most common congenital anomalies seen in adolescents and young adults, occurring in 1 of 1500 live births and constituting 6% to 10% of all congenital heart defects.

There are four main types of ASDs. Ostium secundum defects are the most common, accounting for 75% of all ASDs. This defect occurs in the region of the fossa ovalis and results from excessive absorption of the septum primum or insufficient development of the septum secundum, or both.

Ostium primum defects represent about 20% of all ASDs and represent a form of atrioventricular septal defect (i.e., partial or incomplete atrioventricular canal). These defects are located in the inferior aspect of the atrial septum adjacent to the mitral and tricuspid valves. The defects result from lack of closure of the ostium primum by the endocardial cushions, which are embryologic swellings in the heart that form the primum atrial septum, the inlet portion of the ventricular septum, and parts of the mitral and tricuspid valve. The lesions often are associated with clefts in the mitral and tricuspid valves.

Sinus venosus ASDs represent 5% of all ASDs and are located at the entry of the superior vena cava or inferior vena cava into the right atrium. Frequently, there is associated partial anomalous drainage of the right upper pulmonary vein with the superior sinus venosus defect. This type of defect results from resorption of the wall between the vena cava and pulmonary veins.

An unroofed coronary sinus is a rare form of ASD, representing less than 1% of all ASDs. The coronary sinus is in apposition to the posterior aspect of the left atrium, but the orifice is in the right atrium. When a defect exists in the roof of the coronary sinus, a communication between the left atrium and right atrium exists, allowing shunting.

Pathology

All four types of ASDs allow oxygenated blood to pass from the left atrium into the right atrium, resulting in volume overload of the right atrium and right ventricle (Fig. 5.1). The degree of shunting is determined by the size of the ASD and the compliance of the left and right cardiac chambers. Comorbidities that increase left-sided filling pressures (i.e., left ventricular [LV] diastolic dysfunction, myocardial infarction, and mitral stenosis) may result in an increased left-to-right shunt. Over time, significant left-to-right shunting can cause enlargement of the right atrium and right ventricle, eventually leading to right ventricular (RV) systolic dysfunction and failure. Pulmonary hypertension may occur in approximately 26% of patients with a secundum ASD. However, significant elevation in pulmonary vascular resistance is rare.

Clinical Presentation

Although most individuals with an ASD are diagnosed during childhood after a murmur is noticed, a few patients have symptoms for the first time as adults. Most patients are asymptomatic during the first and second decades of life. In the third decade, increasing numbers of patients develop exercise intolerance, palpitations due to atrial arrhythmias, and cardiac enlargement on the chest radiograph. In patients with ASDs, the RV impulse at the left lower sternal border often has increased force compared with normal. On auscultation, the second heart sound typically is widely split and fixed (i.e., does not vary with inspiration).

All patients have a systolic ejection murmur, which is best heard at the left upper sternal border and is related to increased flow across a usually normal pulmonary valve. When there is a large left-to-right shunt, a mid-diastolic murmur can be heard at the left lower sternal border; it is related to increased flow across a normal tricuspid valve. When a mid-diastolic murmur is identified, the degree of left-to-right shunt is considered to be 1.5 times normal. In the setting of a primum

先天性心脏病

张恒 译 郑哲 张斌 审校 任景怡 通审

引言

先天性心脏缺陷是最常见的出生缺陷,在新生儿中发生率约为9/1000。如果未经治疗,大部分患儿在婴儿期或儿童期死亡,仅5%～15%能存活至成年。随着外科手术和药物治疗的进步,约90%的患儿能存活至成年。据估算,美国成年先天性心脏病患者数量超过儿童,而且成年患者还在以每年5%的速度增长。

大部分成年先天性心脏病患者曾接受过手术或介入治疗(表5.1)。尽管大部分经手术治疗的患儿能存活至成年,但外科手术并不能使所有缺陷完全修复。随着成年先天性心脏病患者生存期较过去延长,即使最简单的先天性心脏病,其长期心脏并发症(如心律失常、传导异常、心室功能不全、残余分流、瓣膜损害、高血压、动脉瘤)和非心脏并发症(如肾功能不全、限制性肺疾病、认知功能异常、焦虑、抑郁、肝功能不全)也逐渐显现。大部分成年先天性心脏病患者需要终身随访。

非发绀型心脏病

房间隔缺损

定义和流行病学

房间隔缺损(ASD)是心房间的通道,使血液从一个心房分流到另一个心房。它是青春期和青年人中最常见的先天性异常之一,新生儿发生率为1/1500,占所有先天性心脏缺陷的6%～10%。

房间隔缺损主要有4种类型。继发孔型房间隔缺损是最常见的一种,占全部房间隔缺损的75%。这种缺损出现在卵圆窝区,源于第一房间隔的过度吸收或第二房间隔发育不全,或两者均有。

原发孔型房间隔缺损占全部房间隔缺损的20%,是房室间隔缺损的一种(如部分或不完全性房室通道)。这种缺损位于房间隔下部毗邻二尖瓣和三尖瓣处。这种缺损由心内膜垫对原发孔封闭不全所致。心内膜垫是心脏内胚胎期的肿胀组织,其发育形成第一房间隔、室间隔入口部、部分二尖瓣和三尖瓣。这种缺损常伴有二尖瓣裂和三尖瓣裂。

静脉窦型房间隔缺损占全部房间隔缺损的5%,位于上腔静脉或下腔静脉进入右心房的入口处,经常伴有右上肺静脉部分异位引流。这种缺损源于腔静脉和肺静脉间血管壁的吸收。

无顶冠状窦是房间隔缺损的少见类型,在所有房间隔缺损病例中占比不足1%。冠状窦位于左心房后方,但开口于右心房。当冠状窦顶部缺损时,左心房和右心房之间就有了一个分流的通道。

病理学

四种房间隔缺损均导致氧合的血液从左心房分流至右心房,从而加重右心房和右心室的容量负荷(图5.1)。分流程度取决于房间隔缺损的大小和左右心腔的顺应性。导致左心充盈压增加的合并症(如左心室舒张功能不全、心肌梗死和二尖瓣狭窄)可能会加重左向右分流。随着时间的推移,显著的左向右分流会造成右心房和右心室增大,最终导致右心室收缩功能不全和右心衰竭。约26%的继发孔型房间隔缺损患者会出现肺动脉高压。但肺血管阻力显著升高少见。

临床表现

尽管大部分房间隔缺损患者是在儿童期发现杂音后诊断的,仍然有少数患者是在成年期出现症状后才被发现。大部分患者在20岁之前没有症状。在20岁以后,越来越多的患者出现运动耐量下降、房性心律失常导致的心悸、胸部X线片发现心脏增大。房间隔缺损患者与正常人相比,胸骨左下缘右心室搏动增强。听诊时的典型表现是第二心音固定分裂(不随呼吸变化)。

所有患者均有收缩期喷射样杂音,在胸骨左上缘听诊最清楚,这与通过肺动脉瓣(通常结构正常)的血流量增大有关。当左向右分流量大时,在胸骨左下缘能听到舒张中期杂音,这与通过结构正常的三尖瓣的血流量增大有关。当听到舒张中期杂音时,左向右分流程度可达到正常的1.5倍。原发孔型房间隔缺损,

TABLE 5.1 Most Common Congenital Heart Defects Surviving to Adulthood Without Surgery or Interventional Catheterization
Mild pulmonary valve stenosis
Bicuspid aortic valve
Small to moderate size atrial septal defect
Small ventricular septal defect
Small patent ductus arteriosus
Mitral valve prolapse
Partial atrioventricular canal (ostium primum atrial septal defect and cleft mitral valve)
Marfan syndrome
Ebstein's anomaly
Congenitally corrected transposition (atrioventricular and ventriculoarterial discordance)

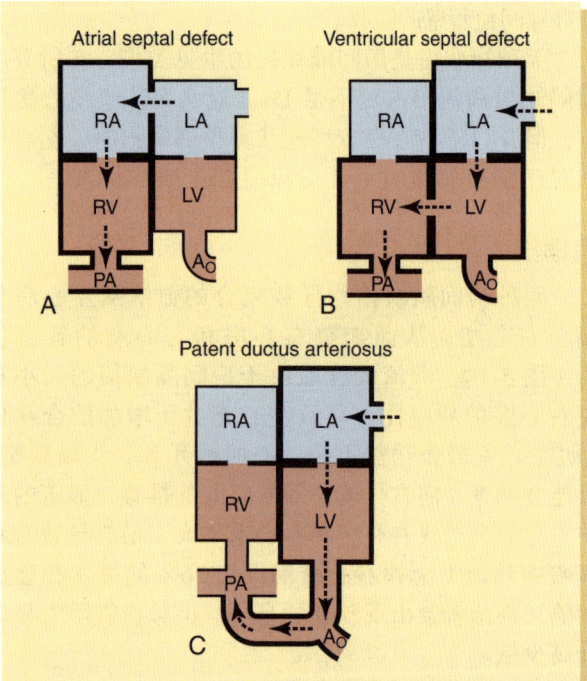

Fig. 5.1 The diagram shows three types of shunt lesions that commonly survive until adulthood and their effects on chamber size. (A) Uncomplicated atrial septal defect with left-to-right shunt flow across the interatrial septum, resulting in dilation of the right atrium (RA), right ventricle (RV), and pulmonary artery (PA). (B) Uncomplicated ventricular septal defect, resulting in dilation of the RV, left atrium (LA), and left ventricle (LV). (C) Uncomplicated patent ductus arteriosus, resulting in dilation of the LA, LV, and PA. *Ao*, Aorta. (From Liberthson RR, Walkdman H: Congenital heart disease in the adult. In Kloner RA, editor: Guide to cardiology, ed 3, Greenwich, Conn., 1991, Le Jacq Communications, pp 24-27.)

ASD, an additional holosystolic murmur at the apex may be caused by a cleft in the anterior leaflet of the mitral valve, resulting in mitral regurgitation.

Diagnosis

On the electrocardiogram (ECG), the features of ASD depend on the size and type of defect. In the setting of a large ostium secundum, sinus venosus, or unroofed coronary sinus defect, the ECG typically demonstrates evidence of right atrial (RA) enlargement, RV hypertrophy, and right axis deviation. In the setting of an ostium primum ASD, like other forms of atrioventricular defects, there is a superior axis. The chest radiograph is helpful for evaluating the degree of left-to-right shunting. With a small shunt, the radiograph will be normal. As the shunt increases in size, the heart size and pulmonary vascular markings also increase.

The diagnosis of an ASD and its location are confirmed by transthoracic echocardiography in most cases. A sinus venosus ASD is the exception. In this setting, transesophageal echocardiography may be necessary. Cardiac catheterization is rarely performed to diagnose an ASD. CT scan or cardiac MRI may be useful in defining the pulmonary venous anatomy especially in defects associated with anomalous pulmonary veins.

Treatment

The treatment of ASDs involves surgical or transcatheter device closure and is indicated in the setting of impaired functional capacity, right atrial and/or right ventricular enlargement or a Qp:Qs (pulmonary to systemic blood flow) ratio of 1.5:1 or greater. Individuals with an ASD and a PA systolic pressure greater than two-thirds of systemic, pulmonary vascular resistance greater than two-thirds of systemic, and/or a net right to left shunt should not undergo ASD closure. However, individuals with significantly elevated PA systolic pressure or pulmonary vascular resistance can be assessed for reversibility during a hemodynamic catheterization (usually with nitric oxide) and if found to have reversible pulmonary vascular disease they can be considered for repair. Those that are not reversible can be placed on pulmonary hypertension targeted therapy and undergo a hemodynamic reassessment after 6 months. A reduction in pulmonary vascular resistance of greater than 20% is associated with a favorable prognosis after ASD closure, and closure with a pulmonary vascular resistance of 6.5 Wood units or less has been associated with improved RV function. For a secundum ASD, surgical closure and transcatheter device closure are accepted treatment options. Device closure is the most commonly used technique for closure of secundum defects. This technique, however, requires an adequate rim of septal tissue around the entire defect to allow for device stabilization. For ostium primum, sinus venosus, and unroofed coronary sinus forms of ASDs, surgical closure remains the only option.

Prognosis

Most patients who have undergone early closure of a defect have excellent long-term survival rates with low morbidity rates if repair is undertaken before 25 years of age. Older age at repair is associated with decreased late survival rates and an associated increased risk of atrial arrhythmias, thromboembolic events, and pulmonary hypertension. After the age of 40 years for patients with unrepaired ASDs, the mortality rate increases by 6% per year, and more than 20% of patients develop atrial fibrillation. By 60 years of age, the number of patients with atrial fibrillation increases to more than 60%. In asymptomatic patients, it is reasonable to close a hemodynamically significant ASD in the absence of significant pulmonary hypertension; however, comorbidities (especially in older adults) may impact the benefit of ASD closure on improving symptoms and functional capacity. Long-term rates of late complications and survival after transcatheter device closure remain unknown.

Ventricular Septal Defects
Definition and Epidemiology

Ventricular septal defects (VSDs) occur in 1.5 to 3.5 of 1000 live births. They constitute 20% of congenital heart defects.

表 5.1　未经手术或导管介入治疗能存活至成年的常见先天性心脏缺陷
轻度肺动脉瓣狭窄
主动脉瓣二叶畸形
小至中等大小的房间隔缺损
小型室间隔缺损
小型动脉导管未闭
二尖瓣脱垂
部分型房室通道（原发孔型房间隔缺损和二尖瓣裂）
马方综合征
埃布斯坦畸形
先天性矫正型转位（房室和心室动脉连接不一致）

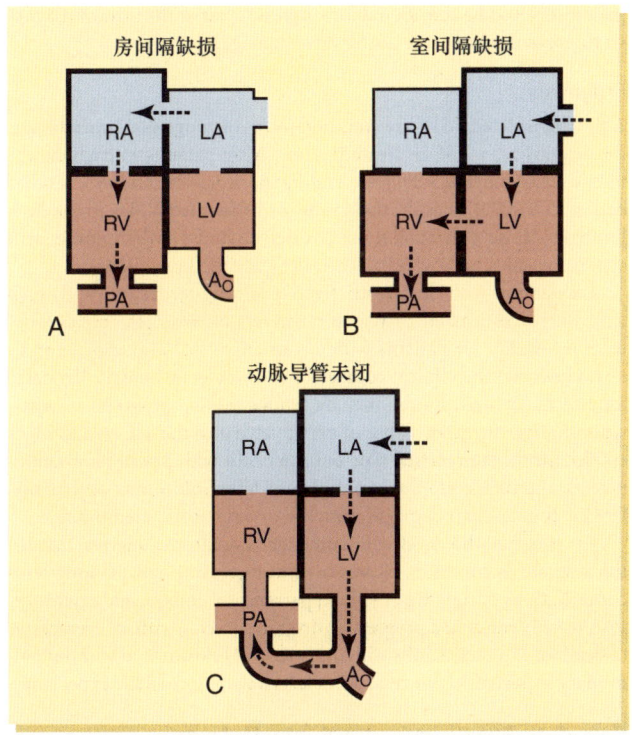

图 5.1　此图显示了三种常见的能存活至成年的分流病变及其对心腔大小的影响。A. 伴有左向右分流的单纯房间隔缺损，导致右心房（RA）、右心室（RV）和肺动脉（PA）扩张。B. 单纯室间隔缺损，导致右心室、左心房（LA）和左心室（LV）扩张。C. 单纯动脉导管未闭，导致左心房、左心室、肺动脉扩张。Ao，主动脉（引自 Liberthson RR, Walkdman H: Congenital heart disease in the adult. In Kloner RA, editor: Guide to cardiology, ed 3, Greenwich, Conn., 1991, Le Jacq Communications, pp 24-27.）

在心尖部能听到额外的全收缩期杂音，可能是二尖瓣前叶裂引起的二尖瓣反流导致的。

诊断

房间隔缺损的心电图表现取决于缺损的大小和类型。在大的继发孔型、静脉窦型或无顶冠状窦型房间隔缺损中，心电图的典型表现是右心房扩大、右心室肥厚和电轴右偏。在原发孔型房间隔缺损中，与其他类型房室缺损相似，存在电轴极度右偏。胸部 X 线片有助于评估左向右分流的程度。分流量较小时，胸部 X 线片可以表现正常。随着分流量增大，心影增大，肺血管纹理增多。

大部分病例由经胸超声心动图确诊房间隔缺损及其位置。而静脉窦型房间隔缺损除外，可能需要经食管超声心动图确诊。心导管检查很少被用于房间隔缺损的诊断。CT 或心脏 MRI 可能有助于明确肺静脉解剖结构，尤其是合并肺静脉异常的情况时。

治疗

房间隔缺损的治疗包括外科手术和经导管封堵，适用于活动耐量下降、右心房和（或）右心室扩大或 Qp：Qs（肺血流与体循环血流比值）为 1.5：1 或更大的情况。肺动脉（PA）收缩压大于体循环收缩压 2/3、肺血管阻力大于体循环阻力 2/3 和（或）右向左分流的房间隔缺损患者不应接受缺损封堵术。然而，肺动脉收缩压或肺血管阻力显著升高的患者可以在血流动力学导管检查（通常使用一氧化氮）期间评估其可逆性，如果发现患有可逆性肺血管疾病，则可以考虑进行手术。不可逆者可进行肺动脉高压靶向治疗，并在 6 个月后重新进行血流动力学评估。肺血管阻力降低超过 20% 提示房间隔缺损修补术后预后良好，而肺血管阻力不超过 6.5 Wood 单位则提示房间隔缺损修补后右心室功能可能得到改善。对于继发孔型房间隔缺损，手术封堵和经导管封堵均可选择。经导管封堵是治疗继发孔型房间隔缺损最常用的技术。但是这项技术需要整个缺损周围都有足够的隔组织以固定封堵器。对于原发孔型、静脉窦型和无顶冠状窦型房间隔缺损，手术封堵是唯一选择。

预后

大部分 25 岁之前接受封堵的患者长期生存率高，并发症发生率低。较晚修补者生存率下降，并且发生房性心律失常、血栓栓塞事件和肺动脉高压的风险增加。40 岁后仍未接受修补治疗的房间隔缺损患者，死亡率每年增加 6%，并且超过 20% 的患者发生心房颤动。到 60 岁时，心房颤动发生率超过 60%。对于无症状患者，在没有严重肺动脉高压的情况下修补分流显著的房间隔缺损是合理的。然而，合并症（尤其是老年人）可能会影响房间隔缺损修补在改善症状和功能方面的获益。经导管封堵后的远期并发症发生率和生存率尚未知。

室间隔缺损

定义和流行病学

室间隔缺损（VSD）在新生儿中发生率为（1.5～3.5）/1000，占先天性心脏病的 20%。

There are four types of VSD: perimembranous, muscular, supracristal, and inlet. Perimembranous VSDs are the most common, comprising 70% of all VSDs. The membranous septum is relatively small and sits directly under the aortic valve. Perimembranous VSDs involve the membranous septum and typically extend into the muscular tissue adjacent to the membranous septum. If not large, these defects may close spontaneously by tissue from the septal leaflet of the tricuspid valve.

Muscular VSDs are the second most common VSD and account for 5% to 20% of all VSDs. Multiple muscular VSDs commonly are found at the time of diagnosis. Muscular VSDs have the highest rate of spontaneous closure.

Supracristal VSDs represent 5% to 8% of all VSDs. These defects are located superior to the crista supraventricularis (i.e., within the RV outflow tract directly below the right cusp of the aortic valve). These defects are associated with prolapse of the right aortic cusp, which can lead to progressive aortic regurgitation. In some cases, the prolapsed right aortic cusp may restrict the defect, but rarely do they spontaneously close.

Inlet VSDs are located in the posterior ventricular septum, just inferior to the tricuspid and mitral valve. They account for 5% to 8% of all VSDs and never close spontaneously.

Pathology

Shunting through a VSD is typically left to right and can cause overcirculation of the pulmonary vasculature and increased pulmonary venous return, resulting in left-sided chamber enlargement (see Fig. 5.1). The degree of shunting depends on the size of the defect and the pulmonary vascular resistance. Small defects (i.e., restrictive defects) typically have a small degree of shunting and normal pulmonary artery pressure. Moderate-sized defects have enough left-to-right shunting to cause mildly elevated pulmonary artery pressures and some left-sided chamber enlargement. Large defects (i.e., nonrestrictive defects) allow LV systolic pressures to be transmitted to the pulmonary circulation. This can cause irreversible obstructive pulmonary vascular disease early in childhood. Eventually, if the pulmonary vascular resistance exceeds the systemic vascular resistance, the shunt may reverse to right to left (i.e., Eisenmenger's physiology).

Clinical Presentation

The physical findings for a patient with a VSD depend on the size of the VSD, magnitude of the shunt, and the level of pulmonary artery hypertension. For patients with a small VSD, the apical impulses of the right ventricle and left ventricle typically have normal intensity on palpation, but there may be a palpable thrill. The first and second heart sounds typically are normal, and in most cases, there is a holosystolic murmur of moderate intensity at the left lower sternal border.

Patients with Eisenmenger's syndrome have cyanosis and secondary erythrocytosis. The RV impulse usually is increased at the left lower sternal border, and the pulmonary component of the second heart sound may be palpable. Typically, no systolic murmur is detected, but a diastolic murmur is often heard at the left upper sternal border due to a severely dilated main pulmonary artery and resultant pulmonary regurgitation.

Diagnosis

The ECG should be normal for patients with small VSDs. For those with Eisenmenger's syndrome, the ECG usually demonstrates RV hypertrophy with right axis deviation. Patients with a small VSD have a normal chest radiograph. Patients with Eisenmenger's syndrome may have mild cardiac enlargement with enlarged proximal pulmonary arteries and peripheral pruning with oligemic lung fields. Echocardiography allows confirmation of the diagnosis, localization of defect, identification of long-term complications, and estimation of pulmonary artery pressure. Cardiac catheterization allows direct measurement of the degree of left-to-right shunting, pulmonary artery pressure, and pulmonary vascular reactivity.

Treatment

Because the majority of adult patients with an isolated VSD have no significant hemodynamic abnormalities, closure of the VSD is typically not needed. Closure of a VSD is indicated if there is evidence of left ventricular volume overload and a hemodynamically significant shunt (Qp:Qs >1.5). Small VSDs that are asymptomatic should be followed conservatively. Because of the long-term risks, they need intermittent follow-up for life to monitor for the development of late complications. The exceptions to this rule are those with small supracristal or perimembranous VSDs with associated prolapse of the aortic cusp into the defect that results in progressive aortic regurgitation. These patients should be considered for surgical repair at the time of diagnosis to prevent progressive aortic valve damage.

Prognosis

Although isolated VSDs are common forms of congenital heart disease, the diagnosis of a VSD in an adult is rare. Most patients with a hemodynamically significant VSD have undergone repair in childhood or died earlier in life. As a result, the spectrum of isolated VSDs in adults is limited to those with small restrictive defects, those with Eisenmenger's syndrome, and those who had their defects closed in childhood.

For patients with small restrictive VSDs, long-term survival is excellent, with an estimated 25-year survival rate of 96%. The rate of long-term morbidity for patients with a restrictive VSD also appears to be low. However, the clinical course is not completely benign. Reported long-term complications include endocarditis, progressive aortic regurgitation due to prolapse of aortic valve into the defect (i.e., highest risk for the supracristal type but can occur with a perimembranous defect), and the development of right and left outflow tract obstruction from a double-chamber right ventricle or a subaortic membrane.

For patients who develop Eisenmenger's syndrome, survival into the third decade is common. However, with increasing age, the long-term complications of right heart failure, paradoxical emboli, and erythrocytosis usually result in a progressive drop in survival, with an average age of death of 37 years. Adults with previous VSD closure and without pulmonary hypertension or residual defects have a normal life expectancy.

Complete Atrioventricular Septal Defects
Definition and Epidemiology

Complete atrioventricular septal defects (AVSDs) consist of several cardiac malformations that result from abnormal development of the endocardial cushions. AVSDs account for 4% to 5% of congenital heart defects. Down syndrome is a common association; 40% of Down syndrome patients have congenital heart disease, and 40% of these have some form of AVSD.

AVSDs are categorized as partial (or incomplete) or complete. Both forms share common structural abnormalities—ostium primum ASD, inlet VSD, and cleft anterior mitral and septal tricuspid leaflet—in various combinations.

Pathology

A combination of the previously described defects results in interatrial and interventricular shunts, LV-to-RA shunt, and atrioventricular regurgitation. Because these defects include deficiency of the inlet portion of the ventricular septum, the LV outflow tract is lengthened and may be narrowed, producing the characteristic goose-neck deformity.

室间隔缺损有四种类型：膜周部型、肌部型、嵴上型和漏斗部型。膜周部型室间隔缺损最为常见，占全部室间隔缺损的70%。室间隔膜部区域相对较小，位于主动脉瓣正下方。膜周部型室间隔缺损累及膜部间隔，并常向邻近的肌部组织延伸。如果缺损较小，三尖瓣隔瓣组织可能自发覆盖缺损使其闭合。

第二常见的类型是肌部型室间隔缺损，占全部室间隔缺损的5%～20%。确诊时常见多发性肌部缺损，此类缺损的自发闭合率最高。

嵴上型室间隔缺损占所有室间隔缺损的5%～8%。缺损位于室上嵴上方（即右心室流出道内主动脉瓣右冠瓣的正下方）。这种缺损可引起主动脉瓣右冠瓣脱垂，导致进行性主动脉瓣反流。在某些病例中，主动脉瓣右冠瓣脱垂可能会减轻缺损，但很少使缺损自行愈合。

漏斗部室间隔缺损位于室间隔后部，在三尖瓣和二尖瓣下方。占室间隔缺损的5%～8%，无法自行闭合。

病理学

典型的室间隔缺损分流是从左向右的，导致肺循环血量增加、肺静脉回流增加和左心腔增大（图5.1）。分流程度取决于缺损大小和肺血管阻力。小的缺损（如限制性缺损）一般分流少且肺动脉压正常。中等大小缺损的左向右分流量足以引起轻度肺动脉高压和一定程度的左心腔扩大。大的缺损（如非限制性缺损）使左心室收缩压传递至肺循环。这会在儿童期引起不可逆的阻塞性肺血管病。如果肺血管阻力最终超过体循环阻力，会逆转为右向左分流（如艾森门格综合征）。

临床表现

室间隔缺损患者的体格检查结果取决于缺损大小、分流程度、肺动脉压力水平。对于小的室间隔缺损，触诊时右心室和左心室心尖搏动正常，但可能有震颤。第一心音和第二心音一般正常；在大多数病例，胸骨左下缘能听到中等强度的全收缩期杂音。

艾森门格综合征患者有发绀和继发性红细胞增多症。胸骨左下缘右心室搏动常增强，可闻及第二心音的肺动脉瓣成分。一般没有收缩期杂音，但由于主肺动脉严重扩张及其造成的肺动脉瓣反流，在胸骨左上缘常可听到舒张期杂音。

诊断

小室间隔缺损患者心电图正常。有艾森门格综合征的患者，心电图常表现为右心室肥厚和电轴右偏。小室间隔缺损患者胸部X线片正常。有艾森门格综合征的患者，胸部X线片表现为心影轻度增大，近段肺动脉扩张及肺血流减少。超声心动图有助于明确诊断、确定缺损位置、发现长期并发症、评估肺动脉压力。心导管检查能直接测量左向右分流程度、肺动脉压力和评估肺血管反应性。

治疗

由于大多数成年患者为单纯性室间隔缺损，不伴有明显的血流动力学异常，因此通常不需要修补缺损。如果有左心室容量超负荷和血流动力学显著分流的证据（Qp：Qs＞1.5），则存在修补室间隔缺损的指征。小室间隔缺损无症状，应保守治疗；但由于存在远期风险，应当终身定期随访以监测晚期并发症的发生。但小嵴上型或膜周部型室间隔缺损伴主动脉瓣叶脱垂进入缺损区的患者例外，因为其会导致进行性主动脉瓣反流；这类患者在确诊后应当考虑外科修补以防止进行性主动脉瓣损害。

预后

尽管单纯室间隔缺损是常见的先天性心脏病，但成年人诊断为室间隔缺损者少见。显著影响血流动力学的室间隔缺损患者大部分在儿童时期接受修补治疗或早年夭折。因此，成年的单纯室间隔缺损患者仅限于小的限制性缺损、艾森门格综合征及儿童期自行闭合这三种形式。

对于小的限制性室间隔缺损患者，长期生存率很高，25年生存率约为96%。限制性室间隔缺损患者的远期并发症发生率也较低。然而临床过程并不完全良好。已报道的限制性室间隔缺损的远期并发症包括心内膜炎、主动脉瓣脱垂进入缺损处导致的进行性主动脉瓣反流（嵴上型风险高，但膜周部型也可能发生）、由双腔右心室或主动脉瓣下膜导致的右侧和左侧流出道梗阻。

艾森门格综合征患者通常能存活至30岁。但随着年龄增长，右心衰竭、反常栓塞、红细胞增多症等远期并发症使生存率迅速下降，平均寿命为37岁。接受过VSD修补术的成人患者，在没有肺动脉高压或残余缺损的情况下，预期寿命与正常人无异。

完全性房室间隔缺损

定义和流行病学

完全性房室间隔缺损（AVSD）包括由心内膜垫发育异常导致的一系列心脏畸形，占先天性心脏病的4%～5%。其与唐氏综合征具有相关性，40%的唐氏综合征患者存在先天性心脏病，其中40%为某种类型的房室间隔缺损。

房室间隔缺损分为部分型（或不完全型）和完全型两种类型。两种类型具有共同的结构异常，包括原发孔型房间隔缺损、漏斗部型室间隔缺损、二尖瓣前叶裂和三尖瓣隔叶裂，这些异常以不同组合的形式出现。

病理学

上述各种缺损组合后会导致心房间分流、心室间分流、左心室向右心房分流和房室间反流。由于这些缺损包括室间隔漏斗部缺陷，左心室流出道延长并有可能狭窄，形成特征性的鹅颈样畸形。

The natural history for patients with complete AVSD is characterized by the early development of pulmonary vascular disease, leading to irreversible damage that often occurs by 1 year of age, particularly for patients with Down syndrome. Surgery needs to be undertaken early if it is to be successful. Patients who are diagnosed in adulthood can be categorized in two groups: those with Eisenmenger's syndrome and those who had their defects closed in childhood.

Clinical Presentation

On physical examination, most previously repaired patients are cardiovascularly normal. However, patients with significant left atrioventricular (AV) valve regurgitation have a grade 3 or 4 (of 6) holosystolic regurgitant murmur at the apex. For the rare patient with subaortic stenosis, a grade 2 or 3 systolic murmur can be detected at the left midsternal border and radiating to the neck. The physical examination findings for patients with Eisenmenger's syndrome are similar to those for patients with unoperated VSDs.

Diagnosis

On the ECG, first-degree heart block is a common finding for patients with AVSD. All patients have a superior, leftward QRS axis. For those with Eisenmenger's syndrome, the chest radiograph demonstrates cardiomegaly, large proximal pulmonary arteries, and small peripheral pulmonary arteries (i.e., peripheral pruning). Patients who underwent previous repair and have significant systemic left AV valve regurgitation have cardiomegaly with increased vascular markings.

Treatment

Patients who underwent previous repair with significant left AV valve regurgitation causing symptoms, atrial arrhythmias, or deterioration in ventricular function should undergo elective repair or replacement. Previously repaired patients who develop significant subaortic stenosis (i.e., peak cardiac catheterization or echo gradient of ≥50 mm Hg or less in the presence of heart failure or moderate to severe mitral regurgitation) should undergo surgical repair.

Prognosis

Overall, for patients who underwent early repair before the development of pulmonary vascular disease, the long-term prognosis is good. The most common long-term complication is left AV valve regurgitation, with approximately 5% to 10% of patients requiring surgical revision for left AV valve repair or replacement during follow-up. The second most common long-term complication for this group is subaortic stenosis, occurring in up to 5% of patients after repair. Other long-term complications include residual atrial- or ventricular-level shunts, complete heart block, atrial and ventricular arrhythmias, and endocarditis.

Patients with Eisenmenger's syndrome are symptomatic with exertional dyspnea, fatigue, palpitations, edema, and syncope. Survival is similar to that for other forms of Eisenmenger's syndrome, with a mean age at death of 37 years. In retrospective studies, strong predictors for death included syncope, age at presentation of symptoms, poor functional class, low oxygen saturation (≤85%), increased serum creatinine and serum uric acid concentrations, and Down syndrome.

Coarctation of the Aorta
Definition

Coarctation of the aorta is an abnormal narrowing of the aortic lumen. It constitutes 5% of congenital heart defects. Coarctation of the aorta may occur anywhere along the descending aorta, even below the diaphragm, but in more than 95% of cases, the narrowing is just below the takeoff of the left subclavian artery. In 50% to 85% of cases, there is an associated bicuspid aortic valve. Other associated lesions include VSDs, subaortic stenosis, and mitral valve stenosis.

Pathology

Coarctation of the aorta is an aortopathy of the entire aorta rather than a localized abnormality. In the young, significant coarctation can decrease blood flow to the kidneys, gut, and lower extremities, resulting in severe acidosis and shock requiring immediate treatment. Unrepaired coarctation of the aorta can be seen in adults, but it is rare. Affected individuals develop extensive arterial collateralization to maintain distal perfusion. Most patients seen in adulthood are patients who have had previous coarctation of the aorta repair using a variety of different techniques.

Even after successful repair to relieve the obstruction, multiple studies have demonstrated that patients have persistent abnormalities in the media of the aorta proximal and distal to the coarctation repair site. The stiff aortic wall is characterized by decreased distensibility and endothelial and vascular dysfunction. These can result in resting and exercise-induced hypertension, increased carotid intimal thickness, and abnormal peripheral arterial responses to augmented blood flow and nitroglycerin.

Clinical Presentation

The clinical presentation of coarctation of the aorta depends on the severity of obstruction and the associated anomalies. Unrepaired coarctation of the aorta typically manifests with symptoms before adulthood. Symptoms include headaches related to hypertension, leg fatigue or cramps, exercise intolerance, and systemic hypertension. Untreated patients surviving to adulthood typically have only mild coarctation of the aorta.

Cardinal clinical features in the setting of a significant coarctation of the aorta include upper body hypertension, weak and delayed femoral pulses, and a blood pressure gradient between the right arm and right leg determined by blood pressure cuff. On auscultation, the aortic valve closure sound is usually loud; in the setting of a bicuspid aortic valve, an ejection click, often with a crescendo-decrescendo systolic murmur, is heard at the right upper sternal border. Often, a continuous systolic murmur is heard over the left scapula. It is related to continuous flow across the coarctation of the aorta.

Diagnosis

Patients with significant coarctation of the aorta typically show various degrees of left atrial (LA) and LV enlargement on an ECG. The chest radiograph typically demonstrates normal heart size with dilation of the ascending aorta and kinking or double contouring in the region of the descending aorta in the area of the coarctation, producing the characteristic figure-3 sign.

Most adult patients have rib notching. It is caused by the dilated intercostal collateral arteries eroding the undersurface of the ribs. Echocardiography is used to identify site, structure, and degree of stenosis or restenosis. Echocardiography is valuable for identifying other lesions, LV systolic function, and degree of LV hypertrophy.

Magnetic resonance imaging (MRI) and CT angiography are quite good for imaging the coarctation, defining the arch vessel anatomy, and identifying collaterals. Cardiac catheterization remains the gold standard for determining the anatomy and absolute degree of stenosis.

Treatment

Patients with hypertension and a significant native or residual coarctation of the aorta (i.e., upper extremity/lower extremity resting peak to peak gradient >20 mm Hg or mean Doppler systolic gradient >20 mm Hg, upper extremity/lower extremity gradient >10 mm Hg or mean

完全性房室间隔缺损的自然病程表现如下：早期出现肺血管疾病，1岁时即发生不可逆性损伤，唐氏综合征患者更是如此。如有条件，应早期手术治疗。成年期诊断的患者包括两种，已经发生艾森门格综合征和儿童期缺损自行愈合的患者。

临床表现

大部分经修复治疗的患者心血管体格检查正常。但有明显左房室瓣反流的患者心尖部有3/6级或4/6级全收缩期反流性杂音。在少见的主动脉瓣下狭窄的患者中，在胸骨中段左缘可闻及2/6～3/6级收缩期杂音并向颈部放射。艾森门格综合征患者的体格检查所见与未经治疗的室间隔缺损类似。

诊断

房室间隔缺损患者的心电图常有一度房室传导阻滞。所有患者均有电轴极度左偏。有艾森门格综合征的患者，胸部X线片表现为心影增大、近端肺动脉增宽、外周肺动脉减少（如肺纹理减少）。经修复并有明显左房室瓣反流的患者存在心脏扩大和肺纹理增多。

治疗

曾做过修复但仍有明显左房室瓣反流，并且有临床症状、房性心律失常或心室功能受损的患者，应择期进行修复或瓣膜置换。曾做过修复并发生明显主动脉瓣下狭窄（心导管或超声测得峰值压差＞50 mmHg或存在心力衰竭或中重度二尖瓣反流）者应行外科修复。

预后

总体而言，在发展至肺血管疾病之前行早期修复的患者远期预后较好。最常见的远期并发症是左房室瓣反流，其中5%～10%的患者在随访中需要行左房室瓣膜修复或置换。第二常见的远期并发症是主动脉瓣下狭窄，修复术后的发生率达5%。其他远期并发症包括残余心房或心室水平分流、完全性心脏传导阻滞、房性或室性心律失常和心内膜炎。

艾森门格综合征患者有劳力性呼吸困难、乏力、心悸、水肿和晕厥等症状。生存率与其他原因所致的艾森门格综合征相似，平均寿命为37岁。在回顾性分析中，死亡的强预测因子包括晕厥、出现症状的年龄、功能分级差、低血氧饱和度（≤85%）、血肌酐和血尿酸升高及唐氏综合征。

主动脉缩窄

定义

主动脉缩窄是主动脉腔的异常狭窄，占先天性心脏病的5%。主动脉缩窄可以出现在降主动脉的任何位置甚至是在膈下，但超过95%的病例缩窄位于左锁骨下动脉发出处下方。50%～85%的患者伴有二叶主动脉瓣。其他伴发情况包括室间隔缺损、主动脉瓣下狭窄和二尖瓣狭窄。

病理学

主动脉缩窄是整个主动脉的疾病，而不是一个局部性异常。在年轻人，明显的主动脉缩窄会减少肾脏、肠道和下肢的血流，导致严重的酸中毒和休克，需要立即处理。成年人可以见到未修复的主动脉缩窄，但很少见。患者会产生大量动脉侧支以维持远端灌注。成年期见到的大部分主动脉缩窄患者都是经过各种方式修复过的。

大量研究证实，即使修复成功解除阻塞，患者仍然在缩窄修复处近端和远端持续存在主动脉中膜异常。主动脉僵硬表现为主动脉扩张性下降、内皮和血管功能异常。临床表现为静息和活动诱发高血压、颈动脉内膜增厚、外周动脉对血流增加调节和硝酸甘油反应异常。

临床表现

主动脉缩窄的临床表现取决于梗阻的严重性及伴发的畸形。未经修复的主动脉缩窄一般在成年前出现症状。症状包括高血压相关性头痛、下肢乏力或痉挛、运动耐力下降、体循环高血压。未经治疗存活至成年的患者一般只有轻度主动脉缩窄。

显著主动脉缩窄患者的主要临床特征包括上半身高血压、股动脉搏动减弱和延迟，以及袖带式血压计测得的右侧上下肢血压差。听诊时，主动脉瓣关闭音增强；存在二叶主动脉瓣时，胸骨右上缘可闻及喷射性喀喇音，常伴有递增-递减型收缩期杂音。在左侧肩胛上区常可闻及持续性收缩期杂音，这与经过主动脉缩窄处的持续血流有关。

诊断

显著主动脉缩窄患者的心电图典型表现为不同程度的左心房和左心室增大。胸部X线片典型表现为心影大小正常，升主动脉增宽，缩窄区域降主动脉扭曲或重影，产生特征性的3字征。

大部分成年患者有肋骨切迹。它是由扩张的肋间侧支动脉侵蚀肋骨所致。超声心动图可以明确缩窄的位置、结构及狭窄或再狭窄的程度，对于评估其他病变、左心室收缩功能及左心室肥厚程度亦有价值。

磁共振成像（MRI）和增强CT在显示缩窄、明确主动脉弓解剖和评估侧支方面很有帮助。心导管检查仍然是明确解剖形态和评估狭窄程度的金标准。

治疗

患有高血压且主动脉显著缩窄的患者（即上肢/下肢静息峰值压差＞20 mmHg或平均多普勒收缩压差＞20 mmHg，上肢/下肢压差＞10 mmHg或平均多普勒压差＞10 mmHg伴有主动脉瓣反流导致的左心室收缩功能下降，上肢/下肢压差＞10 mmHg或平均多普勒

Doppler gradient >10 mm Hg plus either decreased LV systolic function of aortic regurgitation, upper extremity/lower extremity gradient >10 mm Hg or mean Doppler gradient >10 mm Hg with collateral flow) should be considered for surgical repair or catheter intervention with balloon angioplasty with or without stent placement. Surgical repair in the adult patient is technically difficult and is associated with high rates of morbidity. As a result, catheter-based intervention has become the preferred method in most experienced congenital heart disease centers, and balloon angioplasty for a native or recurrent coarctation of the aorta should be considered if stent placement or surgery is not an option.

Prognosis

After surgical repair, long-term survival is good but directly correlates with the age at repair. Those repaired after 14 years of age have a lower 20-year survival rate than those repaired earlier (79% vs. 91%). Long-term outcome data for catheter-based treatment is limited, but studies suggest that stented patients have lower acute and long-term complications at 60 months (25% for surgery vs. 12.5% for stents). Irrespective of the type of repair, the most common long-term complication is persistent or new systemic hypertension at rest or during exercise. Other long-term complications include aneurysms of the ascending or descending aorta (especially after Dacron patch repair), recoarctation at the site of previous repair, coronary artery disease, aortic stenosis or regurgitation (in the setting of a bicuspid aortic valve), and endarteritis. Intracranial aneurysms are seen in approximately 10% of patients with a coarctation, and increasing age and hypertension have been identified as risk factors.

Patent Ductus Arteriosus
Definition and Epidemiology

Patent ductus arteriosus (PDA) represents 9% to 12% of congenital heart defects. It is patent in the fetus but normally closes within several days of birth. However, it remains open in about 1 of 2500 to 5000 births. In infants born prematurely, the incidence is even higher, occurring in 8 of 1000 live births. The incidence of PDA is 30 times greater for babies born at high altitudes than for those born at sea level.

Pathology

A PDA allows transit of blood from the aorta into the pulmonary artery and recirculation through the pulmonary vasculature and the left side of the heart. This can result in left-sided chamber enlargement (see Fig. 5.1). As with VSDs, the size of the defect is the primary determinant of the clinical course in the adult patient. PDAs can be clinically categorized as silent PDAs; small, hemodynamically insignificant PDAs; moderate-size PDAs; large PDAs; and previously repaired PDAs.

Clinical Presentation

A silent PDA is a tiny defect that cannot be heard by auscultation and is detected only by other nonclinical means such as echocardiography. Life expectancy is always normal for this population, and the risk of endocarditis is extremely low.

Patients with a small PDA have an audible, long-ejection or continuous murmur that is heard best at the left upper sternal border and radiating to the back. They have normal peripheral pulses. Because there is negligible left-to-right shunting, these patients have normal LA and LV sizes and normal pulmonary artery pressure. Like those with silent PDAs, these patients are asymptomatic and have a normal life expectancy. However, they do have a higher risk of endocarditis.

Patients with moderate-size PDAs may be diagnosed during adulthood. These patients often have wide, bouncy peripheral pulses and an audible, continuous murmur. They have significant volume overload and develop some degree of LA and LV enlargement and some degree of pulmonary hypertension. These patients are symptomatic with dyspnea, palpitations, and heart failure. Patients with large PDAs typically have signs of severe pulmonary hypertension and Eisenmenger's syndrome. By adulthood, the continuous murmur is typically absent, and there is differential cyanosis (i.e., lower extremity saturations are lower than the right arm saturation).

Diagnosis

Patients with silent and small PDAs appear normal by echocardiography and chest radiography. Calcifications may be seen on the posteroanterior and lateral films of an older patient with a PDA. In patients with significant left-to-right shunting, there typically is dilation of the central pulmonary arteries with increased pulmonary vascular markings. On an ECG, broad P waves and tall QRS complexes suggest LA and LV volume overload. A tall R wave in lead V_1 with a right axis deviation suggests significant pulmonary hypertension. Measurement of oxygen saturation should be performed in feet and both hands in adults with moderate or large PDAs to assess for the presence of right to left shunting. Echocardiography is important to estimate the size of the defect, degree of LA or LV enlargement, and degree of pulmonary artery hypertension.

Treatment

PDA closure is recommended if there is left atrial or left ventricular enlargement present that is attributable to a PDA with left-to-right shunting. Patients with a PDA and severe, irreversible pulmonary hypertension should not have their PDA closed. Catheter device closure is the preferred method in most centers. Surgical closure is reserved for patients with PDAs too large for device closure and for distorted anatomy such as a large ductal aneurysm. Because patients with clinical evidence of a PDA are at increased risk for endocarditis and the low risk of catheter-based device closure, a small audible PDA should be considered for device closure.

Prognosis

Patients with a large PDA who have developed Eisenmenger's syndrome have a prognosis similar to that of other patients with Eisenmenger's syndrome. Patients who underwent PDA repair before the development of pulmonary hypertension have a normal life expectancy without restrictions.

Pulmonary Valve Stenosis
Definition and Epidemiology

Pulmonary valve stenosis occurs in approximately 4 of 1000 live births and constitutes 5% to 8% of congenital cardiac defects. It is one of the most common adult forms of unoperated congenital heart disease. It can occur in isolation or with other congenital heart defects, such as an ASD.

Pathology

In congenital pulmonary valve stenosis, the pulmonary valve leaflets are often fused or thickened, which obstructs blood flow out of the right ventricle. The obstruction elevates RV pressure, and compensatory RV hypertrophy develops. Pulmonary stenosis is often tolerated better than aortic stenosis. Over time, RV dilation and dysfunction may occur.

Clinical Presentation

Most patients with pulmonary valve stenosis are asymptomatic and have a cardiac murmur at presentation. Most unoperated adults with

压差＞10 mmHg 伴侧支血流）应考虑行手术修复或经导管介入球囊血管成形术，必要时植入支架。成年患者外科修复技术上困难且并发症发生率高。因此，经导管介入治疗是大部分有经验的先天性心脏病中心的首选，如果无法选择支架植入或手术，则应考虑对主动脉原发或复发性缩窄行球囊血管成形术。

预后

外科修复后，长期生存率很高，但其与修复时的年龄直接相关。14 岁后修复者 20 年生存率低于早期修复者（79% vs. 91%）。导管治疗的远期预后数据有限，但研究显示植入支架者急性期和 60 个月远期并发症发生率更低（外科手术 25% vs. 植入支架 12.5%）。无论何种修复方式，最常见的长期并发症是持续的或新发的静息或活动时体循环高血压。其他长期并发症包括升主动脉瘤或降主动脉瘤（特别是涤纶补片修复后）、修补处再狭窄、冠状动脉疾病、主动脉瓣狭窄或反流（存在二叶主动脉瓣时）、动脉内膜炎。大约 10% 的缩窄患者会出现颅内动脉瘤，已知的危险因素包括年龄增长和高血压。

动脉导管未闭

定义和流行病学

动脉导管未闭（PDA）占先天性心脏缺陷的 9%～12%。动脉导管在胎儿阶段正常存在，正常情况下出生后数日闭合。但是，2500～5000 名新生儿中就有 1 名患儿动脉导管在出生后持续开放。早产儿中发生率更高，每 1000 名活婴中就有 8 名。高海拔地区动脉导管未闭发生率比海平面水平地区高 30 倍。

病理学

动脉导管未闭使血液从主动脉流入肺动脉并通过肺血管再循环至左心，可能导致左心房和左心室扩大（图 5.1）。其与室间隔缺损相似，缺损大小是成年患者临床病程的主要决定因素。动脉导管未闭临床上分为静默型动脉导管未闭；小型、对血流动力学无显著影响的动脉导管未闭；中型动脉导管未闭；大型动脉导管未闭；已修复的动脉导管未闭。

临床表现

静默型动脉导管未闭是一种微小缺损，听诊没有异常，只有用超声心动图等非临床手段才能发现。这类患者的预期寿命正常，心内膜炎风险极低。

小型动脉导管未闭可以在胸骨左上缘听到长程喷射性或持续性杂音，并向背部放射。其周围脉搏正常。由于其左向右分流量小，患者左心房和左心室大小正常，肺动脉压力正常。与静默型动脉导管未闭相似，这类患者没有症状且预期寿命正常。但他们存在较高的心内膜炎风险。

中型动脉导管未闭患者可以在成年期诊断。这类患者外周脉搏宽大、有力，并可闻及持续性杂音。有明显容量超负荷，并有一定程度的左心房和左心室扩大及一定程度的肺动脉高压。这类患者有呼吸困难、心悸、心力衰竭等症状。大型动脉导管未闭患者常伴有严重肺动脉高压和艾森门格综合征的表现。到成年期，一般没有连续性杂音，会出现差异性发绀（下肢血氧饱和度低于右上肢）。

诊断

静默型和小型动脉导管未闭患者超声心动图和胸部 X 线片正常。老年动脉导管未闭患者可能在后前位或侧位片上看到钙化。在明显左向右分流的患者常表现为中心肺动脉增宽和肺血管纹理增加。在心电图上，P 波增宽、QRS 波群高尖，提示左心房和左心室容量负荷增加。V_1 导联 R 波增高伴电轴右偏提示明显肺动脉高压。对于中型或大型动脉导管未闭的成年患者，应测量脚部和双手的氧饱和度，以评估是否存在右向左分流。超声心动图对评估缺损大小、左心房和左心室增大程度及肺动脉高压程度很重要。

治疗

如果存在由于动脉导管未闭左向右分流而导致左心房或左心室增大，则建议进行动脉导管闭合。合并重度、不可逆肺动脉高压的动脉导管未闭患者，不应考虑封闭动脉导管。大部分中心首选经导管器械封堵。外科手术封堵用于动脉导管太大，器械无法封堵的患者和解剖扭曲如大的导管动脉瘤的患者。由于具有明确动脉导管未闭临床证据的患者发生心内膜炎的风险增加，并且经导管器械封堵的风险较低，因此对小型无症状动脉导管未闭也应考虑行器械封堵。

预后

发生艾森门格综合征的大型动脉导管未闭患者预后与其他艾森门格综合征患者近似。肺动脉高压出现前接受手术治疗的患者预期寿命正常且无活动限制。

肺动脉瓣狭窄

定义和流行病学

每 1000 个活婴中大约有 4 个出现肺动脉瓣狭窄，占先天性心脏缺陷的 5%～8%。它是成人未经手术治疗的先天性心脏病最常见类型之一。它可以单独存在，或与其他先天性心脏缺陷如房间隔缺损等同时存在。

病理学

在先天性肺动脉瓣狭窄中，肺动脉瓣常融合或增厚，阻碍了血液从右心室流出。血流阻塞使右心室压力升高，出现代偿性右心室肥厚。肺动脉狭窄常比主动脉瓣狭窄耐受性好。经过一段时间，其可能出现右心室扩大和功能不全。

临床表现

大多数肺动脉瓣狭窄患者是无症状的，可以有心脏杂音。大部分未经手术治疗的重度狭窄成年患者会

severe stenosis have jugular venous distention, and on palpation, an RV lift at the left lower sternal border and a thrill at the left upper sternal border can be identified. On auscultation, the second heart sound is widely split, and a systolic ejection click may or may not be heard, depending on the mobility of the pulmonary valve leaflets. In most cases, there is a harsh, crescendo-decrescendo systolic ejection murmur, which is heard best at the left upper sternal border; it radiates to the back and varies with inspiration.

Diagnosis

With moderate to severe pulmonary valve stenosis, the ECG demonstrates right axis deviation, RV hypertrophy, and RA enlargement. The ECG is usually normal for patients with mild pulmonary valve stenosis. On the chest radiograph, a prominent main pulmonary artery caused by poststenotic dilatation is a common finding regardless of the degree of stenosis. In patients with severe pulmonary valve stenosis, cardiomegaly due to RA and RV enlargement is often seen.

Echocardiography is the diagnostic method of choice. It allows visualization of the valve anatomy and degree of stenosis and enables estimation of the valve gradient.

Treatment

Survival into adult life and the need for intervention directly correlate with the degree of obstruction. In the Second Natural History Study of Congenital Heart Disease, patients with trivial stenosis (i.e., peak gradient ≤25 mm Hg) who were followed for 25 years remained asymptomatic and had no significant progression of obstruction over time. For those with moderate pulmonary valve stenosis (i.e., peak gradient between 25 and 49 mm Hg), there was an approximately 20% chance of requiring intervention by 25 years of age. Most patients with severe stenosis (i.e., peak gradient of ≥50 mm Hg) require intervention (i.e., surgery or balloon valvuloplasty) by age 25 years. Patients with moderate to severe pulmonary stenosis may be considered for intervention even in the absence of symptoms.

Since 1985, percutaneous balloon valvuloplasty has been the accepted treatment for patients of all ages. Before 1985, surgical valvotomy had been the gold standard. Today, adults with moderate or severe valvular pulmonary stenosis and otherwise unexplained symptoms of heart failure, cyanosis from interatrial right to left shunting, or exercise are recommended to undergo balloon valvuloplasty if feasible; otherwise surgical valvotomy is recommended (if the valve is extremely dysplastic or calcified).

Prognosis

After surgical valvotomy for isolated pulmonary stenosis, long-term survival is excellent. However, with longer follow-up the incidence of late complications and the need for reintervention do increase. The most common indication for reintervention is pulmonary valve replacement for severe pulmonary regurgitation. Other long-term complications include recurrent atrial arrhythmias, endocarditis, and residual subpulmonary obstruction.

Aortic Valve Stenosis
Definition and Epidemiology

Aortic valve stenosis is a common abnormality in adults with congenital heart disease. It is usually caused by a bicuspid aortic valve, which occurs in 1% to 2% of adults and is three times more common in males. It typically is an isolated lesion but can be associated with a dilated ascending aorta and other defects such as coarctation of the aorta or VSD.

Pathology

Aortic valve stenosis results in pressure overload of the left ventricle, which increases wall stress and causes compensatory LV hypertrophy. Diastolic dysfunction and oxygen delivery-demand mismatch ensues. The patient may remain well compensated and asymptomatic for many years, but compensatory mechanisms eventually begin to fail and LV dysfunction can develop. Patients with a bicuspid aortic valve have abnormal structure of the aortic wall that often leads to ascending aortic dilation.

Clinical Presentation

Most patients with aortic valve stenosis are asymptomatic and are diagnosed after a murmur is detected. The severity of obstruction at the time of diagnosis correlates with the pattern of progression. Symptoms are rare until patients have severe aortic valve stenosis (i.e., mean gradient by echocardiography of ≥40 mm Hg). Symptoms include chest pain, exertional dyspnea, near-syncope, and syncope. With any of these symptoms, the risk of sudden cardiac death is very high, and surgical intervention is mandated.

Patients with moderate to severe stenosis typically have decreased peripheral pulses, an increased apical impulse, and a palpable thrill at the base of the heart. On auscultation, these patients have an ejection click followed by a crescendo-decrescendo systolic murmur, which is heard best at the left midsternal border and radiating to the right upper sternal border and the neck. Correlation between the degree of stenosis and the intensity of the murmur is not good. However, it is rare for a murmur of 2/6 or less to be associated with severe stenosis. Some patients with aortic stenosis also have aortic regurgitation, in which case a decrescendo diastolic murmur at the left midsternal border that radiates to the apex is detected at presentation.

Diagnosis

Many patients with significant aortic stenosis have LV hypertrophy identified on the ECG. However, the correlation between the severity of stenosis and the finding of LV hypertrophy on the ECG is unreliable. On chest radiography, most patients with severe aortic stenosis have a normal heart size unless there is concurrent aortic regurgitation. Post-stenotic dilation of the ascending aorta is common irrespective of degree of stenosis, and ascending aorta dilation is a common finding. It appears on the chest radiograph as a widened mediastinum.

Echocardiography is the gold standard for evaluation of the severity of aortic valve stenosis and the anatomic morphology of the aortic valve. Cardiac catheterization is primarily indicated to evaluate coronary artery disease before surgical intervention, because approximately one-half of adults with symptomatic aortic valve stenosis have concurrent coronary artery disease.

Treatment

Patients with severe aortic stenosis and symptoms or asymptomatic patients with severe aortic valve stenosis and reduced LV systolic function (<50%) should be considered for intervention. Treatment involves manipulating the valve to reduce stenosis. This can be accomplished by transvenous balloon dilation of the valve, open surgical valvotomy, or surgical or catheter-based valve replacement. In absence of significant aortic regurgitation, most centers favor balloon dilation or surgical valvotomy for children who have pliable valves with fusion of the commissures. In adults, aortic valve replacement is the treatment of choice. Aortic valve replacement may be done with a mechanical valve, bioprosthetic valve, or the Ross procedure (placing the pulmonary autograft in the aortic position and putting a new valve in the pulmonary position). The ascending aorta may be replaced if it is 5.5 cm (5.0 cm in the setting of high-risk features, such as growth >0.5 cm/year or family history of dissection) or 4.5 cm at the time of an aortic valve replacement.

有颈静脉怒张，触诊可以发现胸骨左下缘右心室抬举样搏动和胸骨左上缘震颤。听诊时，第二心音广泛分裂，肺动脉瓣叶活动度决定是否可闻及收缩期喷射性喀喇音。多数情况下，胸骨左上缘可闻及粗糙的递增-递减型收缩期喷射性杂音，可放射至背部，且随呼吸变化。

诊断

中到重度的肺动脉瓣狭窄，心电图表现为电轴右偏，右心室肥厚和右心房扩大。轻度狭窄的患者心电图常正常。胸部 X 线片上，无论狭窄程度如何，都可以看到狭窄后扩张导致的主肺动脉凸出。严重肺动脉瓣狭窄的患者，常可以看到由右心房和右心室扩大引起的心脏扩大。

超声心动图是可供选择的诊断方法，可以看到瓣膜解剖和狭窄程度，估测跨瓣压差。

治疗

患者成年后的生存率及干预需求与阻塞程度直接相关。根据《先天性心脏病二次自然史研究》，轻度狭窄（峰值压差 ≤ 25 mmHg）患者随访 25 年仍无症状且狭窄无显著进展；中度狭窄（峰值压差 25～49 mmHg）者 25 岁前约 20% 需干预；重度狭窄（峰值压差 ≥ 50 mmHg）者多数需在 25 岁前接受手术或球囊瓣膜成形术。中重度狭窄患者即使无症状也可考虑干预。

从 1985 年开始，经皮球囊瓣膜成形术被认为适用于所有年龄的患者。1985 年以前，外科瓣膜切开术是金标准。如今，中度或重度肺动脉瓣狭窄以及有其他无法解释的心力衰竭症状、存在右向左分流引起的发绀或有锻炼需求的成年人，如果可行，建议行球囊瓣膜成形术；否则建议行瓣膜切开术（如瓣膜严重发育不良或钙化）。

预后

单纯的肺动脉瓣狭窄患者经外科瓣膜切开术治疗后，能长期存活。然而，随着更长时间的随访，晚期并发症和需要再治疗的发生率有所增加。再治疗最常见的情况是因出现重度肺动脉瓣反流而进行肺动脉瓣置换。其他长期并发症包括反复的房性心律失常、心内膜炎和残存的肺动脉瓣下梗阻。

主动脉瓣狭窄

定义和流行病学

主动脉瓣狭窄是成人先天性心脏病的常见畸形。其通常由二叶主动脉瓣引起，二叶主动脉瓣在成人中的发生率为 1%～2%，男性比女性高 3 倍。主动脉瓣狭窄通常单独存在，但也可伴随降主动脉扩张以及主动脉缩窄或室间隔缺损等其他缺损同时存在。

病理学

主动脉瓣狭窄导致左心室压力负荷增加，使室壁应力增加，产生代偿性的左心室肥厚，随后出现舒张功能不全和氧供需失调。患者可以很好地处于代偿状态、无症状很多年，但是代偿机制最终失效，出现左心室功能不全。二叶主动脉瓣患者存在主动脉壁结构异常，常导致升主动脉扩张。

临床表现

大多数主动脉瓣狭窄患者没有症状，在发现杂音后被诊断。诊断时梗阻的严重程度与进展方式相关。患者在出现重度主动脉瓣狭窄（如超声心动图评估的平均跨瓣压差 ≥ 40 mmHg）之前很少有症状。症状包括胸痛、劳力性呼吸困难、晕厥前兆和晕厥。出现上述任何症状时，猝死的风险极高，必须进行外科治疗。

中重度主动脉瓣狭窄的患者通常外周脉搏减弱、心尖搏动增强、心底部可触及震颤。听诊时，这些患者听诊有喷射性喀喇音，之后伴随递增-递减型收缩期杂音，在胸骨中部左缘最清楚，并向胸骨右上缘及颈部放射。狭窄程度和杂音强度的相关性并不好。但如果杂音不超过 2/6 级，很少有严重狭窄。一些主动脉瓣狭窄患者也伴有主动脉瓣反流，这些病例表现为胸骨中部左缘的递减型舒张期杂音并向心尖部放射。

诊断

许多有明显主动脉瓣狭窄的患者可以在心电图上发现左心室肥厚。然而狭窄程度和心电图上左心室肥厚的相关性并不可靠。大部分重度主动脉瓣狭窄患者胸部 X 线片上心脏大小正常，除非同时伴有主动脉瓣反流。无论狭窄程度如何，升主动脉的狭窄后扩张为常见表现，其在胸部 X 线片上表现为纵隔增宽。

超声心动图是评估主动脉瓣狭窄严重程度和解剖形态的金标准。外科治疗前建议行心导管检查评估冠状动脉情况，因为有症状的主动脉瓣狭窄成年患者中大约有 50% 同时伴有冠状动脉疾病。

治疗

有症状的重度主动脉瓣狭窄患者或无症状但合并左心室收缩功能减低（< 50%）的重度主动脉瓣狭窄患者应该进行干预治疗。治疗目的是减轻瓣膜狭窄，可以通过经静脉瓣膜球囊扩张、开放的外科瓣膜切开术、外科或导管为基础的瓣膜置换术治疗。如果没有显著的主动脉瓣反流，对于儿童如果其瓣膜联合部融合、柔韧，大多数中心更倾向于球囊扩张或外科瓣膜切开术。对于成人，可以选择主动脉瓣置换，包括使用机械瓣膜、生物瓣膜或 ROSS 手术（将自体肺动脉瓣移植物放置在主动脉瓣位置并将新瓣膜放置在肺动脉瓣位）。如果升主动脉超过 5.5 cm［在高风险特征的情况下（如每年扩张 > 0.5 cm 或具有夹层家族史）为 5.0 cm］或 4.5 cm（主动脉瓣置换时），则可以考虑行升主动脉置换。

Prognosis

The natural history of aortic valve stenosis in adults varies but is characterized by progressive stenosis over time. By 45 years of age, approximately 50% of bicuspid aortic valves have some degree of stenosis. Most patients requiring surgical valvotomy to relieve the stenosis before adulthood do well. However, by the 25-year follow-up, up to 40% of patients required a second operation for residual stenosis or regurgitation.

CYANOTIC HEART DISEASE

Tetralogy of Fallot

Definition and Epidemiology

Tetralogy of Fallot (TOF) is the most common cyanotic heart disease seen in adulthood, and it represents 10% of congenital heart defects. It consists of a large VSD, pulmonary stenosis (which may be valvular, subvalvular, and or supravalvular), an aorta that overrides the VSD, and RV hypertrophy.

Pathology

Newborns with TOF are cyanotic because of the right-to-left shunt through the VSD and decreased pulmonary blood flow. The amount of pulmonary blood flow depends on the severity of the obstruction through the RV outflow tract. By the time TOF patients reach adulthood, most have had complete repair or palliative surgery.

Many adults with repaired TOF have had a transannular patch (i.e., synthetic patch across the pulmonary annulus) placed to relieve the RV outflow tract obstruction. This patch causes obligatory free pulmonary regurgitation. Free pulmonary regurgitation can be well tolerated by the right ventricle for many years, but usually in the third or fourth decades, the right ventricle begins to dilate, and it may become dysfunctional. Significant RV dilation and dysfunction can lead to LV dysfunction, significant tricuspid regurgitation, and atrial or ventricular arrhythmias. Almost 29% of adults with repaired TOF also have a dilated ascending aorta due to increased blood flow through the aorta before repair.

Clinical Presentation

Patients with repaired TOF typically have normal oxygen saturation levels. On palpation, there often is an RV lift at the left lower sternal border. On auscultation, there typically is a widely split second heart sound with a to-and-fro murmur in the pulmonary area due to significant pulmonary regurgitation or, less commonly, aortic regurgitation. A holosystolic murmur due to tricuspid regurgitation may be heard at the left lower sternal border. Symptoms in the adult with repaired TOF may include exertional dyspnea, palpitations, syncope, and sudden cardiac death.

Diagnosis

The ECG almost universally reveals a right bundle branch block pattern in patients who underwent repair of TOF. The QRS duration from the standard surface ECG correlates with the degree of RV dilation and dysfunction. A maximum QRS duration of 180 milliseconds or more is a highly sensitive and relatively specific marker for sustained ventricular tachycardia and sudden cardiac death. Patients with significant pulmonary regurgitation often have cardiomegaly with dilated central pulmonary arteries identified on the chest radiograph. A right aortic arch occurs in 25% of cases, and it can be detected by close observation of the chest radiograph. An echocardiogram is useful for evaluating the RV outflow tract (e.g., pulmonary regurgitation, residual stenosis), biventricular size and function, tricuspid valve function, and ascending aortic size. MRI is the gold standard for assessing RV size and function (Fig. 5.2). It can also give an accurate assessment of the degree of pulmonary insufficiency and branch pulmonary artery anatomy.

Treatment

Treatment for TOF is surgical repair. Repair is typically performed between 3 to 12 months of age and consists of patch closure of the VSD and relief of the pulmonary outflow tract obstruction by patch augmentation of the RV outflow tract or pulmonary valve annulus, or both. Reintervention is necessary in approximately 10% of adults with repaired TOF after 20 years of follow-up. With longer follow-up, the incidence of reintervention continues to increase. The most common indication for reintervention is pulmonary valve replacement in patients with moderate or greater pulmonary valve regurgitation and symptoms. Pulmonary valve replacement is also reasonable for preservation of ventricular size and function in asymptomatic patients with repaired tetralogy of Fallot and ventricular enlargement or dysfunction and moderate or greater pulmonary regurgitation. Pulmonary valve replacement can be performed surgically, or in some patients, percutaneously. Patients with repaired tetralogy of Fallot may be considered for an ICD for primary prevention if multiple risk factors for sudden death are present, including LV systolic or diastolic dysfunction, nonsustained ventricular tachycardia, QRS greater than 180 ms, extensive right ventricular scarring or inducible sustained ventricular tachycardia at an electrophysiologic study.

Prognosis

In the developed world, the unoperated adult with TOF has become a rarity because most patients undergo palliation (i.e., stenting) or repair in childhood. Survival of the unoperated patient to the seventh decade has been described but is rare. Only 11% of unrepaired patients are alive at 20 years of age and only 3% at 40 years.

Late survival after repair of TOF is excellent. Survival rates at 32 and 35 years are 86% and 85%, respectively, compared with 95% for age- and sex-matched controls. Importantly, most patients live an unrestricted life. However, many patients over time develop late symptoms related to numerous, long-term complications after TOF repair. Late complications include endocarditis, aortic regurgitation with or without aortic root dilation (typically due to damage of the aortic valve during VSD closure or to an intrinsic aortic root abnormality), LV dysfunction (from inadequate myocardial protection during previous repair or chronic LV volume overload due to long-standing palliative arterial shunts), residual pulmonary obstruction, residual pulmonary valve regurgitation, RV dysfunction (due to pulmonary regurgitation or pulmonary stenosis), atrial arrhythmias (typically atrial flutter), ventricular arrhythmias, and heart block.

Transposition of the Great Arteries

Definition and Epidemiology

Transposition of the great arteries (TGA) represents 3.8% of all congenital heart disease. In complete TGA, the aorta arises from the right ventricle and the pulmonary artery from the left ventricle. As a result, the systemic venous flow (i.e., blood with low oxygen content) is returned to the right ventricle and is then pumped to the body through the aorta without passing through the lungs for gas exchange. The pulmonary venous flow (i.e., oxygenated blood) returning to the left ventricle is then pumped back to the lungs. As a result, the systemic and pulmonary circulations run in parallel. Oxygenation and survival depend on mixing between the systemic and pulmonary circulations at the atrial, ventricular, or PDA level. In 50% of cases, there are other anomalies: VSD (30%), pulmonary stenosis (5% to 10%), aortic stenosis, and coarctation of the aorta (≤5%).

The first definitive operations for TGA (i.e., atrial switch procedures) were described by Senning in 1959 and Mustard in 1964. In these procedures, the systemic and pulmonary venous returns are

预后

成人主动脉瓣狭窄的自然病程差异很大，但是均有进行性狭窄的特征。至45岁，约50%二叶主动脉瓣会有一定程度的狭窄。成年之前需要外科瓣膜切开术来减轻狭窄的大多数患者能良好生活。然而，随访至25年时，约40%的患者因残存狭窄或反流需要再次手术。

发绀型心脏病

法洛四联症

定义和流行病学

法洛四联症是成年人最常见的发绀型先天性心脏病，占先天性心脏缺陷的10%。其包括大的室间隔缺损、肺动脉狭窄（可能是瓣膜型、瓣下型或瓣上型）、骑跨于室间隔缺损的主动脉和右心室肥厚。

病理学

法洛四联症的新生儿出现发绀是由于经过室间隔的右向左分流和肺血流的减少。肺血流量取决于右心室流出道梗阻的严重程度。法洛四联症患者至成年期，大多数已经接受完全或姑息性的外科修补手术。

大部分经过修补的成年人放置了一个跨环补片（如穿过肺动脉环的合成补片）来减轻右心室流出道梗阻。补片会导致肺动脉瓣不受限的反流，右心室可以很好地耐受很多年。但是通常在30～40年时，右心室开始扩大，并出现功能不全。显著的右心室扩大和功能不全导致左心室功能不全、严重的三尖瓣反流和房性或室性心律失常。29%经修复的成人法洛四联症患者也会有升主动脉扩张，这是由修复前通过升主动脉的血流增多引起的。

临床表现

修复后的法洛四联症患者通常氧合水平正常。胸骨左下缘常可触诊到右心室抬举。听诊时肺动脉瓣听诊区由于肺动脉瓣反流（或不太常见的主动脉瓣反流）常有广泛分裂的第二心音并伴有拉锯样杂音。胸骨左下缘可以听到三尖瓣反流产生的全收缩期杂音。经修复的成年法洛四联症患者的症状包括劳力性呼吸困难、心悸、晕厥和心源性猝死。

诊断

经过修补的法洛四联症患者心电图普遍表现为右束支传导阻滞图形。标准体表心电图的QRS间期与右心室扩张和功能不全的程度相关。QRS间期180 ms及以上是持续性室性心动过速和心源性猝死的高度敏感和相对特异的指标。显著肺动脉瓣反流患者常可以在胸部X线片上看到心脏扩大和主肺动脉扩张。右侧主动脉弓出现在25%的病例，在胸部X线片上仔细观察可以发现。超声心动图对于评估右心室流出道（如肺动脉瓣反流、残余狭窄）、双心室大小和功能、三尖瓣功能和升主动脉大小非常有用。磁共振成像是评估右心室大小和功能的金标准（图5.2），也可以精确评估肺动脉异常的程度和肺动脉分支的解剖。

治疗

法洛四联症的治疗方法是外科修补。修补常在患者3～12个月时进行，包括补片封闭室间隔缺损，补片扩张右心室流出道或肺动脉瓣环或两者同时进行以减轻肺动脉流出道梗阻。在20年的随访中，约有10%修补后的法洛四联症成人需要再治疗。随着随访时间的延长，需要再次治疗的概率持续增加。最常见的再次手术指征是因中重度肺动脉瓣反流伴随临床症状需要进行肺动脉瓣置换。对于法洛四联症修复后心室扩大或心室功能不全以及中度或以上肺动脉瓣反流的无症状患者，为了保留心室大小和功能，肺动脉瓣置换术也是合理的。肺动脉瓣置换术可以通过常规外科手术进行，或者在某些患者中也可以通过经皮介入置换的方式完成。如果存在猝死的多种危险因素，包括左心室收缩或舒张功能障碍、非持续性室性心动过速、QRS间期大于180 ms、广泛的右心室瘢痕或电生理试验中诱发的持续性室性心动过速，法洛四联症修复术后患者可考虑使用ICD进行一级预防。

预后

在发达国家，因多数患者在儿童期已接受姑息治疗（如支架植入）或修复手术，未经手术治疗的成人TOF患者已较为少见。文献记载未手术患者可存活至70岁，但极为罕见；未手术患者20年生存率为11%，40年生存率仅为3%。

修复后的法洛四联症患者晚期存活率很高。与年龄和性别匹配度95%的对照人群相比，32岁和35岁的存活率分别为86%和85%。重要的是，大多数患者生活不受限制。然而随着时间推移，很多患者在修补术后出现了与大量长期并发症相关的晚期症状。晚期并发症包括心内膜炎、伴或不伴主动脉根部扩张（常由于关闭室间隔缺损时损害了主动脉瓣或本身就有的主动脉根部异常）的主动脉瓣反流、左心室功能不全（由于之前修补时不充分的心肌保护或由于长期姑息性动脉分流引起的左心室容量超负荷）、残存的肺动脉阻塞、残存的肺动脉瓣反流、右心室功能不全（由于肺动脉瓣反流或狭窄）、房性心律失常（常为心房扑动）、室性心律失常和心脏传导阻滞。

大动脉转位

定义和流行病学

大动脉转位（TGA）占所有先天性心脏病的3.8%。完全大动脉转位的主动脉起源于右心室，肺动脉起源于左心室。因此，体循环静脉血（低氧含量血）回到右心室，然后未经肺部气体交换通过主动脉泵入全身。肺静脉血（氧合血）回到左心室然后泵回肺部。结果使体循环和肺循环并行。氧合和存活依赖于体循环和肺循环血液在心房、心室或未闭合的动脉导管水平进行混合。50%的病例还有其他畸形，包括室间隔缺损（30%）、肺动脉狭窄（5%～10%）、主动脉瓣狭窄和主动脉缩窄（≤5%）。

第一批明确的大动脉转位手术（如心房转流术）

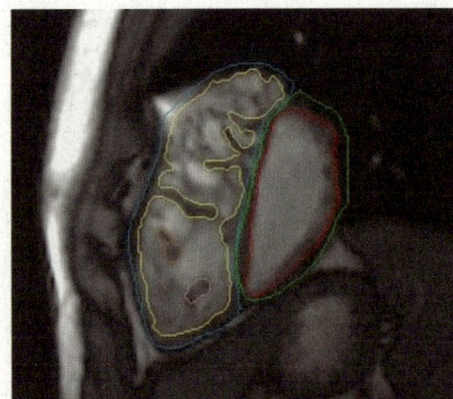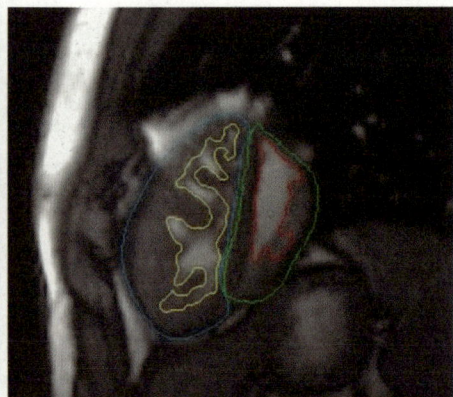

Fig. 5.2 Short axis magnetic resonance images of the right and left ventricles with epicardial and endocardial tracings of both ventricular cavities. There are a predefined number of slices through the heart with a constant thickness. The volumes of the left and right ventricles in each slice are calculated and summed together in end diastole and end systole to determine the total right and left ventricular volumes (i.e., Simpson's method).

rerouted in the atrium by constructing baffles. The systemic venous return from the superior and inferior vena cavae is directed through the mitral valve and into the left ventricle, which is connected to the pulmonary artery. The pulmonary venous return is then directed through the tricuspid valve into the right ventricle, which is connected to the aorta. These procedures leave the left ventricle as the pulmonary ventricle and the right ventricle as the systemic ventricle.

Over the past 20 years, the arterial switch procedure has gained popularity. During the procedure, the great arteries are transected and reanastomosed to the correct ventricle (i.e., left ventricle to the aorta and right ventricle to the pulmonary artery) along with coronary artery transfer. Operative survival after the arterial switch procedure is very good, with a surgical mortality rate of 2% to 5%.

Pathology

Most infants who do not have surgical intervention die in the first few months of life. For adults born with complete TGA who have had an atrial switch procedure, the right ventricle continues to be the systemic ventricle, and the left ventricle is the subpulmonic ventricle. Long-term follow-up series have demonstrated that the right ventricle can function as the systemic ventricle for 30 to 40 years, but with longer follow-up, systemic ventricular dysfunction continues to increase. At the 35-year follow-up, approximately 61% of patients have developed moderate or severe RV dysfunction.

Another common postoperative problem is the tricuspid valve. After the atrial switch procedure, the tricuspid valve remains the systemic atrioventricular valve and must tolerate systemic pressures. Due to changes in RV morphology and abnormal chordal attachments, the tricuspid valve is prone to become dysfunctional and develop significant regurgitation.

Significant coronary lesions, such as occlusions or stenoses, occur in 6.8% of patients who have had the arterial switch procedure. These lesions are likely related to suture lines or kinking at the time of reimplantation of the coronary arteries into the neo-aorta. Systemic LV function is usually normal. LV dysfunction is associated with coronary anomalies.

Clinical Presentation

In the repaired adult with an atrial switch procedure, the physical examination may reveal a murmur consistent with tricuspid valve insufficiency and a prominent second heart sound due to the anterior position of the aorta. Patients who have had an atrial switch procedure tend to have worsening functional status as the length of follow-up increases. They often have resting sinus bradycardia or a junctional rhythm. Palpitations due to atrial arrhythmias are common, occurring in up to 48% of patients 23 years after the atrial switch procedure.

In those who undergo the arterial switch procedure, the physical examination may reveal a murmur of neo-aortic or neo-pulmonic regurgitation. These patients usually have normal function status, but because of denervation of the heart, myocardial ischemia may manifest as atypical chest discomfort.

Diagnosis

After the atrial switch procedure, the ECG may show a loss of sinus rhythm with evidence of RV hypertrophy. Ambulatory monitors are important to monitor for bradyarrhythmias, sinus node dysfunction, and atrial arrhythmias. Chest radiographs may show an enlarged cardiac silhouette in those with a dilated systemic right ventricle. An echocardiogram can demonstrate qualitative systemic RV size and function and the degree of tricuspid regurgitation. MRI is often used to accurately quantify systemic RV size and function, tricuspid valve function, and atrial baffle anatomy.

After the arterial switch, echocardiography is used to assess pulmonary artery and branch pulmonary artery stenosis, neo-aortic and neo-pulmonic valve regurgitation, and ventricular function. MRI or computed tomography may be used to assess the anatomy of the branch pulmonary arteries. An exercise stress test is often used to evaluate myocardial ischemia.

Treatment

Treatment options are limited for adults with complete TGA repaired by atrial switch who have failing systemic right ventricles or significant tricuspid regurgitation, and evidence of significant benefit is lacking. However, potential treatments include medical therapy, revision of atrial baffles, pulmonary artery banding, resynchronization therapy, ventricular assist devices, and possible transplantation. Medical therapy, including consideration of anticoagulation, in patients with atrial tachyarrhythmias is recommended.

After the arterial switch procedure, catheter-based or surgical reintervention for pulmonary artery stenosis may be required in 5% to 25% of patients. Coronary artery revascularization is rarely required (0.46% of patients), as is neo-aortic valve repair or replacement (1.1%

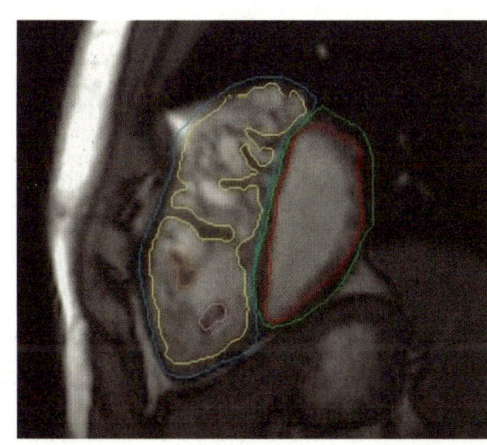 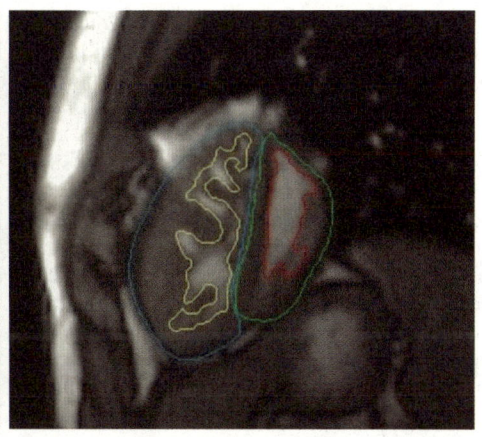

图 5.2 带有双心室腔心外膜和心内膜描记的右心室和左心室的短轴磁共振成像。采用固定厚度对心脏进行预定数目的切面观测。在舒张末期和收缩末期于每一切面计算左右心室的容量并总合在一起来确定右心室和左心室的总容量（即 Simpson 法）

分别由 Senning 在 1959 年和 Mustard 在 1964 年报道。在这些手术中，通过放入隔板使体循环和肺循环的静脉血在心房内改变流向，来自上下腔静脉的体循环静脉血通过二尖瓣直接进入与肺动脉相连的左心室。肺静脉血通过三尖瓣进入与主动脉相连的右心室。这些操作使左心室作为肺循环的心室，右心室作为体循环的心室。

在过去的 20 年，动脉调转术已经普及。手术中，大动脉被横断重新吻合至正确的心室（左心室连接主动脉，右心室连接肺动脉），同时冠状动脉也重新吻合。动脉调转术的围术期存活率很高，外科死亡率为 2%～5%。

病理学

如果没有接受外科治疗，大多数患儿在最初的几个月就会死亡。对于一出生就接受了心房转流术的大动脉转位成年患者，右心室继续为体循环心室，左心室是肺循环心室。长期随访表明，右心室作为体循环心室可以工作 30～40 年，但是随着随访时间延长，体循环心室功能不全持续增加。在 35 年的随访中，大约 61% 的患者发生中到重度的右心室功能不全。

另一个常见的术后问题发生在三尖瓣。心房转流术后，三尖瓣仍然是体循环的房室瓣，必须耐受体循环压力。由于右心室形态改变和异常腱索附着，三尖瓣容易发生功能不全而出现严重反流。

显著的冠状动脉病变，如闭塞或狭窄，占动脉调转术后患者的 6.8%。病变可能与冠状动脉再植入新主动脉时的缝线或打结有关。左心室功能常正常，左心室功能不全的发生与冠状动脉病变有关。

临床表现

心房转流术后的成年患者，体检可以发现与三尖瓣关闭不全相关的杂音和前位主动脉产生的显著的第二心音。心房转流术后患者随着随访时间延长功能状态会逐渐恶化。通常会有静息的窦性心动过缓或交界区节律。房性心律失常导致的心悸常见，在心房转流术后 23 年时发生率达 48%。

动脉调转术后的患者，体格检查可能会有新主动脉或新肺动脉瓣膜反流的杂音。这些患者通常功能状态正常，但是由于心脏的去神经化，心肌缺血可以表现为不典型的胸部不适。

诊断

心房转流术后，心电图上可能有窦性节律缺失，并伴有右心室肥厚的表现。动态监护仪对于监测缓慢性心律失常、窦房结功能障碍和房性心律失常非常重要。在体循环右心室扩张的患者，胸部 X 线片可以表现为心脏扩大。超声心动图可以定性评估体循环右心室的大小和功能及三尖瓣反流的程度。磁共振成像（MRI）常用于准确定量评估体循环右心室大小和功能，三尖瓣功能和心房隔板的解剖。

动脉调转术后，超声心动图用于评估肺动脉和分支的狭窄、新主动脉和新肺动脉瓣膜的反流和心室功能。MRI 或 CT 可用于评估肺动脉分支的解剖。运动负荷试验常用于评估心肌缺血。

治疗

心房转流术修复术后的成年完全性大动脉转位患者，如果出现体循环右心室功能不全或严重的三尖瓣反流，治疗选择有限且缺乏显著获益的证据。可能的治疗包括药物治疗、心房隔板修复、肺动脉环束术、再同步化治疗、心室辅助装置及可能进行移植术。建议对房性快速性心律失常患者进行包括抗凝治疗在内的药物治疗。

动脉调转术修复后，5%～25% 的患者需要导管或外科再干预治疗肺动脉狭窄。很少需要冠状动脉血运重建（0.46%）或新主动脉瓣膜修复或置换（1.1%）。

of patients). Guideline-directed recommendations for aortic valve replacement are reasonable to follow for patients with d-TGA and severe neo-aortic valve regurgitation.

Prognosis

Long-term follow-up studies after the atrial switch procedure show a small but ongoing attrition rate, with numerous intermediate- and long-term complications. Long-term complications include systemic RV dysfunction and tricuspid valve regurgitation, loss of sinus rhythm with the development of atrial arrhythmias (50% incidence by age 25), endocarditis, baffle leaks, baffle obstruction, and sinus node dysfunction requiring pacemaker placement. Intermediate-term complications related to the arterial switch procedure include coronary artery compromise, pulmonary outflow tract obstruction (at the supravalvular level or takeoff of the peripheral pulmonary arteries), neo-aortic valve regurgitation, endocarditis, and neo-aorta dilation.

As a result of the long-term complications associated with the atrial switch procedure, the arterial switch operation has been the procedure of choice since 1985. Long-term data on the survival after the arterial switch operation do not exist, but intermediate-term results are promising: 88% at 10 and 15 years.

❖ For a deeper discussion on this topic, please see Chapter 61, "Congenital Heart Disease in Adults," in *Goldman-Cecil Medicine*, 26th Edition.

SUGGESTED READINGS

Bradley EA, Ammash N, Martinez SC: "Treat to close": Non-repairable ASD-PAH in the adult, Int J Card 291:127–133, 2019.

Campbell M: Natural history of atrial septal defect, Br Heart J 32:820–826, 1970.

Cohen M, Fuster V, Steele PM, et al: Coarctation of the aorta. Long-term follow-up and prediction of outcome after surgical correction, Circulation 80:840–845, 1989.

Cohen SB, Ginde S, Bartz PJ, et al: Extracardiac complications in adults with congenital heart disease, Congenit Heart Dis 8:370–380, 2013.

Co-Vu JG, Ginde S, Bartz PJ, et al: Long-term outcomes of the neoaorta after arterial switch operation for transposition of the great arteries, Ann Thorac Surg 95:1654–1659, 2013.

Cramer JW, Ginde S, Bartz PJ, et al: Aortic aneurysms remain a significant source of morbidity and mortality after use of Dacron patch aortoplasty to repair coarctation of the aorta: results from a single center, Pediatr Cardiol 34:296–301, 2013.

Crumb SR, Dearani JA, Fuller S, et al: 2018 AHA/ACC guideline for the management of adults with congenital heart disease, J Am Coll Cardiol 1–175.

Earing MG, Connolly HM, Dearani JA, et al: Long-term follow-up of patients after surgical treatment for isolated pulmonary valve stenosis, Mayo Clin Proc 80:871–876, 2005.

Earing MG, Webb GD: Congenital heart disease and pregnancy: maternal and fetal risks, Clin Perinatol 32:913–919, 2005.

Gatzoulis MA, Freeman MA, Siu SC, et al: Atrial arrhythmia after surgical closure of atrial septal defects in adults, N Engl J Med 340:839–846, 1999.

Gunther T, Mazzitelli D, Haehnel CJ, et al: Long-term results after repair of complete atrioventricular septal defects: analysis of risk factors, Ann Thorac Surg 65:754–759, 1998, discussion 759-760.

Hickey EJ, Gruschen V, Bradely TJ, et al: Late risk of outcomes for adults with repaired tetralogy of Fallot from an inception cohort spanning four decades, Eur J Cardiothorac Surg 35:156–164, 2009.

Khairy P, Van Hare GF, Balaji S: PACES/HRS expert consensus statement on the recognition and management of arrhythmias in adult congenital heart disease, *Can J Cardiol* e1–e63, 2014.

Losay J, Touchot A, Serraf A, et al: Late outcome after arterial switch operation for transposition of the great arteries, Circulation 104(Suppl 1):I121–I1126, 2001.

Perloff JK, Warnes CA: Challenges posed by adults with repaired congenital heart disease, Circulation 103:2637–2643, 2001.

Soto B, Becker AE, Moulaert AJ, et al.: Classification of ventricular septal defects, Br Heart J 43:332–343, 1980.

Stout KK, Daniels CJ, Aboulhosn JA, et al.: Transposition of the great arteries, Circulation 114:2699–2709, 2006.

对于严重新主动脉瓣反流的完全性大动脉转位患者，遵循指南推荐的主动脉瓣置换是合理的。

预后

心房转流术后的长期随访显示很低但会不断增加的退出率，伴有大量的中长期并发症。长期并发症包括体循环右心室功能不全和三尖瓣反流、窦性节律消失并出现房性心律失常（至 25 岁时有 50% 的发生率）、心内膜炎、隔板漏、隔板阻塞和窦房结功能不全需要起搏器植入。中期并发症包括冠状动脉损害、肺动脉流出道梗阻（在瓣上水平或发出周围肺动脉处）、新主动脉的瓣膜反流、心内膜炎和新主动脉扩张。

由于心房转流术的长期并发症，从 1985 年开始动脉调转术成为治疗首选。尚没有动脉调转术存活率的长期数据，但是中期数据令人振奋：10～15 年生存率为 88%。

❖ 有关此专题的深入讨论，请参阅 *Goldman-Cecil Medicine* 第 26 版第 61 章 "成人先天性心脏病"。

推荐阅读

Bradley EA, Ammash N, Martinez SC: "Treat to close": Non-repairable ASD-PAH in the adult, Int J Card 291:127–133, 2019.

Campbell M: Natural history of atrial septal defect, Br Heart J 32:820–826, 1970.

Cohen M, Fuster V, Steele PM, et al: Coarctation of the aorta. Long-term follow-up and prediction of outcome after surgical correction, Circulation 80:840–845, 1989.

Cohen SB, Ginde S, Bartz PJ, et al: Extracardiac complications in adults with congenital heart disease, Congenit Heart Dis 8:370–380, 2013.

Co-Vu JG, Ginde S, Bartz PJ, et al: Long-term outcomes of the neoaorta after arterial switch operation for transposition of the great arteries, Ann Thorac Surg 95:1654–1659, 2013.

Cramer JW, Ginde S, Bartz PJ, et al: Aortic aneurysms remain a significant source of morbidity and mortality after use of Dacron patch aortoplasty to repair coarctation of the aorta: results from a single center, Pediatr Cardiol 34:296–301, 2013.

Crumb SR, Dearani JA, Fuller S, et al: 2018 AHA/ACC guideline for the management of adults with congenital heart disease, J Am Coll Cardiol 1–175.

Earing MG, Connolly HM, Dearani JA, et al: Long-term follow-up of patients after surgical treatment for isolated pulmonary valve stenosis, Mayo Clin Proc 80:871–876, 2005.

Earing MG, Webb GD: Congenital heart disease and pregnancy: maternal and fetal risks, Clin Perinatol 32:913–919, 2005.

Gatzoulis MA, Freeman MA, Siu SC, et al: Atrial arrhythmia after surgical closure of atrial septal defects in adults, N Engl J Med 340:839–846, 1999.

Gunther T, Mazzitelli D, Haehnel CJ, et al: Long-term results after repair of complete atrioventricular septal defects: analysis of risk factors, Ann Thorac Surg 65:754–759, 1998, discussion 759-760.

Hickey EJ, Gruschen V, Bradely TJ, et al: Late risk of outcomes for adults with repaired tetralogy of Fallot from an inception cohort spanning four decades, Eur J Cardiothorac Surg 35:156–164, 2009.

Khairy P, Van Hare GF, Balaji S: PACES/HRS expert consensus statement on the recognition and management of arrhythmias in adult congenital heart disease, Can J Cardiol e1–e63, 2014.

Losay J, Touchot A, Serraf A, et al: Late outcome after arterial switch operation for transposition of the great arteries, Circulation 104(Suppl 1):I121–I1126, 2001.

Perloff JK, Warnes CA: Challenges posed by adults with repaired congenital heart disease, Circulation 103:2637–2643, 2001.

Soto B, Becker AE, Moulaert AJ, et al.: Classification of ventricular septal defects, Br Heart J 43:332–343, 1980.

Stout KK, Daniels CJ, Aboulhosn JA, et al.: Transposition of the great arteries, Circulation 114:2699–2709, 2006.

6

Valvular Heart Disease

Christopher Song

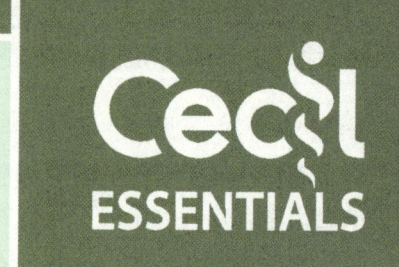

INTRODUCTION

In developing countries, rheumatic heart disease (RHD) remains a common cause of valvular heart disease (VHD). In industrialized countries, the burden of rheumatic disease has significantly decreased, and the most common etiology is degenerative disease. The prevalence of VHD in the US adult population is 2.5%. Prevalence increases with age to as high as 13.3% in those 75 years and older. Moderate or severe VHD is associated with excess mortality. Therefore, with an aging population, valvular heart disease is and will continue to be a major public health problem.

The "2014 AHA/ACC Guideline for the Management of Patients with Valvular Heart Disease" provides a classification of the progression of VHD with 4 stages, A through D (Table 6.1). Timing of intervention for most VHD is guided by the onset of symptoms, severity of VHD, and evidence of adverse cardiac remodeling. Therefore, a thorough history and physical examination along with a comprehensive transthoracic echocardiogram (TTE) are essential in the evaluation of patients with known or suspected VHD. Other cardiac testing modalities can help to determine the severity of VHD and the presence of symptoms. Once intervention is contemplated, each individual patient's surgical risk should be assessed. If surgical risk is high or prohibitive, transcatheter approaches may be an option.

AORTIC STENOSIS

Definition and Etiology

Valvular aortic stenosis (AS) is defined by restriction in leaflet motion resulting in left ventricular (LV) outflow obstruction. Less common causes of LV outflow obstruction include lesions at the supravalvular or subvalvular level. There are three primary etiologies of valvular AS: congenital, rheumatic, and calcific disease.

The etiology often dictates age at presentation. Patients with congenital aortic stenosis and unicuspid aortic valves usually present before the age of 30. Those with a bicuspid aortic valve or rheumatic valve disease typically present between the age of 40 and 60. Patients with calcific trileaflet valve typically present after age 70. However, patients with Paget disease or end-stage renal disease may present at a younger age.

Pathophysiology

The initiation phase of calcific aortic valve disease is similar to atherosclerosis. The process is thought to begin with mechanical stress and endothelial damage leading to inflammation and lipid deposition. The propagation phase is dominated by calcification leading to progressive restriction of the valve leaflets and eventual LV outflow obstruction.

In bicuspid aortic valves there is an associated increase in mechanical stress which leads to accelerated calcification of the valve leaflets. Bicuspid aortic valve occurs in about 1% of the population and it is twice as common in males as in females. Patients with a bicuspid aortic valve often have an associated aortopathy such as coarctation or aortic aneurysm.

Once AS becomes hemodynamically significant, it leads to resistance in LV ejection and an increase in LV systolic pressure and wall stress. In order to maintain normal wall stress, wall thickness increases resulting in concentric hypertrophy. The left ventricle can remain in this compensated state for a prolonged period. However, as valvular stenosis and hypertrophy progress, LV end-diastolic pressure increases and, eventually, LV dilation and systolic dysfunction ensue.

Natural History and Clinical Presentation

Patients with AS are usually asymptomatic for a prolonged period. Symptom onset occurs when valve obstruction is severe and usually prior to the onset of LV systolic dysfunction. In fact, LV chamber size and systolic function can remain normal until the AS is end-stage. The onset of symptoms in AS indicates a significant increase in mortality risk. This was first described by Ross and Braunwald in their seminal paper in 1968. They also found that specific symptoms were associated with different survival rates. The average survival of patients with symptoms of angina, syncope, and heart failure was 5, 3, and 2 years, respectively (Fig. 6.1).

These "classic" symptoms are now thought to be symptoms of end-stage disease. With the advent of echocardiography and close follow-up of patients, the most common presenting symptoms are dyspnea on exertion or decreased exercise tolerance, exertional dizziness, and exertional angina. Given the nonspecific nature of these symptoms along with the prognostic and therapeutic implications of diagnosing a patient with severe symptomatic AS, one must be thorough in screening patients for these symptoms but also be cautious in attributing these symptoms to AS.

Physical Examination

The physical examination is useful in the initial detection of AS and correlates with severity (Table 6.2). However, no physical examination findings can reliably exclude severe AS.

When palpating the carotid artery, a delayed, low amplitude pulse may be appreciated (*pulsus parvus et tardus*). With precordial palpation, a heaving and sustained apical impulse may be noted due to LV hypertrophy or systolic dysfunction. A fourth heart sound (S_4) can be palpable in the setting of a noncompliant left ventricle. In addition, a

心脏瓣膜病

张斌 译 吴永健 张恒 审校 任景怡 通审

引言

在发展中国家，风湿性心脏病（RHD）仍然是心脏瓣膜病（VHD）的主要病因。而在工业化国家，风湿性疾病的负担已显著减轻，最常见的病因逐渐演变为退行性疾病。美国成人中心脏瓣膜病的患病率为 2.5%，且随年龄增长而增加，75 岁及以上人群的患病率已高达 13.3%。中重度心脏瓣膜病与死亡率增加相关。因此，随着人口老龄化，心脏瓣膜病已经并将持续成为一个重大的公共卫生问题。

2014 年美国心脏协会/美国心脏病学会（AHA/ACC）发布的《心脏瓣膜病患者管理指南》将心脏瓣膜病的进展分为 A 到 D 期四个阶段（表 6.1）。大多数心脏瓣膜病的干预时机取决于症状的出现、疾病的严重程度以及心脏不良重构的客观证据。因此，对已知或疑似心脏瓣膜病患者进行详尽的病史和体格检查以及全面的经胸超声心动图（TTE）评估至关重要。其他心脏检查可协助判定心脏瓣膜病的严重程度和症状的存在。一旦考虑干预治疗，应个体化评估患者的外科手术风险。如果外科手术风险高或不适合手术，可考虑经导管治疗。

主动脉瓣狭窄

定义和病因

主动脉瓣狭窄（AS）是指由于瓣叶运动受限，导致左心室（LV）流出道梗阻。其他较少见的左心室流出道梗阻原因包括瓣上或瓣下病变。主动脉瓣狭窄的病因主要有三种：先天性、风湿性以及钙化性疾病。

病因通常决定了出现症状的年龄。先天性主动脉瓣狭窄和单叶瓣主动脉瓣的患者通常在 30 岁前出现症状。二叶主动脉瓣或风湿性瓣膜病的患者通常在 40～60 岁出现症状。而钙化性三叶瓣的患者通常在 70 岁以后出现症状。然而，患有佩吉特病或终末期肾病的患者可能在较年轻时出现症状。

病理生理学

钙化性主动脉瓣疾病的启动阶段病程类似于动脉粥样硬化。目前认为这个过程始于机械应力和内皮损伤，继而引发炎症反应及脂质沉积。进展阶段主要由钙化主导，导致瓣叶进行性受限，并最终导致左心室流出道梗阻。

在二叶主动脉瓣中，机械应力的增加会加速瓣叶钙化。二叶主动脉瓣在人群中发生率约 1%，男性的发生率是女性的 2 倍。具有二叶主动脉瓣的患者通常伴有主动脉病变，如主动脉缩窄或主动脉瘤。

当主动脉瓣狭窄出现血流动力学显著改变时，将引发左心室射血阻力上升，并导致左心室收缩压及室壁应力增加。为维持正常室壁应力，心室壁代偿性增厚，逐渐形成向心性肥厚。左心室可长期维持这种代偿状态。但随着瓣膜狭窄程度加重及心肌肥厚进展，左心室舒张末压逐渐升高，最终出现左心室扩张及收缩功能障碍。

自然病程与临床表现

主动脉瓣狭窄患者通常在较长时间内无症状。症状多于瓣膜梗阻严重时出现，并且通常早于左心室收缩功能障碍的发生阶段。实际上，左心室腔室大小和收缩功能可以在主动脉瓣狭窄进入晚期之前保持正常。主动脉瓣狭窄症状的出现表明死亡风险显著增加。这一点最早在 1968 年由 Ross 和 Braunwald 在其具有开创意义的论文中描述。他们还发现，特定症状与不同的生存率相关。出现心绞痛、晕厥和心力衰竭症状的患者，其平均生存时间分别为 5 年、3 年和 2 年（图 6.1）。

这些"典型"症状现在被认为是晚期疾病的症状。随着超声心动图的出现和对患者的密切随访，最常见的初始症状是运动后呼吸困难或运动耐量下降、劳力性头晕和劳力性心绞痛。鉴于此类症状的非特异性，加之诊断严重症状性主动脉瓣狭窄对患者预后及治疗决策的重要影响，临床医师必须对患者症状进行全面筛查，同时审慎评估症状与主动脉瓣狭窄的因果关系。

体格检查

体格检查在主动脉瓣狭窄的初步评估中有重要价值，并且与疾病的严重程度相关（表 6.2）。然而，没有任何体格检查结果能够明确地排除重度主动脉瓣狭窄的存在。

在触诊颈动脉时，可表现为脉搏延迟、幅度低（细迟脉）。在触诊心前区时，由于左心室肥厚或收缩功能障碍，可触及抬举样心尖搏动。当左心室顺应性下降

TABLE 6.1 Stages of Progression of VHD

Stage	Definition	Description
A	At risk	Patients with risk factors for development of VHD
B	Progressive	Patients with progressive VHD (mild-moderate severity and asymptomatic)
C	Asymptomatic severe	Asymptomatic patients who have the criteria for severe VHD: C1: asymptomatic patients with severe VHD in whom the left and right ventricle remain compensated C2: asymptomatic patients with severe VHD with decompensation of the left or right ventricle
D	Symptomatic severe	Patients who have developed symptoms as a result of VHD

Data from Nishimura R, Otto C, Bonow RO, et al: 2014 AHA/ACC guideline for the management of patients with valvular heart disease. J Am Coll Cardiol 2014;63:e57-e185.

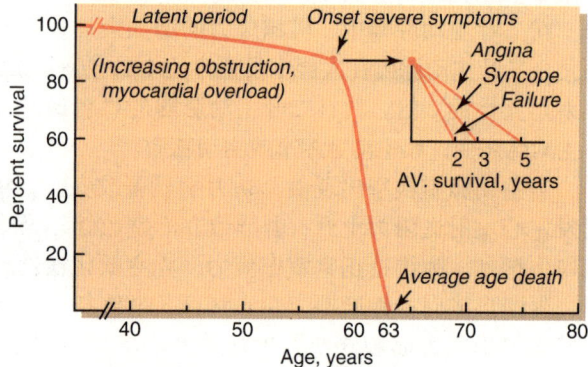

Fig. 6.1 Natural history of severe aortic stenosis without surgery once symptoms develop. (Data from Ross J Jr, Braunwald E: Aortic stenosis, Circulation 38:61, 1968.)

precordial thrill may be appreciated due to turbulent blood flow across a stenotic aortic valve.

The findings on cardiac auscultation are reflective of reduced mobility and delayed closure of the aortic valve leaflets and resistance to flow. The aortic component (A_2) of the second heart sound (S_2) becomes delayed to occur simultaneously with the pulmonic component (P_2) forming a single S_2. In severe AS, A_2 may become inaudible or paradoxical S_2 can be observed. An aortic ejection click can be heard in mild to moderate AS, when the leaflets are stiff but still mobile. The classic murmur AS is described as a harsh crescendo-decrescendo systolic murmur that is best heard at the right upper sternal border that radiates to the carotid arteries. The murmur begins after the first heart sound (S_1) and ends before S_2. Like the carotid pulse, the timing of the murmur correlates with severity of AS. An early peaking murmur is indicative of mild or moderate AS whereas a late peaking murmur is typically a sign of severe AS. The murmur may also radiate to the apex where a distinct musical quality can be appreciated. This is known as Gallavardin's phenomenon and often mistaken as the presence of concomitant mitral regurgitation (MR).

Diagnosis

An electrocardiogram (ECG) and chest radiograph are commonly obtained and can have nonspecific findings such as LV hypertrophy or cardiomegaly, respectively. The primary tool for diagnosing AS is echocardiography. TTE can accurately assess the aortic valve structure, the severity of AS, and the effects of AS on the cardiac chambers. Doppler imaging can be used to estimate the gradients across a stenotic aortic valve and calculate an aortic valve area. Criteria for mild, moderate, and severe AS are well established (Table 6.3).

In most cases the severity of AS by TTE correlates with the clinical evaluation. If there is a discrepancy, further testing can be considered.

An exercise treadmill study can be done to objectively assess functional capacity. A cardiac catheterization with hemodynamic measurements provides an alternative assessment of the severity of AS. Computed tomography can quantify aortic valve calcium, which has been shown to correlate with AS severity by TTE and with clinical outcomes.

In patients with LV systolic dysfunction, it may be unclear if a patient has true severe AS or pseudosevere AS. A low-dose dobutamine stress echocardiogram can help to differentiate between the two. In true severe AS the valve area is fixed, regardless of dobutamine. In pseudosevere AS the aortic valve opening is limited by the low LV outflow and the valve area will increase with dobutamine. This test can also provide information about the contractile reserve of the left ventricle, which has prognostic implications when considering valve replacement.

Treatment

The management of asymptomatic AS involves close monitoring, early detection of symptoms, and treatment of cardiovascular risk factors and comorbidities such as hypertension, hyperlipidemia, and coronary artery disease. No treatments have been shown to prevent the progression of AS.

Once a patient develops severe symptomatic AS, medical therapy has limited benefit and aortic valve replacement (AVR) is recommended. Medical therapy should focus on preventing and optimizing concomitant cardiovascular conditions and treating symptoms. Nonetheless, AVR has been shown to improve symptoms and survival and it is the only effective treatment in severe symptomatic AS. Those with severe asymptomatic AS may also meet indications for AVR if they have concurrent LV systolic dysfunction, very severe AS, rapidly progressing AS, or if they are undergoing another cardiac surgery.

There are two broad approaches to AVR: surgical and transcatheter. For decades, surgical AVR was the mainstay of therapy for severe AS. With surgical AVR, either a mechanical or bioprosthetic valve can be considered. With favorable flow characteristics, mechanical valves can last for the patient's lifetime (Fig. 6.2). However, these valves require anticoagulation with warfarin. While bioprosthetic valves, made from bovine or porcine material, do not require anticoagulation, they are less durable and typically require re-replacement after 10 to 20 years (Fig. 6.3).

Rather than an open procedure requiring sternotomy, transcatheter aortic valve implantation (TAVI) most commonly involves accessing the femoral artery and using a catheter to deliver a bioprosthetic valve into position by expanding a balloon and effectively crushing the native aortic valve against the aortic wall (Fig. 6.4). Less common approaches include transapical, transaortic, and subclavian. The role of TAVI was initially established in patients with severe symptomatic AS and prohibitive surgical risk. TAVI led to significant mortality benefit

表 6.1	心脏瓣膜病进展分期	
分期	定义	描述
A	风险期	有心脏瓣膜病发展危险因素的患者
B	进展期	心脏瓣膜病进展中的患者（轻度至中度且无症状）
C	无症状重度期	符合重度心脏瓣膜病标准但无症状的患者
		C1：无症状且左心室和右心室仍处于代偿状态的重度心脏瓣膜病患者
		C2：无症状但左心室或右心室出现失代偿的重度心脏瓣膜病患者
D	症状性重度期	因心脏瓣膜病出现症状的患者

引自 Nishimura R, Otto C, Bonow RO, et al: 2014 AHA/ACC guideline for the management of patients with valvular heart disease. J Am Coll Cardiol 2014；63：e57-e185.

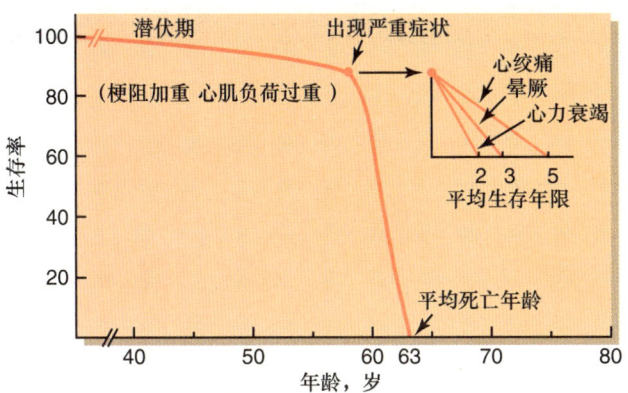

图 6.1 症状发作后未经手术治疗的重度主动脉瓣狭窄自然病程（引自 Ross J Jr, Braunwald E: Aortic stenosis, Circulation 38: 61, 1968.）

时，听诊可闻及第四心音（S_4）。此外，由于狭窄的主动脉瓣导致血流湍流，有时可触及心前区震颤。

心脏听诊发现的体征反映了主动脉瓣叶活动受限和关闭延迟以及血流阻力的增加。第二心音（S_2）的主动脉瓣成分（A_2）延迟，与肺动脉瓣成分（P_2）同时出现并形成单一的 S_2。在重度主动脉瓣狭窄中 A_2 可能消失，或者出现在 P_2 之后形成 S_2 反常分裂。当轻到中度主动脉瓣狭窄时，可闻及主动脉喷射音，这是因为瓣叶僵硬但仍可活动。经典的主动脉瓣狭窄杂音是粗糙的递增-递减型收缩期杂音，杂音始于第一心音（S_1）之后，结束于第二心音（S_2）之前。最佳听诊位置在胸骨右缘第二肋间，杂音向颈动脉传导。类似于颈动脉搏动，杂音达峰的时机与主动脉瓣狭窄的严重程度相关。早期峰值杂音提示轻至中度主动脉瓣狭窄，而晚期峰值杂音通常是重度主动脉瓣狭窄的标志。杂音还可能传导至心尖处，呈独特的乐性杂音，这被称为 Gallavardin 现象，常被误认为是伴随二尖瓣反流（MR）的存在。

诊断

心电图和胸部 X 线片是常规检查手段，可发现左心室肥厚、心脏扩大等非特异性表现。超声心动图是诊断主动脉瓣狭窄的主要工具。TTE 可以准确评估主动脉瓣的结构、主动脉瓣狭窄的严重程度及其对心脏腔室的影响。多普勒成像可以用来估算狭窄主动脉瓣的压力梯度，并计算主动脉瓣口面积。轻度、中度和重度主动脉瓣狭窄的判定标准目前已建立完善（表 6.3）。

在大多数情况下，通过 TTE 评估的主动脉瓣狭窄的严重程度与临床评估一致。若存在不一致的情况，应考虑进一步的检查。运动平板试验可用来客观评估运动耐量。通过心导管检查进行的血流动力学测量提供了评估主动脉瓣狭窄严重程度的替代方法。计算机断层成像可以量化主动脉瓣钙化程度，目前已证实主动脉瓣钙化与 TTE 评估的主动脉瓣狭窄严重程度及临床结局相关。

对于左心室收缩功能障碍的患者，区分真性或假性重度主动脉瓣狭窄可能存在临床不确定性。低剂量多巴酚丁胺负荷的超声心动图可协助鉴别。在真性重度主动脉瓣狭窄中，瓣口面积是固定的，不受多巴酚丁胺影响。而在假性重度主动脉瓣狭窄中，主动脉瓣开口受到左心室低流量的限制，瓣口面积会随多巴酚丁胺的使用而增加。该检查还可评估左心室收缩储备功能，这对瓣膜置换术的预后评估具有重要价值。

治疗

无症状的主动脉瓣狭窄的管理包括密切监测、早期发现症状以及心血管危险因素和伴随疾病的管理，如高血压、高脂血症和冠心病。目前尚无明确的治疗方法能够有效延缓主动脉瓣狭窄的进展。

一旦患者发展为重度症状性主动脉瓣狭窄，药物治疗的效果有限，推荐行主动脉瓣置换术（AVR）。药物治疗应侧重于预防和优化伴随的心血管疾病以及缓解症状。主动脉瓣置换术已被证明能够改善症状和预后，是治疗重度症状性主动脉瓣狭窄的唯一明确有效的治疗手段。对于重度无症状主动脉瓣狭窄患者，若同时存在左心室收缩功能障碍、极重度主动脉瓣狭窄、快速进展的主动脉瓣狭窄或计划进行其他心脏手术，也符合主动脉瓣置换术的指征。

主动脉瓣置换术有两种主要途径：外科手术和经导管介入治疗。数十年来，外科主动脉瓣置换术一直是治疗重度主动脉瓣狭窄的主要手段。对于外科主动脉瓣置换术，可选择机械瓣或生物瓣。机械瓣具有良好的血流动力学特性，耐久性优异（图 6.2），但要求长期华法林抗凝治疗。生物瓣由牛或猪的心包或者瓣膜材料制成，不要求长期抗凝治疗，但相较于机械瓣，其耐久性较差，植入后 10～20 年可能需要再次手术置换（图 6.3）。

经导管主动脉瓣置入术（TAVI）是一种不需要开胸的微创介入手术。手术常采用经股动脉路径，经由导管将生物瓣送至理想位置后通过球囊扩张释放生物瓣，扩张的生物瓣会将原位主动脉瓣压至主动脉壁上（图 6.4）。较少见的手术入路包括经心尖、经主动脉和

TABLE 6.2	AS Exam Findings by Severity		
Exam Finding	Mild	Moderate	Severe
Carotid pulse	Normal	Slow rising	Parvus et tardus
Apical impulse	Normal	Heaving	Heaving and sustained
S_4 gallop	Absent	May be present	Present
Systolic ejection click	Present	May be present	Absent
Systolic murmur peak	Early systole	Mid systole	Mid or late systole
S_2	Normal	Normal or single	Single or paradoxical

TABLE 6.3	Measures of AS Severity on Echocardiography			
Indicator	Normal	Mild	Moderate	Severe
Aortic valve area (cm^2)	>2.0	1.5-2.0	1.0-1.5	<1.0
Mean gradient (mm Hg)		<25	25-40	>40
Peak jet velocity (m/s)	<2.0	2-3	3-4	>4

Data from Baumgartner H, Hung J, Bermego J, et al: Echocardiographic assessment of valve stenosis: EAE/ASE recommendations for clinical practice. J Am Soc Echocardiogr 2009;22:1-22.

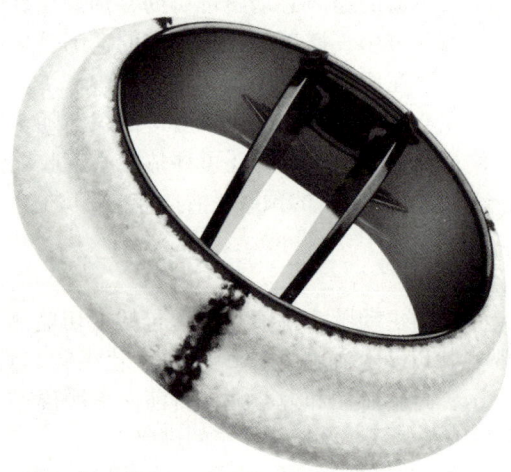

Fig. 6.2 Medtronic bileaflet mechanical prosthetic valve. (Modified from Medtronic, Inc.)

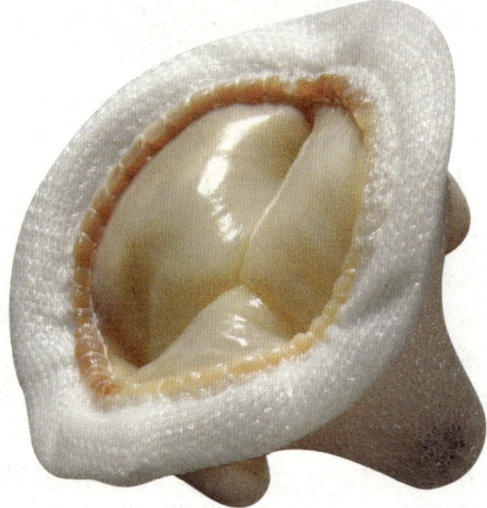

Fig. 6.3 Medtronic Hancock II bioprosthetic valve. (Modified from Medtronic, Inc.)

in this patient population when compared to standard therapy. Since the landmark trial in 2010, TAVI has emerged as an effective therapy for severe symptomatic AS in patients across the entire spectrum of surgical risk, from extreme risk to low risk.

Patients being considered for AVR should undergo a thorough individualized evaluation by a multidisciplinary heart valve team. The patient's life expectancy, surgical risk, comorbidities, frailty, anatomy, quality of life, values, and preferences should all be considered before making an informed shared decision on treatment strategy.

MITRAL STENOSIS

Definition and Etiology

Mitral stenosis (MS) is defined by the restriction of blood flow from the left atrium (LA) to the left ventricle during diastole. RHD is by far the most common cause of MS. In developed nations, rheumatic MS has become less common with the decreasing incidence of rheumatic fever. However, in developing nations, RHD remains a significant public health problem. Less common causes of MS include mitral annular calcification, radiation exposure, congenital, or mechanical obstruction from an atrial myxoma, vegetation, or thrombus.

Pathophysiology

Rheumatic fever is the result of an abnormal immune response usually occurring after 10 days to 3 weeks after untreated group A streptococcal pharyngitis. It typically affects children between the ages of 6 and 15 years. The diagnosis can be made based on clinical manifestations and the revised Jones criteria (Table 6.4).

In RHD, there is inflammatory process thought to be due to cross-reactivity between streptococcal antigen and valve tissue. This along with chronic turbulent flow through a deformed valve results in thickening and calcification of the mitral leaflets, thickening and shortening of the chordae tendineae, and fusion of the leaflet commissures (Fig. 6.5). This ultimately leads to a reduced orifice through which blood can flow from the LA to the left ventricle during diastole.

表 6.2 主动脉瓣狭窄的体征（按疾病严重程度）

体征	轻度	中度	重度
颈动脉搏动	正常	上升缓慢	脉搏微弱且迟缓
心尖搏动	正常	搏动强劲	搏动强劲且持续
第四心音奔马律	无	可能存在	存在
收缩期开瓣音	存在	可能存在	不存在
收缩期杂音峰值	收缩早期	收缩中期	收缩中晚期
第二心音	正常	正常或单一	单一或反常分裂

表 6.3 主动脉瓣狭窄严重程度的超声心动图分度

指标	正常	轻度	中度	重度
主动脉瓣口面积（cm²）	>2.0	1.5~2.0	1.0~1.5	<1
平均压差（mmHg）		<25	25~40	>40
峰值流速（m/s）	<2.0	2~3	3~4	>4

引自 Baumgartner H, Hung J, Bermego J, et al: Echocardiographic assessment of valve stenosis: EAE/ASE recommendations for clinical practice. J Am Soc Echocardiogr 2009; 22: 1-22.

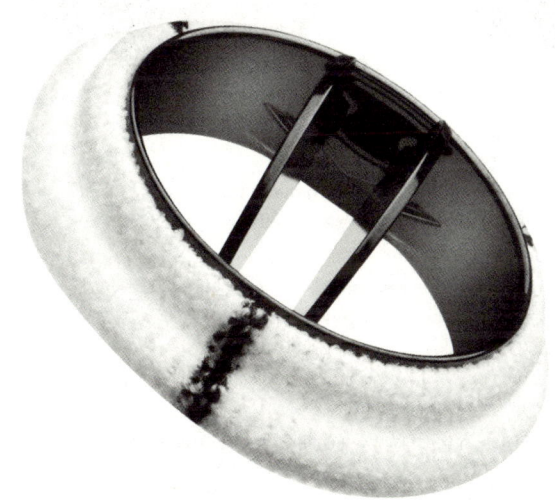

图 6.2 美敦力二叶式机械瓣（改编自 Medtronic, Inc.）

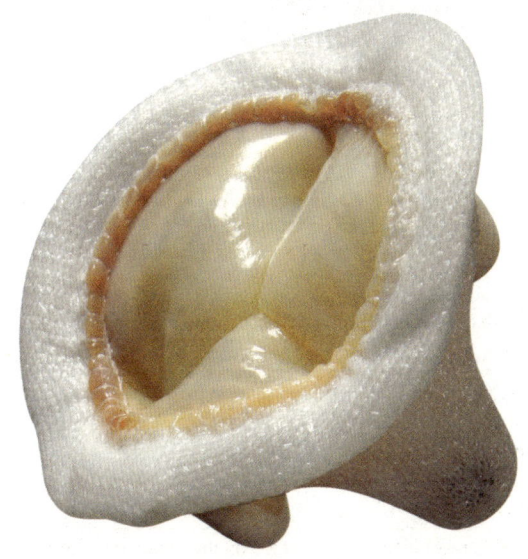

图 6.3 美敦力 Hancock II 生物瓣（改编自 Medtronic, Inc.）

经锁骨下动脉路径。经导管主动脉瓣置入术最初应用于外科手术禁忌的重度症状性主动脉瓣狭窄患者。与标准药物治疗相比，经导管主动脉瓣置入术可显著降低死亡率。2010 年首项临床试验实施以来，经导管主动脉瓣置换术（TAVR）的适应证范围已覆盖外科手术风险从低危到高危的全谱系重度症状性主动脉瓣狭窄患者。

考虑进行主动脉瓣置换术的患者应由多学科心脏瓣膜团队进行全面的个体化评估。在共同决策和知情同意之前，应全面评估患者的预期寿命、手术风险、伴随疾病、虚弱程度、解剖结构、生活质量、价值观和偏好。

二尖瓣狭窄

定义和病因

二尖瓣狭窄（MS）定义为舒张期从左心房（LA）到左心室的血流受限。风湿性心脏病是目前最常见的二尖瓣狭窄病因。在发达国家，由于风湿热的发病率下降，风湿性二尖瓣狭窄变得较为少见。然而，在发展中国家，风湿性心脏病仍然是一个重大的公共卫生问题。其他较少见的二尖瓣狭窄病因包括二尖瓣环钙化、放射暴露、先天性因素，或由于心房黏液瘤、赘生物或血栓引起的机械性梗阻。

病理生理学

风湿热由异常免疫反应介导，通常发生在未经治疗的 A 组溶血性链球菌咽炎后 10 天至 3 周内。它通常影响 6~15 岁的儿童。诊断主要根据临床表现和修订后的琼斯（Jones）标准（表 6.4）。

在风湿性心脏病中，炎症过程被认为是由于链球菌抗原与瓣膜组织之间的交叉反应所致。这种反应加上通过变形瓣膜的长期的血液湍流，导致二尖瓣叶的增厚和钙化、腱索的增厚和缩短以及瓣叶交界处的融合（图 6.5）。最终导致舒张期从左心房到左心室的血流口径缩小。

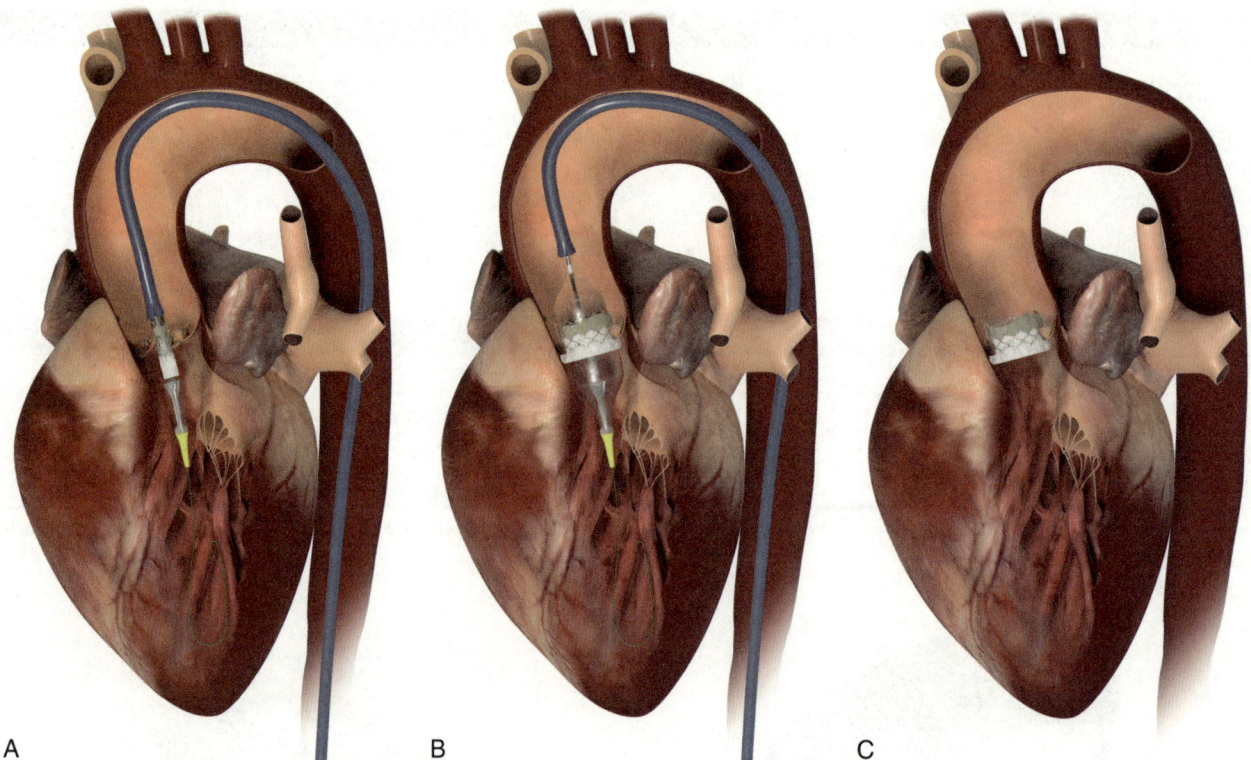

Fig. 6.4 Edwards SAPIEN transcatheter heart valve. (A) Valve is delivered retrograde from the femoral artery and positioned at the level of the aortic annulus. (B) Balloon inflated, deploying the valve. (C) Deployed valve. (With permission from Edwards Lifesciences LLC, Irvine, CA)

TABLE 6.4 Revised Jones Criteria[a]

Major Criteria	Minor Criteria
Carditis (pleuritic chest pain, friction rub, heart failure)	Fever
Polyarthritis	Arthralgia
Chorea	Previous rheumatic fever or known rheumatic heart disease
Erythema marginatum	
Subcutaneous nodules	

[a]Rheumatic fever is diagnosed based on the presence of two major criteria or one major and two minor criteria after a recent documented group A streptococcal infection.

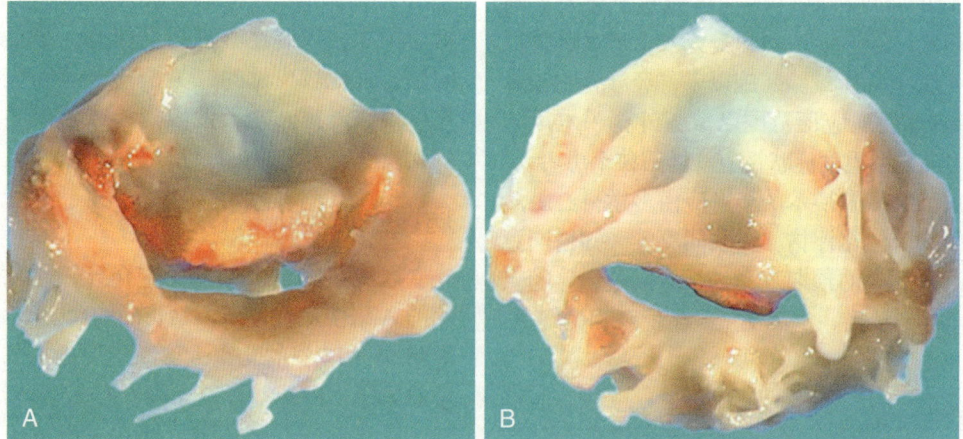

Fig. 6.5 Commissural fusion in mitral stenosis. (A) Left atrial aspect. (B) Left ventricular aspect. (From Cardiovascular Pathology, Fourth Ed, Elsevier, 2016.)

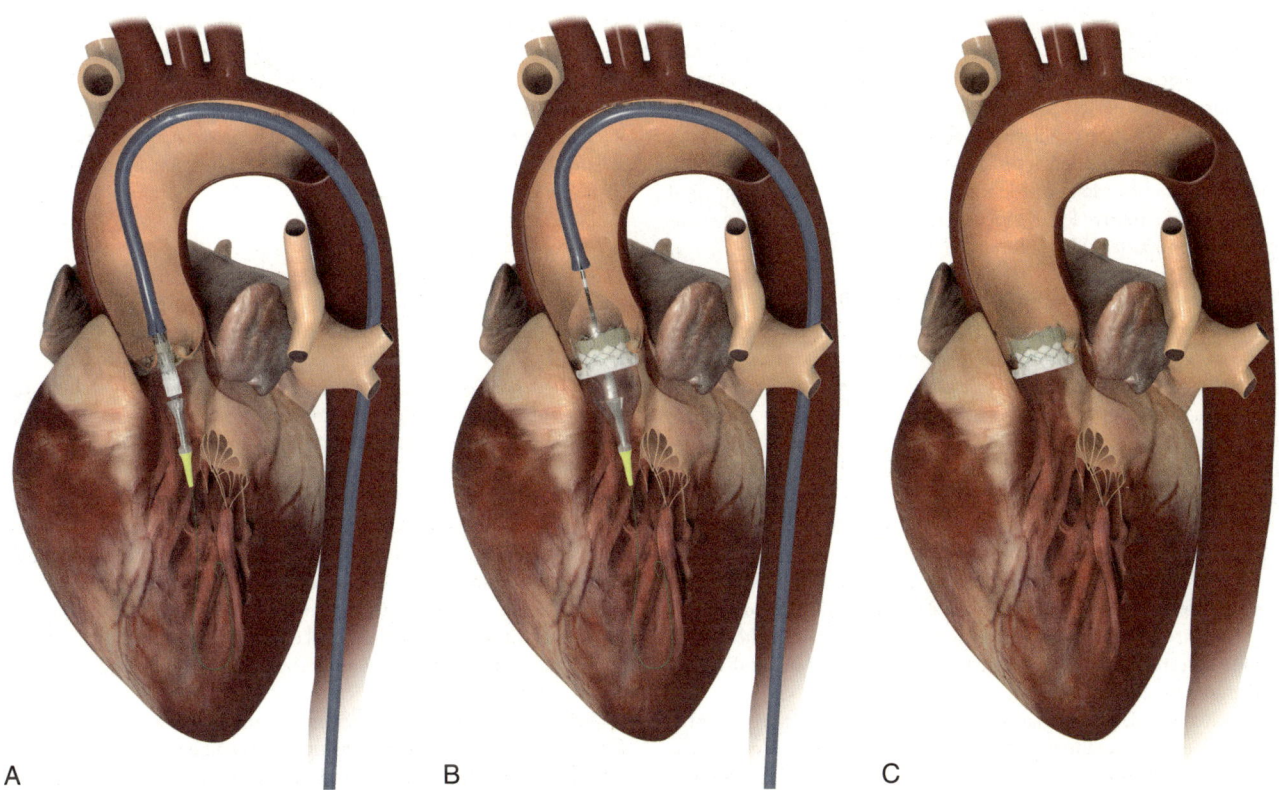

图 6.4 Edwards SAPIEN 经导管心脏瓣膜。(A) 瓣膜经股动脉逆行输送并定位在主动脉环水平。(B) 球囊充气及瓣膜释放。(C) 释放后的瓣膜 (经允许引自 Edwards Lifesciences LLC, Irvine, CA)

表 6.4　修订的 Jones 标准 [a]	
主要标准	次要标准
心脏炎（胸膜性胸痛、摩擦音、心力衰竭）	发热
多关节炎	关节痛
舞蹈症	既往风湿热史或已知风湿性心脏病
环形红斑	
皮下结节	

[a] 风湿热的诊断基于近期确诊的 A 组链球菌感染后，满足两项主要标准或一项主要标准加两项次要标准。

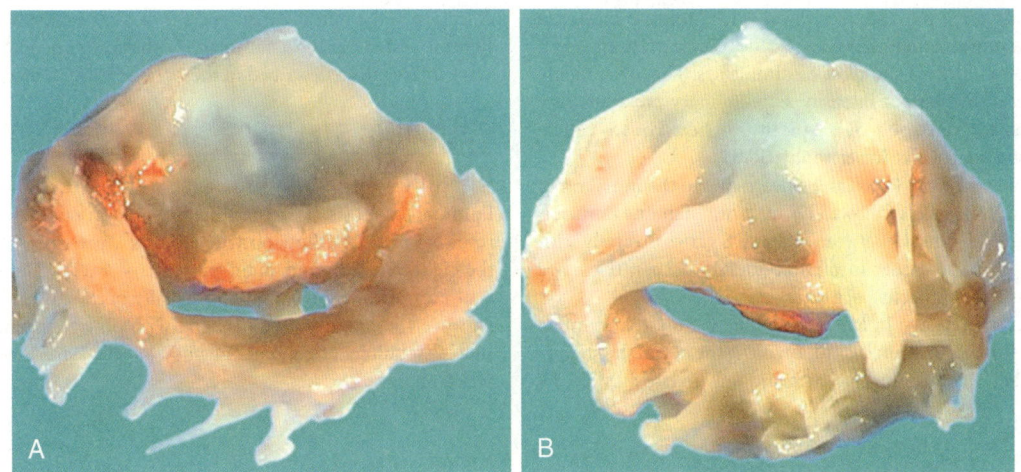

图 6.5　二尖瓣狭窄中的交界处融合。(A) 左心房面。(B) 左心室面 (引自 Cardiovascular Pathology, Fourth Ed, Elsevier, 2016.)

The hemodynamic consequences of MS primarily affect the pulmonary capillary bed, pulmonary artery, and right ventricle. In pure MS, the left ventricle remains unaffected. With resistance to left atrial emptying during diastole, left atrial pressure (LAP) increases. This pressure is reflected back to the capillary bed and pulmonary artery, which can result in pulmonary edema and pulmonary hypertension. This can lead to pressure overload of the right ventricle with subsequent right ventricle hypertrophy (RVH), tricuspid regurgitation (TR), and eventual right ventricular (RV) failure.

Natural History and Clinical Presentation

In developed countries, rheumatic MS is usually a slow progressive disease with a prolonged asymptomatic period of up to several decades. In developing countries, the disease course can be more rapid with symptoms in young adults and children. Symptom onset occurs once the mitral valve area is less than 1.5 cm^2. Once symptom onset occurs, the prognosis becomes worse. Mortality has been linked to New York Heart Association (NYHA) functional class. The presence of atrial fibrillation (AF) and pulmonary hypertension has also been established as a poor prognostic indicator.

Patients often present with dyspnea on exertion and decreased exercise tolerance. This is a consequence of elevated LAP and pulmonary pressures. Additionally, with exertion, an increase in heart rate leads to a decrease in diastolic filling time and increase in the diastolic gradient across the mitral valve.

Elevated LAP leads to left atrial dilation and AF. This can often precipitate or exacerbate the symptoms of MS in two possible ways. First, in AF, there is the loss of atrial contraction which further impedes diastolic flow across a stenotic mitral valve. Second, AF often leads to high heart rates and decreases diastolic filling time. Also, with AF associated with MS, there is an increased thromboembolic risk. If the LA becomes severely dilated, it can compress the recurrent laryngeal nerve and cause hoarseness (Ortner syndrome) or coughing.

Increases in pulmonary pressures and vascular congestion can lead to hemoptysis. As pulmonary hypertension progresses, it affects the right heart and right-sided filling pressures, ultimately leading to symptoms of right heart failure such as ascites and peripheral edema.

Symptoms can be provoked with any state causing an increase in cardiac output or heart rate such as exertion, stress, illness, infection, or arrhythmia. Symptoms may be unmasked in previously asymptomatic women with MS who become pregnant given the increase in heart rate and cardiac output associated with pregnancy.

Physical Examination

Several components of the physical examination need to be carefully assessed when evaluating patients with MS. The patient should be examined in a quiet room and positioned in the left lateral decubitus position because certain characteristic findings of MS may be difficult to appreciate.

S_1 is loud early on in the disease as elevated LAP leads to increased excursion of the mitral leaflets. However, as the disease progresses and the leaflets become calcified and rigid, S_1 diminishes. The S_2 is initially normal but P_2 can increase in intensity as pulmonary pressures rise. Eventually a single S_2 can result. S_3 is typically not heard but S_4 can be heard due to right ventricular hypertrophy (RVH).

A diastolic opening snap (OS) can be heard due to the initial rapid opening of the mitral leaflets followed by an abrupt halt due to fusion of the leaflet tips. The interval between S_2 and OS varies inversely with the severity of MS. The earlier in diastole the OS occurs, the more severe the MS as this is reflective of higher LAP.

The murmur appreciated in MS is a low-pitched diastolic rumble best heard at the apex and at end expiration using the bell of the stethoscope. In mild MS, the murmur may be heard only in late diastole. As MS progresses the murmur may be heard throughout diastole, and if the MS is very severe the murmur may be very soft or absent due to slow flow across the mitral valve.

Patients with symptomatic MS may have signs of heart failure such as rales, jugular venous distension, hepatomegaly, and peripheral edema. If there is significant pulmonary hypertension, a parasternal lift or RV heave may be appreciable.

Diagnosis

ECG and chest radiograph can have nonspecific findings. ECG can show left atrial enlargement, AF, or RVH. Chest radiograph may demonstrate pulmonary vascular congestion, RV dilation, pulmonary artery dilation, or left atrial enlargement ("double density" sign).

TTE is the diagnostic test for MS. TTE is also used to evaluate the severity of MS, assess the effects of the MS on the cardiac chambers and pulmonary pressures, assess for concomitant valvular disease, and assess for suitability of valve anatomy for percutaneous mitral balloon valvotomy (PMBV). On TTE, the mitral leaflets appear thickened and deformed. In rheumatic MS, leaflet motion during diastole is restricted and results in a characteristic "hockey stick" appearance. Doppler interrogation can provide an estimation of mitral valve area and pulmonary artery pressure. The TTE can also assess for the other findings associated with MS such as left atrial dilation, RVH or RV dilation, and TR. With the findings on TTE and the patient's symptoms, MS severity can be staged (Table 6.5).

When there is a discrepancy between the TTE findings and clinical findings, exercise stress echocardiography can be performed to evaluate the mitral valve gradients and pulmonary pressures during exercise. Alternatively, cardiac catheterization can be considered to obtain direct measurements of the cardiac chambers and mitral gradients.

Treatment

There is a limited role for medical therapy in the treatment of MS. If patients have symptoms of heart failure, diuretics can be used to alleviate symptoms. Slowing the heart rate with β-blockers or calcium-channel blockers will increase diastolic filling time and decrease mitral gradients. Rate control is particularly important in AF. Anticoagulation with a vitamin K antagonist is recommended in patients with MS and AF, prior embolic event, or left atrial thrombus. Direct oral anticoagulants have not been approved for this indication.

The decision to proceed with an intervention of the mitral valve depends on the severity of MS and the presence of symptoms, AF, and pulmonary hypertension. Valve morphology, presence of concomitant MR, presence of left atrial thrombus, and the patient's surgical risk will guide whether the patient undergoes a surgical mitral valve replacement or PMBV. Contraindications for PMBV include the presence of left atrial thrombus and more than moderate MR. TTE can be used to assess the suitability for PMBV by assessing the mobility, thickening, and calcification of the mitral leaflets and the degree of subvalvular thickening. Refer to Table 6.6 for a summary of the recommendations for mitral valve intervention described in the 2014 AHA/ACC valve guidelines.

PULMONIC STENOSIS

Definition and Etiology

Pulmonic stenosis (PS) is defined by a restriction in leaflet motion resulting in RV outflow obstruction and a pressure gradient between the right ventricle and main pulmonary artery. The etiology of PS is almost always congenital and usually occurs as an isolated lesion. However, it can also be associated with other congenital conditions such as tetralogy of Fallot, congenital rubella syndrome, and Noonan syndrome.

二尖瓣狭窄的血流动力学后果主要影响肺毛细血管床、肺动脉和右心室。在单纯二尖瓣狭窄中，左心室不受影响。由于舒张期左心房排空受阻，左心房压力升高。该压力传导至肺毛细血管床和肺动脉，可引起肺水肿和肺动脉高压，会进一步导致右心室压力过载，引起右心室肥厚、三尖瓣反流和右心室衰竭。

自然病程与临床表现

在发达国家，风湿性二尖瓣狭窄通常是一种缓慢进展的疾病，可能有长达数十年的无症状期。在发展中国家，疾病进程可能更快，症状可在年轻成人和儿童中出现。一旦二尖瓣瓣口面积< 1.5 cm^2，即可出现症状。症状的出现提示不良预后。死亡率与纽约心脏协会（NYHA）心功能分级有关。心房颤动和肺动脉高压也是预后不良的指标。

患者通常表现为活动后呼吸困难和活动耐量下降。这是由于左心房压力和肺动脉压力升高所致。此外，运动时心率增快导致舒张期充盈时间减少，增加二尖瓣的舒张期压力梯度。

左心房压力升高会导致左心房扩张和心房颤动，诱发或加重二尖瓣狭窄的症状。首先，心房颤动导致心房收缩功能丧失，进一步阻碍通过狭窄的二尖瓣的舒张期血流。其次，心房颤动引起心室率加快，减少了舒张期充盈时间。此外，二尖瓣狭窄合并心房颤动显著增加血栓栓塞风险。若左心房严重扩张，可能压迫喉返神经，导致声音嘶哑（奥特纳综合征）或咳嗽。

肺动脉压升高和肺淤血可导致咯血症状。肺动脉高压的进展会影响右心及右侧的充盈压力，最终导致右心衰竭的症状，如腹水和外周水肿。

任何引起心输出量或心率增快的情况都可能诱发症状，如运动、压力、感染或心律失常。在之前无症状的女性二尖瓣狭窄患者中，怀孕后心率和心输出量的增加，也会导致症状发作。

体格检查

在评估二尖瓣狭窄患者时，需要进行仔细完整的体格检查。由于二尖瓣狭窄的一些特征性发现可能难以察觉，体格检查应在安静的房间中进行，建议患者取左侧卧位。

早期由于左心房压力升高使二尖瓣叶的活动度增加，从而导致第一心音（S$_1$）增强。然而随着疾病进展，瓣叶钙化僵硬，可引起S$_1$减弱。第二心音（S$_2$）初期正常，但随着肺动脉压升高，肺动脉瓣成分（P$_2$）可能增强，最终形成单一的S$_2$。第三心音（S$_3$）通常不可闻及，但由于右心室肥厚，常可闻及第四心音（S$_4$）。

当二尖瓣叶快速打开后因瓣叶尖端融合而突然停止时，听诊可闻及舒张期开瓣音（OS）。S$_2$与开瓣音之间的间隔与二尖瓣狭窄的严重程度成反比。开瓣音出现越早，二尖瓣狭窄越严重，这反映了升高的左心房压力。

二尖瓣狭窄的杂音是低调的舒张期隆隆样杂音，使用听诊器的钟件在心尖区于呼气末听诊效果最好。在轻度二尖瓣狭窄中，杂音可能仅在舒张末期闻及。随着二尖瓣狭窄的进展，杂音可充斥整个舒张期。而若二尖瓣狭窄极重，由于通过二尖瓣的血流缓慢，杂音可能非常轻甚至消失。

有症状的二尖瓣狭窄患者可能有心力衰竭的体征，如双肺湿啰音、颈静脉怒张、肝大和外周水肿。若存在显著的肺动脉高压，可见胸骨旁抬举样搏动或右心室抬举。

诊断

心电图和胸部X线可见非特异性改变。心电图常见左心房扩大、心房颤动、右心室肥厚。胸部X线可见肺淤血、右心室扩张、肺动脉扩张、左心房扩大（"双密度"征）。

经胸超声心动图（TTE）是诊断二尖瓣狭窄的主要工具。TTE还用于评估二尖瓣狭窄的严重程度、狭窄对心脏腔室和肺动脉的影响、是否存在伴随的瓣膜疾病，以及瓣膜解剖结构是否适合行经皮二尖瓣球囊成形术（PMBV）。TTE可探及二尖瓣叶增厚、变形。在风湿性二尖瓣狭窄中，舒张期瓣叶活动受限，表现为特征性的"曲棍球棒"外观。多普勒检查可估算二尖瓣瓣口面积和肺动脉压力。TTE还可评估二尖瓣狭窄继发的病理生理改变，如左心房扩张、右心室肥厚或扩张、三尖瓣反流等。根据TTE的发现和临床症状，可对二尖瓣狭窄的严重程度进行分期（表6.5）。

当TTE的发现与临床表现不一致时，可通过运动负荷超声心动图评估运动期间的二尖瓣压力梯度和肺动脉压。也可考虑进行心导管检查，对心脏腔室和二尖瓣压力梯度进行直接测量。

治疗

药物治疗在二尖瓣狭窄的治疗中效果有限。如果患者有心力衰竭的症状，可以使用利尿剂来缓解。β受体阻滞剂或钙通道阻滞剂可以减慢心率，从而增加舒张期充盈时间并降低二尖瓣压力梯度。在心房颤动患者中，控制心率尤为重要。对于合并心房颤动、有过栓塞事件史或左心房血栓的二尖瓣狭窄患者，推荐使用维生素K拮抗剂进行抗凝治疗。直接口服抗凝剂尚未被批准用于二尖瓣狭窄合并心房颤动的患者。

二尖瓣手术干预治疗的决定因素包括二尖瓣狭窄的严重程度、临床症状以及是否合并心房颤动和肺动脉高压。手术方式的选择，即外科二尖瓣置换术或PMBV，需要考虑患者瓣膜形态、合并症（二尖瓣反流、左心房血栓）以及手术风险。PMBV的禁忌证包括：左心房血栓、中度以上的二尖瓣反流。TTE可以通过评估二尖瓣叶活动度及增厚程度、瓣叶钙化水平、瓣下结构增厚的程度来评估是否适合进行PMBV。（参考表6.6中2014年AHA/ACC《心脏瓣膜病患者管理指南》中关于二尖瓣介入治疗的建议总结。）

肺动脉瓣狭窄

定义和病因

肺动脉瓣狭窄（PS）定义为肺动脉瓣叶运动受限引起右心室流出道受阻，导致右心室和主肺动脉之间形成压力差。肺动脉瓣狭窄的病因以先天性为主，并且通常独立出现。该疾病也可能与其他先天性疾病有关，如法洛四联征、先天性风疹综合征和努南综合征。

TABLE 6.5 Stages of MS

Stage	Definition	Valve Anatomy	Hemodynamic Consequences	Symptoms
A	At risk of MS	Doming of mitral leaflets during diastole	None	None
B	Progressive MS	Rheumatic valve changes with commissural fusion and diastolic doming of the mitral leaflets MVA >1.5 cm^2	Mild to moderate LA enlargement Normal pulmonary pressure at rest	None
C	Asymptomatic severe MS	Rheumatic valve changes with commissural fusion and diastolic doming of the mitral leaflets MVA ≤1.5 cm^2 (MVA <1.0 cm^2 with very severe MS)	Severe LA enlargement Elevated pulmonary artery pressure	None
D	Symptomatic severe MS	See Stage C	See Stage C	Decreased exercise tolerance Exertional dyspnea

Modified from Nishimura R, Otto C, Bonow RO, et al: 2014 AHA/ACC guideline for the management of patients with valvular heart disease. J Am Coll Cardiol 2014;63:e57-e185.

TABLE 6.6 Summary of Recommendations for Mitral Valve Intervention in MS

Recommendation	Class of Recommendation
PMBV is recommended for symptomatic patients with severe MS (MVA ≤1.5 cm^2, stage D) and favorable valve morphology in the absence of contraindications	I
MVR is indicated in severely symptomatic patients (NYHA class III/IV) with severe MS (MVA ≤1.5 cm^2, stage D) who are not high risk for surgery and who are not candidates for or failed previous PMBV	I
Concomitant MVR is indicated for patients with severe MS (MVA ≤1.5 cm^2, stage C or D) undergoing other cardiac surgery	I
PMBV is reasonable for asymptomatic patients with very severe MS (MVA ≤1.0 cm^2, stage C) and favorable valve morphology in the absence of contraindications	IIa
MVR is reasonable for severely symptomatic patients (NYHA class III/IV) with severe MS (MVA ≤1.5 cm^2, stage D), provided there are other operative indications	IIa
PMBV may be considered for asymptomatic patients with severe MS (MVA ≤1.5 cm^2, stage C) and favorable valve morphology who have new onset of AF in the absence of contraindications	IIb
PMBV may be considered for symptomatic patients with MVA >1.5 cm^2 if there is evidence of hemodynamically significant MS during exercise	IIb
PMBV may be considered for severely symptomatic patients (NYHA class III/IV) with severe MS (MVA ≤1.5 cm^2, stage D) who have suboptimal valve anatomy and are not candidates for surgery or at high risk for surgery	IIb
Concomitant MVR may be considered for patients with moderate MS (MVA 1.6 to 2.0 cm^2) undergoing other cardiac surgery	IIb
MVR and excision of the left atrial appendage may be considered for patients with severe MS (MVA ≤1.5 cm^2, stages C and D) who have had recurrent embolic events while receiving adequate anticoagulation	IIb

Modified from Nishimura R, Otto C, Bonow RO, et al: 2014 AHA/ACC guideline for the management of patients with valvular heart disease. J Am Coll Cardiol 2014;63:e57-e185.

Pathophysiology

In PS, the valve is typically trileaflet with thickening and fusion of the commissures resulting in restricted leaflet opening during systole. Post-stenotic dilation of the main pulmonary artery can occur due to eccentric flow through the stenotic valve. Over time, RVH can occur due to increased afterload.

Natural History and Clinical Presentation

Isolated PS is generally well tolerated and survival is comparable to the general population. Patients with mild PS are asymptomatic and may not be diagnosed with PS until adulthood. Moderate PS is usually identified in childhood and patients are usually symptomatic due to RV pressure overload. Decreasing right-sided cardiac output leads to symptoms of dyspnea on exertion and fatigue. In more advanced disease, patients can have RV failure and cyanosis.

Physical Examination

On physical examination, patients with PS can have a parasternal lift as a result of RVH. The jugular veins may demonstrate prominent *a* waves. The murmur of PS is a systolic ejection murmur best heard at the left upper sternal border radiating to the back with the duration correlating with severity. A late peaking murmur indicates more severe disease. A systolic ejection click may be heard in mild to moderate PS. S_2 can have wide splitting due to prolonged ejection time of the right ventricle. Fixed splitting of S_2 occurs in severe disease when the RV output becomes fixed.

表 6.5 二尖瓣狭窄分期

分期	定义	瓣膜解剖	血流动力学结局	症状
A	二尖瓣狭窄风险期	舒张期二尖瓣叶隆起	无	无
B	二尖瓣狭窄进展期	风湿性瓣膜改变伴有交界处融合 舒张期二尖瓣叶隆起 MVA > 1.5 cm^2	左心房轻中度扩大 静息肺动脉压正常	无
C	无症状性重度二尖瓣狭窄	风湿性瓣膜改变伴有交界处融合 舒张期二尖瓣叶隆起 MVA ≤ 1.5 cm^2（极重度 MVA < 1 cm^2）	左心房显著扩大 肺动脉压升高	无
D	症状性重度二尖瓣狭窄	同 C 期	同 C 期	活动耐量减低、劳力性呼吸困难

MVA，二尖瓣瓣口面积。

改编自 Nishimura R, Otto C, Bonow RO, et al: 2014 AHA/ACC guideline for the management of patients with valvular heart disease. J Am Coll Cardiol 2014; 63: e57-e185.

表 6.6 二尖瓣狭窄患者二尖瓣干预的指南推荐总结

推荐	推荐类别
对于有症状的重度二尖瓣狭窄（MVA ≤ 1.5 cm^2，D 期）且瓣膜形态良好的患者，如果没有禁忌证，推荐进行经皮球囊二尖瓣成形术。	I
对于症状严重（NYHA Ⅲ/Ⅳ级）的重度二尖瓣狭窄（MVA ≤ 1.5 cm^2，D 期）患者，如果其手术风险不高且不适合或未成功进行经皮球囊二尖瓣成形术，建议进行二尖瓣置换术。	I
对于进行其他心脏手术的重度二尖瓣狭窄（MVA ≤ 1.5 cm^2，C 期或 D 期）患者，建议同时进行二尖瓣置换术。	I
对于无症状但极重度二尖瓣狭窄（MVA ≤ 1.0 cm^2，C 期）且瓣膜形态良好的患者，如果没有禁忌证，进行经皮球囊二尖瓣成形术是合理的。	Ⅱa
对于症状严重（NYHA Ⅲ/Ⅳ级）的重度二尖瓣狭窄（MVA ≤ 1.5 cm^2，D 期）患者，如果有其他手术指征，进行二尖瓣置换术是合理的。	Ⅱa
对于无症状的重度二尖瓣狭窄（MVA ≤ 1.5 cm^2，C 期）且瓣膜形态良好的新发心房颤动患者，如果没有禁忌证，可以考虑进行经皮球囊二尖瓣成形术。	Ⅱb
对于症状性二尖瓣狭窄（MVA > 1.5 cm^2）的患者，如果在运动时有血流动力学显著的二尖瓣狭窄证据，可以考虑进行经皮球囊二尖瓣成形术。	Ⅱb
对于症状严重（NYHA Ⅲ/Ⅳ级）的重度二尖瓣狭窄（MVA ≤ 1.5 cm^2，D 期）且瓣膜解剖结构不理想、不适合手术或手术风险高的患者，可以考虑进行经皮球囊二尖瓣成形术。	Ⅱb
对于进行其他心脏手术的中度二尖瓣狭窄（MVA 1.6～2.0 cm^2）患者，可以考虑同时进行二尖瓣置换术。	Ⅱb
对于重度二尖瓣狭窄（MVA ≤ 1.5 cm^2，C 期和 D 期）且在接受充分抗凝治疗期间仍有复发性栓塞事件的患者，可以考虑进行二尖瓣置换术并切除左心耳。	Ⅱb

改编自 Nishimura R, Otto C, Bonow RO, et al: 2014 AHA/ACC guideline for the management of patients with valvular heart disease. J Am Coll Cardiol 2014; 63: e57-e185.

病理生理学

肺动脉瓣狭窄的典型病理特征为三叶瓣瓣叶交界处增厚融合，致使收缩期瓣叶开放受限。狭窄处形成的偏心性高速湍流可引发主肺动脉狭窄后扩张。随着时间推移，后负荷增加会导致右心室肥厚。

自然病程与临床表现

孤立性肺动脉瓣狭窄患者通常能耐受，其生存率与普通人群类似。轻度肺动脉瓣狭窄患者通常无症状，可能直到成年才被发现。中度肺动脉瓣狭窄通常在儿童时期诊断，患者因右心室压力负荷过重而出现症状。右心输出量减少会导致劳力性呼吸困难和疲劳。在病情较重时会出现右心室衰竭和发绀。

体格检查

在体格检查中，肺动脉瓣狭窄患者可能因右心室肥厚而出现胸骨旁抬举样搏动。颈静脉可见明显的 a 波。肺动脉瓣狭窄的杂音表现为收缩期喷射样杂音，最佳听诊位置在左上胸骨缘（胸骨左缘第二肋间），杂音向背部传导，杂音的持续时间与疾病的严重程度相关。晚峰杂音提示病情较为严重。轻至中度肺动脉瓣狭窄患者可闻及收缩期喷射音。由于右心室射血时间延长，第二心音可能出现较宽的分裂。在右心输出量明显减少的重度病例中可出现第二心音固定分裂。

Diagnosis

TTE can be used to diagnose PS, assess the severity of PS, and evaluate the right ventricle. Using Doppler measurements, the gradients across a stenotic pulmonic valve can be estimated. If TTE is inconclusive or for patients with complex anatomy, cardiac magnetic resonance imaging (CMR) can be considered as an alternative imaging modality to assess the severity of valve disease and quantitatively measure RV size and function.

Treatment

Intervention is guided by the valve anatomy, gradients measured on TTE, and the presence of symptoms. Percutaneous balloon valvotomy is recommended in asymptomatic patients with a peak gradient of greater than 60 mm Hg or a mean gradient of 40 mm Hg, or in symptomatic patients with a peak gradient of 50 mm Hg or a mean gradient of 30 mm Hg. A surgical approach is usually recommended for dysplastic valves, in the presence of severe pulmonic regurgitation, or if there is another indication for surgery.

TRICUSPID STENOSIS

Definition and Etiology

In tricuspid stenosis (TS), there is restriction of blood flow between the right atrium and right ventricle. The etiology of TS is most commonly rheumatic and is generally associated with MS. Isolated TS is rare but can be seen in congenital tricuspid valve atresia, right heart tumors, carcinoid syndrome, and endocarditis.

Pathophysiology

TS causes flow obstruction at the level of the tricuspid valve resulting in a diastolic pressure gradient between the right atrium and right ventricle. This leads to elevated right atrial pressure (RAP) and systemic venous congestion. With exertion or tachycardia, diastolic filling time decreases and the diastolic pressure gradient increases. With inspiration, the decrease in intrathoracic pressure results in increased venous return which also increases the pressure gradient across the tricuspid valve. Conversely, expiration leads to a decrease in the pressure gradient.

Natural History and Clinical Presentation

The natural history of patients with TS is variable. Most patients with rheumatic TS have concomitant significant aortic and/or mitral valve disease. Tricuspid valve atresia is managed with multiple surgeries starting in the neonatal period into early childhood.

Patients present with signs and symptoms of systemic venous congestion including ascites, peripheral edema, and hepatomegaly. Patients may report a fluttering sensation in the neck from prominent *a* waves.

Physical Examination

With an increase in RAP there is jugular venous distension. A prominent *a* wave can often be appreciated. A rise in jugular venous pressure with inspiration (Kussmaul sign) may also be seen. Other signs of systemic venous congestion can be present including hepatomegaly, ascites, peripheral edema, and anasarca. The murmur of TS is described as a low-frequency, diastolic murmur best heard at the left lower sternal border. There may also be an opening snap. These sounds are difficult to distinguish from the murmur and opening snap of MS. However, with right-sided murmurs, the intensity of the TS murmur should increase with inspiration (Carvallo sign).

Diagnosis

TS can be diagnosed using TTE. In rheumatic TS, as seen in MS, the leaflets are restricted, thickened, and calcified. TTE is also used to assess for concomitant valve disease and to estimate the right atrial size and pressure. Using Doppler, the diastolic pressure gradients can be measured across the tricuspid valve and the tricuspid valve area can be estimated. A valve area of 1.0 cm^2 or less is considered to be severe TS.

Treatment

There are limited data to guide treatment in TS. Options include medical therapy such as diuretics to help with systemic venous congestion, surgical intervention, or percutaneous balloon valvotomy. The decision for surgical versus percutaneous approach should be individualized and based on valve anatomy, surgical risk, and operator experience. A surgical approach is typically reserved for symptomatic patients with severe TS or asymptomatic patients with severe TS requiring cardiac surgery for another indication.

AORTIC REGURGITATION

Definition and Etiology

Aortic regurgitation (AR) is the result of inadequate coaptation of the aortic valve leaflets during diastole leading to regurgitant flow of blood from the aorta to the left ventricle. The ability of the left ventricle to accommodate this additional volume is dependent on the chronicity of the disease. Therefore, acute severe AR and chronic AR should be considered as separate disease processes.

The two most common causes of acute severe AR in a native aortic valve are endocarditis and aortic dissection. Endocarditis can lead to leaflet destruction, leaflet perforation, or perivalvular abscess that can rupture into the left ventricle. Aortic dissection can result in AR by dilation of the sinuses, involvement of the commissures or leaflets, or prolapse of the dissection flap across the aortic valve.

In developing countries, chronic AR is usually due to rheumatic heart disease. In developed countries, aortic root dilation, calcific degeneration, and bicuspid aortic valve are the most common causes. However, many other disease processes can affect the aortic valve or the ascending aorta and lead to chronic AR (Table 6.7).

Pathophysiology

In acute severe AR, a large regurgitant volume enters an unprepared left ventricle which results in a decrease in effective stroke volume and rapid increase in LV end-diastolic pressure with subsequent pulmonary edema, cardiogenic shock, and possible hemodynamic collapse.

In chronic AR, the left ventricle is able to make compensatory changes to maintain cardiac output. The regurgitant flow from the aorta into the left ventricle results in an increase in LV end-diastolic volume and wall stress. In response, there is eccentric hypertrophy, chamber dilation, and an increase in ventricular compliance. Therefore, LV end-diastolic pressure can remain normal despite a significant increase in LV volume. In addition, these compensatory changes can lead to an increase in total stroke volume, which results in an elevation in systolic pressure. During diastole, there is rapid equalization of pressures between the aorta and left ventricle resulting in a low diastolic pressure. This accounts for the wide pulse pressure and several of the characteristic physical examination findings seen in chronic AR.

Natural History and Clinical Presentation

Patients with acute severe AR often present with pulmonary edema and cardiogenic shock. Other presenting symptoms will depend on the etiology, which is usually aortic dissection or endocarditis.

In contrast, there is a prolonged asymptomatic period in chronic AR. Even with severe AR, exercise tolerance can be preserved as an increase in heart rate during exercise leads to shorter diastolic filling times, and thus less AR. However, with progressive LV dilation,

诊断

TTE 可用于诊断肺动脉瓣狭窄，评估狭窄严重程度和右心室状态。多普勒超声可以估算狭窄肺动脉瓣的压力梯度。如果 TTE 结果不明确或患者解剖结构复杂，心脏磁共振成像（CMR）可作为替代的影像学方法，评估瓣膜病变的严重程度并对右心室结构和功能进行定量测量。

治疗

瓣膜干预治疗的决策依据主要包括瓣膜解剖结构、TTE 测量的压力阶差以及临床症状。对于无症状但峰值压差超过 60 mmHg 或平均压差超过 40 mmHg 的患者，或有症状且峰值压差超过 50 mmHg 或平均压差超过 30 mmHg 的患者，推荐进行经皮瓣膜球囊成形术。对于瓣膜发育不良、存在严重肺动脉瓣反流或有其他手术指征的患者，通常推荐外科手术。

三尖瓣狭窄

定义和病因

三尖瓣狭窄（TS）是指三尖瓣病变导致右心房与右心室之间的血流受限，其最常见的病因是风湿性疾病，通常合并二尖瓣狭窄。孤立性三尖瓣狭窄较为罕见，可见于先天性三尖瓣闭锁、右心肿瘤、类癌综合征和心内膜炎。

病理生理学

三尖瓣狭窄在三尖瓣水平造成血流梗阻，引起右心房和右心室之间产生舒张期压力阶差，导致右心房压力（RAP）升高和体循环静脉淤血。运动或心动过速时，舒张期充盈时间减少，舒张期压力梯度增加。吸气时由于胸腔内压降低，静脉回流增加，也会增加三尖瓣的压力阶差，反之呼气时压力阶差下降。

自然病程与临床表现

三尖瓣狭窄患者的自然病程因人而异。大多数风湿性三尖瓣狭窄患者常合并显著的主动脉瓣和（或）二尖瓣疾病。三尖瓣闭锁的患者新生儿期到儿童早期即需进行多次手术治疗。

患者可表现为体循环静脉淤血的症状和体征：腹水、周围水肿和肝大。由于颈静脉 a 波增强，部分患者有颈部扑动感。

体格检查

由于右心房压力升高，患者可出现颈静脉怒张，常可见明显的 a 波和吸气时颈静脉压升高（Kussmaul 征）。其他体循环静脉淤血的体征包括肝大、腹水、周围及全身性水肿。三尖瓣狭窄的杂音为低频的舒张期杂音，最佳听诊位置在左下胸骨缘，可能伴有开瓣音。杂音与二尖瓣狭窄的杂音和开瓣音难以区分。不过三尖瓣狭窄的杂音作为右心杂音，吸气时杂音的强度增加（Carvallo 征）。

诊断

TTE 可用于诊断三尖瓣狭窄。在风湿性三尖瓣狭窄中，瓣叶活动受限、增厚、钙化。TTE 还能够评估合并的瓣膜病变，并估算右心房的大小和压力。超声多普勒可测量三尖瓣的舒张期压力阶差并计算三尖瓣瓣口面积。若瓣口面积小于或等于 $1.0\ cm^2$，则诊断重度三尖瓣狭窄。

治疗

目前关于三尖瓣狭窄治疗的指南数据有限。治疗方式包括药物治疗、外科手术、经皮球囊成形术。药物治疗主要指利尿剂的使用以缓解体循环静脉淤血。外科手术和经皮介入治疗的选择应基于瓣膜解剖结构、手术风险和操作经验进行个体化评估。通常外科手术适用于有症状的重度三尖瓣狭窄患者或因其他原因需行心脏手术的无症状重度三尖瓣狭窄患者。

主动脉瓣反流

定义和病因

主动脉瓣反流（AR）是由于舒张期主动脉瓣叶不能完全闭合，导致血流从主动脉反流到左心室。左心室适应额外增加的容量负荷的能力取决于疾病的慢性程度。因此，急性重度主动脉瓣反流和慢性主动脉瓣反流应视为不同的病程。

急性重度主动脉瓣反流的两个最常见原因是心内膜炎和主动脉夹层。心内膜炎可导致瓣叶破坏、穿孔或瓣周脓肿破裂入左心室。主动脉夹层可导致主动脉窦扩张，也可累及瓣叶或瓣膜接合缘，或撕裂的内膜片脱垂至主动脉瓣，最终引发急性主动脉瓣反流。

在发展中国家，慢性主动脉瓣反流通常由风湿性心脏病引起。在发达国家，主动脉根部扩张、钙化退行性变和二叶主动脉瓣是最常见病因。然而，其他疾病也可通过影响主动脉瓣或升主动脉导致慢性主动脉瓣反流（表 6.7）。

病理生理学

在急性重度主动脉瓣反流中，大量反流血液进入尚未适应的左心室，有效心搏出量减少，并导致左心室舒张末期压力迅速增加，继而引发肺水肿、心源性休克，甚至血流动力学崩溃。

在慢性主动脉瓣反流中，左心室通过代偿变化以维持心输出量。反流的血液进入左心室可导致左心室舒张末期容积和室壁应力增加，左心室相应地发生离心性肥厚、心腔扩张以增加室壁顺应性。因此尽管左心室容积显著增大，舒张末期压力仍可保持正常。以上代偿性改变也导致心输出量增加，引起收缩压升高，而舒张期时主动脉和左心室之间的压力迅速平衡，引起舒张压降低。以上改变是慢性主动脉瓣反流中脉压增大和出现特征性体征的基础。

自然病程与临床表现

急性重度主动脉瓣反流患者通常表现为肺水肿和心源性休克。其他症状则取决于病因，常与主动脉夹层或心内膜炎相关。

TABLE 6.7 Causes of Chronic Aortic Regurgitation

Mechanism	Etiology
Congenital/leaflet abnormalities	Bicuspid, unicuspid, or quadricuspid aortic valve
	Ventricular septal defect
Acquired leaflet abnormalities	Senile calcification
	Infective endocarditis
	Rheumatic disease
	Radiation-induced valvulopathy
	Toxin-induced valvulopathy: anorectic drugs, 5-hydroxytryptamine
Congenital/genetic aortic root abnormalities	Annuloaortic ectasia
	Connective tissue disease: Loeys Dietz, Ehlers-Danlos, Marfan syndrome, osteogenesis imperfecta
Acquired aortic root abnormalities	Idiopathic aortic root dilation
	Systemic hypertension
	Autoimmune disease: systemic lupus erythematosus, ankylosing spondylitis, reactive arthritis
	Aortitis: syphilis, Takayasu arteritis
	Aortic dissection
	Trauma

Modified from: Zoghbi W, Adams D, et al: Recommendations for noninvasive evaluation of native valvular regurgitation. JASE 2017;30:303-371.

patients can develop LV systolic dysfunction and symptoms of heart failure.

Physical Examination

Patients with acute severe AR will have physical examination findings consistent with cardiogenic shock and pulmonary edema such as hypotension, pallor, peripheral vasoconstriction, and rales. Wide pulse pressures and the characteristic findings seen in chronic AR are typically not appreciated.

With regards to the heart sounds in acute severe AR, A_2 may be diminished, P_2 is more prominent due to pulmonary hypertension, and S_3 can be heard. The murmurs heard in acute AR include an early, low-pitched, diastolic murmur and a soft systolic murmur due to increased flow across the aortic valve. The presence of both results in a characteristic "to-and-fro" murmur. However, depending on the diastolic gradient between the aorta and left ventricle, these murmurs may be inaudible.

The wide pulse pressure seen in chronic AR can lead to several physical findings (Table 6.8). The murmur of chronic AR is a blowing early diastolic murmur best heard at the left upper sternal border with the patient sitting up, leaning forward, and at end-expiration. As AR progresses, this murmur can become holodiastolic and harsher in quality. In very severe AR, the murmur can become soft or even absent.

An Austin-Flint murmur, a mid to late diastolic rumble best heard at the apex in severe AR and due to vibration of the anterior mitral leaflet as it is struck by the jet of AR, may also be appreciated. Additionally, a short midsystolic ejection murmur radiating to the neck can be heard as a result of increased stroke volume.

Diagnosis

In both acute and chronic AR, echocardiography can evaluate the presence, severity, and mechanism of AR, the effect of AR on the other cardiac chambers, and the presence of concomitant valve disease. In the case of acute severe AR with suspected aortic dissection or endocarditis, a transesophageal echocardiogram (TEE) should be considered over TTE given its superior sensitivity and specificity for these diagnoses. Computed tomography (CT) imaging has similar sensitivity and specificity for diagnosing aortic dissection. However, TEE also allows for concomitant evaluation of the aortic valve structure, AR, and the other cardiac structures.

In the assessment of chronic AR, when the TTE results are inconclusive or discrepant from clinical findings, alternative imaging modalities can be considered. TEE generally provides superior image quality compared to TTE. CMR can accurately quantify the severity of AR as well as chamber sizes and LV systolic function. Aortography and cardiac catheterization may also be considered to evaluate AR, aortic root, and left-sided filling pressures. However, their role has diminished because of the availability and accuracy of noninvasive imaging.

Treatment

In acute severe AR, emergent or urgent surgical intervention is usually indicated in the setting of aortic dissection or infective endocarditis. Prior to surgery, the mainstay of medical therapy is afterload reduction. This can be achieved with intravenous nitroprusside. Diuretics and ionotropic agents may be helpful in the setting of cardiogenic shock and pulmonary edema. Beta-blockers, while helpful for aortic dissection, can lead to further hemodynamic deterioration as the increase in diastolic filling time leads to more AR. Vasopressors and intra-aortic balloon pumps are contraindicated in this setting.

With chronic AR, there is a limited role for medical therapy. Vasodilators such as hydralazine, angiotensin-converting enzyme (ACE) inhibitors, and calcium-channel blockers can be used in patients who are asymptomatic and hypertensive. There is conflicting evidence for their use to delay surgery. AVR is recommended once a patient has severe symptomatic AR or severe asymptomatic AR with a LV systolic dysfunction (left ventricular ejection fraction (LVEF) of less than 50%) or chamber dilation (LV end systolic diameter (LVESD) of greater than 50 mm or LV end diastolic diameter (LVEDD) of greater than 65 mm). AVR is also indicated in patients with severe asymptomatic AR if there is another indication for cardiac surgery.

The options for mechanical and biologic prostheses are similar to those for surgical AVR for AS. However, a percutaneous approach is not available.

MITRAL REGURGITATION

Definition and Etiology

Mitral regurgitation (MR) is defined by the inadequate coaptation of the mitral leaflets during systole resulting in regurgitant flow from the left ventricle to the left atrium. Similar to AR, MR leads to LV volume overload

表 6.7 慢性主动脉瓣反流的原因	
机制	病因
先天性/瓣叶异常	二叶、单叶或四叶瓣主动脉瓣
	室间隔缺损
获得性瓣叶异常	老年性钙化
	感染性心内膜炎
	风湿性疾病
	辐射引起的瓣膜病变
	毒素引起的瓣膜病变：食欲抑制剂、5-羟色胺
先天性主动脉根部异常	主动脉瓣环扩张
	结缔组织病：Loeys-Dietz 综合征、Ehlers-Danlos 综合征、马方综合征、成骨不全症
获得性主动脉根部异常	特发性主动脉根部扩张
	系统性高血压
	自身免疫性疾病：系统性红斑狼疮、强直性脊柱炎、反应性关节炎
	主动脉炎：梅毒、Takayasu 动脉炎
	主动脉夹层
	创伤

改编自 Zoghbi W, Adams D, et al: Recommendations for noninvasive evaluation of native valvular regurgitation. JASE 2017; 30: 303-371.

相较之下慢性主动脉瓣反流患者有较长的无症状期。即使在重度主动脉瓣反流的情况下，患者的活动耐量也可保持正常，因为运动时心率增快引起左心室舒张充盈时间缩短，反而减少了主动脉瓣反流。然而随着左心室进行性扩张，患者会出现左心室收缩功能障碍和心力衰竭的症状。

体格检查

急性重度主动脉瓣反流患者常表现为心源性休克和肺水肿的体征，如低血压、面色苍白、外周血管收缩和湿啰音。慢性主动脉瓣反流中常见的脉压增大和特征性体征在急性反流中通常不明显。

在急性重度主动脉瓣反流中，听诊可闻及第二心音 A_2 减弱及 P_2 增强（肺动脉高压引起），有时亦可闻及第三心音。急性主动脉瓣反流的杂音包括低调的舒张早期杂音以及因主动脉瓣血流增加而引起的轻度的收缩期杂音，两者形成了特征性的"往复"杂音。但由于主动脉和左心室之间舒张期的压力阶差决定了杂音的性质及程度，特征性的杂音可能很难闻及。

慢性主动脉瓣反流中的脉压增大可以引起多种体征（表 6.8）。慢性主动脉瓣反流的杂音表现为舒张早期吹风样杂音，最佳听诊位置在左上胸骨缘。杂音在患者坐起、前倾、呼气末时明显。随着主动脉瓣反流的进展，杂音可拓展至全舒张期，音质更加尖锐。在极重度的主动脉瓣反流中，杂音反而可能变得轻微甚至消失。

在严重主动脉瓣反流时亦可闻及 Austin-Flint 杂音，这是心尖区的舒张中晚期隆隆样杂音，产生机制是由于主动脉瓣的反流束撞击二尖瓣前叶所引起的振动。此外由于心脏搏出量增加，还可闻及短促的收缩中期喷射样杂音，杂音可放射至颈部。

诊断

在急性和慢性主动脉瓣反流中，超声心动图可评估反流的严重程度和产生机制，并了解反流对心脏腔室的影响，以及合并的瓣膜病变。在怀疑主动脉夹层或心内膜炎引起的急性重度主动脉瓣反流时建议优先选择经食管超声心动图（TEE）而非 TTE，因为 TEE 在这些疾病中具有更高的敏感性和特异性。计算机断层成像（CT）在诊断主动脉夹层方面也具有较高的敏感性和特异性。然而，TEE 的优势还在于可同时评估主动脉瓣结构、主动脉瓣反流以及其他心脏结构。

在评估慢性主动脉瓣反流时，如果 TTE 的结果不明确或与临床表现不一致，可考虑其他影像学检查。与 TTE 相比，TEE 可提供更高质量的图像。CMR 可以准确量化反流的严重程度、心腔大小和左心室收缩功能。主动脉造影和心导管检查也可用来评估主动脉瓣反流、主动脉根部和左心室充盈压力。然而随着非侵入性影像学技术的普及和应用，侵入性检查的应用需求已明显减少。

治疗

主动脉夹层或感染性心内膜炎引起的急性重度主动脉瓣反流通常需急诊手术干预。术前药物治疗的主要目的是减少后负荷，通常予静脉应用硝普钠。心源性休克和肺水肿时应用利尿剂和正性肌力药物有益。尽管 β 受体阻滞剂对主动脉夹层有益，但在急性主动脉瓣反流时，应用 β 受体阻滞剂可通过延长舒张期充盈时间加重反流进而导致血流动力学恶化。血管升压药和主动脉内球囊反搏在此类情况下禁忌。

对于慢性主动脉瓣反流，药物治疗的作用有限。对于无症状且血压升高的患者可给予血管扩张剂如肼屈嗪、血管紧张素转换酶抑制剂、钙通道阻滞剂等。药物治疗在延缓病情进展至需进行手术中的作用目前存在争议。重度症状性主动脉瓣反流、重度无症状性主动脉瓣反流伴左心室收缩功能障碍（左心室射血分数 < 50%）或左心室扩张（左心室收缩末期内径 > 50 mm 或左心室舒张末期内径 > 65 mm）建议行主动脉瓣置换术。若存在其他心脏手术指征，重度无症状性主动脉瓣反流患者也应同期进行主动脉瓣置换术。

机械瓣和生物瓣的选择与在主动脉瓣狭窄中的外科主动脉瓣置换术类似。目前经皮介入治疗在主动脉瓣反流中的证据尚缺乏。

二尖瓣反流

定义和病因

二尖瓣反流（MR）是指在收缩期二尖瓣叶未能完全闭合，导致血液从左心室反流到左心房。类似于

TABLE 6.8 Signs of Chronic Aortic Regurgitation

Name	Description
Corrigan pulse	Rapid upstroke and collapse of pulses; "water hammer pulses"
Musset sign	Head bob with each heartbeat
Traube sign	Systolic and diastolic sounds heard over femoral arteries; "pistol shot pulse"
Duroziez sign	Systolic and diastolic bruit heard with compression of femoral artery
Quincke pulses	Capillary pulsations
Mueller sign	Pulsation of uvula
Becker sign	Pulsation of retinal arteries and pupils
Hills sign	Popliteal systolic cuff pressure exceed brachial pressure by >20 mm Hg
Mayne sign	>15 mm Hg decrease in diastolic blood pressure with arm elevation
Rosenbach sign	Pulsations of liver
Gerhard sign	Pulsations of spleen

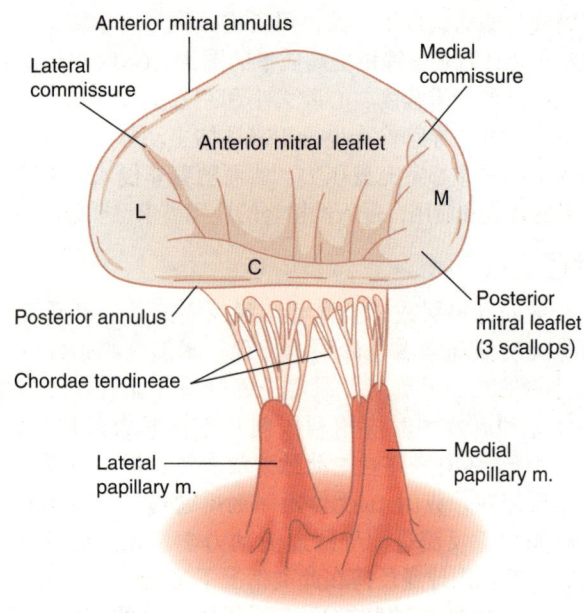

Fig. 6.6 Mitral apparatus. (From Otto C: Textbook of Clinical Echocardiography, 6th ed., Elsevier, 2018.)

and the ability of the left ventricle to compensate for this additional volume is dependent upon chronicity. Therefore, like AR, acute severe MR and chronic MR should be considered as two distinct disease processes.

The mitral apparatus consists of the left atrial wall, mitral annulus, anterior and posterior leaflets, chordae tendineae, papillary muscles, and the LV myocardium underlying the papillary muscles (Fig. 6.6). Disturbance to any component of the mitral apparatus can result in MR.

Acute MR can be caused by ischemic and nonischemic etiologies. Papillary muscle rupture or displacement can be seen in the setting of an acute myocardial infarction or ischemia. Nonischemic causes include infective endocarditis, ruptured chordae tendineae, trauma, RHD, and dynamic LV outflow obstruction.

Given the complexity of the mitral apparatus, it is useful to categorize the causes of MR as primary or secondary (Table 6.9). Primary MR is due to an intrinsic abnormality of the mitral leaflets. Secondary MR is a result of distortion of the mitral annulus in the setting of ventricular remodeling. Distinguishing between primary and secondary MR is important because the management and outcomes differ. Alternatively, MR can be classified based on leaflet motion using the Carpentier classification (Fig. 6.7).

Pathophysiology

The pathophysiology of MR and the differences in the pathophysiology between acute and chronic MR are illustrated in Fig. 6.8. In acute severe MR, there is a sudden increase in preload and decrease in afterload. This leads to an increase in the total stroke volume (TSV) and LVEF. However, the forward stroke volume (FSV) decreases resulting in reduced cardiac output. Simultaneously, there is an acute rise in LAP causing pulmonary edema. This ultimately leads to cardiogenic shock.

In chronic compensated MR, the progressive rise in LV preload leads to increased wall stress. In response, there is eccentric hypertrophy of the left ventricle and an increase in the LV end diastolic volume. This not only increases LVEF and TSV, but it also allows for the maintenance of a normal FSV. However, as MR progresses, LV systolic dysfunction and dilation occur. In this setting, LVEF, TSV, and FSV all decrease, resulting in chronic decompensated MR.

In chronic MR, the compliant left atrium is able to accommodate a large regurgitant volume from the left ventricle. However, this eventually results in left atrial dilation and pulmonary hypertension.

Natural History and Clinical Presentation

Patients with acute severe MR are acutely ill and often in cardiogenic shock. Along with hemodynamic instability, patients may have symptoms related to the etiology of MR. For example, in the setting of an acute myocardial infarction with papillary muscle rupture, a patient may present with chest pain along with ischemic ECG changes and elevated cardiac enzymes. Patients with infective endocarditis may have fevers, positive blood cultures, vascular phenomena, immunologic phenomena, or a predisposing condition such as intravenous drug use.

With chronic MR, the natural history and clinical presentation are quite different because the left ventricle has time to remodel and compensate via the mechanisms noted above. Often times, patients have a prolonged asymptomatic phase. Over time, as the left-sided filling pressures increase, patients may develop fatigue or decreased exercise tolerance. Eventually, patients can have signs and symptoms of congestive heart failure (CHF) such as dyspnea on exertion, orthopnea, paroxysmal nocturnal dyspnea, and/or peripheral edema. With left atrial dilation, patients may develop AF.

Physical Examination

Patients with acute severe MR are often in pulmonary edema and cardiogenic shock. Physical examination may be remarkable for pallor, cool extremities due to peripheral vasoconstriction, rales, jugular venous distension, and diminished peripheral pulses. The murmur of acute severe MR is usually soft, low-pitched, decrescendo, and early systolic. However, in about half of the patients, no murmur may be appreciated due to the low-pressure gradient between the left ventricle and the left atrium. Therefore, the absence of a systolic murmur does not necessarily rule out acute severe MR.

In chronic MR, S_1 is diminished due to inadequate coaptation of the mitral leaflets. S_2 is widely split with a reduced forward stroke volume leading to an early A_2 and pulmonary hypertension delaying P_2. An S_3 can also be appreciated with the increased diastolic flow across the mitral valve into a left ventricle. The murmur of chronic MR is

表 6.8	慢性主动脉瓣反流的体征
体征	描述
Corrigan 脉搏	脉搏的快速上升和下降;"水冲脉"
Musset 征	随心脏搏动的点头征
Traube 征	在股动脉上闻及收缩期和舒张期声音;"手枪脉"
Duroziez 征	压迫股动脉时听到的收缩期和舒张期杂音
Quincke 脉搏	毛细血管搏动征
Mueller 征	悬雍垂的搏动
Becker 征	视网膜动脉和瞳孔的搏动
Hills 征	腘动脉收缩压超过肱动脉压 20 mmHg 以上
Mayne 征	举臂时舒张压降低超过 15 mmHg
Rosenbach 征	肝脏的搏动
Gerhard 征	脾脏的搏动

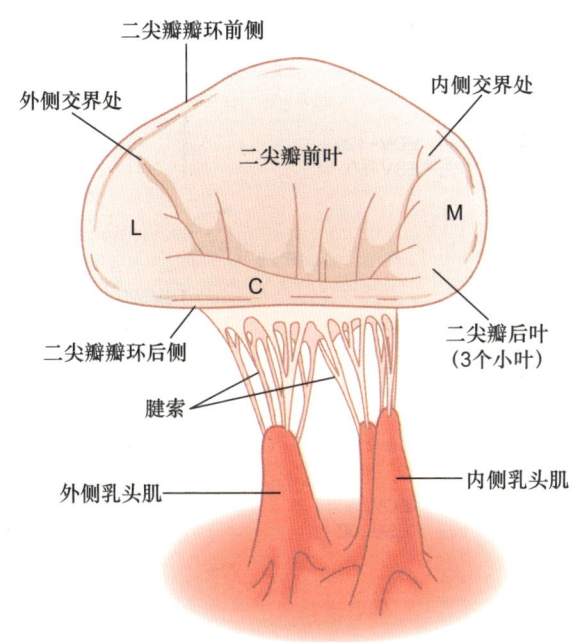

图 6.6 二尖瓣复合体 (引自 Otto C: Textbook of Clinical Echocardiography, 6th ed., Elsevier, 2018.)

主动脉瓣反流,二尖瓣反流导致左心室容量负荷过重,左心室适应额外容量负荷的能力取决于疾病的慢性程度。因此,急性重度二尖瓣反流和慢性二尖瓣反流应被视为两种不同的病程。

二尖瓣复合体包括左心房壁、二尖瓣环、二尖瓣前叶和后叶、腱索、乳头肌和乳头肌下方的左心室心肌(图 6.6)。二尖瓣复合体任何部件异常都可能导致二尖瓣反流。

急性二尖瓣反流的原因包括缺血和非缺血性。急性心肌梗死或缺血时可出现乳头肌断裂或移位。非缺血性原因包括感染性心内膜炎、腱索断裂、外伤、风湿性心脏病和左心室流出道梗阻。

鉴于二尖瓣复合体的复杂性,区分二尖瓣反流病因的原发性和继发性有益于临床实践(表 6.9)。原发性二尖瓣反流由二尖瓣叶的固有异常引起。继发性二尖瓣反流则是由于心室重塑过程中二尖瓣环的变形所致。区分原发性和继发性二尖瓣反流十分重要,因为

两者的管理和预后不同。临床亦可根据瓣叶活动参照 Carpentier 分型对二尖瓣反流进行分类(图 6.7)。

病理生理学

二尖瓣反流的病理生理学以及急性和慢性二尖瓣反流之间的差异见图 6.8。在急性重度二尖瓣反流中,前负荷快速增加的同时后负荷减小,导致总搏出量(TSV)和左心室射血分数增加,然而前向搏出量(FSV)的减少导致有效心输出量下降。同时左心房压力的急剧上升可引起肺水肿,严重可致心源性休克。

在代偿性慢性二尖瓣反流中,左心室前负荷的逐渐增加导致室壁应力增加,左心室相应地发生离心性肥厚,左心室舒张末期容积增加,增加了左心室射血分数和总搏出量,同时维持了相对正常的前向搏出量。然而随着反流的进展,左心室收缩功能障碍和左心室进行性扩张,左心室射血分数、总搏出量和前向搏出量都随之减少,导致失代偿性慢性二尖瓣反流。

在慢性二尖瓣反流中,顺应性较好的左心房能够容纳来自左心室的大量反流。然而这最终可导致左心房扩大和肺动脉高压。

自然病程与临床表现

急性重度二尖瓣反流患者通常病情恶化迅速,常可致心源性休克。除血流动力学不稳定外,患者还可能表现出与二尖瓣反流病因相关的症状。例如在急性心肌梗死伴乳头肌破裂的情况下,会出现胸痛、缺血性心电图改变和心肌酶升高。感染性心内膜炎患者会有发热、血培养阳性、血管损害表现、免疫学表现、高危因素诸如静脉注射毒品等。

慢性二尖瓣反流的自然病程和临床表现则不同于急性二尖瓣反流,因为左心室有时间通过上述机制进行重塑和代偿。患者通常无症状期较长。随时间推移,左心充盈压升高,患者会出现疲劳或活动耐量下降。最终出现充血性心力衰竭的症状和体征,如活动后呼吸困难、端坐呼吸、夜间阵发性呼吸困难、外周水肿。左心房扩大的患者会发展为心房颤动。

体格检查

急性重度二尖瓣反流患者常表现为肺水肿和心源性休克。体格检查可见面色苍白、四肢湿冷(外周血管收缩)、肺湿啰音、颈静脉怒张和外周脉搏减弱。急性重度二尖瓣反流的杂音出现在收缩早期,通常较轻、低调、呈递减型。约一半的患者听不到杂音,原因是左心室和左心房之间的压力阶差较低。因此,收缩期未闻及杂音不能排除急性重度二尖瓣反流。

慢性二尖瓣反流中,由于收缩期二尖瓣叶未完全闭合,第一心音减弱。前向搏出量减少引起第二心音 A_2 提前,同时肺动脉高压引起 P_2 延迟,最终导致第二心音分裂增宽。由于反流增加了舒张期左心室的血流量,可闻及第三心音。慢性二尖瓣反流的杂音最常见

TABLE 6.9 Mechanisms of Mitral Regurgitation

	Valvular Abnormality
Primary Mitral Regurgitation	
Degenerative	Mitral valve prolapse, thickening/calcification
Rheumatic	Leaflet thickening/restriction
Infectious endocarditis	Vegetations, tissue destruction, leaflet perforation
Systemic inflammatory conditions	Libman-Sacks lesions
Malignancy associated	Marantic endocarditis
Genetic connective tissue disorders (Marfan syndrome, Ehlers-Danlos syndrome)	Elongated, redundant leaflet tissue
Irradiation	Diffuse leaflet thickening/calcification
Drug-induced (anorexigen, ergotamine)	Diffuse leaflet thickening
Congenital	Cleft/parachute mitral valve
Secondary Mitral Regurgitation	
	Ventricular distortion of mitral apparatus (coronary artery disease, cardiomyopathy)
	Mitral annular dilation (usually with atrial fibrillation)

Modified from Otto C: Practice of Clinical Echocardiography, Fifth Edition. Philadelphia, Elsevier, 2017.

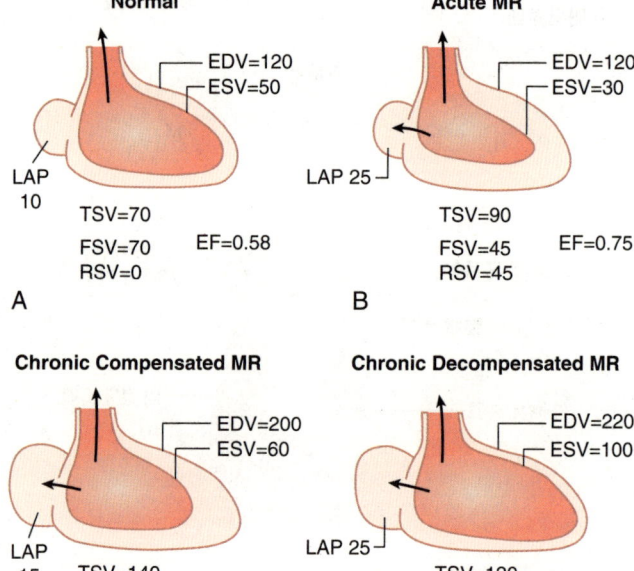

Fig. 6.8 Pathophysiology of mitral regurgitation. (From Otto C: Textbook of Clinical Echocardiography, 5th ed., Elsevier, 2013.)

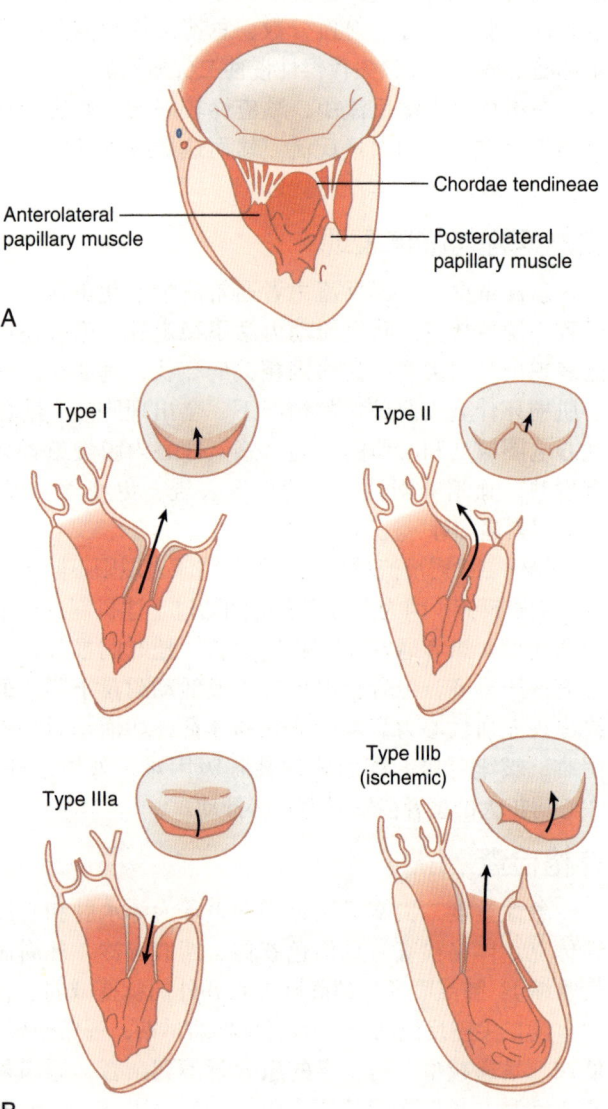

Fig. 6.7 (A) Mitral apparatus. (B) Carpentier classification of mitral regurgitation. (From Interventional Cardiology Clinics, Volume 5, Issue 1, 2016.)

most commonly a blowing, high-pitched, holosystolic murmur best heard at the apex. Depending on the direction of the MR jet, the murmur may radiate toward the axilla or the neck. In MR due to mitral valve prolapse, a midsystolic click can be heard followed by a mid or late systolic murmur.

Diagnosis

An electrocardiogram (ECG) and chest radiograph may have nonspecific findings such as left atrial enlargement or cardiomegaly, respectively. Pulmonary edema can be seen on chest radiograph in the setting of CHF. However, the diagnosis of MR is ultimately made by TTE, which can assess for the presence and severity of MR, the effect of MR on the other cardiac chambers, the presence of concomitant valve disease, and possibly the etiology of MR. If TTE is inadequate, there are other imaging modalities that are useful. CMR can be used to accurately

表 6.9 二尖瓣反流的机制

	瓣膜异常
原发性二尖瓣反流	
退行性	二尖瓣脱垂、增厚或钙化
风湿性	瓣叶增厚、受限
感染性心内膜炎	赘生物、组织破坏、瓣叶穿孔
系统性炎症性疾病	Libman-Sacks 病变
恶性肿瘤相关	消耗性心内膜炎
遗传性结缔组织病（马方综合征、Ehlers-Danlos 综合征）	瓣叶组织冗长
放射性	弥漫性瓣叶增厚、钙化
药物诱导（食欲抑制剂、麦角胺）	弥漫性瓣叶增厚
先天性	二尖瓣裂，降落伞状二尖瓣
继发性二尖瓣反流	心室扩大形变导致二尖瓣复合体异常（冠状动脉疾病，心肌病）
	二尖瓣环扩张（常伴心房颤动）

改编自 Practice of Clinical Echocardiography, Fifth Edition. Philadelphia, Elsevier, 2017.

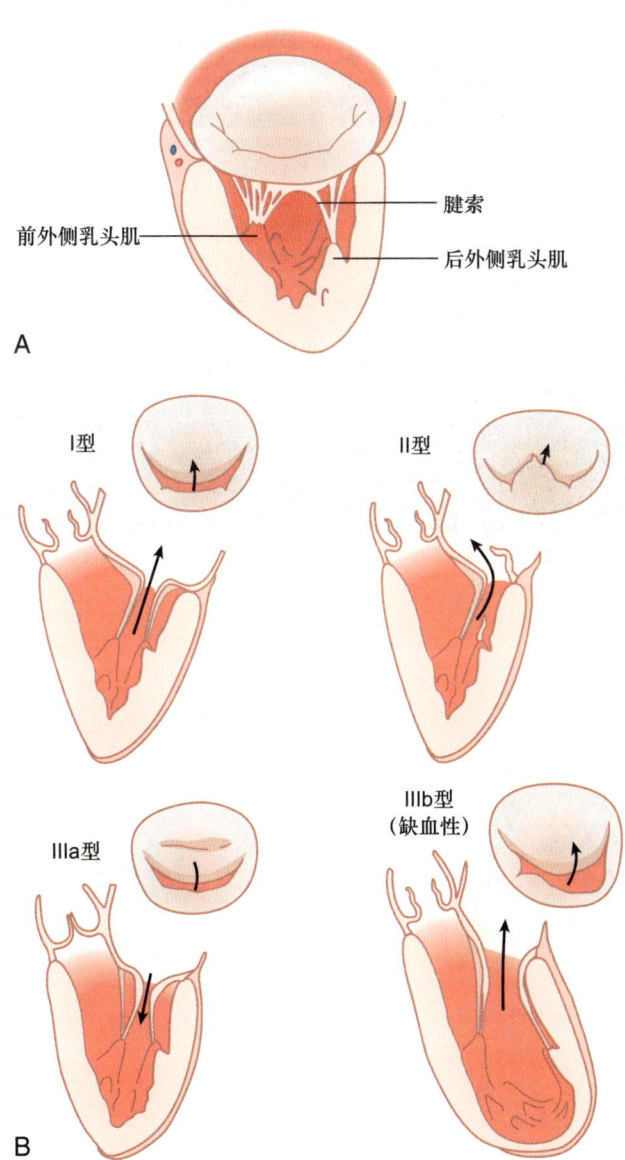

图 6.7 （A）二尖瓣复合体 （B）二尖瓣反流的 Carpentier 分型（引自 Interventional Cardiology Clinics, Volume 5, Issue 1, 2016.）

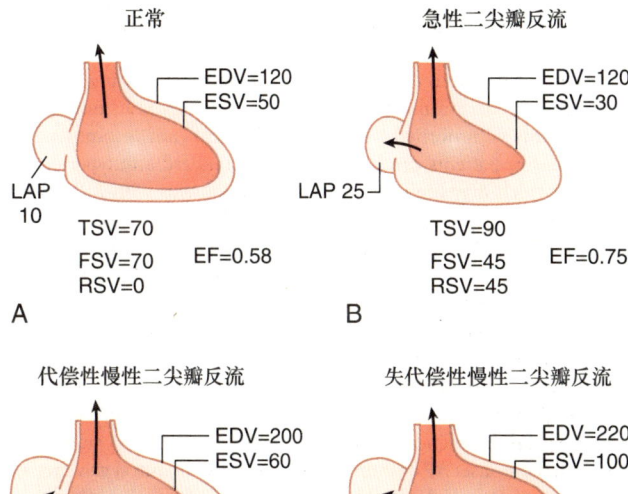

图 6.8 二尖瓣反流的病理生理学。EDV，舒张末期容积；ESV，收缩末期容积；TSV，总搏出量；FSV，前向搏出量；RSV，反流量；LAP，左心房压。（引自 Otto C: Textbook of Clinical Echocardiography, 5th ed., Elsevier, 2013.）

为高调的全收缩期吹风样杂音，最佳听诊部位是心尖区。根据二尖瓣反流束的方向，杂音可向腋下或颈部传导。二尖瓣脱垂引起的二尖瓣反流可闻及收缩中期喀喇音，继之为中晚期收缩期杂音。

诊断

心电图和胸部 X 线可有非特异性表现，如左心房扩大、左心室扩大。充血性心力衰竭时胸部 X 线可见肺水肿。二尖瓣反流的诊断依赖于 TTE，该检查可评估二尖瓣反流的严重程度、反流对心脏腔室的影响、合并的瓣膜病变并提示可能的病因。如果 TTE 评估不充分，可选择其他影像学检查。CMR 可准确量化心脏

quantify the chamber sizes, LVEF, and the severity of MR. TEE can provide superior image quality to TTE, including three-dimensional imaging, and help to clarify the severity and anatomic mechanism of MR. In the case of acute severe MR, if the level of suspicion is high and the TTE does not show significant MR, a TEE can be performed. Alternatively, a right heart catheterization can be considered. In the presence of significant MR, the pulmonary capillary wedge waveform would have prominent v waves from the regurgitant flow from the left atrium. Finally, in patients who have symptoms that are out of proportion to the severity of MR, exercise echocardiography can be considered to assess for changes in MR and pulmonary artery pressure with exercise.

Treatment

In acute severe MR, emergent or urgent surgical intervention is usually indicated. Until surgery can be performed, afterload reduction is essential. This is achieved with an intra-aortic balloon pump which not only reduces afterload but also improves cardiac output and coronary blood flow. Nitroprusside can also be given to reduce afterload and ionotropic agents can be given for hemodynamic support. In the absence of hypotension, diuretics can be given to treat pulmonary edema.

There is no clear role for medical therapy in treating the primary process of chronic MR. The use of vasodilators in normotensive patients with normal LV systolic function is not recommended. Hypertensive patients can be treated with standard antihypertensive therapy which may limit worsening of MR. Patients with LV systolic dysfunction can be given guideline-directed medical therapy (ACE inhibitors/angiotensin-receptor blockers/angiotensin receptor–neprilysin inhibitor, β-blocker, aldosterone antagonist, and diuretics).

The indication for mitral valve intervention depends on several factors. If a patient has severe symptomatic MR, mitral valve surgery is recommended. If a patient has severe asymptomatic MR and LVEF between 30% and 60%, LVESD 40 mm or greater, or if there is a progressive decrease in LVEF or increase in LVESD, then mitral valve surgery is also recommended. Also, in patients with severe asymptomatic MR with new onset AF or pulmonary hypertension, mitral valve repair can be considered if the likelihood of successful repair is greater than 95% and the expected mortality is less than 1%. In general, there is a higher chance of successful repair in primary MR involving the posterior leaflet. Mitral valve repair is preferred over mitral valve replacement, when possible.

For patients with prohibitive surgical risk, transcatheter mitral valve repair (TMVR) can be considered (Figs. 6.9 and 6.10). Patients with prohibitive surgical risk, at least moderate to severe primary MR with NYHA class III or IV symptoms despite optimal medical therapy, favorable anatomy, and reasonable life expectancy (≥2 years), should be referred to a heart valve team for evaluation for TMVR. Trials assessing the benefit of TMVR in secondary MR have yielded conflicting results. Nonetheless, TMVR has been approved for moderate to severe or severe secondary MR.

PULMONIC REGURGITATION

Definition and Etiology

Pulmonic regurgitation (PR) is a result of inadequate coaptation of the pulmonic leaflets resulting in diastolic flow from the pulmonary artery to the right ventricle. Physiologic to mild PR is common in normal adults. Primary PR is due to an abnormality of the valve leaflets. Causes of primary PR include iatrogenic, endocarditis, RHD, carcinoid syndrome, and congenital. Secondary PR occurs in the setting of normal valve leaflets and can be seen in patients with pulmonary artery dilation or severe pulmonary arterial hypertension. Severe PR is most

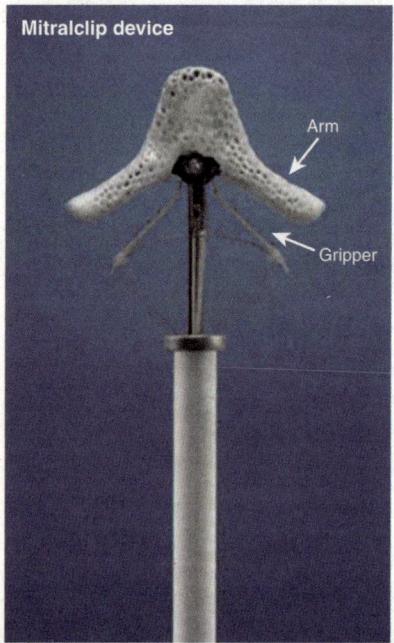

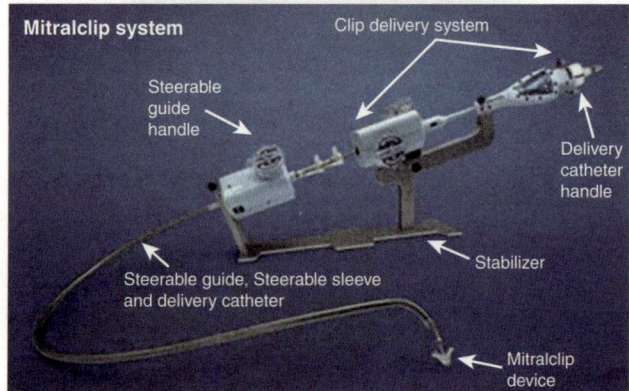

Fig. 6.9 Mitralclip delivery system. (Modified from Abbott Vascular.)

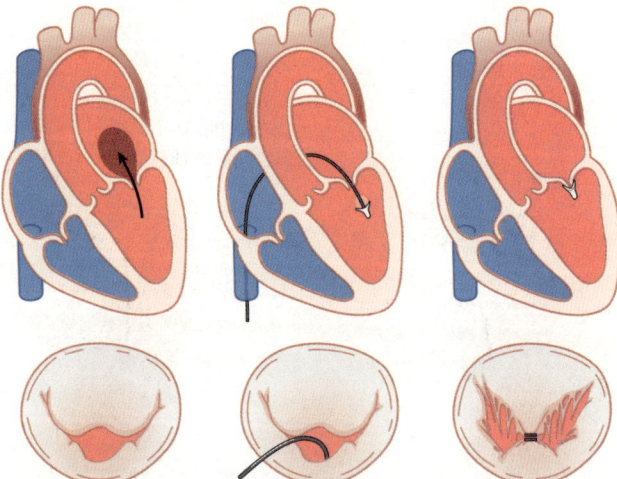

Fig. 6.10 Transcatheter mitral valve repair. (From Interventional Cardiology Clinics, Volume 5, Issue 1, 2016.)

腔室大小、左心室射血分数、二尖瓣反流的严重程度。TEE 相比 TTE 能提供更优质的图像，包括三维成像，有助于判断二尖瓣反流的严重程度和可能的解剖机制。当高度怀疑急性重度二尖瓣反流时，若 TTE 无阳性发现，可行 TEE 检查。右心导管检查也可提示二尖瓣反流。若存在显著的二尖瓣反流，肺毛细血管楔压波形会显示反流血流引起的明显 v 波。若临床症状与二尖瓣反流严重程度不成比例，可考虑行运动负荷超声心动图评估运动时二尖瓣反流和肺动脉压力的变化。

治疗

急性重度二尖瓣反流通常需要急诊手术干预。术前管理的关键是减轻后负荷，可行主动脉内球囊反搏。主动脉内球囊反搏不仅可减轻后负荷，还能改善心输出量和冠状动脉血流量。硝普钠也可用来减轻后负荷。正性肌力药物的使用能够提供血流动力学支持。若无低血压表现，可使用利尿剂缓解肺水肿。

尚无明确的药物治疗能够延缓慢性二尖瓣反流进展。不推荐在血压及左心室收缩功能正常的患者中使用血管扩张剂。高血压患者可接受标准降压药物治疗，可能有助于延缓二尖瓣反流的恶化。左心室收缩功能障碍的患者可使用指南推荐的药物治疗（血管紧张素转换酶抑制剂/血管紧张素受体阻滞剂/血管紧张素受体-脑啡肽酶抑制剂、β 受体阻滞剂、醛固酮受体拮抗剂和利尿剂）。

二尖瓣干预的指征取决于多个因素。症状性重度二尖瓣反流患者建议行二尖瓣手术。无症状性重度二尖瓣反流若左心室射血分数在 30%～60% 之间、左心室收缩末期内径 ≥ 40 mm，或左心室射血分数进行性下降、左心室收缩末期内径进行性增大，也建议行二尖瓣手术。此外，对于无症状性重度二尖瓣反流伴新发心房颤动或肺动脉高压的患者，若修复成功率 > 95% 且预期死亡率 < 1%，可考虑行二尖瓣修复。通常累及后叶的原发性二尖瓣反流的修复成功率较高。在符合指征的情况下二尖瓣修复优于二尖瓣置换。

外科手术高危的患者可考虑经导管二尖瓣修复（TMVR）（图 6.9，图 6.10）。对于外科手术高危、接受指南指导的最佳药物治疗但心功能仍维持 NYHA Ⅲ 或 Ⅳ 级症状，中至重度的原发性二尖瓣反流患者，若解剖结构合适且预期寿命合理（≥ 2 年），应将患者转诊至心脏瓣膜团队评估是否适合行 TMVR。目前评估 TMVR 在继发性二尖瓣反流中的获益的临床试验结果不一致。尽管如此，TMVR 已获批用于中至重度继发性二尖瓣反流。

肺动脉瓣反流

定义和病因

肺动脉瓣反流（PR）是由于肺动脉瓣叶无法完全闭合导致舒张期血流从肺动脉回流到右心室。生理性到轻度的肺动脉瓣反流可见于正常成年人。原发性肺动脉瓣反流由瓣叶异常引起，原因包括医源性损伤、心内膜炎、风湿性心脏病、类癌综合征和先天异常。继发性肺动脉瓣反流发生在瓣叶正常的情况下，常见于肺动脉扩张或严重肺动脉高压患者。最严重的肺动

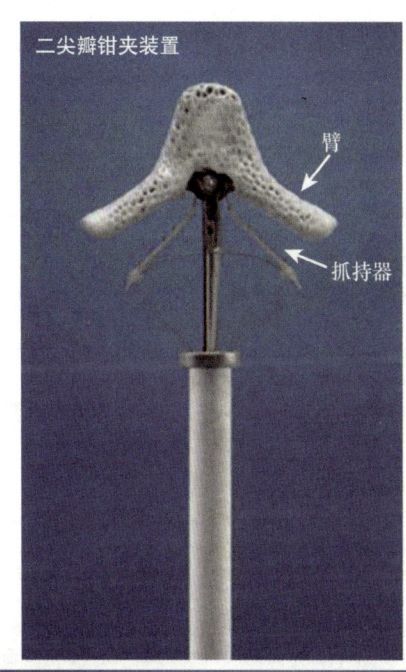

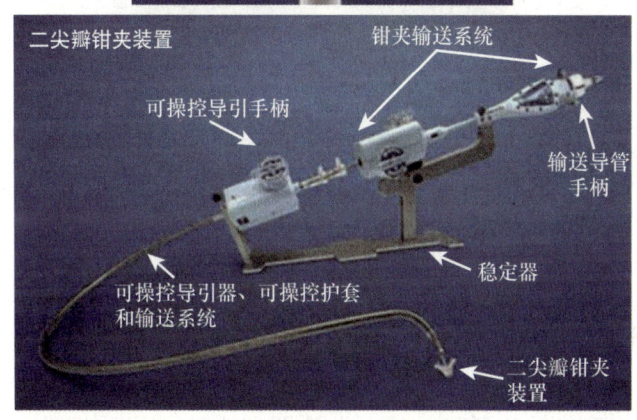

图 6.9　二尖瓣钳夹输送系统（改编自 Abbott Vascular.）

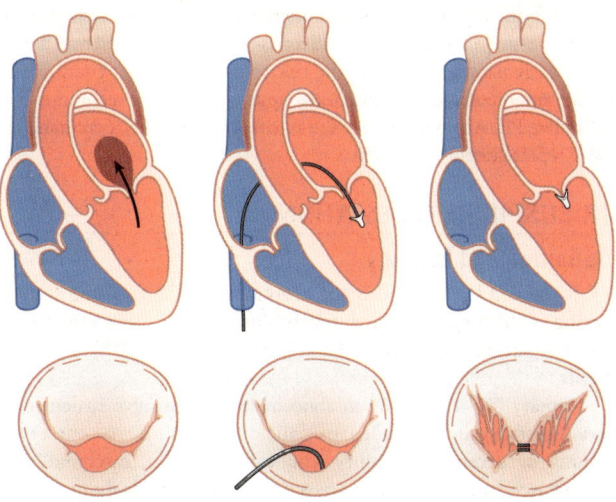

图 6.10　经导管二尖瓣修复（引自 Interventional Cardiology Clinics，Volume 5，Issue 1，2016.）

commonly seen in patients with of tetralogy of Fallot who underwent surgical valvotomy or balloon valvuloplasty.

Pathophysiology

Regurgitant diastolic flow from the main pulmonary artery to the right ventricle leads to RV volume overload. Eventually, patients may develop RV dilation, RV dysfunction, and TR.

Natural History and Clinical Presentation

Patients with PR typically have a prolonged asymptomatic phase. As RV systolic function declines, cardiac output decreases and patients can develop fatigue or decreasing exercise tolerance. With RV dilation, TR and elevated right-sided filling pressure may develop along with signs and symptoms of right-sided heart failure such as ascites, peripheral edema, and hepatosplenomegaly.

Physical Examination

The murmur of PR is an early diastolic murmur best heard over the left upper sternal border that increases in intensity with inspiration. A systolic ejection murmur may also be heard with more significant amounts of PR due to increased RV flow. With concomitant pulmonary hypertension, a high frequency, blowing, diastolic murmur (Graham-Steell murmur) may be present. On examination of the neck veins, a prominent *a* wave can be seen in pulmonary hypertension and a prominent *v* wave in TR.

Diagnosis

ECG may have nonspecific findings such as RVH or arrhythmias. A right bundle branch block with intraventricular conduction delay can be observed in patients with a history of tetralogy of Fallot repair and severe PR. RV dilation may be seen on chest radiograph.

TTE can confirm the diagnosis of PR and also evaluates the severity, etiology, and, hemodynamic effects of PR, as well as concomitant valvular disease or pulmonary hypertension. CMR can also provide a quantitative assessment of PR and RV size and function.

Treatment

Medical therapy of secondary PR should target the underlying cause. Patients with right-sided heart failure can be given diuretics. However, surgical intervention is recommended for severe symptomatic PR. Surgery can also be considered for patients with severe asymptomatic PR with RV dilation or dysfunction, symptomatic arrhythmias, or progressive TR. In general, patients with native PR undergo surgical valve replacement. Due to the risk of prosthesis regurgitation and device embolization, a percutaneous approach is rarely recommended for native PR. Alternatively, for those with prosthetic PR, percutaneous valve replacement is an option.

TRICUSPID REGURGITATION

Definition and Etiology

TR is defined by the inadequate coaptation of the tricuspid leaflets during systole resulting in regurgitant flow from the right ventricle to the right atrium. Physiologic TR is present in about 70% of healthy adults.

Primary TR, a result of an abnormality of the valve structure, is rare. Possible causes include iatrogenic direct valve injury, chest wall trauma or deceleration injury, endocarditis, RHD, carcinoid syndrome, ischemic heart disease (causing papillary muscle dysfunction), myxomatous degeneration, Marfan syndrome, or drug-induced (fenfluramine, phentermine). The most common congenital heart disease affecting the tricuspid valve is Ebstein's anomaly.

Secondary TR occurs in the setting of normal valve anatomy and is much more common. TR is most often a result of RV dilation, annular dilation, or leaflet tethering. This can occur in any condition with increased right-sided filling pressures or pulmonary hypertension such as left-sided heart failure, mitral valve disease, stenosis of the pulmonic valve or pulmonary artery, primary pulmonary disease, left-to-right shunting, and Eisenmenger syndrome.

Pathophysiology

With regurgitant systolic flow into the right atrium, there is a progressive increase in RAP and RV volume. This leads to signs and symptoms of right-sided heart failure and low cardiac output due to RV systolic dysfunction.

Natural History and Clinical Presentation

Since the right atrium is a compliant chamber, it is able to accommodate the regurgitant volume when TR is mild or moderate. Therefore, patients are usually asymptomatic. Once severe, patients may have symptoms of venous congestion and right-sided heart failure such as hepatosplenomegaly, ascites, and peripheral edema. Patients with significant pulmonary hypertension may have signs of reduced cardiac output such as fatigue and dyspnea on exertion.

Physical Examination

TR leads to elevated RAP. This is demonstrated on physical examination by distended jugular veins. A prominent *c-v* wave due to the regurgitant flow may be observed. Kussmaul sign, a paradoxical rise in jugular venous pressure with inspiration, can be seen in the setting of RV dysfunction. With right-sided heart failure, peripheral edema, ascites, anasarca, and painful hepatosplenomegaly may be present.

On cardiac exam, wide splitting of S_2 and a loud P_2 can be heard with pulmonary hypertension. S_3 or S_4 may also be present in the setting of RV dilation or hypertrophy. The murmur of TR is holosystolic and best heard at the mid left sternal border. The intensity of the murmur will increase with maneuvers that increase venous return such as inspiration, leg raise, and hepatic compression. An RV heave may be appreciated on palpation in the setting of RV dilation.

Diagnosis

TR is diagnosed by TTE. Echocardiography can help to determine the severity and etiology of TR and RV size and function. In addition, Doppler can be used to estimate the pulmonary artery systolic pressure. If the TTE is inconclusive, CMR can quantify TR, RV size, and RV function. Right heart catheterization can provide direct measurements of right-sided pressures, pulmonary pressures, and pulmonary vascular resistance.

Treatment

Medical therapy for severe TR and right-sided heart failure consists of diuretics to treat volume overload. If possible, the primary disease process should be treated such as in ischemic heart disease, left-sided heart failure, mitral valve disease, and pulmonary arterial hypertension.

Isolated tricuspid valve surgery is only recommended in patients with severe symptomatic primary TR or severe asymptomatic TR with progressive RV dysfunction. If a patient is undergoing left-sided valve surgery, tricuspid valve surgery is recommended for those with concomitant severe TR or at least mild functional TR with tricuspid annular dilation or right-sided heart failure.

脉瓣反流通常见于接受过外科瓣膜切开术或球囊瓣膜成形术的法洛四联症患者。

病理生理学

从主肺动脉回流到右心室的血液可导致右心室容量负荷过重。最终患者会出现右心室扩张、右心室功能障碍和继发的三尖瓣反流。

自然病程与临床表现

肺动脉反流患者通常有较长的无症状期。随右心室收缩功能下降，心输出量减少，患者会出现疲劳、活动耐量下降。右心室扩张可能继发三尖瓣反流和右侧充盈压升高，出现腹水、周围水肿和肝脾肿大等右心衰竭的症状和体征。

体格检查

肺动脉瓣反流的杂音表现为舒张早期杂音，最佳听诊位置为左上胸骨缘（胸骨左缘第二肋间），吸气时杂音增强。显著的肺动脉瓣反流亦可闻及收缩期喷射样杂音，这是由于右心室血流量增加所致。合并明显的肺动脉高压时，可能会出现高频的舒张期吹风样杂音（Graham-Steell 杂音）。进行颈静脉检查时，肺动脉高压患者亦可见明显的颈静脉 a 波，三尖瓣反流时可见明显的 v 波。

诊断

心电图可提示非特异性表现如右心室肥厚、心律失常。有法洛四联症修复、严重肺动脉瓣反流病史的患者可出现右束支传导阻滞伴室内传导延迟。胸部 X 线可见右心室扩张。

TTE 可用于诊断肺动脉瓣反流并评估其严重程度、病因、对血流动力学的影响以及伴随的瓣膜病变或肺动脉高压。CMR 也可以对肺动脉瓣反流及右心室结构和功能进行定量评估。

治疗

继发性肺动脉瓣反流的药物治疗应针对其潜在病因。对于右心衰竭患者可使用利尿剂。对于有症状的重度肺动脉瓣反流患者推荐进行手术干预。对于伴有右心室扩张或功能障碍、症状性心律失常、三尖瓣反流持续进展的无症状重度肺动脉瓣反流患者，也可考虑手术干预。原发性肺动脉瓣反流患者通常行外科瓣膜置换。原发性肺动脉瓣反流患者很少推荐经皮介入治疗，因为存在生物瓣反流和栓塞的风险。而对于肺动脉生物瓣反流的患者，经皮瓣膜置换是一种选择。

三尖瓣反流

定义和病因

三尖瓣反流（TR）是指由于收缩期三尖瓣未能完全闭合，导致血液从右心室反流到右心房。约 70% 的健康成年人存在生理性三尖瓣反流。

原发性三尖瓣反流较为罕见，通常由瓣膜结构异常引起。可能的原因包括医源性损伤、胸壁创伤、心内膜炎、风湿性心脏病、类癌综合征、缺血性心脏病（引起乳头肌功能障碍）、黏液变性、马方综合征或药物（如芬氟拉明、芬特明）。最常见的先天性三尖瓣病变是 Ebstein 畸形。

继发性三尖瓣反流发生于瓣膜解剖结构正常的情况下，并且比原发性三尖瓣反流更加常见。继发性三尖瓣反流最常见的原因是右心室扩张、瓣环扩张或瓣叶牵拉，可发生于任何导致右侧充盈压升高或肺动脉高压的情况，如左心衰竭、二尖瓣疾病、肺动脉瓣或肺动脉狭窄、原发性肺部疾病、左向右分流和艾森-门格综合征。

病理生理学

收缩期反流束进入右心房导致右心房压力和右心室容量增加，当出现右心室收缩功能障碍时，可引起右心衰竭和低心输出量的症状。

自然病程及临床表现

由于右心房是一个顺应性较高的心腔，能够适应轻至中度的反流，因此患者通常无症状。一旦反流进展至严重，患者可能会出现静脉淤血和右心衰竭的症状，如肝脾肿大、腹水和外周水肿。严重肺动脉高压患者会出现心输出量减少体征，如疲劳和活动后呼吸困难。

体格检查

三尖瓣反流导致右心房压力升高，体格检查中可见颈静脉怒张。反流束的存在可引起明显的 c-v 波。Kussmaul 征（吸气时颈静脉压矛盾性升高）可见于右心功能障碍的情况。右心衰竭时可出现水肿、腹水和痛性肝脾肿大。

对肺动脉高压患者进行心脏查体时，可闻及第二心音分裂增宽和 P_2 增强。右心室扩张或肥厚时可闻及第三心音或第四心音。三尖瓣反流杂音表现为全收缩期杂音，最佳听诊位置在胸骨左缘中段。吸气、抬腿和压迫肝脏等增加静脉回流的动作可增强杂音的强度。右心室扩张时可触及右心室抬举。

诊断

三尖瓣反流可由 TTE 诊断。超声心动图可评估三尖瓣反流的严重程度、病因、右心室的结构和功能。此外，超声多普勒可估算肺动脉收缩压。如 TTE 结果不明确，可行 CMR 定量评估三尖瓣反流、右心室结构和功能。右心导管则可对右心压力、肺动脉压力和肺血管阻力进行直接测量。

治疗

重度三尖瓣反流和右心衰竭的药物治疗主要包括利尿剂的使用以减轻容量负荷。应积极治疗原发病如缺血性心脏病、左心衰竭、二尖瓣疾病和肺动脉高压。

目前仅推荐在有症状的重度原发性三尖瓣反流患者，无症状但伴有右心室功能进行性恶化的重度三尖瓣反流患者中进行单纯三尖瓣手术。对于拟行左心瓣膜手术的患者，若并存重度三尖瓣反流或至少轻度功能性三尖瓣反流伴瓣环扩张或右心衰竭，建议同期行三尖瓣手术干预。

SUGGESTED READINGS

Mack M, Leon M, et al: Transcatheter aortic-valve replacement with a balloon-expandable valve in low risk patients, NEJM 380:1695–1705, 2019.

Nishimura R, Otto C, Bonow RO, et al.: 2014 AHA/ACC Guideline for the management of patients with valvular heart disease, J Am Coll Cardiol 63:e57–e185, 2014.

Nishimura R, Otto C, Bonow RO, et al.: 2017 AHA/ACC focused update of the 2014 AHA/ACC Guideline for the management of patients with valvular heart disease, J Am Coll Cardiol 70:252–289, 2017.

Nkomo V, Gardin J, et al.: Burden of valvular heart diseases: a population-based study, Lancet 368:1005–1011, 2006.

Obadia J, Messika-Zeitoun D, et al.: Percutaneous repair or medical treatment for secondary mitral regurgitation, NEJM 379:2297–2306, 2018.

推荐阅读

Mack M, Leon M, et al: Transcatheter aortic-valve replacement with a balloon-expandable valve in low risk patients, NEJM 380:1695–1705, 2019.

Nishimura R, Otto C, Bonow RO, et al.: 2014 AHA/ACC Guideline for the management of patients with valvular heart disease, J Am Coll Cardiol 63:e57–e185, 2014.

Nishimura R, Otto C, Bonow RO, et al.: 2017 AHA/ACC focused update of the 2014 AHA/ACC Guideline for the management of patients with valvular heart disease, J Am Coll Cardiol 70:252–289, 2017.

Nkomo V, Gardin J, et al.: Burden of valvular heart diseases: a population-based study, Lancet 368:1005–1011, 2006.

Obadia J, Messika-Zeitoun D, et al.: Percutaneous repair or medical treatment for secondary mitral regurgitation, NEJM 379:2297–2306, 2018.

Coronary Heart Disease

David E. Lewandowski, Michael P. Cinquegrani

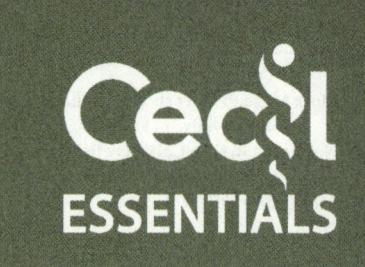

DEFINITION AND EPIDEMIOLOGY

The term *coronary heart disease* (CHD) describes a number of cardiac conditions that result from the presence of atherosclerotic lesions in the coronary arteries. The development of atherosclerotic plaque within the coronary arteries can result in obstruction to blood flow, producing ischemia, which can be acute or chronic in nature. Atherosclerosis is a disease process that starts at a young age and can be present for years in an asymptomatic form until the degree of vessel obstruction leads to ischemic symptoms. Obstructive atherosclerotic lesions can cause chronic symptoms of exercise- or stress-related angina; or, in the case of plaque rupture and acute thrombosis, sudden death, unstable angina, or myocardial infarction (MI) may ensue.

In the United States, more than 18 million people experience some form of CHD. Approximately 10 million suffer from symptoms of angina, and at least 360,000 deaths occur each year from acute MI or CHD-related sudden death. Despite progress in therapy and overall reductions in CHD-related mortality, CHD remains the number one cause of death in both men and women, accounting for 27% of deaths in women (more than deaths due to cancer). The incidence of CHD increases with age for both men and women. There are at least 1.3 million MIs per year in the United States and many more cases of unstable angina. CHD frequently results in lifestyle-limiting symptoms due to angina or impairment of left ventricular (LV) function. The cost of care related directly to CHD and indirectly to lost productivity from CHD is in the range of $156 billion per year. CHD remains a major life-threatening disease process associated with significant economic impact.

RISK FACTORS FOR ATHEROSCLEROSIS

There are a number of well-known risk factors for coronary artery disease (CAD), some of which are modifiable (Table 7.1). Although women ultimately also carry a significant atherosclerotic burden, men develop CAD at younger ages, and the prevalence of the disease also increases as men age. Another potent risk factor for the development of CAD is a family history of premature CAD. This speaks to a nonmodifiable, genetically based risk. Commonly, multiple family members develop symptomatic CAD before the age of 55 years (65 years for women). Risks are additive, making it very important to appreciate the modifiable risk factors such as hyperlipidemia, hypertension, diabetes mellitus, metabolic syndrome, cigarette smoking, obesity, sedentary lifestyle, and heavy alcohol intake. Patients are risk-stratified for the likelihood of developing clinically significant coronary artery disease through the ASCVD (atherosclerotic cardiovascular disease) score. Taking into account multiple patient-specific factors, the score estimates the patient's 10-year probability of experiencing an adverse event such as nonfatal MI, cardiovascular death, or stroke. The score can help guide blood pressure goals, the need for statin therapy, and other key preventative measures against CAD.

Metabolic syndrome deserves particular attention given that up to 25% of the adult US population may satisfy the definition of the disorder as laid out by the National Cholesterol Education Program Adult Treatment Panel. The definition of metabolic syndrome requires the presence of at least three of the following five criteria: waist circumference greater than 102 cm in men or 88 cm in women, triglyceride level 150 mg/dL or higher, high-density lipoprotein (HDL) cholesterol level lower than 40 mg/dL in men or 50 mg/dL in women, blood pressure 130/85 mm Hg or higher, and fasting serum glucose level 110 mg/dL or higher. The features of metabolic syndrome are largely modifiable risk factors for CAD.

Hyperlipidemia, in particular elevated levels of low-density lipoprotein (LDL) cholesterol, plays a pivotal role in the development and evolution of atherosclerosis. HDL-cholesterol is believed to be protective, likely due to its role in transporting cholesterol from the vessel wall to the liver for degradation. Increased levels of HDL are inversely proportional to the risk of CAD-related problems. The interplay among circulating lipids is complex. Elevated levels of triglycerides are a risk factor for CAD and are frequently associated with reduced levels of protective HDL. Hyperlipidemia is highly modifiable, and clinical trials have shown that drug treatment directed at lowering LDL-cholesterol significantly reduces the risk of CAD-related complications or death.

As with hyperlipidemia, hypertension contributes to the risk of CAD-related complications. Hypertension, probably through sheer stress, causes vessel injury that supports the development of atherosclerotic plaque. Increasing severity of hypertension is associated with greater risk of CAD. Control of hypertension is associated with a reduced risk of CAD. Recent guidelines advise more aggressive blood pressure goals for patients at high risk for coronary artery disease. Antihypertensive medications are advised for patients with a blood pressure greater than 130/80 and diabetes, chronic kidney disease, or an ASCVD 10-year risk of greater than 10%.

Diabetes mellitus is a prominent risk factor for CAD, and the disease is becoming epidemic. Diabetes mellitus typically is associated with other risk factors, such as elevated triglycerides, reduced HDL, and hypertension, which accounts for the enhanced risk of CAD-related problems in diabetic patients. It is not clear that control of hyperglycemia in diabetic patients translates into a reduced risk of CAD, but the presence of diabetes mellitus drives the need to ensure good treatment

冠心病

盛兆雪　李依珂　译　郑金刚　曾和松　审校　郑金刚　通审

定义和流行病学

冠心病（CHD）是指由冠状动脉发生动脉粥样硬化导致的一类心脏疾病。冠状动脉粥样硬化性斑块的进展可导致冠状动脉血流受阻，进而引起急性或慢性心肌缺血。动脉粥样硬化的病理过程年轻时即开始启动，可以无症状存在很多年，直至进展为引起缺血症状的阻塞性病变。阻塞性动脉粥样硬化病变可以引起运动或应激相关心绞痛等慢性症状；当出现斑块破裂和急性血栓形成时则可能导致猝死、不稳定型心绞痛或心肌梗死（MI）。

美国有超过 1800 万人罹患不同形式的冠心病。大约 1000 万人发作过心绞痛，每年至少有 36 万人死于急性心肌梗死或冠心病相关性猝死。尽管在治疗方面有所进展，冠心病相关的总体死亡率也有所降低，但不论男性还是女性，冠心病仍然是其首位死亡原因，冠心病相关的死亡占女性死亡人数的 27%（超过癌症死亡人数）。不论男性还是女性，冠心病的发病率都随年龄的增长而升高。美国每年至少发生 130 万例心肌梗死，不稳定型心绞痛的发病人数更多。冠心病患者经常由于心绞痛症状或左心室功能受损导致日常生活受限。每年因治疗冠心病产生的直接费用和由冠心病相关生产力损失引起的间接经济损失总合达 1560 亿美元左右。因此，冠心病仍然是一种威胁生命安全并且有显著经济影响的重大疾病。

动脉粥样硬化的危险因素

已知有多种危险因素与冠状动脉疾病（CAD）发病有关，其中一些危险因素是可逆的（表 7.1）。虽然女性最终也可能会发生严重的冠状动脉粥样硬化，但男性发生 CAD 的年龄更早，且患病率也会随男性年龄的增长而升高。早发 CAD 家族史是另一项由遗传因素决定的且不可逆转的强大危险因素，通常该家族会有多位成员在 55 岁之前（女性在 65 岁之前）即可表现出症状性 CAD。

考虑到危险因素具有叠加效应，识别可逆转的危险因素就显得尤为重要。这些可逆转的危险因素通常包括高脂血症、高血压、糖尿病、代谢综合征、吸烟、肥胖、缺乏运动和酗酒。ASCVD（atherosclerotic cardiovascular disease）评分可用来评估发生 CAD 的可能性并进行危险分层。该评分综合了多种患者特定危险因素，可以估算出未来 10 年发生诸如非致死性心肌梗死、心血管死亡或卒中等不良事件的概率，有助于指导血压控制、他汀类药物使用以及其他预防 CAD 的关键措施。

代谢综合征值得特别注意，因为多达 25% 的美国成人符合"国家胆固醇教育项目成人治疗小组（National Cholesterol Education Program Adult Treatment Panel）"制定的该疾病定义。代谢综合征应至少满足以下五项标准中的三项：男性腰围 > 102 cm、女性腰围 > 88 cm；甘油三酯水平 ≥ 150 mg/dl；高密度脂蛋白（HDL）胆固醇水平男性 < 40 mg/dl、女性 < 50 mg/dl；血压 ≥ 130/85 mmHg；空腹血糖水平 ≥ 110 mg/dl。这些特征大部分是可逆转的 CAD 危险因素。

高脂血症，尤其是低密度脂蛋白（LDL）胆固醇的升高，在动脉粥样硬化的发展和演变中起关键作用。而 HDL 胆固醇的作用是将胆固醇由血管壁转运至肝降解，因此被认为是 CAD 的保护因素。HDL 水平与 CAD 发病风险呈负相关。血液中脂质成分间相互作用非常复杂。甘油三酯升高也是 CAD 的危险因素，通常与保护性 HDL 降低有关。高脂血症具有高度可逆转性，临床试验证实，通过药物治疗降低 LDL 胆固醇水平可以显著降低 CAD 相关并发症或死亡风险。

与高脂血症类似，高血压也增加了 CAD 相关并发症的发生风险。高血压可能通过剪切应力造成血管损伤，从而促进动脉粥样硬化斑块的形成。高血压的严重程度与 CAD 的发病风险呈正相关，有效地控制血压能够降低 CAD 发生风险。最新指南建议对 CAD 高风险患者采用更为积极的血压控制目标值。对于血压超过 130/80 mmHg 且合并糖尿病、慢性肾脏病或 ASCVD 10 年风险超过 10% 的患者建议使用降压药物。

糖尿病是 CAD 发病的突出危险因素，其发病也呈现增长趋势。糖尿病常常伴发其他 CAD 危险因素，如甘油三酯升高、HDL 降低和高血压，因此糖尿病患者 CAD 风险更高。目前尚不明确控制糖尿病患者的高血糖能否降低 CAD 的发病风险，但是需要加强糖尿病患者的其他 CAD 可逆危险因素的治疗。尽管二甲双胍仍

TABLE 7.1 Risk Factors and Markers for Coronary Artery Disease
Nonmodifiable Risk Factors
Age
Male sex
Family history of premature coronary artery disease
Modifiable Independent Risk Factors
Hyperlipidemia
Hypertension
Diabetes mellitus
Metabolic syndrome
Cigarette smoking
Obesity
Sedentary lifestyle
Heavy alcohol intake
Markers
Elevated lipoprotein(a)
Hyperhomocysteinemia
Elevated high-sensitivity C-reactive protein (hsCRP)
Coronary arterial calcification detected by EBCT or MDCT

EBCT, Electron beam computed tomography; *MDCT,* multidetector computed tomography.

of other modifiable risk factors. Although metformin remains the first-line agent for glycemic control, the new sodium-glucose cotransporter-2 (SGLT-2) inhibitors and the glucagon-like peptide-1 (GLP-1) receptor agonists have shown improvements in ASCVD outcomes in patients with diabetes and established CAD.

Chronic kidney disease (CKD) is increasingly being recognized as a unique risk factor in the development of CAD. Although not recognized as a CAD risk equivalent to diabetes, patients with CKD, particularly end-stage renal disease (ESRD) on dialysis, have dramatically elevated risks of CAD compared to the general population. In addition, outcomes of acute coronary syndrome (ACS) in CKD patients are worse compared to the general population.

Cigarette smoking has long been known as a significant risk factor for both CAD and lung cancer. Cigarette smoking is associated with increased platelet reactivity and increased risk of thrombosis, as well as lipid abnormalities. This addictive habit is modifiable, and smoking cessation can lead to a decrease in CAD event rates by 50% in the first 2 years of cessation.

Similar to diabetes mellitus, obesity (body mass index >30 kg/m^2) is associated with risk factors such as hypertension, hyperlipidemia, and glucose intolerance. Although multiple risk factors are frequently present in obese people, obesity itself carries some independent risk for CAD. The location and type of adipose tissue appear to influence CAD risk, with abdominal obesity posing a greater risk for CAD in men and women.

Numerous clinical studies have shown the benefit of regular aerobic exercise in decreasing the risk for CAD-related problems, both in the people without known CAD and in those with the disease. Sedentary lifestyles carry an increased risk that is modifiable through exercise.

Another common attribute of life, alcohol consumption, can influence the risk of CAD in both directions. One to two ounces of alcohol per day may reduce the risk for CAD-related events, but more than 2 ounces of alcohol per day is associated with an increased risk of events. Lower levels of alcohol consumption can increase HDL levels, although it is not clear that this is the mechanism of benefit. In contrast, excessive alcohol consumption is associated with hypertension, a definite risk for CAD, although other effects of high-dose alcohol may also be at play.

Additional factors that may have some role in adding CAD risk include lipoprotein(a) and homocysteine. Lipoprotein(a) is structurally similar to plasminogen and may interfere with the activity of plasmin, thus contributing to a prothrombotic state. Hyperhomocysteinemia has been associated with increased vascular risks, including coronary, cerebral, and peripheral vascular disease. It is not clear that a causal link exists, and the use of folic acid supplementation to lower homocysteine levels has not been shown to reduce the risk of MI or stroke.

C-reactive protein (CRP) is a marker of systemic inflammation, and it indicates an increased risk for coronary plaque rupture. High-sensitivity assays for CRP (hsCRP) have measured elevated levels that correlate with risk for MI, stroke, peripheral vascular disease, and sudden cardiac death. Another marker for the presence of CAD is coronary calcification. The process of atherosclerosis is often associated with deposition of calcium within the plaque.

Coronary artery calcification can be detected by fluoroscopy during cardiac catheterization as well as by computed tomography (CT) scanning using multidetector computed tomography (MDCT). CT technology allows for a quantitative measure of coronary calcium deposits that correlates with the probability of having significant obstructive lesions. Advantages to this method include low cost and relatively low radiation exposure. This technology can be used in conjunction with ASCVD score stratification to identify patients at elevated risk for MI. Patients in whom coronary calcification is identified should be approached with aggressive risk-factor modification.

Historically, low-dose aspirin therapy (75-162 mg daily) has been recommended for patients deemed "high-risk" for CAD for the prevention of CAD-related adverse events. More recently, several trials looking at aspirin use for patients without CAD (primary prevention) failed to find a mortality benefit. Furthermore, in patients over age 70 there was a significantly increased risk of bleeding associated with aspirin use that outweighed any small reduction in ASCVD events. Given these findings, the use of aspirin for patients without established CAD is no longer routinely recommended. Aspirin use in patients with established CAD (secondary prevention) is still highly recommended.

PATHOLOGY

The process of atherosclerosis is known to begin at a young age. Autopsies of teenagers frequently demonstrate the presence of atherosclerotic changes in coronary arteries. Atherosclerosis is a process linked to the subintimal accumulation of small lipoprotein particles that are rich in LDL. Subintimal deposits of LDL are oxidized, setting off a cascade of events that culminate in not only the development of atherosclerotic plaque but also vascular inflammation. Vascular inflammation drives progression of atherosclerosis as well as the potential rupture of plaque leading to vessel occlusion. The process of lipoprotein uptake by the vessel wall is enhanced by vascular endothelial injury, which may be triggered by hypercholesterolemia, the toxic effects of cigarette smoking, sheer stresses associated with hypertension, or vascular effects of diabetes mellitus.

Oxidized LDL aggregates trigger the expression of endothelial cell surface adhesion molecules, including vascular adhesion molecule-1, intracellular adhesion molecule-1, and selectins, which results in the binding of circulating macrophages to the endothelium. In response to cytokines and chemokines released by endothelial and smooth muscle cells, macrophages migrate into the subintimal region, where they ingest oxidized LDL aggregates. These LDL-laden macrophages are also called foam cells (based on the microscopic appearance),

表7.1 CAD的危险因素和标志物
不可逆的危险因素
年龄
男性
早发CAD家族史
可逆的独立危险因素
高脂血症
高血压
糖尿病
代谢综合征
吸烟
肥胖
缺乏运动
酗酒
标志物
脂蛋白（a）升高
高同型半胱氨酸血症
高敏C反应蛋白升高
冠状动脉钙化（可由EBCT或MDCT识别）

注：EBCT，电子束计算机断层成像；MDCT，多排螺旋计算机断层成像。

然是血糖控制的一线药物，但新型药物包括钠-葡萄糖共转运蛋白-2（SGLT-2）抑制剂和胰高血糖素样肽-1（GLP-1）受体激动剂显示可以改善糖尿病合并CAD患者的ASCVD结局。

慢性肾脏病（CKD）促进CAD发生发展的独特作用已被普遍认可。尽管目前认为CKD并不具有糖尿病同等致CAD的风险，但CKD患者，尤其是接受透析治疗的终末期肾脏病（ESRD）患者的CAD发病风险显著高于普通人群。此外，CKD患者发生急性冠脉综合征（ACS）的预后也比普通人群更差。

吸烟长期以来都被认为是CAD和肺癌的重要危险因素。吸烟不仅增加血小板活性和血栓形成风险，还能引起血脂异常。吸烟是一种成瘾性习惯，因此是一种可逆转的危险因素。戒烟可以在2年内使CAD发病风险下降50%。

与糖尿病类似，肥胖（体重指数>30 kg/m²）也与高血压、高脂血症和糖耐量异常等危险因素相关。虽然肥胖人群中常常存在多种CAD危险因素，但是肥胖本身也是CAD的独立危险因素。脂肪组织的分布及类型似乎也影响CAD的发病，不论男性还是女性，腹型肥胖都具有更高的CAD风险。

大量临床研究表明，不论是否罹患CAD，规律的有氧运动能够降低CAD风险。相反，缺乏运动增加CAD风险，这一风险可以通过运动得到改善。

饮酒作为一种常见的生活方式，对CAD发病的影响具有双向性。每日饮酒1~2盎司（约30~60 ml）可以降低CAD发病风险，但是超过2盎司（约60 ml）则增加CAD发病风险。少量饮酒可以升高HDL水平，但是，目前还不清楚少量饮酒带来的获益是否与此有关；相反，过量饮酒与高血压这一明确的CAD发病危险因素密切相关，同时还可能存在其他机制参与CAD发病。

其他可能增加CAD发病风险的因素包括脂蛋白（a）和同型半胱氨酸。脂蛋白（a）的结构与纤溶酶原类似，因此可能干扰纤溶酶活性，引发血栓前状态。高同型半胱氨酸血症与CAD、脑血管疾病及周围血管疾病等血管性疾病的发生密切相关，但目前尚未明确两者存在因果关系，而且补充叶酸降低同型半胱氨酸的水平并没有降低心肌梗死或卒中的风险。

C反应蛋白（CRP）是全身炎症标志物，提示冠状动脉斑块破裂的风险增加。高敏C反应蛋白（hsCRP）的升高与心肌梗死、卒中、周围血管疾病及心源性猝死等疾病发生相关。冠状动脉钙化是CAD的另一标志，动脉粥样硬化的进程常伴随着斑块内钙盐沉积。

冠状动脉钙化可在心导管检查中通过X线透视或者使用多探测器计算机断层成像（MDCT）进行CT检查来检测。CT技术能够定量分析冠状动脉钙化，而冠状动脉钙化积分与严重阻塞性冠状动脉病变密切相关。这种方法的优点包括低廉的医疗成本和较低的辐射暴露剂量。该技术可以与ASCVD评分相结合，用以识别心肌梗死高风险患者。存在冠状动脉钙化的患者应更加积极地控制相关危险因素。

低剂量阿司匹林治疗（75~162 mg/d）通常被推荐用于CAD"高风险"患者，以预防CAD相关的不良事件。然而，最近一些临床试验发现阿司匹林未能降低非CAD患者（一级预防）的死亡率。此外，阿司匹林显著增加70岁以上患者的出血风险，这一风险超过了阿司匹林小幅降低ASCVD事件带来的获益。基于这些研究结论，阿司匹林不再常规推荐用于未确诊CAD的患者；仍高度推荐用于已确诊CAD的患者（二级预防）。

病理学

动脉粥样硬化在年轻时即可发病。尸检研究显示青少年阶段的冠状动脉就已存在动脉粥样硬化性改变。动脉粥样硬化的形成过程与低密度脂蛋白里富含的微小脂蛋白颗粒在内膜下积累有关。血管内膜下沉积的低密度脂蛋白被氧化后引起级联反应，不仅促进动脉粥样硬化斑块的进展，还能引起血管炎症。血管炎症又能加快动脉粥样硬化的发展，并促使斑块破裂，最终导致血管堵塞。由高胆固醇血症、吸烟的毒性效应、高血压相关的剪切应力、糖尿病血管损伤等引发的血管内皮损伤都能够促进血管壁对脂蛋白的摄取。

氧化型LDL聚集物可诱导血管黏附分子-1、细胞间黏附分子-1、选择素等内皮细胞黏附分子的表达，促进循环系统中巨噬细胞与内皮细胞结合。此外，内皮细胞和平滑肌细胞释放的细胞因子和趋化因子也可促使巨噬细胞迁移至内膜下，在此，巨噬细胞吞噬氧化型LDL聚集物。这些富含LDL的巨噬细胞又称泡沫细胞（基于显微镜下细胞特点命名），泡沫细胞的聚集标

and the accumulation of foam cells represents the development of atherosclerosis.

Foam cells break down, releasing pro-inflammatory substances that promote ongoing accumulation of both macrophages and T lymphocytes. This process potentiates the development of atherosclerotic plaque. Growth factors are also released that promote smooth muscle cell and fibroblast proliferation. The net result is the development of a fibrous cap, which covers a lipid-rich core.

Important contributors to the pathologic evolution of atherosclerotic plaque include impaired endothelial synthesis of nitric oxide and prostacyclin, both of which play major roles in vascular homeostasis. The loss of these vasodilators leads to abnormal regulation of vascular tone and also plays a role in evolving a local prothrombotic state. Platelets adhere to areas of vascular injury and are not only prothrombotic but also release growth factors that help drive the aforementioned proliferation of smooth muscle cells and fibroblasts. A key structural constituent of the fibrous cap is collagen, and its synthesis by fibroblasts is inhibited by cytokines elaborated by accumulating T lymphocytes. Foam cell degradation also releases matrix metalloproteinases that break down collagen, leading to weakening of the fibrous core and making it prone to rupture. T lymphocytes tend to accumulate at the border of plaque, which is the frequent site of plaque rupture.

As the fibrous cap thins through collagen degradation and eventually ruptures, blood is exposed to the thrombogenic triggers of collagen and lipid. In this setting, platelets are activated and begin to aggregate at the site of rupture. Platelets release vasoconstrictor substances thromboxane and serotonin, but more importantly, they serve as the trigger for thrombin formation, which leads to local thrombosis. Thrombin accumulation along with ongoing platelet activation can lead to rapid accumulation of thrombus in the vessel lumen. The combination of platelet-mediated thrombus accumulation and vasoconstriction can significantly limit blood flow, leading to myocardial ischemia. The degree of ischemia and its duration can culminate in MI. Complete vessel occlusion by thrombus leads to the greatest degree of myocardial ischemia and infarction, typically resulting in an ST elevation myocardial infarction (STEMI). Incomplete vessel occlusion limits blood flow enough to cause symptomatic myocardial ischemia and lesser degrees of MI, resulting in the syndromes of unstable angina or non–ST segment elevation myocardial infarction (NSTEMI).

MI is the most profound consequence of atherosclerotic plaque pathology, but significant disability can also develop when atherosclerotic plaques expand in size, leading to obstruction of blood flow and resultant myocardial ischemia. Plaque growth, driven by smooth muscle cell proliferation, initially causes the vessel to expand toward the adventitia (Glagov remodeling). Once a limit of lateral expansion is reached, the enlarging plaque encroaches on the vessel lumen. Typically, when the diameter of the lumen is decreased by at least 70%, myocardial ischemia and symptoms of angina can develop under conditions of increasing demand for blood flow. In the case of exercise, increases in heart rate and blood pressure lead to increasing myocardial oxygen demand; when flow-limiting atherosclerotic lesions are present, oxygen demand may not be met by supply and myocardial ischemia ensues. The greater the degree of vessel obstruction, the more likely it is that myocardial ischemia and angina will occur at low workloads, even to the point of angina at rest. Fig. 7.1 shows an angiogram demonstrating a coronary artery obstruction before and after angioplasty. Other forms of stress, such as emotional stress or cold exposure, can also cause symptoms of angina in patients with significant obstructive plaque through mechanisms such as hypertension (increased myocardial oxygen demand) or sympathetically mediated vasoconstriction and tachycardia.

CLINICAL PRESENTATIONS OF CORONARY ARTERY DISEASE

The clinical syndromes that patients experience due to the presence of CAD principally relate to the occurrence of myocardial ischemia. Myocardial ischemia develops when there is a mismatch of oxygen delivery and oxygen demand. Given that extraction of oxygen by the myocardium is very high, any increase in oxygen demand must be met with an increase in coronary blood flow. Oxygen demand is directly related to increases in heart rate, myocardial contractility, and wall stress (which are related to blood pressure and cardiac dimensions). There is a reflex increase in myocardial oxygen demand driven by these factors as the heart is required to deliver more systemic blood flow in the face of various stresses, the most common of which is increased exertion. Coronary blood flow also depends on the vascular tone of arterioles that are under the control of vasodilators derived from normal functioning endothelium and autonomic tone.

Coronary blood flow increases to meet an increase in myocardial oxygen demand through endothelium-mediated vasodilation. In the face of atherosclerosis, endothelial dysfunction may develop, resulting in reduced endothelium-mediated vasodilation. Endothelial dysfunction coupled with a flow-limiting stenosis sets the stage for the development of myocardial ischemia. The coronary vessel distal to a flow-limiting stenosis tends to be maximally dilated. As myocardial oxygen demand increases, the myocardium distal to a flow-limiting stenosis is no longer able to augment flow by additional dilation. An overall limitation in the ability to increase coronary blood flow due to flow-limiting stenosis and endothelial dysfunction results in supply/demand mismatch and myocardial ischemia.

The major clinical manifestation of myocardial ischemia is chest discomfort (angina pectoris), which is usually described as a pressure or sensation of midsternal tightness. It may be quite pronounced in intensity or relatively subtle. Myocardial ischemia produces not only the sensation of angina pectoris but also a number of derangements in myocyte function. As in any tissue, inadequate oxygen delivery leads to a transition to anaerobic glycolysis, increased lactate production causing cellular acidosis, and abnormal calcium homeostasis. The net consequences of these cellular abnormalities include reductions in myocardial contractility and relaxation. Decreased myocardial contractility results in systolic wall motion abnormalities in the area of ischemia, and the abnormality of relaxation causes reduced ventricular compliance. These changes cause an increase in LV filling pressures above the normal range. The cellular abnormalities related to myocardial ischemia also translate into changes in cellular electrical activity that appear as abnormalities in the electrocardiogram (ECG). Myocardial ischemia may result in either ST depression or ST elevation, depending on the duration, severity, and location of the ischemia. The cellular, mechanical, and electrical abnormalities caused by ischemia typically precede the patient's perception of angina.

Myocardial dysfunction due to ischemia may recover quickly to normal if the duration of ischemia is brief. Prolonged myocardial ischemia can lead to conditions of myocardial stunning or myocardial hibernation. In the case of stunning, the mechanical dysfunction induced by prolonged ischemia persists for hours or days until function returns to normal. In the face of chronic ischemia, myocyte viability may be maintained, but because of ischemia, mechanical dysfunction persists; in this condition, known as hibernation, restoration of blood flow can result in recovery of myocardial function.

The heart's conduction system is less prone to ischemic injury, but ischemia can lead to impaired conduction. Ischemic disruption of myocyte electrical homeostasis also sets the stage for potentially life-threatening arrhythmias.

志着动脉粥样硬化的进展。

泡沫细胞裂解所释放的促炎物质可引起巨噬细胞和T淋巴细胞持续积聚，这一过程加快了动脉粥样硬化斑块的形成；其释放的生长因子也能够促进平滑肌细胞和成纤维细胞增殖。上述过程最终形成了覆盖在脂质核心上的纤维帽结构。

由内皮细胞合成的一氧化氮和前列环素具有重要的血管稳态作用；其合成受损大大促进了动脉粥样硬化斑块的病理演变。这些血管舒张剂的缺失导致血管张力调控异常，也促进形成局部血栓前状态。血小板黏附在血管损伤处，不仅可以促进血栓形成，还通过释放生长因子促进平滑肌细胞和成纤维细胞增殖。纤维帽的关键结构成分是胶原蛋白，而聚集的T淋巴细胞释放细胞因子可以抑制成纤维细胞合成胶原蛋白。泡沫细胞裂解释放的基质金属蛋白酶可以降解胶原，削弱纤维帽的稳定性（译者注：原文fibrous core应为fibrous cap），使其更易破裂。T淋巴细胞常在斑块边缘聚集，其聚集处往往是斑块破裂的好发部位。

随着胶原蛋白降解导致纤维帽变薄并最终破裂，具有致栓作用的胶原蛋白和脂质直接暴露于血液。在这种情况下，血小板激活并聚集在斑块破裂口处；血小板释放血栓素和5-羟色胺等缩血管物质，更重要的是激活的血小板可以诱发凝血酶形成，导致局部血栓形成。凝血酶的聚集与持续血小板活化导致血栓在血管腔内快速形成。血小板介导的血栓形成和血管收缩协同作用，显著限制血流并导致心肌缺血。随着缺血程度加重和持续时间延长最终引起心肌梗死。血管被血栓完全阻塞会出现最严重的心肌缺血和梗死，这种心肌梗死通常表现为ST段抬高型心肌梗死（STEMI）。不完全性血管阻塞则会限制血流，引起症状性心肌缺血和程度较轻的心肌梗死，临床表现为不稳定型心绞痛或非ST段抬高型心肌梗死（NSTEMI）。

虽然，心肌梗死是动脉粥样硬化斑块病理学上最严重的后果，但是，当动脉粥样硬化斑块逐渐变大时，也可引起血流受阻及慢性心肌缺血，常常导致日常生活显著受限。由平滑肌细胞增殖引起的斑块生长最初导致血管向外膜方向扩张［Glagov重构现象（译者注：又称正性重构）］。达到正性重构极限后，扩大的斑块就会压缩血管腔（译者注：即负性重构）。通常当管腔直径狭窄超过70%后，在心肌需血量增大时即可诱发心肌缺血和心绞痛症状。以运动为例，运动时心率加快、血压升高导致心肌需氧增加，当存在限制血流的动脉粥样硬化病变时，会出现血氧供应不足，导致心肌缺血。随着血管阻塞程度加重，较低的工作负荷甚至在静息时即可诱发心肌缺血和心绞痛。图7.1展示了血管成形术前后冠状动脉阻塞的血管造影图。情绪紧张、寒冷刺激等其他形式的应激可能通过升高血压（增加了心肌需氧量），或通过交感神经介导的血管收缩和心动过速等机制，也能够导致有严重阻塞性斑块的患者出现心绞痛症状。

CAD的临床表现

CAD患者的临床症状主要与心肌缺血相关。当血氧供应与需求不匹配时就会出现心肌缺血。由于心肌摄氧量已经非常高，心肌需氧量的增加只能通过增加冠状动脉血流来满足。心肌需氧量与心率、心肌收缩力和心室壁张力（与血压和心脏形态相关）增加直接相关。以运动量增加为主的各种应激事件可以增加心率、心肌收缩力和心室壁张力，从而增加心输出量，这也反射性地增加了心肌氧耗。冠状动脉血流还取决于小动脉的血管张力，小动脉的血管张力受具有正常功能的内皮细胞释放的血管舒张剂和自主神经系统张力的调控。

冠状动脉通过内皮介导的血管扩张引起血流增加，以满足心肌需氧量的增加。动脉粥样硬化可能导致内皮功能障碍，使内皮介导的血管扩张作用受损。内皮功能障碍加上限制血流的狭窄，形成了心肌缺血发生的基础。限制血流的狭窄病变以远的冠状动脉血管往往已经处于最大扩张状态。随着心肌需氧量增加，狭窄以远血管所支配的心肌不再能够通过冠状动脉进一步扩张来获得更多的血供。限制血流的狭窄和内皮功能障碍共同导致冠状动脉血流增加受限，最终引起血氧供需失衡和心肌缺血。

心肌缺血的主要临床表现是胸部不适（心绞痛），通常被描述为胸骨中部的压迫或紧缩感。症状可能很明显也可以很轻微。心肌缺血不仅能够引发心绞痛症状，还会导致一系列心肌细胞功能紊乱。像其他组织一样，当供氧不足时心肌细胞会转为无氧糖酵解，造成乳酸产生增加，从而导致细胞酸中毒和钙稳态异常。上述细胞功能紊乱会导致心肌收缩和舒张功能的下降。心肌收缩力降低导致缺血区室壁运动异常，舒张功能异常导致心室顺应性降低，这些变化导致左心室充盈压增加并超过正常范围。心肌缺血导致的细胞功能异常还可以体现在细胞电活动改变，出现异常的心电图表现。心肌缺血可能导致ST段压低或ST段抬高，这取决于缺血的持续时间、严重程度和缺血部位。缺血引起的细胞、机械和电活动的异常通常早于心绞痛症状的出现。

如果缺血时间较短，缺血相关的心肌功能障碍可以快速恢复；而长期心肌缺血可导致心肌顿抑或心肌冬眠。心肌顿抑发生后，长时间缺血导致的心脏机械功能异常可持续数小时或数天，但心肌细胞功能有机会完全恢复正常。更长时间的慢性心肌缺血会使心肌机械功能持续异常，但心肌细胞仍然可以存活，称之为冬眠心肌；冬眠心肌随着血供恢复，心功能也能够恢复。

心脏传导系统不太容易受缺血损伤，但缺血还是会导致心脏传导功能障碍。此外，缺血引发的心肌细胞电活动紊乱也可能导致致命性心律失常。

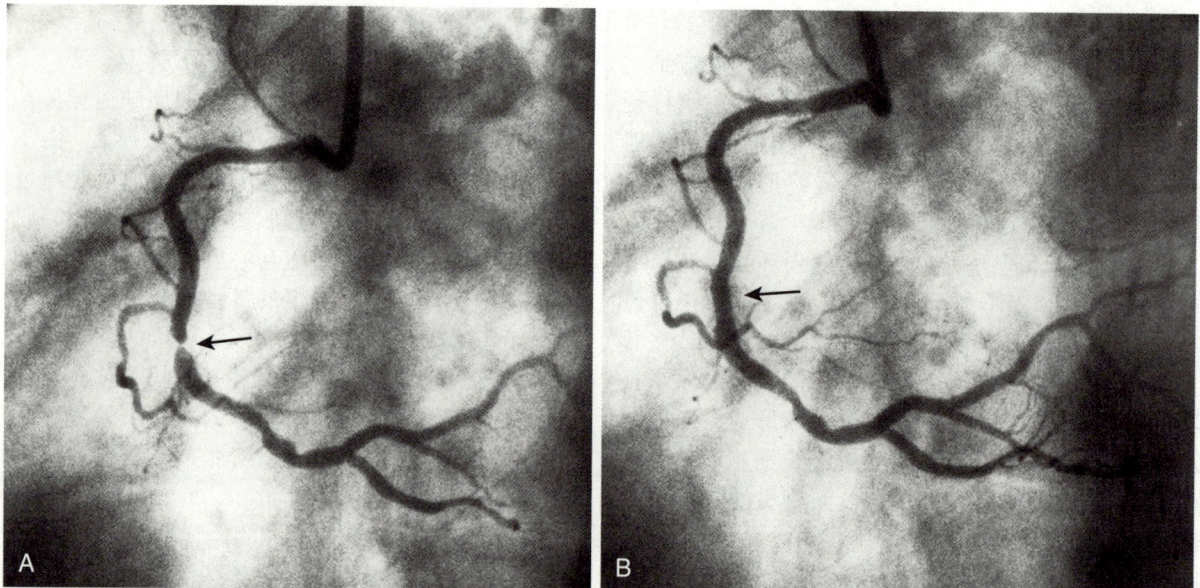

Fig. 7.1 Angiograms of the right coronary artery. (A) Discrete stenosis is observed in the middle segment of the artery *(arrow)*. (B) The same artery is shown after successful balloon angioplasty of the stenosis and placement of an intracoronary stent *(arrow)*.

Angina Pectoris and Stable Ischemic Heart Disease
Definition
Angina pectoris is a clinical manifestation of obstructive CAD, which in turn is usually the result of atherosclerotic plaque formation over a number of years. The term *angina pectoris* refers to the symptom of chest discomfort that may be described by the patient as a sensation of chest tightness or burning. Of the 18,000,000 adults in the United States with heart disease, as many as 9,400,00 have angina pectoris. It is estimated that 785,000 people experience a new ischemic episode annually, and recurrent events occur in at least 470,000 Americans each year.

Pathology
As a symptom, angina pectoris is experienced when myocardial ischemia develops. Myocardial ischemia and angina pectoris may occur in the face of obstructive atherosclerotic plaque that limits blood flow in the face of increased demand such as exertion or emotional excitement. Myocardial oxygen demand is directly related to increases in heart rate and blood pressure; these variables, in turn, can be manipulated with medical therapy to reduce the demand. Restricted oxygen supply, in the form of reduced blood flow, can also induce myocardial ischemia. Blood flow reduction is a prominent feature of acute presentations of CAD such as NSTEMI and STEMI, but atherosclerosis-mediated coronary vasoconstriction, or coronary vasospasm, is also a potential cause of flow limitation leading to myocardial ischemia. Another example of supply limitation is anemia, whereby reduced oxygen-carrying capacity coupled with obstructive lesions leads to myocardial ischemia and symptoms of angina pectoris. The term *stable* angina pectoris refers to myocardial ischemia caused by either plaque-mediated flow limitation in the face of excess demand or supply limitation due to coronary vasospasm.

Clinical Presentation
Angina pectoris may manifest in either stable or unstable patterns (Table 7.2), but the symptom expression is similar. Typically, patients complain of retrosternal discomfort that they may describe as pressure, tightness, or heaviness. The symptom can be subtle in its presentation, and inquiry as to the presence of "chest pain" may lead to a negative response in a patient experiencing angina pectoris. When taking a history aimed at discerning angina pectoris, one needs to seek answers to these more nuanced descriptions of symptoms. In addition to chest discomfort, patients may have associated discomfort in the arm, throat, back, or jaw. They also may experience dyspnea, diaphoresis, or nausea associated with angina pectoris.

There is a good deal of variability in the expression of symptoms related to myocardial ischemia, although each person tends to have a unique signature of symptoms. Some have no chest discomfort but only radiated arm, throat, or back symptoms; dyspnea; or abdominal discomfort. Myocardial ischemia can also manifest in a "silent" form, particularly in the elderly and in patients with long-standing diabetes mellitus. The duration of angina pectoris varies, probably depending on the magnitude of the underlying myocardial ischemia. Exertion-related angina pectoris, the hallmark of stable obstructive CAD, typically resolves with rest or with decreased intensity of exercise. In stable angina pectoris, the duration of events is usually in the range of 1 to 3 minutes. Prolonged symptoms in the 20- to 30-minute range are indicative of a more serious problem such as NSTEMI or STEMI.

The physical examination of patients with CAD is typically normal. However, if the patient is physically examined during an episode of myocardial ischemia, either at rest or after exertion, significant changes may be present. As with any form of discomfort, there may be a reflex increase in heart rate and blood pressure. Elevated heart rate and blood pressure may act to sustain the duration of angina by increasing myocardial oxygen demand in the face of supply-limiting coronary stenosis. Acute mitral regurgitation can develop if the distribution of myocardial ischemia includes a papillary muscle, the supporting structure of the mitral valve. The physical examination in such cases would demonstrate a new systolic murmur consistent with mitral regurgitation. If severe enough in degree, this mitral regurgitation will cause decreased LV compliance and, consequently, an acute elevation in left atrial and pulmonary vein pressure leading to pulmonary congestion. In this setting, the patient will have not only

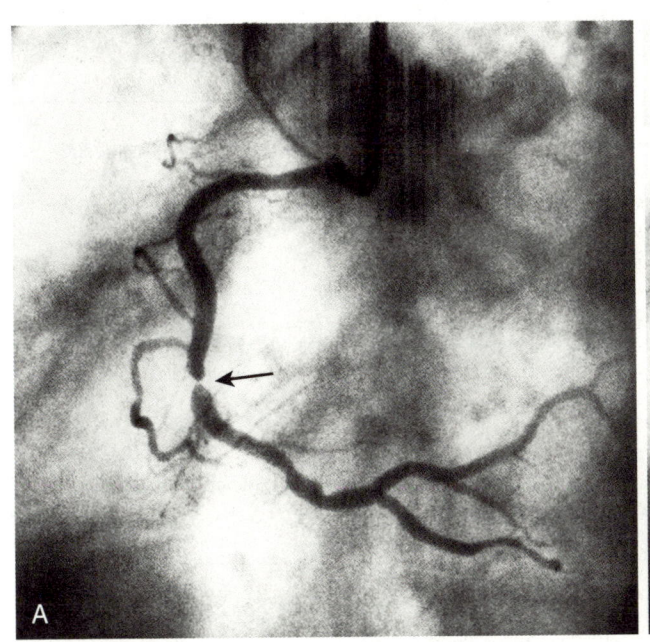 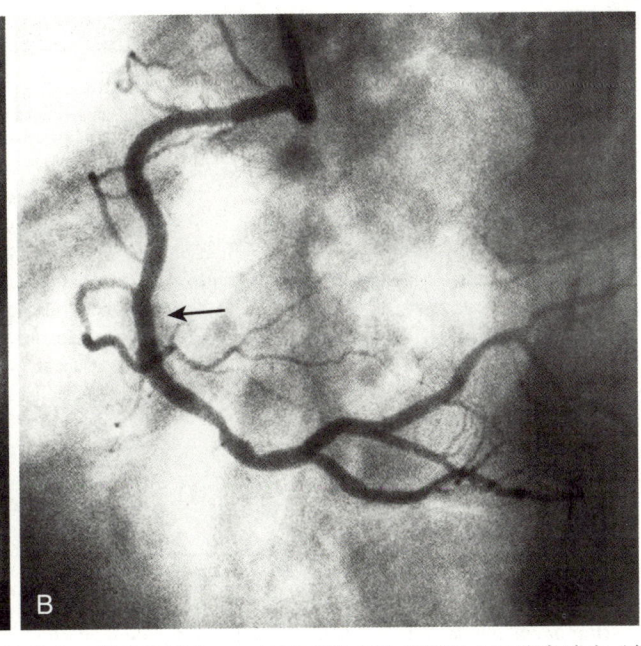

图 7.1 右冠状动脉的血管造影图。**A**.右冠状动脉中间段局限性狭窄（箭头所指）；**B**.球囊成形术及支架置入后狭窄消失（箭头所指）

心绞痛和稳定性缺血性心脏病

定义

心绞痛是阻塞性 CAD 的一种临床表现，通常是经过数年冠状动脉粥样硬化斑块形成的结果。心绞痛这一专业名词指的是胸部不适的症状，患者多描述为胸部紧缩或灼烧感。美国 1800 万例成人心脏病患者中，心绞痛患者高达 940 万例（译者注：原书为 9 400 00 例）。据估计，每年有 78.5 万例新发心脏缺血事件，至少有 47 万例复发性心脏缺血事件。

病理学

心肌缺血会引起心绞痛症状的发作。在动脉粥样硬化狭窄基础上，若出现心肌需氧量增加的情况，如运动或情绪激动时，就会出现心肌缺血和心绞痛症状。心肌需氧量与心率和血压的增加直接相关，因此可以通过药物来控制这些变量，从而减少心肌需氧量。血流量降低导致的血氧供应减少也可以引起心肌缺血。血流量减少是 NSTEMI 和 STEMI 等 CAD 急性表现的一个显著特征，而动脉粥样硬化介导的冠状动脉收缩或痉挛引起血流量减少也是导致心肌缺血的潜在原因。另外一种血氧供应减少的情况是贫血，贫血时血液携氧能力下降，如合并冠状动脉阻塞性病变，则可导致心肌缺血和心绞痛的症状。稳定型心绞痛指的是，心肌需氧量增加时，冠状动脉斑块狭窄限制血流增加或冠状动脉痉挛，导致供氧受限时出现的心肌缺血表现。

临床表现

心绞痛可分为稳定型心绞痛和不稳定型心绞痛（表 7.2），但症状表现相似。通常，患者会主诉胸骨后不适，表现为压迫感、紧缩感或沉重感。心绞痛症状也可以很不典型，当被问及是否有"胸痛"症状时，患者可能会予以否认。在采集病史时需要更详细地询问症状的细节来识别出心绞痛。除了胸部不适外，患者还可能伴有手臂、咽喉部、背部或下颌等部位的不适。患者在心绞痛发作时还可能会出现呼吸困难、出汗、恶心等症状。

心肌缺血相关症状的临床表现存在很大的变异性，但某个患者的症状可以具有独特性。有些患者没有胸部不适，只有手臂、喉部或背部放射性症状，或表现为呼吸困难或腹部不适。心肌缺血还可以表现为"无症状"形式，特别是在老年人和长期糖尿病患者。心绞痛症状持续时间的长短主要取决于心肌缺血的程度。劳力性心绞痛是稳定性阻塞性 CAD 的典型表现，休息或减少活动强度后症状即可缓解。稳定型心绞痛症状持续时间通常在 1～3 min；若症状持续 20～30 min，通常预示着更严重的问题，如可能发生了 NSTEMI 或 STEMI。

CAD 患者的体格检查往往是正常的。但如果在心肌缺血发作（无论是在休息时还是在运动后发作）期间进行体格检查，可能会出现有意义的阳性体征。任何形式的不适都可能反射性地引起心率增快和血压升高，继而在冠状动脉狭窄的情况下增加心肌需氧量，延长心绞痛的持续时间。心肌缺血若影响到乳头肌（二尖瓣的支持结构）时，可发生急性二尖瓣反流，查体可发现二尖瓣反流相关的新发收缩期杂音。重度二尖瓣反流会导致左心室顺应性下降，随后，左心房和肺静脉压急剧升高，从而导致肺淤血；在此情况下，患者不

TABLE 7.2   Angina Pectoris

Type	Pattern	ECG	Abnormality	Medical Therapy
Stable	Stable pattern, induced by physical exertion, exposure to cold, eating, emotional stress	Baseline often normal or non-specific ST-T changes	≥70% Luminal narrowing of one or more coronary arteries from atherosclerosis	Aspirin Sublingual nitroglycerin
	Lasts 5-10 min Relieved by rest or nitroglycerin	Signs of previous MI ST-segment depression during angina		Anti-ischemic medications Statin
Unstable	Increase in anginal frequency, severity, or duration	Same as stable angina, although changes during discomfort may be more pronounced	Plaque rupture with platelet and fibrin thrombus, causing worsening coronary obstruction	Aspirin and clopidogrel Anti-ischemic medications Heparin or LMWH Glycoprotein IIb/IIIa inhibitors
	Angina of new onset or now occurring at low level of activity or at rest			
	May be less responsive to sublingual nitroglycerin	Occasional ST-segment elevation during discomfort		
Prinzmetal or variant angina	Angina without provocation, typically occurring at rest	Transient ST-segment elevation during pain Often with associated AV block or ventricular arrhythmias	Coronary artery spasm	Calcium-channel blockers Nitrates

AV, Atrioventricular; *ECG*, electrocardiography; *LMWH*, low-molecular-weight heparin; *MI*, myocardial infarction.

the symptom of angina pectoris but also the symptom of dyspnea and the physical finding of rales. Ischemia-induced increases in LV filling pressure due to diminished compliance also can occur independently of ischemia-induced mitral regurgitation. Decreased LV compliance can produce the abnormal heart sound S_4; in the case of severe diffuse myocardial ischemia causing LV systolic dysfunction, an S_3 may also be perceived. Resolution of myocardial ischemia results in not only a cessation of angina pectoris but also a return to the patient's baseline physical examination status.

Diagnosis and Differential Diagnosis

Three basic forms of testing have played major roles in assessing patients with chest discomfort possibly due to CAD. All of these tests capitalize on the effect of myocardial ischemia on various aspects of cardiac physiology. First, myocardial ischemia induced by exercise or by spontaneous coronary occlusion results in subendocardial ischemia, which appears on an ECG as diffuse ST depression (Fig. 7.2). Once ischemia resolves, the ECG returns to normal. Second, myocardial ischemia typically affects a segment of heart muscle, and that territory develops a wall motion abnormality that can be detected by either echocardiography or nuclear scintigraphy. Third, the basis for myocardial ischemia is a decrease in coronary and myocardial blood flow. This abnormality can be detected by assessing the distribution of radioactive tracers such as thallium 201 or technetium sestamibi using specialized detectors for imaging myocardial perfusion. All stress test techniques used in diagnosing patients with possible CAD rely on these means of detecting the impact of myocardial ischemia on cardiac electrical activity, mechanical function, or myocardial perfusion.

Stress testing in its various forms frequently plays a pivotal role in the assessment of patients with possible CAD. In using stress testing, it is important to understand the significance of pretest probability of CAD in interpreting the results of any stress test method. For a patient with a high pretest probability of CAD, a positive test is highly predictive of underlying CAD, and a negative test carries the weight of being falsely negative. The opposite is true in a patient with a low pretest probability of CAD: A negative test is associated with a high negative predicative value for the presence of CAD, but a positive test is likely to be falsely positive.

Stress testing is useful not only as a diagnostic tool but also in the long-term management of established CAD. Exercise stress testing, through its ability to quantify exercise capacity, can monitor the effectiveness of medical therapy directed at reducing myocardial ischemia. The findings of an exercise stress test also have predictive value in that patients with ischemia induced at low workloads are more likely to have extensive multivessel disease, whereas those who achieve high workloads are less prone to ischemic complications of CAD. A higher risk for poor outcomes related to CAD is implied by (1) ECG changes of ST depression early during exercise and persisting late into recovery; (2) exercise-induced reduction in systolic blood pressure; and (3) poor exercise tolerance (<6 minutes on the Bruce stress test protocol).

Patients with a normal resting ECG can reliably be assessed by standard exercise stress testing with ECG monitoring (Fig. 7.3). The specificity of ST changes with exertion is significantly reduced in the face of baseline ECG abnormalities related to LV hypertrophy, left bundle branch block (LBBB), preexcitation, or use of digoxin. Various imaging techniques (echocardiography, nuclear scintigraphy, magnetic resonance imaging) have been developed to overcome the impact of baseline ECG abnormalities on the validity of stress testing. Because women also have lower specificity for ECG changes during exercise testing than men, an imaging technique is frequently used in the assessment of women. Overall, the addition of an imaging technique to stress testing significantly improves the sensitivity, specificity, and predictive value of the stress test but also greatly increases its cost.

Radionuclide stress testing is a common form of imaging-based stress test. Near peak exertion, a radionuclide tracer (thallium-201, technetium-99, or tetrofosmin) is administered intravenously. The tracer is distributed to the myocardium in a quantity directly proportional to blood flow. This type of image testing relies on a disparity of tracer uptake to detect an area of ischemia. Thallium-201 redistributes over 4 hours to viable myocardium, allowing for comparison of stress-induced ischemia to a baseline state. The other tracers do not share this redistribution feature, and tests using technetium-99 or tetrofosmin require both "rest" and "stress" injections of tracer to differentiate ischemic myocardium. Patients with normal perfusion studies have a low risk of coronary events (<1%/year). The presence of a positive perfusion study confers a risk of about 7%/year for coronary events, with the risk increasing relative to the extent of perfusion abnormality.

An alternative means of imaging for exercise testing is the use of echocardiography to detect ischemia-induced wall motion abnormalities. This form of testing is increasingly favored because there is no

表 7.2　心绞痛

类型	症状	心电图	异常	药物治疗
稳定型	稳定发作模式，由体力活动、寒冷、进食、情绪压力等诱发	基线通常正常或非特异性 ST-T 改变	一支或多支冠状动脉粥样硬化狭窄 ≥ 70%	阿司匹林 舌下含服硝酸甘油
	持续 5～10 min	既往心肌梗死的表现（译者注：可以有）		抗缺血药物
	休息或舌下含服硝酸甘油缓解	发作时 ST 段压低		他汀类药物
不稳定型	心绞痛频率、严重程度或持续时间增加；轻微运动或休息时即可发生心绞痛；可能对舌下含服硝酸甘油反应较差	和稳定型心绞痛一样，但发作时的心电图变化可能更为明显；发作期偶有 ST 段抬高	斑块破裂伴血小板性和纤维蛋白性血栓形成，导致冠状动脉阻塞恶化	阿司匹林和氯吡格雷 抗缺血药物 肝素或低分子量肝素 糖蛋白 Ⅱb/Ⅲa 抑制剂
变异型心绞痛	无诱发因素发生的心绞痛，通常发生于休息时	发作时短暂的 ST 段抬高 通常伴有房室传导阻滞或室性心律失常	冠状动脉痉挛	钙通道阻滞剂 硝酸盐

但会出现心绞痛的症状，而且会出现呼吸困难和肺部啰音。由于顺应性降低导致的左心室充盈压增加也可以独立于缺血引起二尖瓣关闭不全。另外，左心室顺应性降低还可以产生异常的第四心音；若出现严重广泛的心肌缺血引起左心室收缩功能障碍时，可产生第三心音。心肌缺血的缓解不仅可以终止心绞痛症状，也能使上述阳性体征恢复正常。

诊断和鉴别诊断

在评估患者是否因 CAD 引起的胸部不适时，三种基本检查较为重要。所有这些检查都利用了心肌缺血对心脏生理各方面的影响。首先，运动或自发性冠状动脉闭塞引起的心肌缺血会导致心内膜下缺血，在心电图上表现为弥漫性 ST 段压低（图 7.2）。一旦缺血缓解，心电图就会恢复正常。其次，心肌缺血通常会影响心肌的某一节段，该区域会出现室壁运动异常，可通过超声心动图或核素显像检测到。最后，心肌缺血的基础是冠状动脉和心肌血流量减少。这种异常可通过使用心肌灌注成像专用探测器，通过评估放射性示踪剂（如铊 201 或锝甲氧异腈）的分布来检测。所有用于诊断患者是否患有 CAD 的负荷试验，都是通过检测上述心肌缺血对心电活动、机械功能或心肌灌注的影响来发现的。

在评估患者是否患有 CAD 时，各种形式的负荷试验经常起着关键作用。在使用心脏负荷试验前，需了解患者罹患 CAD 的概率，这对正确解释检查结果较为重要。对于患 CAD 概率较高的患者来说，检测结果呈阳性就很有可能是 CAD，而检测结果呈阴性则有可能是假阴性。而对于 CAD 可能性较低的患者来说，情况则恰恰相反：阴性结果对是否存在 CAD 具有很高的阴性预测价值，但阳性检测结果有可能是假阳性。

负荷试验不仅可作为诊断工具，还可用于已确诊的 CAD 的长期管理。运动负荷试验通过量化运动能力，可以监测改善心肌缺血药物的治疗效果。运动负荷试验的结果还具有预测价值，因为在低负荷下即可诱发心肌缺血的患者更可能存在多支血管疾病，而高负荷诱导缺血的患者则不易出现 CAD 的缺血并发症。出现以下情况时，提示 CAD 患者预后较差：①运动早期心电图出现 ST 段压低变化，并持续到恢复期；②运动导致收缩压降低；以及③运动耐受性较差（Bruce 负荷试验的持续时间小于 6 min）。

静息心电图正常的患者可以通过心电图监测下的标准运动负荷试验进行可靠的评估（图 7.3）。当有左心室肥厚、左束支传导阻滞（LBBB）、预激或使用地高辛等情况时，患者基础心电图存在异常，此时，运动时的 ST 改变对缺血诊断的特异性会明显降低。为了克服基线心电图异常对负荷试验有效性的影响，人们开发了各种成像技术（超声心动图、核素闪烁成像、磁共振成像）。由于女性对运动负荷试验期间心电图变化的特异性也低于男性，因此在对女性进行评估时经常使用成像技术。总之，在负荷试验中引入成像技术，可显著提高负荷试验的敏感性、特异性和预测价值，但同时也极大地增加了成本。

放射性核素负荷试验是一种常见的基于成像的负荷试验。在接近峰值负荷时，静脉注射放射性核素示踪剂（铊 -201、锝 -99 或替曲膦）。示踪剂分布到心肌的量与血流量成正比。这类图像检测技术依靠示踪剂摄取的差异来检测缺血区域。铊 -201 会在 4 h 内重新分布到存活的心肌中，从而可以将负荷诱导的心肌缺血与基线状态进行比较，其他示踪剂不具有这种再分布特征。使用锝 -99 或替曲膦进行检测时，需要分别在"静息"和"负荷"时注射示踪剂才能区分缺血心肌。灌注检查正常的患者发生冠脉事件的风险较低（＜ 1%/年）。灌注检查阳性的患者发生冠脉事件的风险约为 7%/年，风险随灌注异常程度的增加而增加。

运动试验的另一种成像方法是使用超声心动图检测缺血引起的室壁运动异常。因为其没有辐射，这种检测方式越来越受到青睐，而放射性核素示踪剂会使

Boston University Hospital　　　　　　　　　　　　　　　　　　　　　　　　　　　　1 MAR 1999

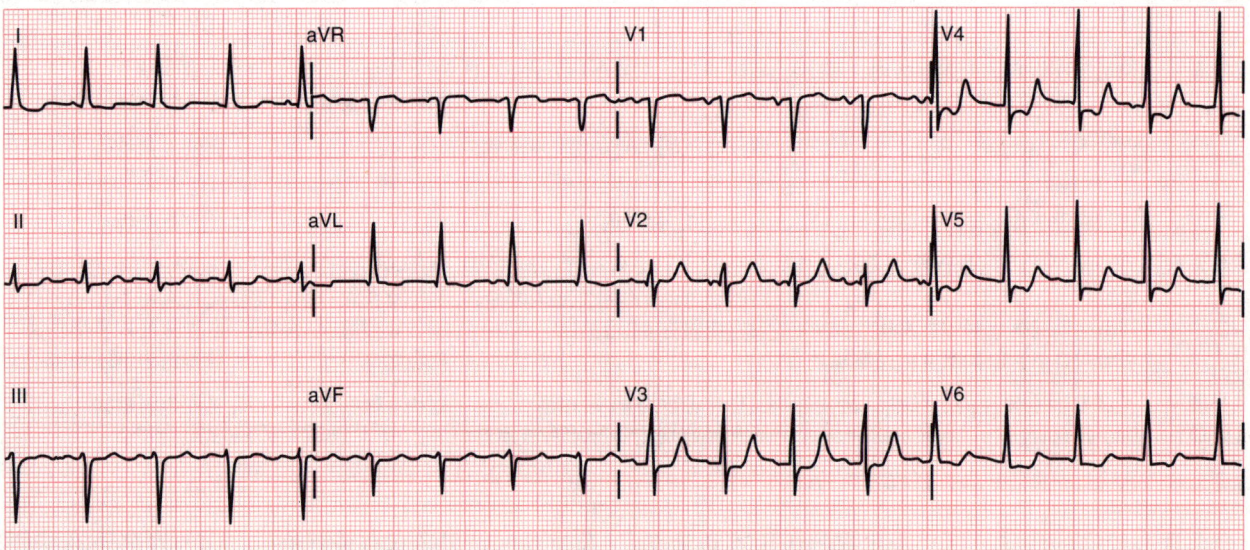

A

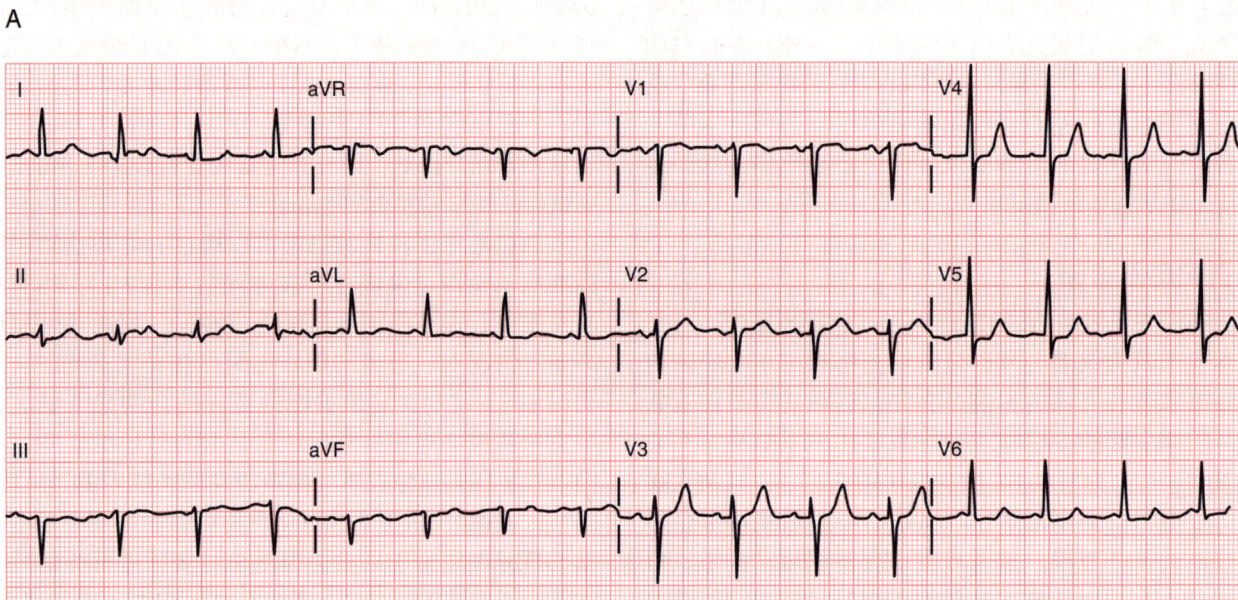

B

Fig. 7.2 Electrocardiogram obtained during angina (A) and after the administration of sublingual nitroglycerin and subsequent resolution of angina (B). During angina, transient ST-segment depression and T wave abnormalities are present.

radiation associated with its use, whereas radionuclide tracers expose the patient to a significant dose of radiation. Stress echocardiography carries with it the same enhancement in sensitivity, specificity, and predictive value as radionuclide imaging. An additional benefit of echocardiography imaging is more discrete anatomic data on valve function. If it is coupled with Doppler flow imaging, information regarding exercise-induced mitral regurgitation can be obtained.

Another means of assessing for exercise-induced wall motion abnormalities is the use of radionuclide ventriculography or multigated acquisition scanning (MUGA). This technique is usually included as part of the interpretation of an exercise stress radionuclide study. This imaging technique does not provide the anatomic detail associated with echocardiography, and it has the negative feature of significant radiation exposure.

An additional imaging technique for stress testing is the use of magnetic resonance imaging. Radiation is not a concern, and cardiac structural imaging can match echocardiography (or exceed it in patients with poor images on echocardiography). The technique is not as easy to execute as echocardiography and is not as frequently utilized.

Not all patients who require noninvasive testing for CAD are able to exercise to a degree sufficient to induce ischemia, and for some patients exercise testing is not an option at all. For these patients,

波士顿大学医院　　　　　　　　　　　　　　　　　　　　　　　　　　　　　　　　1999年3月1日

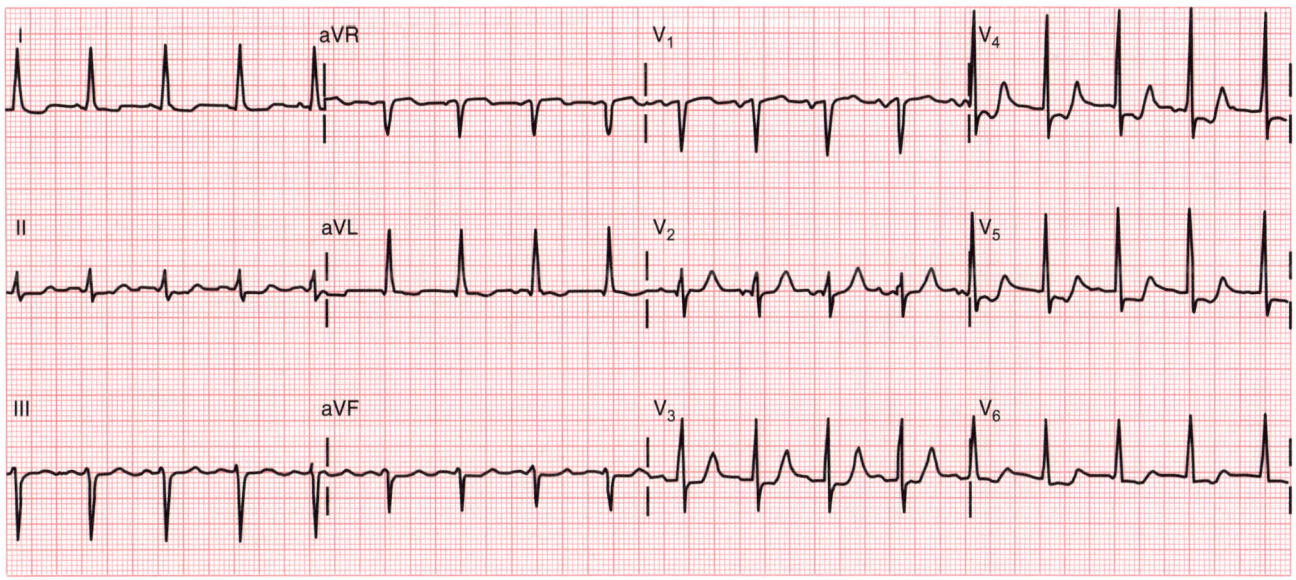

A

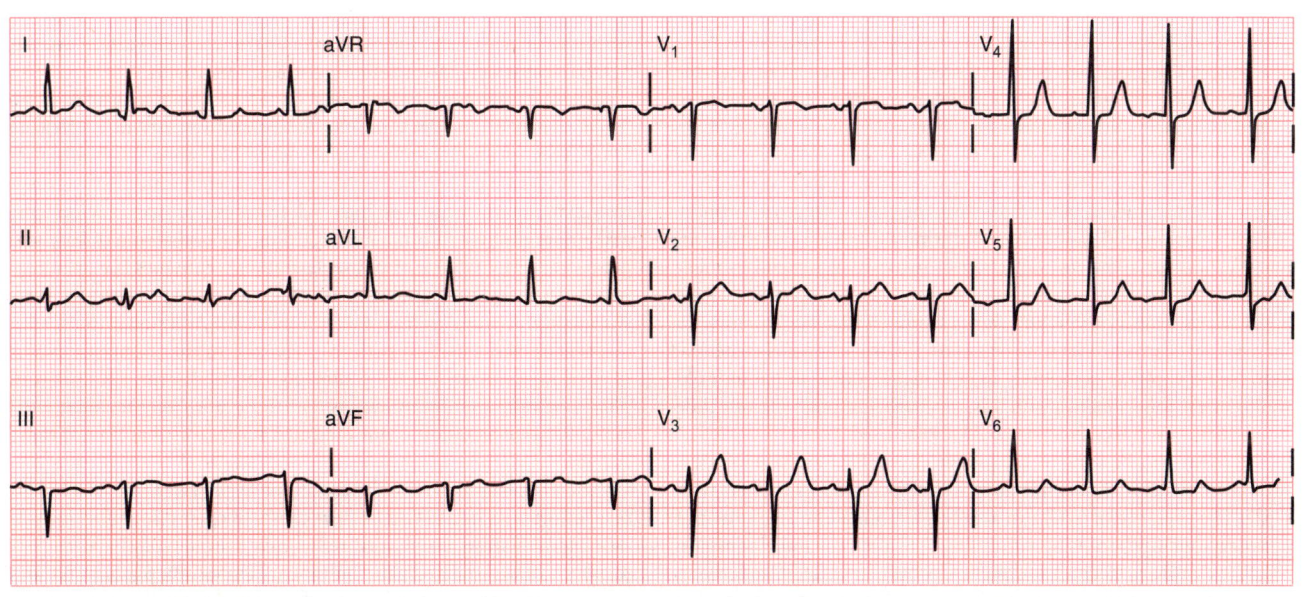

B

图 7.2　在心绞痛期间（A）和舌下含服硝酸甘油心绞痛缓解后（B）的心电图。在心绞痛期间出现短暂的 ST 段压低和 T 波异常

患者暴露在大量辐射中。负荷超声心动图具有与放射性核素成像相同的敏感性、特异性和预测价值。超声心动图成像的另一个好处是可以获得瓣膜功能的解剖数据。如果结合多普勒血流成像，就能获得运动诱发二尖瓣反流的相关信息。

另一种评估运动诱发室壁运动异常的方法是使用放射性核素心室造影或多门控采集扫描（MUGA）。这项技术通常作为心脏运动负荷核医学分析的一部分。这种成像技术无法提供像超声心动图那样的解剖细节，而且存在大量辐射。

另外一种负荷试验是使用磁共振成像技术。磁共振成像不存在辐射问题，而且在心脏结构成像方面可以与超声心动图相媲美（对于超声心动图成像不佳的患者，磁共振成像还能优于超声心动图）。但是该技术不像超声心动图那样容易操作，在临床中也不常用。

并非所有需要进行 CAD 无创检测的患者都能进行到足以诱发缺血的运动量，甚至，有些患者根本无法进行运动检测。对于这些患者，药物负荷试验已成

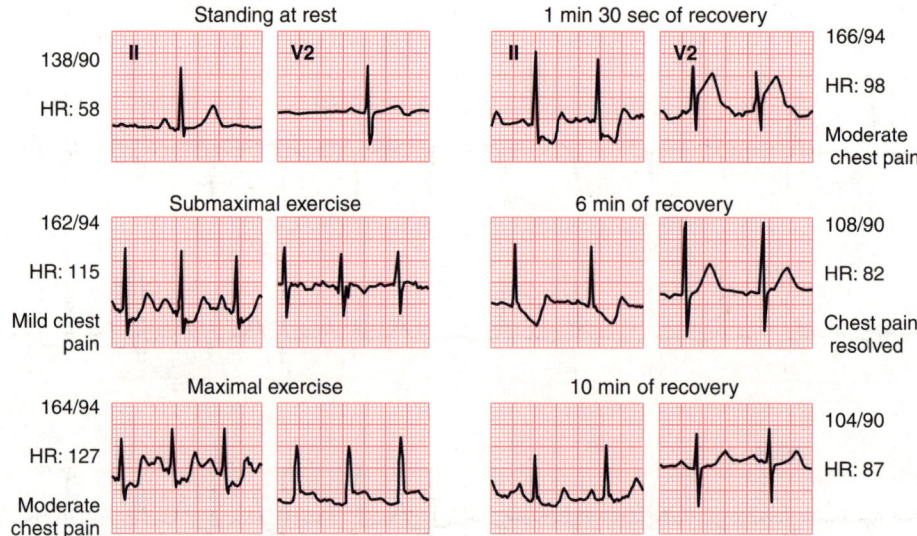

Fig. 7.3 Treadmill exercise test demonstrates a markedly ischemic electrocardiogram (ECG) response. The resting ECG is normal. The test was stopped when the patient developed angina at a relatively low workload, accompanied by ST-segment depression in lead II and ST-segment elevation in lead V_2. These changes worsened early in recovery and resolved after administration of sublingual nitroglycerin. Only leads II and V_2 are shown; however, ischemic changes were seen in 10 of the 12 recorded leads. Severe atherosclerotic disease of all three coronary arteries was documented at subsequent cardiac catheterization.

pharmacologic stress testing has evolved as a viable alternative to exercise testing. The prognostic benefit of exercise workload is not available from this form of testing, but information regarding the presence of ischemia-inducing atherosclerosis is obtainable. One common form of pharmacologic testing relies on inducing coronary vasodilation (as with dipyridamole, adenosine, or regadenoson), which produces a disparity of myocardial blood flow based on the presence of coronary stenosis. Radionuclide administered during the infusion of the coronary vasodilator allows for detection of myocardial ischemia similar to that observed with exercise testing. An alternative pharmacologic approach uses the inotropic and chronotropic effects of dobutamine to increase myocardial oxygen demand and induce segmental ischemia. Echocardiography is commonly used to detect dobutamine-induced wall motion abnormalities with this approach, although radionuclide or magnetic resonance imaging could also be used.

All of the stress testing techniques discussed here are able to assess for the presence of inducible myocardial ischemia associated with CAD. The presence of CAD can also be determined by assessment of coronary calcification using either EBCT or the now more common MDCT. Coronary calcification is present only because of underlying CAD. Although detecting its presence does not directly indicate the presence of obstructive CAD as would an abnormal imaging stress test, studies have shown a direct correlation between the amount of coronary calcification and the probability that a 70% stenosis is present.

Multidetector computed tomography (MDCT) scanners can reliably perform coronary angiography with the use of intravenous contrast agents and specifically timed imaging protocols. This can provide insight into coronary anatomy that stress testing cannot. When this technique is coupled with newer techniques such as CT fractional flow reserve (FFR), it can provide a functional assessment as well. The PLATFORM trial demonstrated that in patients with stable chest pain, CTA + FFR guiding the need for invasive coronary angiography (ICA) resulted in similar outcomes but with lower costs compared to standard of care. A negative study carries a high negative predictive value for the occurrence of coronary events and thus is useful in patients with low-intermediate pretest probability for coronary artery disease. MDCT is also valuable in defining coronary anomalies.

Invasive coronary angiography (ICA) has been considered the "gold standard" for detecting the extent and severity of underlying CAD. This approach carries a small risk of MI, stroke, or death, so it must not be taken lightly. In the case of patients with positive stress tests, particularly those with high-risk features, coronary angiography adds more discrete information regarding the underlying disease and guides the potential use of revascularization techniques (i.e., percutaneous coronary intervention or coronary artery bypass surgery) versus medical therapy to treat CAD (Table 7.3). Additional tools, such as pressure wires used to perform FFR, add to the diagnostic power of invasive catheterization by allowing one to discriminate between physiologically significant lesions and those not likely to cause ischemia. Revascularization is not indicated for lesions that do not cause ischemia.

The physician must also be cognizant of the fact that not all chest discomfort is related to CAD. Other causes of chest discomfort include esophageal disease (esophageal reflux may mimic typical angina pectoris), chest wall–related pain, pulmonary embolism, pneumonia, and trauma. The clinical presentation of the patient usually points in one direction or another, but patients with chest discomfort commonly undergo an evaluation for CAD, typically with the use of stress testing. Once CAD is reliably ruled out, the physician needs to consider alternative causes of the symptom. In the acute setting of severe chest discomfort, particularly in a hemodynamically unstable patient, the differential diagnosis includes acute MI, pulmonary embolism, and aortic dissection. Prompt and accurate diagnostic evaluation, commonly with the use of invasive or CT angiography, can be lifesaving in this situation.

Treatment

Medical management of stable angina. The treatment of CAD and angina pectoris is multifaceted. The presence of CAD with or without angina requires the physician to recommend risk factor modification, frequently associated with lifestyle changes. For

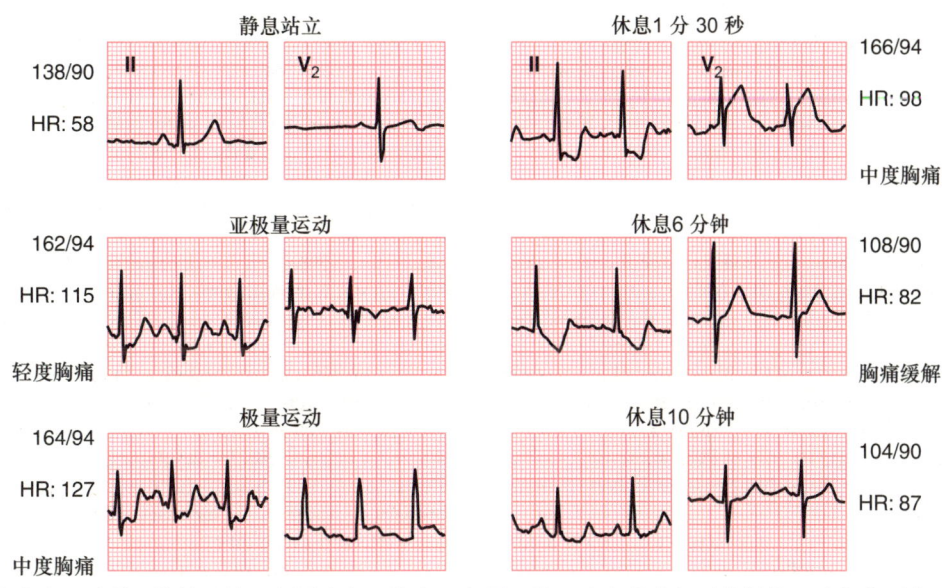

图 7.3 平板运动试验显示明显的缺血性心电图改变。静息心电图正常。当患者在相对较低的运动负荷下发生心绞痛,并伴有 II 导联 ST 段压低和 V_2 导联 ST 段抬高时,试验停止。这些变化在休息早期恶化,并在舌下含服硝酸甘油后缓解。此处只展示 II 和 V_2 导联,然而,在 12 个记录的导联中有 10 个导联观察到缺血性变化。在随后的冠脉造影中显示所有三支冠状动脉均有严重的动脉粥样硬化

为运动试验的可行替代方法。目前还不知道运动负荷试验结果是否有预后预测价值,但可以获知是否存在可诱发缺血的动脉粥样硬化病变。一种常见的药物负荷试验方式是通过药物诱导冠状动脉血管扩张(如使用双嘧达莫、腺苷或瑞加德松等药物),在冠状动脉狭窄的情况下,冠脉扩张会造成心肌血流的差异性分布。在输注冠状动脉血管扩张剂时注入放射性核素,可以检测到与运动试验类似的心肌缺血。另一种药理学方法是利用多巴酚丁胺的正性变力和变时作用来增加心肌需氧量并诱发节段性心肌缺血。使用这种方法时,通常使用超声心动图来检测多巴酚丁胺诱导的室壁运动异常,放射性核素或磁共振成像亦可使用。

本章讨论的所有负荷试验技术都能评估是否存在与 CAD 相关的、可诱发的心肌缺血。通过使用电子束计算机断层成像(EBCT)或现在更常见的多排螺旋计算机断层成像(MDCT)评估冠状动脉钙化,可以判定是否存在 CAD。冠状动脉钙化的存在和潜在的 CAD 风险有关。虽然检测到钙化并不直接提示阻塞性 CAD 的存在(而负荷影像试验异常可以),但研究表明,一定程度的冠状动脉钙化与冠状动脉 70% 狭窄的可能性直接相关。

通过使用静脉注射造影剂和特定时间的成像方案,MDCT 可以可靠地进行冠状动脉成像(CTA)。这样就能深入了解冠状动脉的解剖结构,而负荷试验则无法做到这一点。当这项技术与 CT 血流储备分数(FFR)等新技术相结合时,还能提供功能学评估。PLATFORM 试验表明,在稳定性胸痛患者中,CTA + FFR 策略指导下的有指征的有创性冠状动脉造影(ICA)与标准诊疗策略相比,临床结局类似,但明显减少了需要行 ICA 的患者数量从而降低了医疗费用。阴性结果对冠状动脉事件的发生具有较高的阴性预测值,因此对中低预检概率的 CAD 患者非常有用。MDCT 在确定冠状动脉异常方面也很有价值。

有创的冠状动脉造影(ICA)被认为是检测 CAD 病变的范围和严重程度的"金标准"。但这种方法有发生心肌梗死、卒中或死亡的轻微风险,因此需谨慎选择。对于负荷试验呈阳性的患者,尤其是具有高危特征的患者,冠状动脉造影可获得关于冠状动脉及病变等更多的信息,并指导选择血运重建术(即经皮冠状动脉介入治疗或冠状动脉旁路移植术)还是药物治疗(表 7.3)。其他工具,如用于进行 FFR 的压力导丝,可以区分有生理意义的病变和不太可能导致缺血的病变,从而提高有创检查的诊断效能。对于不会导致缺血的病变,不建议进行血运重建。

医生还必须认识到,并非所有胸部不适都与 CAD 有关。引起胸部不适的其他原因包括食管疾病(胃食管反流可能会和典型的心绞痛症状类似)、胸壁相关疼痛、肺栓塞、肺炎和外伤。患者的临床表现通常指向各异,但胸部不适的患者通常可使用负荷试验的方法进行 CAD 评估。一旦明确地排除了 CAD,医生就需要考虑引起该症状的其他原因。在严重胸部不适的急性期,尤其是血流动力学不稳定的患者,鉴别诊断包括急性心肌梗死、肺栓塞和主动脉夹层。在这种情况下,及时准确的诊断评估(通常使用有创或 CT 血管造影术)可以挽救患者的生命。

治疗

稳定型心绞痛的药物治疗 CAD 和心绞痛的治疗是多方面的。无论 CAD 患者是否有心绞痛,医生都应该建议他们控制危险因素,积极改变生活方式。对于心绞痛,药物治疗通常用于控制症状,从而维持合理

angina pectoris, pharmacologic therapy is typically used to control symptoms, allowing for maintenance of reasonable exercise tolerance. Revascularization is commonly used to control symptoms to a degree better than what can be achieved with medications alone, but only a small group of patients with CAD benefit from revascularization in terms of increased longevity.

Other medical conditions can lower the threshold for angina, causing worsening symptoms and affecting quality of life. Anemia is a common medical problem that, when addressed, can significantly reduce the frequency of angina pectoris. Hyperthyroidism, with its increased metabolic demand and tachycardia, can increase the frequency of angina pectoris. Uncompensated congestive heart failure lowers the anginal threshold through the effects of LV dilation and filling pressure elevation on myocardial oxygen demand. Chronic obstructive pulmonary disease (COPD) and obstructive sleep apnea leading to hypoxemia can trigger angina pectoris. The use of illicit substances such as cocaine can also lead to angina through increased metabolic demand as well as coronary vasospasm.

Attention to the major modifiable risk factors for CAD is a cornerstone of therapy. Poorly controlled diabetes mellitus, hypertension, hyperlipidemia, and ongoing smoking all drive the progression of CAD and increase the risk for catastrophic events such as MI or sudden death. The wealth of clinical research on preventing death and disability from CAD has led to the development of evidence-based guidelines that form the basis of contemporary therapy for CAD (Table 7.4). Complete smoking cessation is a must for patients with CAD regardless of the presence of symptoms. Control of hypertension is also important. The use of statin medications to reduce LDL cholesterol has revolutionized the therapy for CAD and remains the cornerstone of lipid therapy. Statins have been shown to reduce the risk of MI in patients with proven CAD (goal LDL <70 mg/dL) and in those at significant risk (goal to lower LDL levels by >30% in intermediate risk patients and >50% in high-risk patients). If LDL levels do not reach the goal with statin monotherapy, ezetimibe can be utilized as an adjunctive agent. A new class of drug, PCSK-9 inhibitors (alirocumab and evolocumab), can have a dramatic impact on a patient's lipid profile but are somewhat cost-prohibitive. These are considered for secondary prevention in patients who have refractory hyperlipidemia to statin therapy as well as patients with familial hyperlipidemia syndromes who are at extreme risk for developing clinical ASCVD. There is also interest in low HDL levels, which appear to confer increased risk for coronary events. Exercise increases HDL levels and may confer protective effects through other mechanisms. Pharmacologic strategies to elevate HDL including niacin have not been proven to be beneficial.

Antiplatelet therapy is known to reduce the risk of MI in those who have known CAD. Patients should be instructed to take aspirin, 75 to 162 mg/day (clopidogrel 75 mg/day may be used in those who are aspirin intolerant or allergic). Angiotensin-converting enzyme (ACE) inhibitors reduce the risk of recurrent MI and are also beneficial for patients with diabetes mellitus or reduced LV function. Angiotensin receptor blockers (ARBs) can be substituted in those who experience significant side effects from ACE inhibitors.

Regular aerobic exercise can benefit patients with CAD by reducing their risk for complications related to the disease. Aerobic exercise also increases exercise tolerance and may reduce the frequency of exercise-related angina pectoris. Positive benefits also accrue from weight loss related to exercise and improved blood pressure control. In sedentary individuals, isometric activities such as snow shoveling can trigger MI and should be avoided. There may be some benefits to judicious weight training in patients with CAD.

TABLE 7.3 Indications for Coronary Angiography in Patients With Stable Angina Pectoris

Unacceptable angina despite medical therapy (for consideration of revascularization)
Noninvasive testing results with high-risk features
Angina or risk factors for coronary artery disease in the setting of depressed left ventricular systolic function
For diagnostic purposes, in the individual in whom the results of noninvasive testing are unclear

TABLE 7.4 Goals of Risk Factor Modification

Risk Factor	Goal
Dyslipidemia	
Elevated LDL-cholesterol level	
Patients with CAD or CAD equivalent[a]	LDL <70 mg/dL
Without CAD, ≥2 risk factors[b]	LDL <130 mg/dL (or <100 mg/dL[c])
Without CAD, 0-1 risk factors[c]	LDL <160 mg/dL
Elevated TG	TG <200 mg/dL
Reduced HDL-cholesterol level	HDL >40 mg/dL
Hypertension	Systolic blood pressure <140 mm Hg
	Diastolic blood pressure <90 mm Hg
Smoking	Complete cessation
Obesity	<120% of ideal body weight for height
Sedentary lifestyle	30-60 min moderately intense activity (e.g., walking, jogging, cycling, rowing) five times per week

CAD, Coronary artery disease; *CRP*, C-reactive protein; *HDL*, high-density lipoprotein; *hsCRP*, high-sensitivity C-reactive protein; *LDL*, low-density lipoprotein; *TG*, triglycerides.
[a]CAD equivalents include diabetes mellitus, noncoronary atherosclerotic vascular disease, or >20% 10-year risk for a cardiovascular event as predicted by the Framingham risk score.
[b]Risk factors include cigarette smoking, blood pressure ≥140/90 mm Hg or taking antihypertensive medication, HDL-cholesterol level <40 mg/dL, family history of premature coronary atherosclerosis (male, <45 yr; female, <55 yr).
[c]Target of 100 mg/dL should be strongly considered for men ≥60 yr and for individuals with a high burden of subclinical atherosclerosis (coronary calcification >75th percentile for age and sex), hsCRP >3 mg/dL, or metabolic syndrome.

的运动耐量。相较于单纯药物治疗，血运重建能更好地控制症状，但只有一小部分 CAD 患者能因血运重建而延长寿命。

其他疾病会降低心绞痛的阈值，导致症状恶化，影响生活质量。贫血是一种常见的内科疾病，如果得到治疗，可显著降低心绞痛的发生频率。甲状腺功能亢进会导致代谢需求增加和心动过速，从而增加心绞痛的发作频率。失代偿期充血性心力衰竭会通过左心室扩张和充盈压升高，从而影响心肌需氧量，而降低心绞痛阈值。慢性阻塞性肺疾病（COPD）和阻塞性睡眠呼吸暂停导致的低氧血症，可诱发心绞痛。使用可卡因等违禁药物也会因代谢需求增加和冠状动脉血管痉挛而导致心绞痛。

关注可改变的、主要 CAD 危险因素是治疗的基础。控制不佳的糖尿病、高血压、高脂血症和持续吸烟都会导致 CAD 的进展，并增加发生心肌梗死或猝死等灾难性事件的风险。关于预防 CAD 导致的死亡和致残的大量临床研究促进了循证指南制定，这些指南构成了现代 CAD 治疗的基础（表 7.4）。无论有无症状，患有 CAD 的患者都必须彻底戒烟；控制高血压也很重要；使用他汀类药物降低低密度脂蛋白胆固醇彻底改变了心血管疾病的治疗，目前仍是血脂治疗的基石。他汀类药物已被证明可降低 CAD 确诊患者（目标 LDL < 70 mg/dl）和高风险患者（目标是将中危患者的 LDL 水平降低 > 30%，高危患者降低 > 50%）的心肌梗死风险。如果他汀类药物单药治疗后低密度脂蛋白水平不达标，可以使用依折麦布作为辅助药物。PCSK-9 抑制剂（alirocumab 和 evolocumab）是一种新型药物，可显著降低患者的血脂水平，但成本较高。这些药物可用于他汀类药物耐药的难治性高脂血症患者的二级预防，也可用于家族性高脂血症综合征患者的二级预防，这些患者患 ASCVD 的风险极高。高密度脂蛋白水平降低似乎会增加 CAD 事件的风险，这也引起了人们的关注。运动可增加高密度脂蛋白水平，并可能通过其他机制产生保护作用。包括烟酸在内的、旨在提高高密度脂蛋白的药物尚未被证实对 CAD 有益。

抗血小板治疗可降低 CAD 患者的心肌梗死风险。应指导患者服用阿司匹林 75 ~ 162 mg/d（不耐受阿司匹林或对阿司匹林过敏者可使用氯吡格雷 75 mg/d）。血管紧张素转换酶（ACE）抑制剂可降低心肌梗死复发的风险，对糖尿病或左心室功能减退的患者也有好处。应用 ACE 抑制剂出现明显副作用的患者，可以用血管紧张素受体阻滞剂（ARB）替代。

规律的有氧运动可以降低 CAD 患者出现并发症的风险，从而使他们受益。有氧运动还能提高运动耐量，并可减少与运动相关的心绞痛发生频率。运动可以改善血压，减轻体重，带来更多获益。对于缺乏运动的人，铲雪等肌肉等长收缩活动可能会诱发心肌梗死，应尽量避免。对 CAD 患者进行一定程度重量训练可能会有益。

表 7.3　稳定型心绞痛患者行冠状动脉造影的指征

药物治疗后心绞痛仍无法耐受（考虑进行血运重建）
无创检测结果具有高风险特征
左心室收缩功能减退情况下的心绞痛或具有 CAD 危险因素
无创检测结果不明确者，为明确诊断

表 7.4　危险因素控制目标

危险因素	目标
血脂异常	
LDL- 胆固醇升高	
CAD 或 CAD 等危症 [a]	LDL < 70 mg/dl
无 CAD，≥ 2 个危险因素 [b]	LDL < 130 mg/dl（或 < 100 mg/dl [c]）
无 CAD，0 ~ 1 个危险因素	LDL < 160 mg/dl
TG 升高	TG < 200 mg/dl
HDL- 胆固醇减少	HDL > 40 mg/dl
高血压	收缩压 < 140 mmHg
	舒张压 < 90 mmHg
吸烟	完全戒烟
肥胖	< 120% 基于身高的理想体重
缺乏运动	30 ~ 60 min 中等强度体力活动（如走路、慢跑、骑自行车、划船）每周 5 次

CAD，冠状动脉疾病；HDL，高密度脂蛋白；hsCRP，高敏 C 反应蛋白；LDL，低密度脂蛋白；TG，甘油三酯。
[a] CAD 等危症包括糖尿病、非冠状动脉的粥样硬化性血管疾病，或 Framingham 风险评分预测的 10 年心血管事件风险 > 20%。
[b] 危险因素包括：吸烟、血压 ≥ 140/90 mmHg 或服用降压药物、高密度脂蛋白胆固醇水平 < 40 mg/dl、早发 CAD 家族史（男性 < 45 岁，女性 < 55 岁）。
[c] 年龄 ≥ 60 岁的男性、动脉粥样硬化负荷较重（冠状动脉钙化 > 75% 同等性别和年龄人群）亚临床患者、hsCRP > 3 mg/dl 或代谢综合征患者，应考虑目标值为 100 mg/dl。

TABLE 7.5 Medications for Angina Pectoris

Drug Class	Examples	Antianginal Effect	Physiologic Side Effects	Comments
Nitroglycerin	Sublingual Topical Intravenous Oral	Decreased preload and afterload Coronary vasodilation Increased collateral blood flow	Headache Flushing Orthostasis	Tolerance develops with continuous use
β-Adrenergic blocking agents	Metoprolol Atenolol Propranolol Nadolol	Decreased heart rate Decreased blood pressure Decreased contractility	Bradycardia Hypotension Bronchospasm Depression	May worsen heart failure and AV conduction block; avoid in vasospastic angina
Calcium-channel blocking agents (non-dihydropyridine)	Phenylalkylamine (verapamil) Benzothiazepine (diltiazem)	Decreased heart rate Decreased blood pressure Decreased contractility Coronary vasodilation	Bradycardia Hypotension Constipation with verapamil	May worsen heart failure and AV conduction
Calcium-channel blocking agents	Dihydropyridine (nifedipine, amlodipine)	Decreased blood pressure Coronary vasodilation	Hypotension, reflex tachycardia Peripheral edema	Short-acting nifedipine is associated with increased risk for cardiovascular events.
Late sodium current blocking agents	Ranolazine	Inhibits cardiac late I_{Na} Prevents calcium overload	Dizziness Headache Constipation Nausea	No effects on blood pressure or heart rate Modest QTc prolongation

AV, Atrioventricular; I_{Na}, sodium current.

In addition to antiplatelet therapy, the commonly employed medications to control angina pectoris include β-blockers, nitrates, and calcium-channel blockers. These agents work by correcting supply/demand blood flow mismatch that is the cause of myocardial ischemia and angina pectoris (Table 7.5). Interestingly, these drugs principally control symptoms in chronic stable angina pectoris, but they do not reduce mortality risk as therapy with aspirin or statins does.

Nitrates in various forms have a long history of use in patients with symptomatic CAD and can be very effective in controlling exertion-related angina. Nitrates work by venodilating large-capacitance veins and thus shifting blood out of the heart, reducing preload and myocardial oxygen demand. Nitrates are also potent coronary vasodilators and can reverse coronary spasm, allowing for improved perfusion. Short-duration but quick-acting sublingual nitroglycerin has been a mainstay both for treatment of an anginal episode and for prophylaxis against angina in situations where it is likely to occur. Patients who respond well to nitrates are frequently treated with long-acting oral or topical preparations. Both methods can effectively prevent angina pectoris, but continued use can induce tolerance. There is a recognized need for patients to have a nitrate-free period of about 8 hours every day to prevent tolerance. This usually involves cessation of use during sleep. Intravenous nitroglycerin administered by continuous drip is reserved for patients with unstable angina or acute MI.

β-Blocker therapy is very effective at reducing the likelihood of exertion-related angina. β-Blockers bind to cell surface β-receptors and by so doing reduce heart rate, contractility, and blood pressure, all of which tip the balance in favor of reduced oxygen demand and less angina. The use of β-blockers can be limited by the degree of bradycardia they induce or by baseline atrioventricular (AV) conduction abnormalities. In patients with higher degrees of AV block, β-blockers can induce complete heart block. These drugs also vary in their β-receptor selectivity. Blockade of $β_2$-adrenergic receptors can lead to bronchospasm and vasoconstriction. Even selective $β_1$-adrenergic antagonists such as atenolol and metoprolol have some $β_2$ activity at higher doses. Intolerance of β-blockers can limit their use in patients with significant COPD or peripheral vascular disease. β-Blockers may also add to glucose intolerance and may affect lipids by increasing triglycerides or reducing HDL. In general, these effects do not preclude their use if they prove effective in controlling angina pectoris.

Calcium-channel blocking drugs can decrease myocardial oxygen demand by causing arterial vasodilation, bradycardia, and decreased contractility. The magnitude of these effects varies according to the class of agent used. Dihydropyridines such as nifedipine and amlodipine cause arterial vasodilation leading to a blood pressure–lowering effect. In the dose ranges administered, they have no significant effect on contractility or heart rate. In contrast, verapamil, a phenylalkylamine, has significant effects on heart rate, AV conduction, and contractility. Benzothiazepine agents such as diltiazem manifest less vasodilation than dihydropyridines and less effect on contractility than phenylalkylamine drugs. The net effect of calcium-channel blocking drugs is reduced myocardial oxygen demand resulting in less angina pectoris. Diltiazem should be used with caution in patients who are also taking a β-blocker, because severe bradycardia or heart block can occur. Verapamil should not be co-administered with a β-blocker.

A newer class of antianginal drug is represented by ranolazine. This drug is a selective inhibitor of late sodium current and reduces sodium-induced calcium overload in myocytes. Although it has no effect on heart rate or blood pressure, ranolazine demonstrates antianginal properties. It is typically used when other medical therapy is insufficient in controlling angina.

Revascularization therapy for chronic stable angina pectoris. Revascularization therapy is an option to be considered when medical therapy is not sufficiently controlling symptoms leading to impaired lifestyle. It is also frequently pursued in the face of high-risk situations such as unstable angina, STEMI, heart failure complicated by angina, arrhythmias associated with angina, or the presence of large areas of myocardial ischemia documented by noninvasive imaging. The two types of revascularization procedures are coronary bypass grafting (CABG) and percutaneous coronary intervention (PCI).

Percutaneous transluminal coronary angioplasty was the initial mode of catheter-based revascularization introduced in the late 1970s. In this technique, a guidewire is placed through a stenotic segment of artery, after which a balloon-tipped catheter is threaded over the

表 7.5 治疗心绞痛的药物

药物分类	举例	抗心绞痛效果	生理副作用	备注
硝酸甘油	舌下含服 局部用药 静脉注射 口服	减少前负荷和后负荷 扩张冠状动脉 增加侧支血流	头痛 潮红 直立性低血压	连续使用会产生耐受性
β 受体阻滞剂	美托洛尔 阿替洛尔 普萘洛尔 纳多洛尔（Nadolol）	减慢心率 降低血压 减弱收缩力	心动过缓 低血压 支气管痉挛 抑郁	可能加重心力衰竭和房室传导阻滞；血管痉挛性心绞痛患者避免使用
钙通道阻滞剂（非二氢吡啶类）	苯烷胺类（维拉帕米） 苯硫䓬类（地尔硫䓬）	减慢心率 降低血压 减弱收缩力 扩张冠状动脉	心动过缓 低血压 维拉帕米相关便秘	可能加重心力衰竭和房室传导
钙通道阻滞剂	二氢吡啶（硝苯地平、氨氯地平）	降低血压 扩张冠状动脉	低血压、反射性心动过速 周围水肿	短效硝苯地平与心血管事件风险增加有关
晚期钠电流阻滞剂	雷诺嗪	抑制心脏晚期 I_{Na} 防止钙超载	头晕 头痛 便秘 恶心	对血压或心率无影响 轻度 QTc 延长

I_{Na}，钠电流。

除抗血小板治疗外，控制心绞痛的常用药物还包括 β 受体阻滞剂、硝酸酯类和钙通道阻滞剂。这些药物通过纠正血氧供需失衡而发挥作用，而血氧供需失衡正是心肌缺血和心绞痛的原因（表 7.5）。有趣的是，这些药物主要控制慢性稳定型心绞痛的症状，但并不能像阿司匹林或他汀类药物那样，降低死亡风险。

各种形式的硝酸酯类药物用于有症状的 CAD 患者已经有很长的历史了，对控制劳累引起的心绞痛非常有效。硝酸酯类药物的作用原理是扩张大的容量静脉，从而将血液转移出心脏，减轻前负荷和心肌需氧量。其还是强效的冠状动脉血管扩张剂，可逆转冠状动脉痉挛，从而改善灌注。硝酸甘油舌下含服作用时间短但起效快，一直是治疗心绞痛发作和在可能发生心绞痛的情况下预防心绞痛的主要药物。对硝酸盐类药物反应良好的患者经常使用长效口服制剂或局部制剂。这两种方法都能有效预防心绞痛，但持续使用会产生耐药性。患者每天需要有大约 8 h 的无药期，以防止产生耐药性。通常的做法是在睡眠时停止使用。对于不稳定型心绞痛或急性心肌梗死患者，仍可保留使用持续静脉滴注硝酸甘油。

β 受体阻滞剂对劳力相关的心绞痛非常有效。β 受体阻滞剂能与细胞表面的 β 受体结合，从而降低心率、心肌收缩力和血压，所有这些都可通过减少心肌氧需求，改善心肌血氧供需失衡，从而缓解心绞痛。β 受体阻滞剂的使用会受到其诱发的心动过缓的程度或基础的房室传导异常所限制。对于房室传导阻滞程度较高的患者，β 受体阻滞剂可导致完全性传导阻滞。不同药物对 β 受体的选择性也不尽相同。阻断 β$_2$-肾上腺素能受体可导致支气管痉挛和血管收缩。即使是选择性 β$_1$-肾上腺素能阻滞剂，如阿替洛尔和美托洛尔，在剂量较大时也有一定的 β$_2$ 受体阻断作用。对 β 受体阻滞剂的不耐受会限制其在患有严重慢性阻塞性肺疾病或周围血管疾病患者中的使用。β 受体阻滞剂还可能导致胰岛素抵抗，并通过增加甘油三酯或降低高密度脂蛋白，从而影响血脂水平。一般来说，尽管有这些副作用，如果能有效控制心绞痛，并不影响这些药物的使用。

钙通道阻滞药物可导致动脉血管扩张、心动过缓以及收缩力下降，从而降低心肌需氧量。这些影响的程度因所用药物的类别而异。二氢吡啶类药物，如硝苯地平和氨氯地平会导致动脉血管扩张，从而产生降压效果。在合理的剂量范围内，它们对收缩力或心率没有明显影响。相反，苯烷胺类药物维拉帕米对心率、房室传导和收缩力有明显影响。与二氢吡啶类药物相比，地尔硫䓬等苯硫䓬类药物对血管扩张的作用较小；对收缩力的影响也较苯烷胺类药物小。钙通道阻滞药的净效应是降低心肌需氧量，从而减轻心绞痛。已经服用 β 受体阻滞剂的患者应慎用地尔硫䓬，因为可能会出现严重的心动过缓或心脏传导阻滞。维拉帕米不能与 β 受体阻滞剂合用。

最近，出现了以雷诺嗪为代表的一类新型抗心绞痛药物。这种药物是心肌细胞晚期钠电流的选择性抑制剂，可降低钠离子诱导的心肌细胞钙超载。雷诺嗪具有抗心绞痛的特性，与心率和血压没有关系。当其他药物治疗不足以控制心绞痛时，通常会使用这种药物。

慢性稳定型心绞痛的血运重建治疗 当药物治疗无法充分控制症状，导致生活质量受影响时，可以考虑血运重建。出现高风险情况时（如不稳定型心绞痛、STEMI、心绞痛并发心力衰竭、心绞痛伴有心律失常，或无创成像显示存在大面积心肌缺血时）也会经常采用血运重建疗法。血运重建手术分为冠状动脉旁路移植术（CABG）和经皮冠状动脉介入治疗（PCI）两种。

经皮腔内冠状动脉血管成形术是 20 世纪 70 年代末引入的首个经导管血运重建方式。在该技术中，将导丝通过狭窄的冠状动脉，然后将球囊导入血管内。然后将球囊导管穿在导丝上到达狭窄部位，再对其进行扩张。这种形式的血管成形术通过破坏斑块和损伤血管内膜，

wire to the area of stenosis and then inflated. Angioplasty of this form enlarges the vessel lumen in an irregular geometry through disruption of the plaque and injury to the vessel intima. Plain old balloon angioplasty (POBA), as the procedure later became known, was effective at improving myocardial perfusion and reducing exercise-related angina. However, because of plaque disruption, there was a 2% to 5% risk of abrupt vessel closure frequently leading to MI. In addition, there was a high incidence of injury-mediated restenosis (up to 50%) during the first 3 to 6 months after the procedure. The process of restenosis involved intimal hyperplasia and remodeling, yielding a recurrent stenosis sometimes more severe in nature than the original lesion.

The innovation of coronary stents pioneered through the 1980s and clinically available in the early 1990s represented a significant advance in PCI. Coronary stents are expandable metallic mesh tubes that are mounted on an angioplasty balloon, allowing delivery to an area of stenosis, where balloon inflation expands the stent into the vessel wall. The stent becomes permanently embedded in the vessel wall and scaffolds the artery to keep it open. This procedure not only reduces the risk of abrupt vessel occlusion to 1% or less, but it is also associated with a significant reduction in restenosis risk (20% to 25%, compared with 50% for POBA). The benefit of stenting for a patient is clear in terms of less risk of procedure-related acute MI and less need for repeat procedures. Vessels smaller than 2 mm in diameter are not good targets for stenting, because the smallest-diameter stent is 2 mm. Stents do have a risk of thrombosis, necessitating lifelong aspirin therapy and the use of clopidogrel for 4 weeks to 1 year after the procedure (there may be some advantage to longer-duration clopidogrel for 1 year).

Despite the reduction achieved with coronary stents, there was still a significant risk of restenosis, leading investigators to search for a means to lower that risk. Drug-eluting stents (DES) were found to significantly reduce the risk of restenosis compared to bare metal stents. The first DES, released for use in 2003, was coated with either sirolimus or paclitaxel, both of which inhibited the hyperplastic response in the vessel wall triggered by PCI. The current generations of DES are coated with either zotarolimus or everolimus, both very effective at reducing restenosis. The predicted restenosis rate for current-generation DES is in the range of 5% to 10%. Vessel diameter affects restenosis risk, with larger-diameter vessels demonstrating less restenosis. The benefit of inhibiting tissue overgrowth within the stent is also associated with delayed endothelialization of the stent, which increases the risk of stent thrombosis for a longer time than with bare metal stents. For this reason P2Y12 inhibitors, in conjunction with aspirin, are prescribed to patients with stents to prevent stent thrombosis. If a situation arises in which the P2Y12 inhibitor must be discontinued the minimum time post-stent implantation at which it can safely be held depends on the type of stent implanted: 1 month for a bare metal stent (BMS) and 3 to 6 months for a drug-eluting stent. The decision regarding whether to implant a DES or a BMS is based on patient characteristics such as risk of bleeding or need for urgent surgical procedure. However, the use of BMS has declined over recent years as the safety and effectiveness of newer generation DES has been demonstrated. Aspirin should be continued indefinitely, to minimize the risk of late stent thrombosis.

A host of other devices to treat stenotic coronary arteries have come and gone over time. In this era, rotational atherectomy plays a role in treating calcified lesions in about 5% of patients. Routine use of catheter-based aspiration of thrombus led to an increased incidence of stroke and thus is no longer recommended on a routine basis. Intravascular ultrasound is an important imaging adjunct that can be helpful in interrogating lesions or defining the end result of stent placement.

CABG emerged in the 1970s as an effective means of coronary revascularization for the control of angina. Bypass grafts take the form of saphenous vein from the leg, free radial artery segments, or intact left or right internal mammary artery grafts. The vein or radial artery grafts are placed on the ascending aorta and then anastomosed to the coronary vessels distal to the site of obstruction. In contrast, left or right internal mammary arteries are left intact at their origins and anastomosed distal to the obstruction. The left internal mammary artery is typically placed onto the left anterior descending coronary artery. This is the most important vessel to graft because of its size and distribution, and the left internal mammary artery is ideal given an expected patency rate of 90% at 10 years. Saphenous vein grafts degenerate over time, leading to episodes of symptomatic abrupt occlusion and a 50% patency rate at 10 years. Free radial artery grafts perform better than vein grafts but less well than intact mammary artery grafts. CABG is a major cardiac surgical procedure, but in skilled hands the mortality rate is expected to be 1% to 2%, with a similar risk of stroke. Periprocedural MI rates are in the range of 5% to 10%. There has been controversy over whether the use of the heart-lung machine to support CABG causes more problems for patients than "beating heart" surgery does. Recent studies suggest there is no long-term difference in outcomes, such as death, MI, or stroke, for patients undergoing CABG, either on- or off-pump.

Most CABG procedures are performed for symptom control and are not likely to enhance longevity. The categories of patients likely to have life prolonged by CABG include those with a left main coronary artery more than 50% narrowed, those with severe three-vessel obstructive disease associated with a decrease in ejection fraction (EF, 35% to 50%), and those with two- or three-artery disease whose proximal left anterior descending artery is severely stenosed.

Clinical trials comparing CABG and PCI have consistently shown that patients undergoing CABG require fewer repeat procedures during the first 2 years after surgery. In the first 2 years, it is more likely that patients with PCI will experience symptomatic restenosis than that patients with CABG will have graft failure. Over time, this advantage is lost as vein grafts begin to fail 5 to 10 years after surgery. However, there is evidence that a survival advantage exists for diabetic patients with multivessel CAD who undergo CABG as opposed to PCI. A recent study also demonstrated long-term survival benefit for CABG over PCI in the face of multivessel CAD. Some of the survival advantages in favor of CABG may be linked to the use of the left internal mammary artery as a graft.

Despite the use of either revascularization technique, patients remain prone to progressive atherosclerotic disease with the potential to form plaque at previously unaffected sites. This necessitates aggressive long-term medical therapy and risk factor modification to achieve the lowest possible risk of symptomatic progression or MI. Retreatment with CABG is possible but is fraught with higher risk, and the outcome of repeat stenting for in-stent restenosis is never as good as for de novo lesions.

In a small group of patients, PCI and/or CABG fails and the patient has refractory angina. Once medical therapy has been maximized, few truly effective options remain. Transmyocardial laser revascularization in areas of ischemia has been used to reduce symptoms, but this technique is now of uncertain value. External counterpulsation is a technique whereby blood pressure cuffs are placed on each leg, inflated during diastole and deflated during systole. Patients typically have a 1-hour session that may be repeated 35 times. Angina relief has been reported with this procedure and may reflect some beneficial effect on endothelial function. Spinal cord stimulation using electrodes placed in the C7-T1 dorsal epidural space can reduce anginal symptoms in the short term, although the long-term role needs definition.

以不规则的几何形状扩大血管腔。这种后来被称为"单纯球囊血管成形术"(POBA)的手术可有效改善心肌灌注和减少运动性心绞痛。然而，由于斑块被破坏，血管突然闭塞的风险为 2%～5%，这常可导致心肌梗死。此外，在手术后的前 3～6 个月内，损伤介导的再狭窄发生率很高（高达 50%）。再狭窄的过程包括血管内膜增生和重塑，产生的再发狭窄有时比原来的病变更为严重。

冠状动脉支架这一创新始于 20 世纪 80 年代，并于 20 世纪 90 年代初应用于临床，代表了 PCI 的重大进步。冠状动脉支架是安装在血管成形术球囊上的可膨胀金属网管，可输送到狭窄部位，球囊充气后支架膨胀入血管壁。支架会永久嵌入血管壁，为动脉提供支撑，使其保持通畅。这种手术不仅能将血管突然闭塞的风险降到 1% 或更低，还能显著降低血管再狭窄风险（20%～25%，而 POBA 为 50%）。支架置入术对患者的益处显而易见，降低了与手术相关的急性心肌梗死风险，减少了再次手术风险。直径小于 2 mm 的血管不是支架置入的理想目标，因为支架的最小直径是 2 mm。支架置入术后确实存在血栓形成的风险，因此需要终生服用阿司匹林治疗，并在术后 4 周至 1 年内使用氯吡格雷（使用长达 1 年的氯吡格雷可能有一定益处）。

尽管冠状动脉支架置入术降低了再狭窄的风险，但血管再狭窄的风险仍然较大，导致研究人员开始寻找降低再狭窄风险的方法。研究发现，与裸金属支架（BMS）相比，药物洗脱支架（DES）可显著降低再狭窄风险。2003 年上市的第一款 DES 涂有西罗莫司或紫杉醇，这两种药物都能抑制 PCI 引发的血管壁增生反应。目前的新一代 DES 涂有佐他莫司或依维莫司，这两种药物都能很有效地减少再狭窄。目前新一代 DES 的再狭窄率为 5%～10%。血管直径会影响再狭窄风险，直径较大的血管再狭窄率较低。DES 可以抑制支架内组织过度生长，但是也会引起支架内皮化延迟，因此，与裸金属支架相比，DES 将在更长的时间内增加支架内血栓形成的风险。因此，P2Y12 抑制剂与阿司匹林一起被用于支架置入术后患者，以防止支架内血栓形成。如果出现必须停用 P2Y12 抑制剂的情况，支架置入后联合使用的最短时间取决于置入支架的类型：裸金属支架为 1 个月，药物洗脱支架为 3～6 个月。决定置入 DES 还是 BMS 的依据是患者的特点，如出血风险或是否需要紧急手术。不过，随着新一代 DES 的安全性和有效性得到证实，近年来 BMS 的使用量显著下降。阿司匹林应一直服用，以降低晚期支架内血栓形成的风险。

随着时代的发展，治疗冠状动脉狭窄的其他设备层出不穷。目前，冠脉旋磨术在治疗钙化病变中发挥了作用，该类病变的发生率约 5%。常规使用导管抽吸血栓导致卒中发生率增加，因此不再推荐常规使用。血管内超声是一种重要的辅助成像手段，有助于检查病变或确定支架置入的最终结果。

CABG 兴起于 20 世纪 70 年代，是控制心绞痛的有效冠状动脉血运重建手段。旁路移植血管的来源包括腿部大隐静脉、游离桡动脉段或完整的左或右侧乳内动脉。静脉或桡动脉移植物近段连接在升主动脉上，远端与冠状动脉阻塞部位远端的血管吻合。而左或右侧乳内动脉则在其起源处保持完整，远端与冠状动脉阻塞部位远端进行吻合。左乳内动脉通常被置于左前降支冠状动脉上。由于左前降支的大小和分布，它被认为是最重要的、需要被移植的血管，而且左乳内动脉用于移植后的 10 年预期通畅率为 90%，因此左乳内动脉是最理想的、用于给前降支"搭桥"的血管。大隐静脉移植后会逐渐老化，出现有症状的突然闭塞，其 10 年的通畅率仅为 50%。游离桡动脉移植物的表现优于静脉移植物，但不如完整的乳内动脉。CABG 是一项大型心脏外科手术，但由技术熟练的医生操作，死亡率预计为 1%～2%，卒中的风险与此类似。围术期心肌梗死的发生率在 5%～10%。关于使用体外循环支持的 CABG 是否会比"心脏不停跳"手术给患者带来更多问题，一直存在争议。最近的研究表明，接受 CABG 治疗的患者无论在手术时是否"心脏停跳"，其在死亡、心肌梗死或卒中等方面均没有长期的差异。

大多数 CABG 只能控制症状，并不能延长患者寿命。有可能通过 CABG 延长寿命的患者包括左冠状动脉主干狭窄超过 50%、患有严重三支血管阻塞性病变且射血分数下降（EF 35%～50%）的患者，以及患有二或三支动脉疾病且左前降支动脉近端严重狭窄的患者。

诸多比较 CABG 和 PCI 的临床试验均一致表明，接受 CABG 的患者在术后前 2 年内需要再次手术的概率减小。在最初的 2 年中，PCI 患者出现症状性再狭窄的概率要高于 CABG 患者出现移植失败的概率。由于静脉移植物会在术后 5～10 年开始失效，因此随时间推移，这一优势会逐渐丧失。不过，有证据表明，对于多支血管病变的 CAD 合并糖尿病患者，与 PCI 相比，接受 CABG 的治疗更具生存优势。最近的一项研究也证明，多支血管病变的 CAD 患者，接受 CABG 比 PCI 更能在长期生存方面获益。CABG 的生存优势部分可能与使用左乳内动脉作为移植物有关。

尽管使用了血运重建技术，但患者仍容易发生动脉粥样硬化疾病进展，并有可能在以前未受影响的部位形成斑块。这就需要积极的长期药物治疗和控制危险因素，以尽可能降低症状恶化或心肌梗死的风险。CABG 术后因为疾病进展而进行再次旁路移植术是可行的，但风险较高；而针对支架内再狭窄进行的重复支架置入术，其疗效永远比不上对原位血管病变治疗的效果。

在一小部分患者中，PCI 和（或）CABG 治疗失败，患者会出现难治性心绞痛。一旦药物治疗已经调整到最大剂量，其余真正有效的选择就所剩无几。在缺血区域进行经心肌激光血运重建可减轻症状，但这种技术目前的临床价值尚不确定。体外反搏技术是将血压袖带放置在患者的每条腿上，舒张期充气，收缩期放气的一种技术。患者通常每次接受 1 h 的治疗，可重复 35 次。有报告称这种方法可缓解心绞痛，这可能反映了它对内皮功能的一些有益影响。使用放置在 C7～T1 背侧硬膜外腔的电极进行脊髓刺激可在短期内减轻心绞痛症状，但长期作用尚待明确。

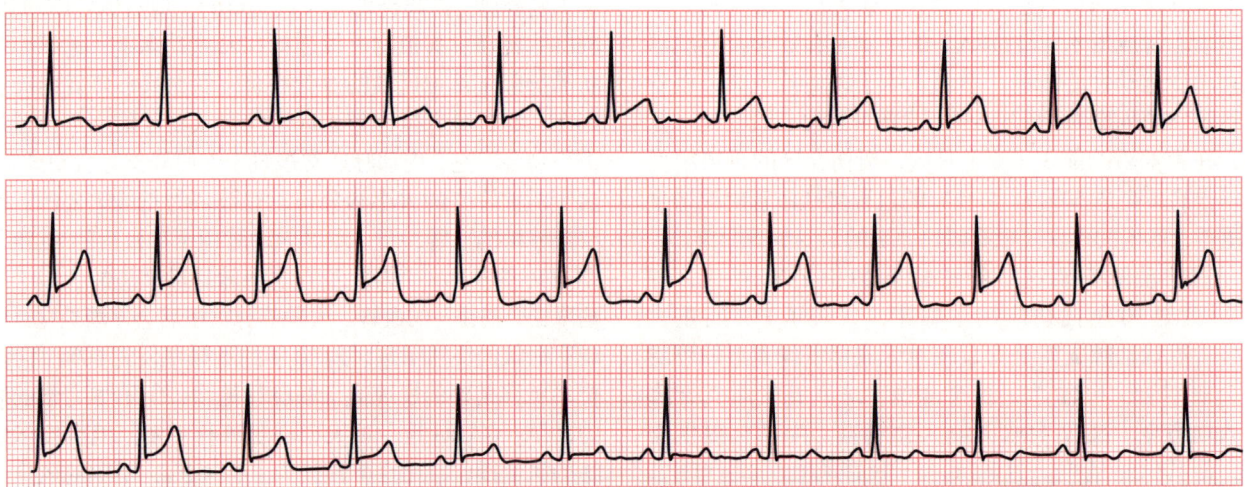

Fig. 7.4 Continuous electrocardiogram recording in a patient with Prinzmetal (variant) angina. The spontaneous onset of chest discomfort began during the top strip, accompanied by transient ST-segment elevation. By the bottom strip, several minutes later, both discomfort and ST-segment elevation had resolved.

Other Anginal Syndromes

Variant angina. Whereas typical angina pectoris is usually triggered by physical or emotional stress, some patients experience a syndrome termed variant angina. Variant angina was first described in 1959 by Prinzmetal and colleagues, who observed patients with chest discomfort at rest, not triggered by physical or emotional stress, and associated with ST-segment elevation (Fig. 7.4). Episodes of AV block and ventricular ectopy were observed, but MI was not a common feature. These patients typically did not have the common CAD risk factors other than smoking. Coronary angiography demonstrated these patients to be experiencing transient coronary vasospasm. The vasospasm tended to occur in an area of atherosclerotic plaque, but some patients had spasm in angiographically normal segments of coronary artery.

In the course of investigating the pathophysiology of variant angina, a number of provocative tests were developed to induce coronary spasm in susceptible individuals. Intracoronary ergonovine or acetylcholine can induce spasm in patients with variant angina, probably as a result of underlying endothelial dysfunction. Other spasm-inducing provocations include the cold pressor test (placing a hand in an ice bath), the induction of alkalosis (hyperventilation or intravenous bicarbonate), and histamine infusion. Provocative testing to induce coronary vasospasm has fallen out of favor in the routine assessment of patients with angina.

Coronary vasospasm usually resolves promptly with the administration of nitroglycerin (sublingual, intravenous, or intra-arterial). The combination of oral nitrates and calcium-channel blockers is often used to prevent spasm. β-Blockers may aggravate coronary spasm by inhibiting the action of vasodilating β2-receptors, allowing for unopposed α-receptor induced vasoconstriction. Rare patients do not respond to vasodilator medical therapy and may benefit from coronary stent placement in spasm-prone atherosclerotic lesions.

Microvascular angina with normal coronary arteries. Angina can occur in some patients in the face of normal-appearing coronary arteries and no provocable spasm. Decreased endothelium-dependent vasodilation may be the underlying pathophysiology of microvascular angina. Patients with this condition may demonstrate an increase in coronary resistance and an inability to increase coronary blood flow sufficiently when challenged by increases in myocardial oxygen demand. Women are more likely to be affected with microvascular angina, and the symptoms not uncommonly occur at rest or with emotional stress. Exercise can also trigger angina.

A host of diagnostic tests can detect the presence of ischemia in patients with microvascular angina. In the case of stress testing, ST changes of ischemia can be detected as well as nuclear perfusion defects and transient wall motion abnormalities on echocardiography. More sophisticated invasive testing may demonstrate the presence of stress-induced metabolic abnormalities characteristic of ischemia and endothelial dysfunction.

Exercise-related ischemic symptoms may respond to β-blocker therapy. Microvascular angina also tends to respond well to nitrates, both short-acting sublingual nitroglycerin and long-acting oral nitrates. Calcium-channel antagonists are sometimes used together with nitrates to control angina related to microvascular ischemia.

Silent myocardial ischemia. Not all episodes of myocardial ischemia are associated with angina. Some patients may only experience episodes of silent myocardial ischemia as evidenced by transient ST depression with ECG monitoring. Such patients can also have silent MI. It is also possible, and probably not uncommon, for patients to have both silent myocardial ischemia episodes and typical angina; this is termed mixed angina. Episodes of silent myocardial ischemia can be observed in all settings of CAD: chronic stable angina, unstable angina, and coronary vasospasm. Silent ischemia is more common in diabetic patients. Medical therapy directed at controlling symptomatic angina also reduces the number of episodes of silent ischemia.

Prognosis

Contemporary therapies for stable ischemic heart disease have significantly reduced the risks of cardiac events and mortality. The annual rate of major ischemic events such as MI is in the range of 1% to 2%, and the yearly mortality rate is 1% to 3%. CAD is frequently associated with systemic vascular disease, making these patients prone to a host of other events. Patients with stable ischemic heart disease have a yearly combined outcome risk for cardiovascular death, MI, or stroke in the range of 4.5%.

Despite advances in medical and revascularization therapies, up to 30% of patients face some limiting symptoms of recurrent angina.

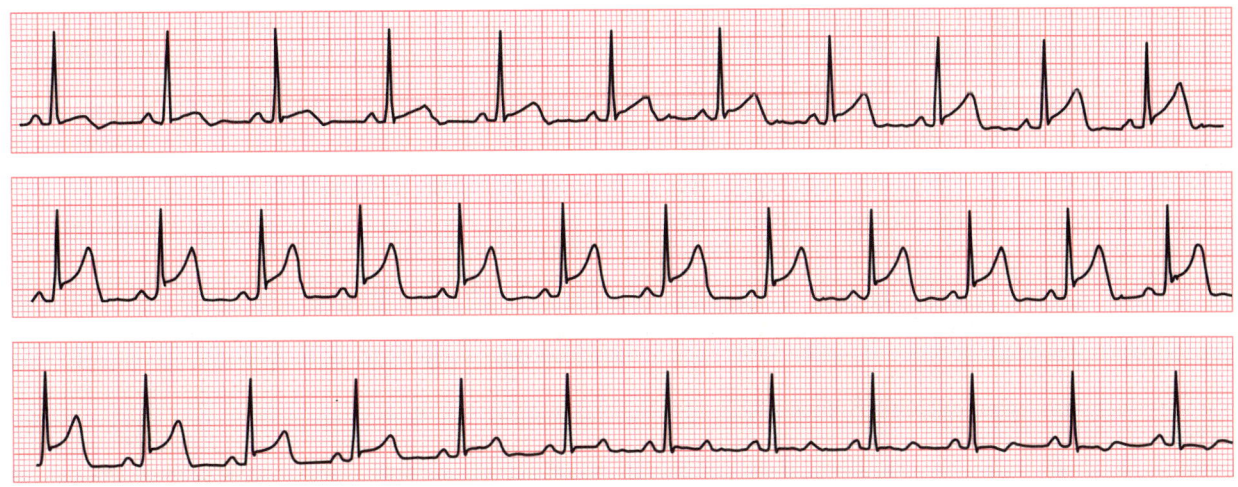

图 7.4 一例变异型心绞痛患者的连续心电图记录。上图中患者自发出现胸部不适，并伴有一过性 ST 段抬高；下图中不适症状和 ST 段抬高在几分钟后消失

其他类型的心绞痛

变异型心绞痛 典型的心绞痛通常由体力活动或情绪应激引发，然而有些患者会发生变异型心绞痛。变异型心绞痛于 1959 年由 Prinzmetal 及其同事首次描述，他们观察到有些患者在休息时出现胸部不适，而不被体力活动或情绪应激诱发，且伴有 ST 段抬高（图 7.4）。变异型心绞痛患者可出现房室传导阻滞和室性异位心律的发作，但发生（急性）心肌梗死者并不多见。除吸烟外，这些患者通常不具备常见的 CAD 危险因素。冠状动脉造影证实这些患者出现一过性冠状动脉血管痉挛。血管痉挛往往发生在动脉粥样硬化斑块区域，但也有一些患者在冠状动脉造影正常的节段出现痉挛。

在研究变异型心绞痛的病理生理过程中，人们开发了许多激发试验来诱发可疑人群的冠状动脉痉挛。冠状动脉内注射麦角新碱或乙酰胆碱可诱发变异型心绞痛患者的冠状动脉痉挛，这可能是潜在内皮功能障碍的结果。其他可诱发痉挛的激发试验包括冷加压试验（将手放入冰浴中）、碱中毒诱导（过度通气或静脉注射碳酸氢盐）和组胺输注。在心绞痛患者的评估中，不建议常规进行诱导冠状动脉血管痉挛的激发试验。

冠状动脉血管痉挛通常在使用硝酸甘油（舌下含服、静脉注射或动脉内注射）后迅速缓解。口服硝酸盐和钙通道阻滞剂的联合使用常用于预防血管痉挛。β 受体阻滞剂会抑制 β₂ 受体的血管舒张作用，使 α 受体诱导血管收缩的作用不受抑制，从而加重冠状动脉痉挛。极少数患者对血管扩张药物治疗无效，在易发生痉挛的动脉粥样硬化病变部位置入冠状动脉支架可能会使患者获益。

冠状动脉正常的微血管性心绞痛 部分患者即使冠状动脉影像学表现正常且无可诱发的血管痉挛，仍可能出现心绞痛。内皮依赖性血管舒张功能下降可能是微血管性心绞痛的潜在病理生理基础。这类患者可表现为冠状动脉阻力增加，并且，当心肌需氧量增加时，不能足够地增加冠状动脉血流量。女性更有可能患微血管性心绞痛，症状往往在休息或情绪应激时发作。运动也会引发心绞痛。

一系列诊断测试可用于检测微血管性心绞痛患者是否存在缺血。在负荷试验中，可以检测到 ST 段的缺血性改变以及核素灌注缺损，超声心动图可发现一过性室壁运动异常。更精细的有创检测，可发现负荷诱导的心肌缺血和内皮功能障碍导致的特征性代谢异常。

运动相关的缺血症状可能会对 β 受体阻滞剂治疗产生反应。微血管性心绞痛也往往对硝酸酯类药物反应良好，包括短效硝酸甘油舌下含服和长效口服硝酸盐。钙通道阻滞剂有时与硝酸酯类一起用于治疗微血管缺血相关的心绞痛。

无症状性心肌缺血 并非所有的心肌缺血事件都伴有心绞痛。有些患者可能仅为无症状性心肌缺血，在心电图监测中表现为一过性 ST 段压低。这类患者也可能出现无症状性心肌梗死。患者可能同时存在无症状心肌缺血发作和典型心绞痛，这种情况称为混合型心绞痛，且并不少见。无症状心肌缺血发作可见于所有类型的冠心病：慢性稳定型心绞痛、不稳定型心绞痛和冠状动脉痉挛。无症状性心肌缺血在糖尿病患者中更为常见。控制症状性心绞痛的药物治疗也能减少无症状性心肌缺血的发作次数。

预后

对于稳定性缺血性心脏病的现代治疗显著降低了心脏事件和死亡的风险。主要缺血事件（如心肌梗死）的年发生率介于 1% 至 2%，年死亡率则为 1% 至 3%。CAD 常常伴发全身性血管疾病，使这些患者容易发生其他一系列事件。患有稳定性缺血性心脏病的患者，每年发生心血管死亡、心肌梗死或卒中复合事件的风险约为 4.5%。

尽管药物和血运重建治疗取得了进展，高达 30% 的患者仍面临一些复发性限制生活的心绞痛症状。80% 的

Revascularization does not abolish the need for ongoing antianginal medical therapy in 80% of patients.

Patients with stable ischemic heart disease should first be treated with medical therapy appropriate to reduce the risk of ischemic events (aspirin, statins) and to control symptoms of angina (nitrates, β-blockers, calcium-channel antagonists). Revascularization therapy with either PCI or CABG is an option for patients who continue to have lifestyle-limiting symptoms despite the use of medical therapy and risk factor modification. The goal of all therapies for patients with stable ischemic heart disease should be individualized, taking advantage of information from controlled trials and directed at improving overall lifestyle and reducing the risk of death and disability due to progressive CAD or systemic vascular disease.

Acute Coronary Syndrome: Unstable Angina and NSTEMI

Definition

Asymptomatic CAD or chronic stable angina may undergo transition to a more aggressive stage of disease called acute coronary syndrome (ACS). ACS comprises a spectrum of clinical presentations, ranging from unstable angina to NSTEMI or STEMI. Unstable angina represents the new onset of angina at rest or on exertion, or an increase in frequency of previously stable anginal symptoms, particularly at rest. ACS manifesting as MI, either NSTEMI or STEMI, is differentiated from unstable angina on the basis of prolonged symptoms, characteristic ECG changes, and the presence of biomarkers in blood. Unstable angina may be a harbinger of either NSTEMI or STEMI, and the diagnosis of unstable angina identifies a patient who requires careful assessment and treatment.

Epidemiology

The occurrence of ACS represents a significant clinical event in up to 1.3 million Americans annually. One third of those categorized as having ACS are diagnosed with NSTEMI. More than half of patients with NSTEMI are 65 years of age or older, and approximately one half are women. NSTEMI is more common in patients with diabetes, peripheral vascular disease, or chronic inflammatory disease (e.g., rheumatoid arthritis).

Primary ACS is the most common form of the disease and reflects underlying plaque rupture leading to intracoronary thrombus formation and limitation of blood flow. This is in contrast to demand ischemia that reflects imbalances in myocardial oxygen supply and demand leading to myocardial ischemia. Examples of decreased oxygen supply include profound anemia, systemic hypotension, and hypoxemia. Increased demand occurs in the face of severe systemic hypertension, fever, tachycardia, and thyrotoxicosis. Demand ischemia not uncommonly unmasks previously asymptomatic obstructive CAD, but it may also occur in the absence of CAD. Treatment of demand ischemia is directed at correcting the underlying medical condition.

Pathology

Most patients who experience NSTEMI do so as a result of plaque rupture with subsequent thrombosis causing subtotal occlusion of the coronary artery. The limitation of coronary blood flow in this situation leads to subendocardial ischemia in the distribution of the affected coronary artery. The same pathology underlies STEMI, although in that case complete vessel occlusion occurs, leading to more extensive MI. It is possible for patients with obstructive CAD to develop collateral support of the affected artery, and in that case plaque rupture with complete vessel occlusion may lead to NSTEMI as opposed to STEMI.

A smaller percentage of patients have ACS due to coronary vasospasm, which, if severe and prolonged, can lead to myocardial necrosis. Vasospasm may occur in regions of endothelial dysfunction induced by atherosclerotic plaque, or it may be triggered by exogenous vasoconstrictors such as cocaine ingestion, the use of serotonin agonists (for migraine therapy), or chemotherapeutic agents (e.g., 5-fluorouracil). A less common cause of ACS is coronary vasculitis.

An alternative coronary artery pathology that can lead to MI is spontaneous coronary artery dissection (SCAD). Less is known about the underlying pathology of SCAD in contrast with MI due to plaque rupture, but its recognition is critical to appropriate treatment. SCAD has a predilection for a younger patient population with a strong bias toward females and is associated in particular with pregnancy and in patients with fibromuscular dysplasia. Rapid diagnosis can be challenging given that the patient population is one with few risk factors for CAD, and so a high index of suspicious is critical. Treatment differs from traditional MI in that a conservative approach is more often taken owing to increased complexity of percutaneous coronary intervention (PCI) on coronary dissection. Medical therapy for SCAD is similar to plaque rupture MI.

Atherosclerotic plaques rich in LDL are prone to develop inflammation, which in turn degrades the collagen-rich fibrous cap, leading to rupture and thrombosis as described previously. Systemic inflammatory conditions may also play a role in plaque rupture in some patients. It is possible to have multiple sites of plaque ulceration or rupture.

Plaque rupture leads to platelet adherence and subsequent activation at the site of rupture. As platelets aggregate, the thrombosis cascade is triggered, leading to progressive accumulation of intravascular thrombus. The severity of myocardial ischemia and MI depends on the degree to which thrombus occludes the vessel. It is also possible for ACS to occur as a result of embolization of platelet aggregates or thrombus.

Clinical Presentation

ACS may manifest as a first symptom of angina pectoris in a previously asymptomatic patient. Alternatively, patients with preexisting angina pectoris experience more frequent angina, angina at lower levels of exertion, or angina at rest. Patients who have developed ACS commonly experience their typical symptom of angina in terms of location and radiation but with increased intensity and duration. Patients with subtotal or total occlusion of a coronary artery may be much less responsive or completely unresponsive to the effects of nitroglycerin.

Physical examination during myocardial ischemia may reveal a patient who is clearly anxious and uncomfortable and who may also be experiencing dyspnea, nausea, or vomiting. Sinus tachycardia and hypertension is a common response to the discomfort of ACS, but in some instances sinus bradycardia and varying degrees of heart block may be observed. Bradyarrhythmias may also be associated with hypotension. Auscultation may reveal the presence of an S_4, reflecting diminished LV compliance, or an S_3 if there is extensive LV dysfunction. In the case of ischemia-induced papillary muscle dysfunction, the systolic murmur of mitral regurgitation can be heard. Patients with large areas of ischemic myocardium develop elevated LV filling pressures leading to pulmonary congestion, dyspnea, and the physical finding of rales on lung auscultation.

Diagnosis

Patients presenting with ACS require urgent care directed at rapid diagnosis and treatment. The ECG is critically important in early diagnosis of presumed ACS. The finding of ST elevation in multiple leads (Fig. 7.5) is diagnostic of STEMI and portends a more extensive MI

患者进行血运重建后仍需接受持续的抗心绞痛药物治疗。

稳定性缺血性心脏病患者应首先接受适当的药物治疗，以降低缺血性事件的风险（阿司匹林、他汀类药物），并控制心绞痛症状（硝酸酯类、β受体阻滞剂、钙通道阻滞剂）。如果患者在接受药物治疗和调整危险因素后仍有限制生活的不适症状，可以选择 PCI 或 CABG 进行血运重建。稳定性缺血性心脏病患者的治疗目标均应个体化制定；需充分参考临床对照试验的循证医学证据，致力于改善患者的整体生活方式，降低因冠心病或全身性血管病变进展而导致的死亡及致残风险。

急性冠脉综合征：不稳定型心绞痛和 NSTEMI

定义

无症状的 CAD 或慢性稳定型心绞痛可能转变为更加严重的疾病阶段，称为急性冠脉综合征（ACS）。急性冠脉综合征包括一系列临床表现，从不稳定型心绞痛到 NSTEMI 或 STEMI。不稳定型心绞痛是指新出现的静息或劳累时心绞痛，或者既往稳定的心绞痛症状发生频率增加，尤其是在静息时出现。表现为心肌梗死（NSTEMI 或 STEMI）的 ACS 可根据症状持续时间延长、特征性心电图变化和血液中生物标志物的升高而与不稳定型心绞痛相鉴别。不稳定型心绞痛可能是 NSTEMI 或 STEMI 的先兆，确诊不稳定型心绞痛需要仔细的评估和治疗。

流行病学

每年有多达 130 万美国人发生 ACS，这是一个重大的临床问题。在被归类为 ACS 的患者中，有 1/3 被诊断为 NSTEMI。一半以上的 NSTEMI 患者年龄在 65 岁及以上，约有一半是女性。NSTEMI 更常见于糖尿病、周围血管疾病或慢性炎症性疾病（如风湿性关节炎）患者。

原发性 ACS 是该病最常见的疾病形式，潜在的机制是斑块破裂导致冠状动脉内血栓形成和血流受限。这与血氧供需失衡型心肌缺血不同，血氧供需失衡型心肌缺血反映的是心肌供氧和需氧失衡导致心肌缺血。供氧减少的情况包括严重贫血、低血压和低氧血症。需氧增加可发生在严重的高血压、发热、心动过速和甲状腺毒症时。血氧供需失衡型心肌缺血通常能够揭示此前虽无症状但已存在的阻塞性 CAD。然而，即便不存在冠状动脉病变，同样可能发生此类心肌缺血。治疗血氧供需失衡型心肌缺血的关键是纠正潜在的病症。

病理学

大多数 NSTEMI 患者是由于斑块破裂，随后血栓形成导致冠状动脉次全闭塞。在这种情况下，冠状动脉血流受限导致受影响的冠状动脉供血区域发生心内膜下心肌缺血。STEMI 的病理机制相同，但在 STEMI 时血管完全闭塞，导致更广泛的心肌梗死。阻塞性 CAD 患者的受累动脉有可能出现侧支循环，在这种情况下，斑块破裂导致的血管完全闭塞可能表现为 NSTEMI，而不是 STEMI。

一小部分的 ACS 患者是由于冠状动脉血管痉挛引起的，如果痉挛严重且持续时间长，可导致心肌坏死。冠脉痉挛可以发生在动脉粥样硬化斑块部位，是该部位的动脉粥样硬化导致的内皮功能障碍所致；冠脉痉挛也可能由外源性血管收缩剂引发，如摄入可卡因、使用血清素激动剂（用于偏头痛治疗）或化疗药物（如 5-氟尿嘧啶）。冠状动脉血管炎是导致 ACS 的一个更少见原因。

可导致心肌梗死的另一种冠状动脉病变是自发性冠状动脉夹层（SCAD）。与斑块破裂导致的心肌梗死相比，人们对 SCAD 的潜在病理生理机制知之甚少，而这些认知对于合理地治疗 SCAD 至关重要。SCAD 的发病人群偏向于年轻患者，且女性患者居多，尤其与妊娠和患有纤维肌性发育不良相关。由于这类患者人群中的 CAD 危险因素较少，快速诊断可能具有挑战性，因此高度警惕是至关重要的。治疗不同于传统的心肌梗死，由于 PCI 在冠状动脉夹层患者中的手术复杂性增加，所以通常会采用保守方法。SCAD 的药物治疗与斑块破裂引起的心肌梗死相似。

富含低密度脂蛋白的动脉粥样硬化斑块容易发生炎症，这反过来又会降解富含胶原蛋白的纤维帽，导致斑块破裂和血栓形成。全身性炎症也可能在某些患者的斑块破裂中起作用。斑块溃疡或破裂有可能发生在多个部位。

斑块破裂导致血小板在破裂部位附着并随后激活。随着血小板聚集，触发了血栓形成级联反应，导致血管内血栓的逐渐堆积。心肌缺血和心肌梗死的严重程度取决于血栓堵塞血管的程度。此外，血小板聚集物或血栓导致的栓塞也可能引起 ACS。

临床表现

急性冠脉综合征的首发症状可能表现为先前无症状的患者出现心绞痛。或者，原有心绞痛的患者会出现更频繁的心绞痛、在较低强度的劳累时出现心绞痛或在静息时出现心绞痛。发生 ACS 的患者通常会在胸痛位置和放射部位出现典型的心绞痛症状，但强度和持续时间有所增加。冠状动脉次全闭塞或完全闭塞的患者对硝酸甘油的治疗反应较弱或完全无反应。

心肌缺血时的体格检查可能会发现患者明显感到焦虑和不适，还可能有呼吸困难、恶心或呕吐。窦性心动过速和高血压是对 ACS 引起的不适的常见反应，但在某些情况下，也会出现窦性心动过缓和不同程度的心脏传导阻滞；缓慢性心律失常还可能伴有低血压。听诊可发现第四心音，反映出左心室顺应性减弱。如果存在严重的左心室功能障碍，则会出现第三心音。在缺血诱发乳头肌功能障碍的情况下，会出现二尖瓣反流引起的收缩期杂音。大面积心肌缺血的患者会出现左心室充盈压升高导致肺淤血、呼吸困难，肺部听诊可发现啰音。

诊断

出现 ACS 的患者需要紧急处理，以快速诊断和治疗。心电图对于早期诊断 ACS 至关重要。多导联 ST 段抬高（图 7.5）是 STEMI 的诊断依据，预示着心肌

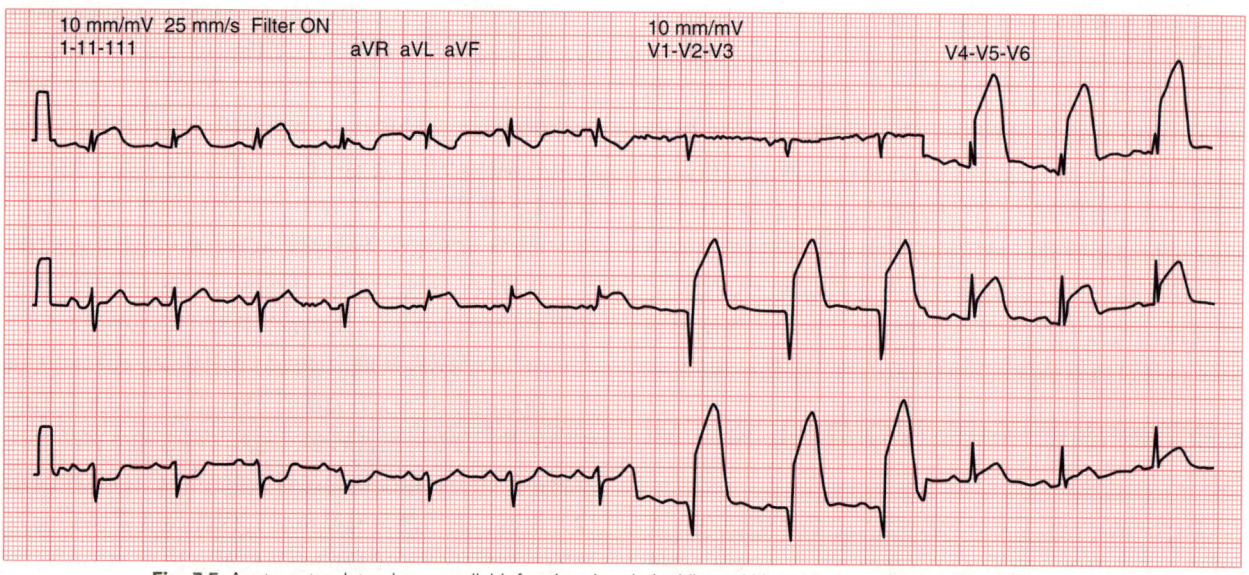

Fig. 7.5 Acute anterolateral myocardial infarction. Leads I, aVL, and V_2 to V_6 demonstrate ST-segment elevation. Reciprocal ST-segment depression is seen in leads II, III, and aVF. Deep Q waves have developed in leads V_2 and V_3.

and the need for prompt revascularization. The distribution of ST elevation reflects the region of myocardium affected by thrombotic coronary occlusion. For example, ST elevation in leads II, III, and aVF reflects an inferior MI due to occlusion of the right coronary artery (or circumflex coronary artery in some cases). ST elevation in leads V_2 through V_6 (see Fig. 7.5) reflects an anterior MI caused by obstruction of the left anterior descending coronary artery.

Unstable angina or NSTEMI is caused by subtotal vessel occlusion by thrombus leading to reduced coronary blood flow. This results in subendocardial ischemia and the characteristic ECG changes of ST depression (Fig. 7.6). It is important to recognize that up to half of patients with acute MI do not have significant ECG abnormalities on the initial study. Sequential ECGs are frequently required to establish a diagnosis. If there is a high index of suspicion for MI and ECGs are persistently nondiagnostic, the use of leads extending to the patient's back (V_7 to V_9) may demonstrate ST changes related to posterior LV ischemia (usually a circumflex coronary artery occlusion). Echocardiography showing regional wall motion abnormalities can also help to establish the diagnosis of acute MI.

Serum biomarkers also play an important role in the diagnosis of acute MI. Myocardial necrosis leads to the release of biomarkers that can be measured in serial fashion to document the occurrence of MI. The presence of specific biomarkers is definitive evidence of MI, and they are particularly helpful to provide prognostic significance when symptoms are mild and ECG changes are minimal. Common biomarkers include creatine kinase (CK), troponin I, troponin T, lactate dehydrogenase (LDH), and aspartate aminotransferase (AST). Sequential measurement of biomarkers demonstrates their various time courses for abnormal elevation after an acute MI (Fig. 7.7). This information can be helpful in retrospectively timing the occurrence of an event. In contemporary practice, troponin has become the most frequently measured biomarker. LDH, CK, and AST are no longer routinely measured for the diagnosis of MI. Some centers are adopting the "high-sensitivity troponin," which can detect more subtle degrees of myocardial injury than its predecessors. In principle this allows for more rapid triaging of patients presenting with chest pain while maintaining high sensitivity as the test will pick up on troponin release very early in the course of ACS.

Troponins I and T are the most sensitive and most specific markers of myocardial necrosis, and as a consequence, they have become the standard in the biochemical diagnosis of acute MI. The myocardial-specific isozyme CK-MB may be in the normal range while concomitant measurement of troponin I or T reveals the presence of myocardial necrosis. Troponins I and T begin to rise within 4 hours of myocardial necrosis and remain elevated for 7 to 10 days after the MI event. Confounding elevations of troponin T occur in patients with renal failure and congestive heart failure not related to ACS. Troponin release also occurs in the case of demand ischemia not related to coronary thrombosis. This requires careful attention to the entire clinical presentation in discerning the likelihood of underlying ACS due to coronary thrombosis.

In the absence of clear evidence of NSTEMI (i.e., normal examination, ECG findings, and biomarkers), patients who present with the diagnosis of unstable angina should undergo stress testing. A negative exercise stress test is very helpful for distinguishing those patients who require more aggressive diagnostic testing (e.g., catheterization) from those who can be monitored as outpatients. Some centers have embraced the use of CT coronary angiography in the assessment of low-risk patients. This technique has a high negative predictive value for ACS by demonstrating the absence of obstructive CAD.

Echocardiography can be helpful in patients with equivocal ECG findings for ischemia and normal biomarkers. The presence of regional wall motion abnormalities, particularly if they correlate with the distribution of ECG abnormalities, raises the risk for underlying CAD as a cause of symptoms. The echocardiogram may also show evidence of other abnormalities as causes of chest discomfort, such as pericarditis, pulmonary embolism, or aortic dissection.

Patients with a high risk for future coronary events should be directed toward coronary angiography. In the absence of contraindications, coronary angiography is indicated for patients with clear evidence of NSTEMI based on clinical presentation of symptoms, ECG changes, and positive biomarkers. Patients undergoing evaluation for unstable angina who have significant stress test abnormalities are also candidates for coronary angiography. Some patients who have ambiguous stress test findings or ongoing symptoms in the absence of other

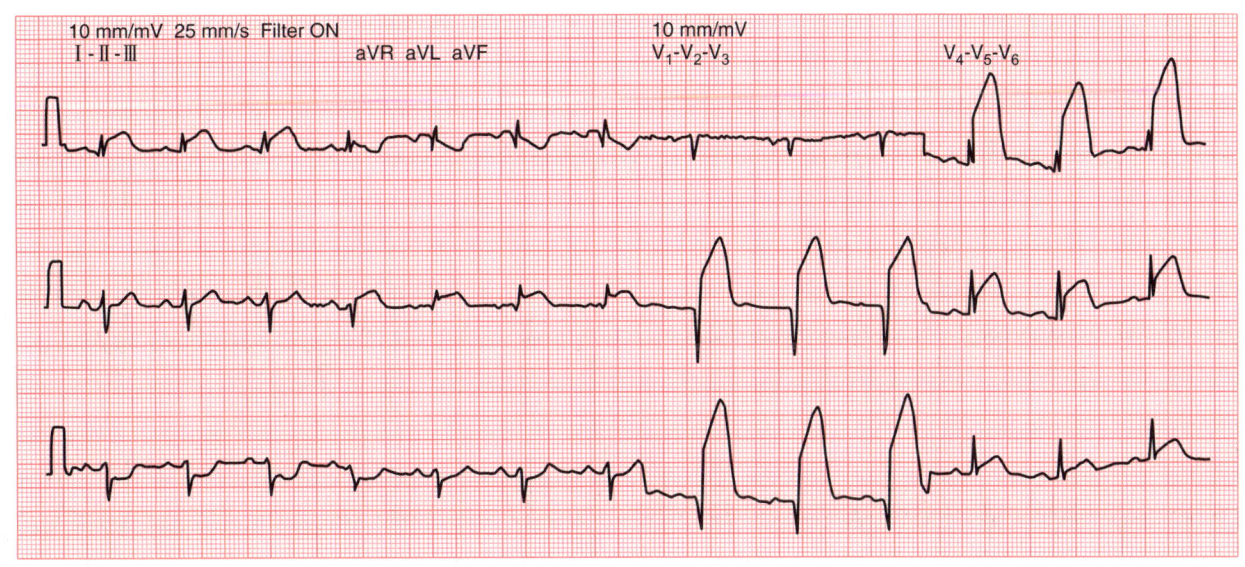

图 7.5 急性前侧壁心肌梗死。Ⅰ、aVL 和 V$_2$～V$_6$ 导联 ST 段抬高。（原文有Ⅱ）Ⅲ和 aVF 导联出现镜像性 ST 段压低。V$_2$ 和 V$_3$ 导联出现深 Q 波

梗死的范围较大，需要即刻进行血运重建。ST 段抬高的导联分布反映了血栓导致的冠状动脉闭塞影响的心肌缺血区域。例如，Ⅱ、Ⅲ和 aVF 导联的 ST 段抬高反映了右冠状动脉（或在某些情况下为回旋支）闭塞导致的下壁心肌梗死。V$_2$～V$_6$ 导联（见图 7.5）ST 段抬高反映左前降支冠状动脉阻塞导致的前壁心肌梗死。

不稳定型心绞痛或 NSTEMI 是由于血栓引起的血管次全闭塞，造成冠状动脉血流减少而引起的。这导致心内膜下缺血和心电图特征性 ST 段压低改变（图 7.6）。重要的是，多达一半的急性心肌梗死患者在初次检查时没有明显的心电图异常。通常需要连续的心电图检查来确定诊断。如果高度怀疑心肌梗死而心电图持续无诊断意义，患者背部导联（V$_7$～V$_9$）的心电图可能会显示与左心室后壁缺血（通常是回旋支闭塞）相关的 ST 段改变。超声心动图显示节段性室壁运动异常也有助于确定急性心肌梗死的诊断。

血清生物标志物在急性心肌梗死的诊断中也发挥着重要作用。心肌坏死会导致生物标志物的释放，通过连续测量这些生物标志物可以明确心肌梗死的发生。特定生物标志物的出现是心肌梗死的确凿证据，尤其是在症状轻微、心电图变化很小的情况下，生物标志物更有助于判断预后。常见的生物标志物包括肌酸激酶（CK）、肌钙蛋白 I、肌钙蛋白 T、乳酸脱氢酶（LDH）和天冬氨酸转氨酶（AST）。通过对生物标志物的连续监测会显示出急性心肌梗死后不同生物标志物异常升高具有不同时程（图 7.7）。这些信息有助于回溯事件发生的时间。在当代实践中，肌钙蛋白已成为最常用的生物标志物。LDH、CK 和 AST 不再是诊断 MI 的常规指标。一些中心正在使用"高敏肌钙蛋白"，它比肌钙蛋白能检测到更微小程度的心肌损伤。因为该检测在 ACS 的早期就可发现肌钙蛋白的升高，并具有高度敏感性，原则上，这就可以更快速地对胸痛患者进行分流。

肌钙蛋白 I 和 T 是心肌坏死最敏感和最特异的标志物，因此已成为急性心肌梗死生化诊断的标准。可能在心肌特异性同工酶 CK-MB 还处于正常范围时，同时测量的肌钙蛋白 I 或 T 即提示心肌坏死的存在。肌钙蛋白 I 和 T 在心肌坏死后 4 h 内开始升高，并持续至心肌梗死发生后 7～10 天。肾衰竭和非 ACS 导致的充血性心力衰竭患者也会出现肌钙蛋白 T 的升高，这有时会造成误导。与冠状动脉血栓形成无关的血氧供需失衡型心肌缺血也会导致肌钙蛋白升高，这就需要关注患者整体的临床表现，以与因冠状动脉血栓形成而导致的 ACS 相区别。

如果没有 NSTEMI 的明确证据（即检查、心电图结果和生物标志物正常），被诊断为不稳定型心绞痛的患者应接受运动负荷试验。运动负荷试验阴性非常有助于区分哪些患者需要进行更积极的诊断性检查（如心导管检查）、哪些患者可以在门诊定期复查。一些中心已开始使用冠状动脉 CTA 对低风险患者进行评估。当 CT 未发现冠状动脉阻塞性病变时，对 ACS 具有很高的阴性预测价值。

对于心电图心肌缺血证据不明确、生物标志物正常的患者，超声心动图检查可能会有所帮助。出现节段性室壁运动异常，尤其部位与心电图异常的分布区域一致时，提示不适症状为 CAD 引起的可能性增加。超声心动图还可能发现导致胸部不适的其他异常证据，如心包炎、肺栓塞或主动脉夹层。

未来发生冠脉事件风险较高的患者应接受冠状动脉造影检查。在没有禁忌证的情况下，冠状动脉造影适用于有明确 NSTEMI 证据的患者，包括临床表现、心电图变化和阳性的生物标志物。不稳定型心绞痛患者如果运动负荷试验明显异常，也有指征进行冠状动脉造影检查。有些患者的运动负荷试验结果不明确，或者没有发现其他 NSTEMI 的证据但症状仍

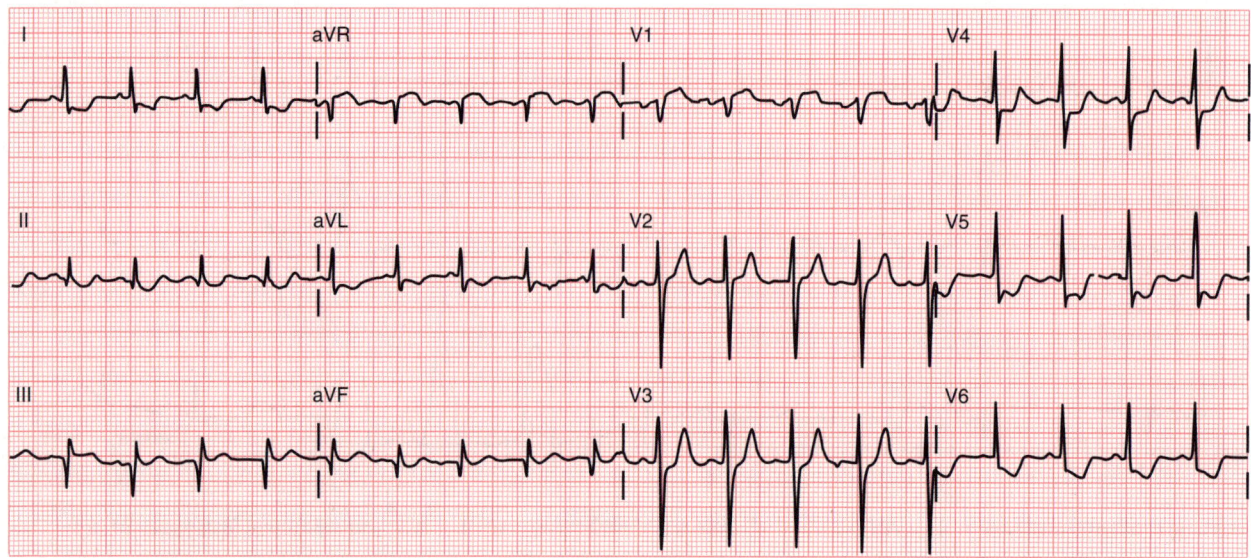

Fig. 7.6 Marked ST-segment depression in a patient with prolonged chest pain resulting from an acute non–ST segment elevation myocardial infarction. Between 1 and 3 mm of ST-segment depression is seen in leads I, aVL, and V_4 to V_6. The patient was known to have had a previous inferior myocardial infarction.

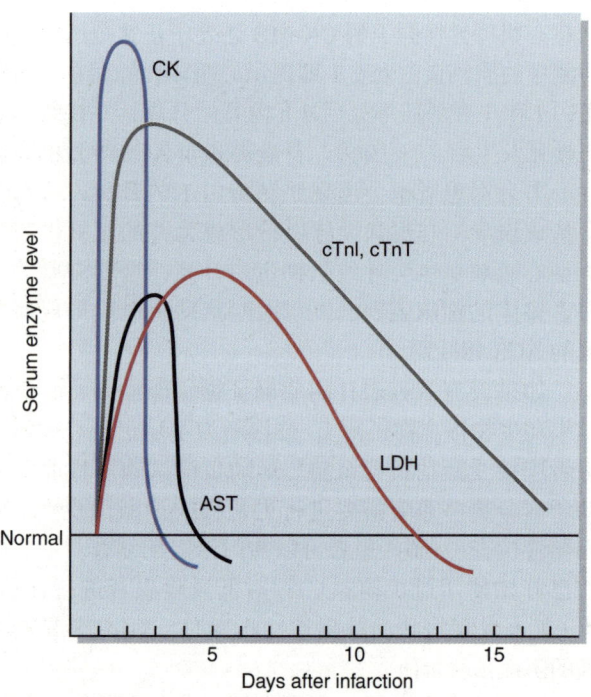

Fig. 7.7 Typical time course for the detection of enzymes released after myocardial infarction. *AST,* Serum aspartate aminotransferase; *CK,* creatine kinase; *cTnI,* cardiac troponin I; *cTnT,* cardiac troponin T; *LDH,* lactate dehydrogenase.

findings of NSTEMI require coronary angiography to resolve the issue as to whether underlying CAD is present.

Up to 15% of patients undergoing coronary angiography for NSTEMI have no significant obstructive CAD. In a number of patients, there will be a clear "culprit" lesion showing the earmarks of plaque rupture with ulceration, associated thrombus, or reduced coronary flow. Lesions that may have played a role in symptoms, ECG findings, or biomarker release that are not clearly stenotic may be assessed for physiologic significance with the use of a fractional flow reserve (FFR) study using a pressure wire device.

Patients who have new-onset chest pain require careful monitoring in an appropriate care setting that allows for rhythm monitoring as well as repeat evaluations of ECG findings and biomarker measurements. Risk assessment is aided by the use of risk scores calculated with either the Thrombolysis in Myocardial Infarction (TIMI) or the Global Registry of Acute Coronary Events (GRACE) algorithms (see Chapter 63, "Acute Coronary Syndrome: Unstable Angina and Non-ST Elevation Myocardial Infarction," in *Goldman-Cecil Medicine,* 26th Edition). The overall assessment in cases of new symptoms of chest discomfort aims to triage patients based on risk for coronary events. Low-risk patients can be spared aggressive anticoagulation protocols and coronary angiography, whereas high-risk patients are likely to benefit from these approaches. The use of appropriate therapies in high-risk patients (medical therapy or revascularization or both) leads to a 20% to 40% decrease in recurrent ischemic events and a 10% reduction in mortality.

Differential Diagnosis

The initial assessment of patients with possible ACS should include consideration of other potentially life-threatening conditions such as pulmonary embolism and aortic dissection. These considerations are particularly important if the patient's presentation does not entirely fit that of ACS. Pulmonary embolism can be associated with ECG changes and troponin elevation, and such findings lead to early use of coronary angiography. If there is no CAD-related explanation of the patient's presentation, prompt investigation for pulmonary embolism is warranted. If the patient has findings suggestive of aortic dissection, that diagnosis should be aggressively pursued with appropriate imaging techniques, given the high risk of mortality associated with that disease. Valvular heart diseases such as aortic stenosis or regurgitation and hypertrophic cardiomyopathy can manifest with symptoms and ECG findings suggestive of ACS. Physical examination should aid in

波士顿大学医院

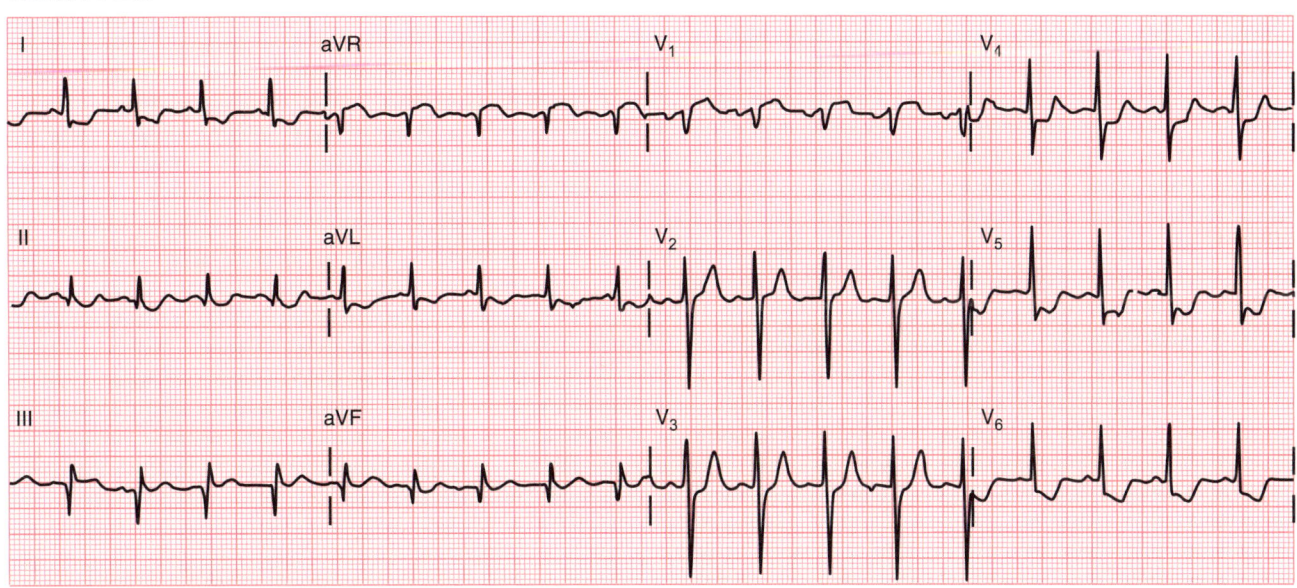

图 7.6 因急性非 ST 段抬高型心肌梗死导致长时间胸痛的患者，可见明显的 ST 段压低。在 Ⅰ、aVL 和 V_4～V_6 导联可见 1～3 mm 的 ST 段压低。患者既往曾发生过下壁心肌梗死

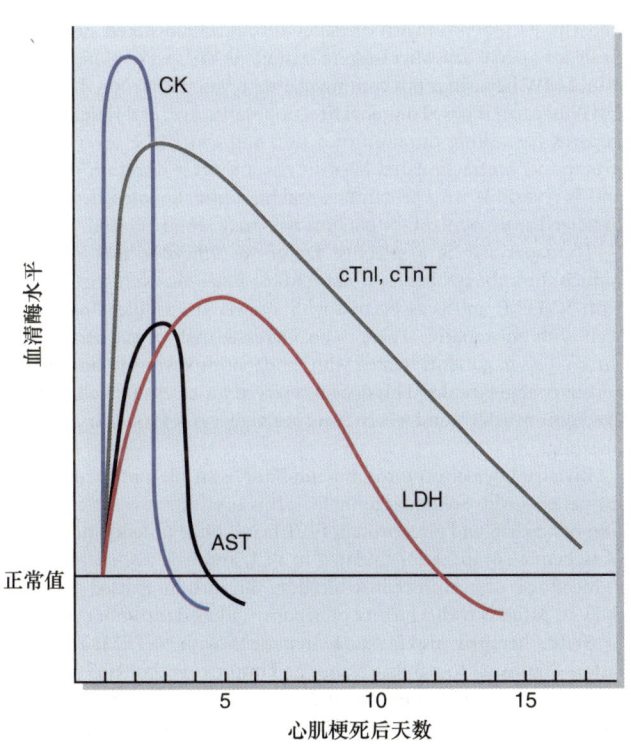

图 7.7 心肌梗死后心肌酶释放的典型时程图。AST：血清天冬氨酸转氨酶；CK：肌酸肌酶；cTnI：心肌肌钙蛋白 I；cTnT：心肌肌钙蛋白 T；LDH：乳酸脱氢酶

持续，也需要进行冠状动脉造影，以确定是否存在潜在的 CAD。

在因 NSTEMI 而接受冠状动脉造影的患者中，多达 15% 的患者没有明显的阻塞性 CAD。在一些患者中，会有一个明显的"罪犯"病变，显示出斑块破裂、溃疡的征兆，伴有血栓形成或冠状动脉血流减少。对于症状、心电图检查结果或生物标志物升高，没法确定是由冠状动脉狭窄引起的时，可以使用压力导丝进行血流储备分数（FFR）检测，以评估其生理意义。

新发胸痛患者需要在适当的病房中接受监测，以便进行心律监测以及反复进行心电图和生物标志物检测。使用 TIMI（Thrombolysis in Myocardial Infarction）评分或 GRACE（Global Registry of Acute Coronary Events）评分可帮助进行风险评估（参见 Goldman-Cecil Medicine 第 26 版第 63 章"急性冠脉综合征：不稳定型心绞痛和非 ST 段抬高型心肌梗死"）。在新出现胸部不适症状时，整体评估的目的是根据患者发生冠状动脉事件的风险对患者进行分级。低风险患者无须接受积极的抗凝治疗和冠状动脉造影，而高风险患者则有可能从中获益。对高风险患者采用适当的治疗方法（药物治疗或血运重建或两者兼用）可使再发缺血事件减少 20%～40%，死亡率降低 10%。

鉴别诊断

对疑诊 ACS 的患者进行初步评估时，应考虑其他可能危及生命的疾病，如肺栓塞和主动脉夹层。如果患者的表现并不完全符合 ACS，这些鉴别就尤为重要。肺栓塞可能发生心电图变化和肌钙蛋白升高，这种发现往往需要尽早行冠状动脉造影以明确。如果患者的表现不能用 CAD 解释，则应立即进行肺栓塞筛查。如果患者的检查结果提示主动脉夹层，考虑到该疾病的高致死风险，应积极使用适当的影像学技术进行诊断。心脏瓣膜病如主动脉瓣狭窄或反流以及肥厚型心肌病的症状和心电图表现均可与 ACS 类似，应针对这些疾病进行体格检查。心包炎和心肌心包炎也会出现胸

consideration of these conditions. Pericarditis and myopericarditis can also present diagnostic dilemmas related to chest pain, ECG abnormalities (ST and T wave changes mimicking ischemia), and positive biomarkers. Stress cardiomyopathy (takotsubo syndrome) also manifests with chest pain, T wave inversion, and positive biomarkers. Patients with this diagnosis frequently undergo urgent catheterization to assess for CAD. The absence of a culprit lesion and findings of characteristic wall motion abnormalities establish the diagnosis.

Treatment

Patients with chest pain suggestive of ACS need urgent evaluation for evidence of ischemia (serial ECGs) and myocardial necrosis (serial biomarkers). Serial biomarker measurements, in the current era usually troponin, establish the diagnosis of MI. Continuous ECG monitoring is important given the risk of ischemia-mediated arrhythmias, and serial ECGs establish a pattern of ST changes consistent with ischemia. Patients are also placed on activity limitations up to and including bedrest for patients with particularly difficult to control angina. Supplemental oxygen is provided to patients who are hypoxemic, but routine administration of supplemental oxygen to patients with ACS has not been shown to provide any benefit. Those with a high index of suspicion for ACS require hospital admission for observation and appropriate diagnostic testing. Chest pain lends itself well to diagnosis and treatment algorithms that guide the clinician through decision trees based on expert opinion and evidence-based medicine (see Chapter 63, "Acute Coronary Syndrome: Unstable Angina and Non-ST Elevation Myocardial Infarction," in *Goldman-Cecil Medicine*, ❖ 26th Edition). STEMI is typically diagnosed at the time of initial presentation. Those without evidence of ST elevation can be risk stratified, as discussed earlier, using the guidance of recurrent symptoms, ECG changes, or abnormal biomarker levels. Treatment of patients who are categorized as having unstable angina or NSTEMI is directed by their allocation to either low- or high-risk status.

Once recognized as having ACS, patients require antiplatelet therapy because plaque rupture and thrombosis is a frequent underlying pathology, and antiplatelet therapy significantly reduces mortality risk in patients with NSTEMI. Patients should be given aspirin (75 to 162 mg per day) and a P2Y12 inhibitor (either clopidogrel or ticagrelor). Given prasugrel and ticagrelor's increased strength and rapidity of platelet inhibition compared to clopidogrel they are favored in the ACS setting. Note that prasugrel is reserved for patients undergoing PCI and is contraindicated in patients with a history of stroke or transient ischemic attack.

The use of these more potent antiplatelet agents must be weighed against an increased risk of bleeding that accompanies this effect. The aspirin/P2Y12 inhibitor combination is indicated as ongoing therapy in the year following diagnosis of NSTEMI.

Symptoms of chest discomfort can be treated with nitrates (sublingual, topical, or intravenous drip) and β-blockers. The latter therapy slows heart rate and reduces blood pressure, effects that translate into reduced myocardial oxygen demand in the face of limited supply. It is important not to give nitrates to patients who have taken phosphodiesterase-5 inhibitors (sildenafil, tadalafil, or vardenafil) within the previous 24 to 48 hours. Attention to this detail minimizes the risk for nitrate-induced hypotension. Calcium-channel antagonists may be used in lieu of β-blockers, particularly if there is a need for blood pressure control, but they should be avoided in patients with reduced EF or overt heart failure. The dihydropyridine calcium-channel blocker nifedipine can be effective in controlling blood pressure and promoting coronary vasodilation, but it should be given in conjunction with a β-blocker because of the potential for the drug to induce reflex tachycardia and thereby increase myocardial oxygen demand.

Glycoprotein IIb/IIIa inhibitors block platelet aggregation and can reduce ischemic events in patients undergoing PCI as treatment for NSTEMI. These drugs are usually reserved for high-risk patients at the time of PCI. They require intravenous administration and are given for 12 to 24 hours after PCI. The use of this class of drugs for PCI has decreased in light of data suggesting advantages of bivalirudin, a direct thrombin inhibitor, over the glycoprotein IIb/IIIa inhibitors.

Heparin, given in its unfractionated form or as a low-molecular-weight (LMW) preparation, has been shown to reduce the risk of ischemic complications in patients with NSTEMI. Heparin acts by activating antithrombin and thereby inhibiting the formation and activity of thrombin. The anti-ischemic effect of heparin is additive to that of aspirin. Unfractionated heparin is given by continuous intravenous drip for up to 48 hours. It is usually not continued after revascularization. Heparin may be associated with mild thrombocytopenia, and 1% to 5% of patients experience profound antibody-mediated thrombocytopenia. These patients usually have been exposed to heparin in the past, and a known diagnosis of heparin-induced thrombocytopenia necessitates the use of alternative antithrombin therapy.

LMW heparins are fragments of unfractionated heparin that are more predictable in their antithrombin activity and are associated with reduced risks for thrombocytopenia and bleeding complications. The drug should be avoided in patients who have a history of heparin-induced thrombocytopenia. Clinical studies of patients with NSTEMI have shown superiority of LMW heparin over unfractionated heparin in reducing the end point of death or MI during hospitalization. LMW heparin, either enoxaparin or dalteparin, is administered subcutaneously for up to 8 days after hospitalization. As with unfractionated heparin, LMW heparin is not continued after revascularization. Dosing of LMW heparin is based on renal function status, age, and weight. LMW heparin has a long duration of action and cannot be reversed with protamine. Unfractionated heparin has a shorter duration of action and is reversible with protamine, making unfractionated heparin the preferred anticoagulant for patients who may require CABG.

Fondaparinux is a selective factor Xa inhibitor that does not induce thrombocytopenia. It can reduce ischemic events in patients with NSTEMI and is associated with a lower risk of bleeding than is seen with enoxaparin. There is an increased risk of catheter-related thrombosis in patients treated with fondaparinux who are undergoing coronary angiography. This drug is reserved for cases that will be managed noninvasively and where there is a higher risk for heparin-related bleeding.

Bivalirudin, a direct thrombin inhibitor, is an alternative to heparin for patients who are undergoing PCI. It is as effective as the combination of heparin and glycoprotein IIb/IIIa inhibitor in reducing the risk of ischemic complications related to PCI, and it is associated with a reduced risk of postprocedure bleeding. Bivalirudin is used preferentially in patients with a history of heparin-induced thrombocytopenia.

Statin therapy is also indicated in patients with NSTEMI at presentation. Statins act to stabilize plaque and improve endothelial function. These drugs should be initiated at the time of admission to the hospital and continued after discharge. There is evidence that high-dose atorvastatin (80 mg/day) given to patients with NSTEMI reduces the risk of subsequent ischemic events.

Risk stratification is important in appropriately evaluating patients with ACS. Low-risk patients (age <75 years, normal troponin levels, 0 to 2 TIMI risk factors) should be evaluated with noninvasive testing, either exercise or pharmacologic stress testing before hospital discharge. Those whose tests are positive for ischemia should be considered for predischarge coronary angiography. This approach leads to selective use of invasive testing and subsequent revascularization. Patients with high-risk ACS profiles (age >75 years, elevated troponin

痛、心电图异常（类似心肌缺血的 ST 段和 T 波变化）和生物标志物阳性，导致诊断困难。应激性心肌病（Takotsubo 综合征）也表现为胸痛、T 波倒置和生物标志物阳性，此类患者通常需要进行紧急的心导管检查，以评估是否存在 CAD。如果没有发现罪犯病变且表现出特征性室壁运动异常，即可确诊。

治疗

出现胸痛怀疑 ACS 的患者需要紧急评估心肌缺血（连续心电图）和心肌坏死（连续生物标志物）的证据。连续生物标志物检测（在当今时代通常是肌钙蛋白）可确定心肌梗死的诊断。鉴于心肌缺血导致心律失常的风险，连续心电监测非常重要，连续心电图检查可确定与心肌缺血一致的 ST 段变化。对于难以控制的心绞痛患者，还要限制其活动，甚至卧床休息。低氧血症患者需要吸氧治疗，但常规吸氧对 ACS 患者并无益处。对于高度怀疑 ACS 的患者需要入院观察并进行适当的诊断检查。胸痛需要根据专家意见和循证医学的证据，通过决策树的方式指导医生进行诊断和治疗（参见 Goldman-Cecil Medicine 第 26 版第 63 章，"急性冠脉综合征：不稳定型心绞痛和非 ST 段抬高型心肌梗死"）。STEMI 通常在初次就诊时即可确诊。对于没有 ST 段抬高证据的患者，可以依据反复的胸痛症状、心电图变化或异常生物标志物水平进行风险分层，如前所述。对被归类为不稳定型心绞痛或 NSTEMI 的患者，其治疗应根据风险分层来决定。

ACS 患者一旦确诊就需要接受抗血小板治疗，因为斑块破裂和血栓形成是常见的病理基础，抗血小板治疗可显著降低 NSTEMI 患者的死亡风险。患者可服用阿司匹林（75～162 mg/d）和 P2Y12 抑制剂（氯吡格雷或替格瑞洛）。与氯吡格雷相比，普拉格雷和替格瑞洛的血小板抑制作用更强、更快，因此更适用于 ACS。需要注意的是，普拉格雷仅推荐用于接受介入治疗的 ACS 患者（换句话说，不推荐普拉格雷用于不接受介入治疗的 ACS 患者），有卒中或一过性脑缺血发作病史的患者禁用。

在使用这些药效更强的抗血小板药物时，必须权衡继发的出血风险。NSTEMI 诊断后 1 年内，适合进行阿司匹林/P2Y12 抑制剂的联合治疗。

胸部不适症状可通过硝酸盐（舌下含服、局部使用或静脉滴注）和 β 受体阻滞剂来治疗。后者可减慢心率和降低血压，从而在血氧供应有限的情况下减少心肌对血氧的需求。重要的是，使用磷酸二酯酶-5 抑制剂（西地那非、他达拉非或伐地那非）后的 24～48 h 内避免使用硝酸盐类药物，这样可以减少硝酸盐诱发低血压的风险。钙通道阻滞剂可以代替 β 受体阻滞剂，尤其是在需要控制血压的情况下。但对于 EF 值降低或有明显心力衰竭的患者，应避免使用钙通道阻滞剂。二氢吡啶类钙通道阻滞剂硝苯地平可有效控制血压并促进冠状动脉血管扩张，但应与 β 受体阻滞剂同时使用，因为该药可能反射性诱发心动过速，从而增加心肌需氧量。

糖蛋白 IIb/IIIa 抑制剂可阻断血小板聚集，减少接受 PCI 治疗的 NSTEMI 患者缺血性事件的发生。这些药物通常用于高风险患者接受 PCI 治疗时；需静脉注射，并在 PCI 后 12～24 h 内使用。鉴于有数据表明比伐卢定（一种直接凝血酶抑制剂）比糖蛋白 IIb/IIIa 抑制剂更有优势，PCI 中这类药物的使用有所减少。

肝素，无论是普通肝素或低分子量（LMW）肝素，已被证明可以降低 NSTEMI 患者发生缺血性并发症的风险。肝素的作用是激活抗凝血酶，从而抑制凝血酶的形成和活性。肝素的抗缺血效应与阿司匹林的效应具有叠加作用。普通肝素可持续静脉滴注长达 48 h，血运重建术后通常不再继续使用。肝素可能会导致轻度血小板减少，1%～5% 的患者会出现抗体介导的严重血小板减少。这些患者过去通常使用过肝素，如果已知确诊为肝素诱导的血小板减少症，就必须使用其他抗凝血酶疗法。

LMW 肝素是普通肝素的片段，其抗血栓活性更易预测，可降低血小板减少和出血并发症的风险。有肝素诱导血小板减少症病史的患者应避免使用该药物。对 NSTEMI 患者进行的临床研究显示，在降低住院期间死亡或心肌梗死终点方面，LMW 肝素优于普通肝素。LMW 肝素（如依诺肝素或达肝素）以皮下注射的方式在住院后使用，最长可达 8 天。与普通肝素一样，LMW 肝素在血运重建后不再继续使用。LMW 肝素的剂量取决于肾功能状况、年龄和体重。LMW 肝素的作用时间较长，不能用鱼精蛋白逆转。普通肝素的作用持续时间较短，并且可用鱼精蛋白逆转，因此普通肝素是可能需要接受 CABG 治疗患者的首选抗凝剂。

磺达肝癸钠是一种选择性 Xa 因子抑制剂，不会诱发血小板减少。它可以减少 NSTEMI 患者的缺血性事件，出血风险低于依诺肝素。进行冠状动脉造影的患者使用磺达肝癸钠时发生导管相关血栓的风险会增加。这种药物适用于非侵入性治疗，且肝素相关出血风险较高的病例。

比伐卢定是一种直接的凝血酶抑制剂，是患者接受 PCI 治疗时肝素的替代品。在降低 PCI 相关缺血性并发症的风险方面，它与肝素和糖蛋白 IIb/IIIa 抑制剂联用的效果相当，而且还能降低术后出血的风险。有肝素诱导的血小板减少症病史的患者优先使用比伐卢定。

他汀类药物治疗也适用于 NSTEMI 的患者。他汀类药物具有稳定斑块和改善内皮功能的作用。这些药物应在入院时开始使用，并在出院后继续使用。有证据表明，给予 NSTEMI 患者大剂量阿托伐他汀（80 mg/d）可降低后续发生缺血性事件的风险。

对 ACS 患者进行风险分层非常重要。低风险患者（年龄＜75 岁、肌钙蛋白水平正常、TIMI 危险因素为 0～2 个）应在出院前接受无创检测，包括运动或药物负荷试验。对于检测结果呈缺血阳性的患者，应考虑在出院前进行冠状动脉造影。这样可以选择性地进行有创检查，同时根据需要进行血运重建。高风险 ACS 患者（年龄＞75 岁、肌钙蛋白水平升高、TIMI 危险因

levels, ≥3 TIMI risk factors) are candidates for coronary angiography and, when appropriate, revascularization. The high-risk ACS patient group will have fewer subsequent ischemic events when approached in this way. Risk stratification occurs early after admission for possible ACS. An early invasive strategy (coronary angiography within 24 hours of admission) for high-risk patients has been shown to reduce the combined end point of death, MI, or stroke compared with a delayed invasive approach. The occurrence of acute heart failure, hypotension, or ventricular arrhythmias in the face of ACS prompts urgent coronary angiography to identify patients with high-risk coronary anatomy that requires urgent revascularization (see video, Cardiac Cath, http://www.heartsite.com/html/cardiac_cath.html).

Invasive coronary angiography always carries with it a risk of bleeding complications that is no doubt enhanced by the concomitant use of potent antiplatelet and antithrombin therapies. Those at increased risk for bleeding complications include patients with female gender, low body weight, diabetes mellitus, renal insufficiency, low hematocrit, and hypertension. The risks of bleeding as well as vascular complications are lower via radial artery catheterization compared to a femoral artery approach at the cost of some increased difficulty in catheter manipulation. Utilization of a radial approach is becoming more commonplace and has become the preferred method of access for a large number of interventional cardiologists.

Prognosis

The extent and magnitude of ST depression noted on ECG in patients with NSTEMI predicts mortality risk. Patients who exhibit 2 mm or more of ST depression in multiple leads have a 10-fold increased mortality rate at 1 year. The degree of elevation in troponin also identifies patients with an increased risk of mortality during the following year. It has also been observed that the combined measurement of troponin, hsCRP, and B-type natriuretic peptide (BNP) predicts an increased mortality risk better than any individual biomarker.

Contemporary practice significantly reduced the risk of mortality for patients with ACS at presentation. Risk stratification with appropriate revascularization and use of antiplatelet therapy, statins, and overall coronary risk factor reduction also contribute to this decrease in mortality risk. Whereas the immediate mortality risk for patients with NSTEMI is lower than for patients with STEMI (5% vs. 7%), those with NSTEMI are more prone to subsequent recurrent coronary events. The cumulative mortality rate for STEMI and NSTEMI is similar at 6 months after presentation (12% vs.13%). NSTEMI identifies a patient group with significant long-term mortality risk who require aggressive attention to modifiable coronary risk factors.

Acute STEMI and Complications of Myocardial Infarction
Definition and Epidemiology

Sustained myocardial ischemia, regardless of its cause, can result in myocardial necrosis, which underlies the clinical syndrome of MI. MI represents a spectrum of myocardial necrosis, from relatively small amounts of muscle in the case of demand ischemia, to more extensive subendocardial MI that characterizes NSTEMI, to typically large transmural MIs commonly manifesting as STEMI. The current accepted definition of acute MI accounts for clinical setting and mechanism. STEMI represents the range of large MIs that are almost always caused by total occlusion of an epicardial coronary artery resulting in extensive transmural myonecrosis (Fig. 7.8). In contrast, NSTEMI reflects subtotal coronary occlusion leading to subendocardial myonecrosis. Whereas both NSTEMI and STEMI are life-threatening, their different underlying mechanisms mandate different therapeutic strategies and affect the urgency with which they are applied.

One half of all deaths in the United States and developed countries are related to cardiovascular disease. In the United States, there are over one million nonfatal or fatal MIs each year. CAD plays a role in 360,000 deaths each year, and 110,000 deaths are caused by acute MI. One half of patients with acute MI at presentation die within 1 hour of onset, before therapy can be instituted. Of the 5 million patients who come to emergency rooms with chest pain, 1.3 million are admitted to hospital with ACS. In this group of patients, the presence of ST elevation on ECG or an LBBB indicates the diagnosis of STEMI and the need for prompt intervention to open an occluded coronary artery. STEMI accounts for 30% of all MIs, but this mechanism of MI is associated with the highest immediate mortality risk, prompting the need for urgent therapeutic intervention.

Pathology

Lipid-rich coronary plaques are subject to inflammation incited by the response to oxidation of LDL-cholesterol within the plaque. A sequence of inflammatory events leads to macrophage accumulation and the elaboration of metalloproteinases that degrade collagen in the fibrous cap of the plaque. Thinning of the fibrous cap makes the plaque vulnerable to rupture and exposure of blood to thrombogenic stimuli, resulting in platelet aggregation and activation, thrombin generation, and the evolution of fibrin-based thrombus. If the occlusion is total, transmural myocardial ischemia and necrosis ensue and the ECG demonstrates ST elevation. In contrast, partially occlusive thrombus can result in unstable angina or NSTEMI (subendocardial MI). The presence of coronary collaterals can limit the extent of ischemia and necrosis in either scenario. Both STEMI and NSTEMI can set the stage for arrhythmias and LV dysfunction. Whereas coronary thrombosis is the cause of most MIs, there are patients who develop MI related to coronary embolization, coronary vasospasm, vasculitis, coronary anomalies, dissection of the aorta or a coronary artery, or trauma.

One key feature of the pathology of MI is its time-dependent nature. Experimental and clinical studies have documented that coronary occlusion leads to ischemia and myonecrosis in a wavefront manner, from endocardium to epicardium. Restoration of flow to the vessel within 6 hours after occlusion is associated with limitation of infarct size and a favorable effect on mortality risk. The principle of time dependency of MI drives the need to aggressively reperfuse occluded coronary arteries, and this is the cornerstone of contemporary therapy for STEMI.

Clinical Presentation

Patients with acute MI usually have a combination of chest discomfort, ECG changes (ST elevation in contiguous leads or LBBB), and elevation in biomarkers such as CK-MB and troponin. The high sensitivity and high specificity of troponin have made it the preferred biomarker in the diagnosis of MI. The chest discomfort associated with MI is similar to angina pectoris but more severe in nature. It is usually described as substernal pressure, tightness, or fullness. Patients may have symptoms of discomfort that radiate to the neck, jaw, one or both arms, or the back. Not uncommonly, patients with symptoms of acute MI also experience nausea, vomiting, diaphoresis, apprehension, dyspnea, or weakness. In contrast to angina pectoris associated with stable CAD, acute MI symptoms last longer than 20 to 30 minutes (up to hours).

Occasionally, patients only have symptoms in the non-chest areas usually associated with radiation. Up to 20% of patients, particularly the elderly and diabetics, do not have typical chest discomfort at presentation. The index of suspicion for acute MI should be high in these groups if the patient exhibits profound weakness, acute dyspnea or pulmonary edema, nausea, vomiting, ventricular arrhythmias, or hypotension. The differential diagnosis for patients with chest

素≥3个)可接受冠状动脉造影，并在适当时接受血运重建术。高风险ACS患者以这种方式进行治疗，会减少后续缺血性事件的发生。因怀疑ACS而入院的患者应尽早进行风险分层，对高风险患者采取早期有创治疗策略（入院后24 h内进行冠状动脉造影）与延迟有创治疗相比，可降低死亡、心肌梗死和卒中的复合终点事件。在ACS时，如果出现急性心力衰竭、低血压或室性心律失常，应立即进行冠状动脉造影检查，以识别那些冠状动脉病变高危、需要紧急血运重建的患者。

侵入性冠状动脉造影始终伴随着出血并发症的风险，同时使用强效抗血小板和抗凝治疗无疑会增加这种风险。出血并发症的高危人群包括女性、低体重、糖尿病、肾功能不全、血细胞比容低和高血压患者。与经股动脉途径相比，经桡动脉插管术引起的出血和血管并发症风险较低，但插管操作难度有所增加。目前桡动脉途径的应用越来越普遍，已成为许多介入医师的首选方法。

预后

通过NSTEMI患者心电图上ST段压低的范围和程度可预测死亡风险。在多个导联中出现ST段压低2 mm或以上的患者，1年死亡率增加10倍。肌钙蛋白升高的程度也可识别未来1年内死亡风险增加的患者。此外，联合测量肌钙蛋白、高敏C反应蛋白和B型利钠肽（BNP）比任一个单一生物标志物更能预测死亡风险的增加。

当代医疗显著降低了以ACS就诊时患者的死亡风险。基于风险分层的策略，通过适当的血运重建、抗血小板治疗、他汀类药物以及全面控制冠状动脉危险因素，均有助于降低死亡风险。虽然NSTEMI患者的急性期死亡风险低于STEMI患者（5% vs. 7%），但NSTEMI患者更容易发生后续的复发性冠脉事件。在初诊后6个月，STEMI与NSTEMI患者的累积死亡率相似（12% vs. 13%）；NSTEMI患者的长期死亡风险更高，需要积极关注可逆的冠状动脉危险因素。

急性ST段抬高型心肌梗死和心肌梗死并发症
定义和流行病学

任何原因导致的持续性心肌缺血都会引起心肌坏死，这是心肌梗死临床综合征的基础。心肌梗死可以表现为一系列不同形式的心肌坏死，从心肌血氧需求增加导致的相对少量的心肌坏死；到表现为NSTEMI的、更广泛的心内膜下心肌坏死；以及典型的表现为STEMI的、大面积透壁性心肌坏死。目前公认的急性心肌梗死定义考虑了临床背景和发病机制。STEMI代表不同范围的大面积MI，多由心外膜冠状动脉完全闭塞引起（图7.8）。相比之下，NSTEMI为冠状动脉次全闭塞导致的心内膜下心肌坏死。尽管两者都具有致命性，但由于发病机制不同，其治疗策略和治疗紧急性也就有所不同。

在美国及其他发达国家，心血管疾病相关死亡占总死亡的50%。在美国，每年有超过100万例非致死性或致死性心肌梗死病例；每年有36万人的死亡与CAD有关，11万人死于急性心肌梗死。约一半的急性心肌梗死患者会在发病1 h内死亡，往往来不及治疗。500万因胸痛急诊就诊的患者中，130万人以急性冠脉综合征收住入院。在这部分患者，如心电图显示ST段抬高或新发左束支传导阻滞提示STEMI，需要急诊介入开通闭塞的冠状动脉。STEMI占所有心肌梗死的30%，该病的发病机制导致极高的短期死亡风险，往往需要紧急的介入治疗。

病理学

斑块内低密度脂蛋白胆固醇的氧化，使富含脂质的冠状动脉斑块易于发生炎症反应。一系列的炎症反应可导致巨噬细胞聚集，并产生金属蛋白酶，使斑块纤维帽中的胶原降解。纤维帽的变薄使斑块容易破裂，暴露出诱发血栓形成的刺激物质，导致血小板聚集和活化、凝血酶生成以及纤维蛋白血栓的形成。如果是完全性血管闭塞，则会导致透壁性心肌缺血和坏死，心电图会显示ST段抬高；而血管非完全性闭塞可导致不稳定型心绞痛或NSTEMI（心内膜下心肌梗死）。不论冠脉血管完全闭塞还是非完全闭塞，如果能够形成侧支循环则可以限制心肌缺血和坏死范围。STEMI和NSTEMI都会导致心律失常和左心功能障碍。冠状动脉内血栓形成是心肌梗死的主要原因，此外冠状动脉栓塞、冠状动脉痉挛、血管炎、冠状动脉畸形、主动脉或冠状动脉夹层及创伤等因素也可引起心肌梗死。

心肌梗死病理学的显著特点是具有时间依赖性。实验和临床研究表明，冠状动脉完全闭塞引起的缺血和心肌坏死以波面形式、从心内膜向心外膜心肌推进。血管在闭塞后6 h内恢复血流可以减少梗死面积和降低死亡风险。心肌梗死的时间依赖性特点要求尽早开通闭塞的冠状动脉，这也是当前STEMI治疗策略的基石。

临床表现

急性心肌梗死患者通常伴有胸部不适、心电图改变（相邻导联ST段抬高或左束支传导阻滞）以及CK-MB和肌钙蛋白等生物标志物的升高等多项表现。肌钙蛋白的高敏感性和高特异性使其成为诊断心肌梗死的首选生物标志物。心肌梗死相关的胸部不适症状与心绞痛相似，但是程度更严重，常表现为胸骨后压榨感、紧缩感或闷胀感。有些患者不适症状可放射至颈部、下颌、单侧或者双侧上肢或背部。其他常见症状包括恶心、呕吐、大汗、濒死感、呼吸困难、乏力等。与稳定性CAD的心绞痛症状相比，急性心肌梗死症状持续时间常超过20～30 min，甚至可达数小时。

急性心肌梗死患者有时仅表现出胸部以外的症状，这通常是放射痛导致的。多达20%的患者，尤其是老年和糖尿病患者，可没有典型的胸部不适症状；如果此类患者表现出明显乏力、急性呼吸困难或肺水肿、恶心、呕吐、室性心律失常或低血压等症状时，应高度

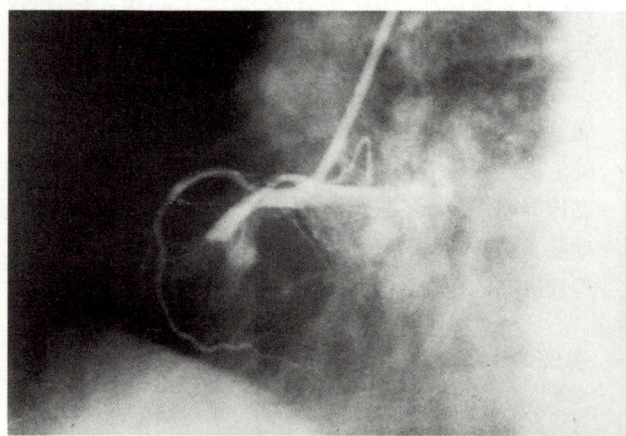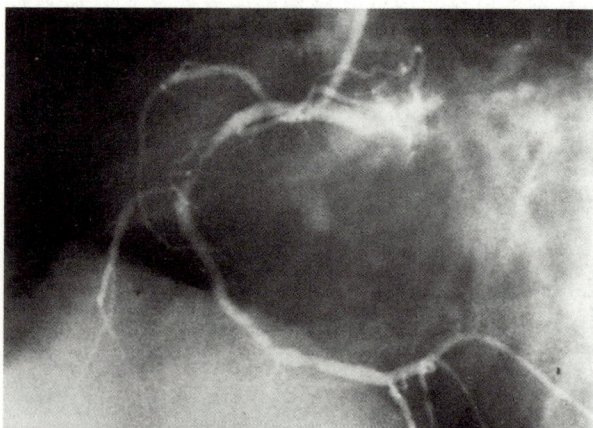

Fig. 7.8 Right coronary artery angiogram in a patient with acute inferior myocardial infarction. The left panel demonstrates total occlusion of the right coronary artery. The right panel depicts restoration of flow 90 minutes after the intravenous administration of tissue-type plasminogen activator.

discomfort suspicious for acute MI includes aortic dissection, pulmonary embolism, chest wall pain, esophageal reflux, acute pericarditis, pleuritis, and panic attacks. Given the life-threatening nature of aortic dissection and pulmonary embolism, these diagnoses should always be paramount, along with acute MI, in patients presenting with chest discomfort.

Physical examination. A comprehensive examination should be undertaken if acute MI is suspected. Attention must be paid to vital signs, because patients may be either hypertensive or hypotensive during the course of an MI. In some cases, such as inferior MI, profound bradycardia may be present. Auscultation of the heart may reveal an S_4. In the case of a large MI, the patient may have symptoms and signs of heart failure such as dyspnea, rales, elevated central venous pressure, and an S_3. Severe heart failure may lead to cardiogenic shock with hypotension and vasoconstriction causing the extremities to be cool to touch. Patients with acute MI are also subject to mechanical problems such as mitral regurgitation due to papillary muscle dysfunction.

Electrocardiogram. The ECG is an important tool in the diagnosis of acute MI. ST elevation of 1 mm or greater in contiguous leads is seen in most patients with acute MI. The initial ECG may be nondiagnostic, so it is important to obtain serial tracings no more than 20 minutes apart to detect the evolutionary changes characteristic of STEMI. The first stage of ECG presentation is ST elevation that subtends the region of the heart affected by transmural ischemia. ST depression may be present in opposing leads, and these are termed reciprocal changes (see Chapter 64, "ST Elevation Acute Myocardial Infarction and Complications of Myocardial Infarction," in *Goldman-Cecil Medicine*, 26th Edition). The presence of reciprocal changes may indicate a larger and more threatening MI. As the MI progresses, ST elevation gives way to T wave inversion. Varying degrees of resolution of ST and T wave changes occur over time, but patients with transmural MI develop pathologic Q waves in the leads subtending the infarcted muscle. Other causes of ST elevation include pericarditis and a chronic repolarization finding of "early repolarization." The presence of either cause of ST elevation can confound the early ECG diagnosis of acute MI.

Approximately 30% of acute MIs originate from the circumflex coronary artery on the posterior wall of the heart. This type of MI appears on the ECG as precordial ST depression. The presence of precordial ST depression should raise suspicion of the presence of "true posterior MI," and additional leads placed through the axilla to the back may reveal the presence of posterior ST elevation. Echocardiography demonstrating posterior hypokinesis is also useful in discriminating true posterior MI. Acute inferior MI due to occlusion of the right coronary artery can also be associated with right ventricular infarction if the right coronary artery's acute marginal branch is compromised. Right ventricular infarction can lead to some challenging management issues, and its diagnosis is aided by the use of right precordial leads to detect ST elevation.

LBBB or ventricular pacing can mask ST elevation due to acute MI. Patients with clinical features of acute MI who have an LBBB (particularly a new LBBB) should be presumed to have STEMI and treated appropriately. Right bundle branch block (RBBB) does not mask the ST elevation of STEMI.

Differential Diagnosis

The diagnosis of STEMI is usually straightforward based on symptoms and ECG findings, but a number of conditions can mimic the ST elevation of STEMI and confound the diagnosis. The ECG changes of early repolarization, takotsubo syndrome, acute myocarditis, or pericarditis can be difficult or impossible to distinguish from those of STEMI. In the face of ST elevation and chest discomfort, it may be necessary to perform coronary angiography in patients who ultimately are diagnosed with a condition other than STEMI so as to not miss this critical diagnosis.

Diagnostic testing. Cardiac troponins (cTnI and cTnT) are sarcomere proteins that, when measured in blood, are specific for myocardial injury. The troponin level becomes elevated 2 to 4 hours after the onset of injury, and the abnormal elevation can persist for up to 2 weeks after the event. The CK-MB isomer is not as specific for heart injury as troponin, but it can still be useful in documenting the presence of MI. CK-MB is found elevated within 4 hours after an acute MI, but it clears more rapidly than troponin. In the case of persistently elevated troponin, a measurable increase in CK-MB may herald another episode of myocardial necrosis. Chronic renal insufficiency is associated with false-positive elevations of troponin T, more so than troponin I. In addition to biomarkers of myocardial injury, other laboratory studies obtained in patients with acute MI include a complete blood count, blood chemistries, lipid panel, prothrombin time (PT), and partial thromboplastin time (PTT). Leukocytosis is a common finding in acute MI, reflecting the inflammatory nature of myocardial necrosis.

At the time of admission, chest radiographs are obtained to assess for the presence of pulmonary edema or mediastinal widening

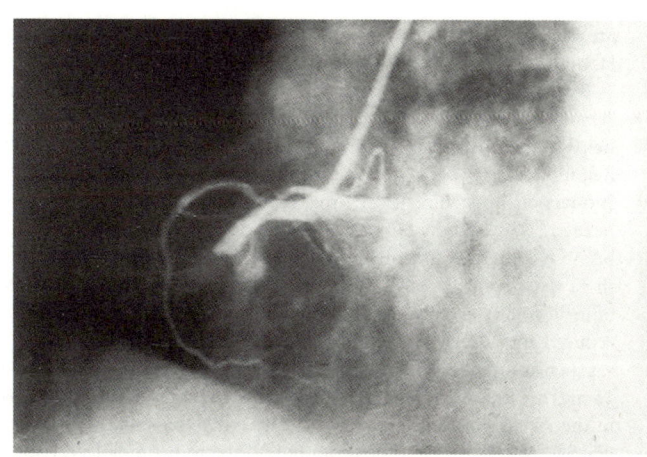 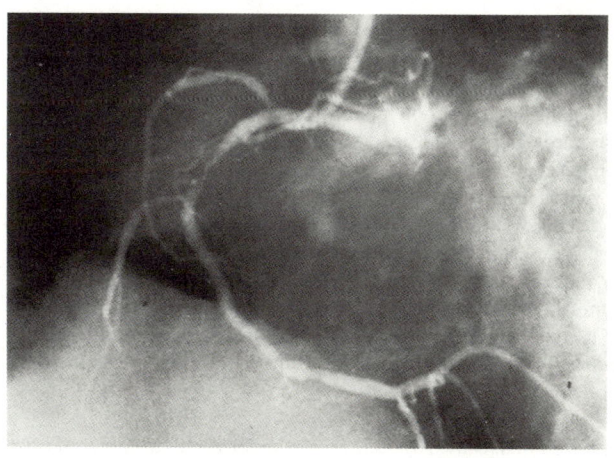

图 7.8 1 例急性下壁心肌梗死患者的右冠状动脉造影图像。左图显示右冠状动脉完全闭塞；右图显示静脉注射组织型纤溶酶原激活剂 90 min 后右冠状动脉血流恢复

警惕急性心肌梗死。需要与心肌梗死导致的胸部不适相鉴别的疾病包括主动脉夹层、肺动脉栓塞、胸壁疼痛、胃食管反流、急性心包炎、胸膜炎和惊恐发作等。主动脉夹层及肺动脉栓塞与急性心肌梗死一样具有致命性，因此胸部不适患者需要首先排查这些疾病。

体格检查 应对疑诊急性心肌梗死患者进行全面的体格检查。首先要关注患者生命体征，心肌梗死患者既可以处于高血压状态也可以出现低血压；如果是下壁心肌梗死等情况，可出现严重心动过缓；心脏听诊可闻及第四心音。大面积心肌梗死患者可出现心力衰竭的症状和体征，如呼吸困难、肺部啰音、中心静脉压升高和出现第三心音。严重心力衰竭可导致心源性休克，表现为低血压和外周血管收缩导致的肢端发冷。急性心肌梗死患者还可能出现机械并发症，如由于乳头肌功能障碍导致的二尖瓣反流。

心电图 心电图是诊断急性心肌梗死的重要工具。大多数急性 STEMI 患者相邻导联的 ST 段抬高达到或超过 1 mm。首份心电图可能没有典型表现而无法明确诊断心肌梗死，这时应每间隔不超过 20 min 多次复查心电图，以发现 STEMI 心电图的特征性演变。早期透壁性心肌缺血的心电图表现为相应导联 ST 段抬高；而在对应导联则可以表现为 ST 段压低，这就是所谓的"镜像改变"（详见 *Goldman-Cecil Medicine* 第 26 版第 64 章"急性 ST 段抬高型心肌梗死和心肌梗死并发症"）。镜像改变的出现往往提示心肌梗死面积更大、死亡风险更高。随着心肌梗死进展，ST 段抬高后出现 T 波倒置；后期抬高的 ST 段可有不同程度回落，T 波也可以出现多种形态改变，但透壁性心肌梗死患者在面向心肌梗死区域的导联可出现病理性 Q 波。除心肌梗死外，其他引起 ST 段抬高的情况包括心包炎和"早复极"，两者均会干扰急性心肌梗死的早期心电图诊断。

约有 30% 的急性心肌梗死是由支配心脏后壁的回旋支闭塞引起的，此类心肌梗死的心电图可表现为胸前导联 ST 段压低。因此，当出现胸前导联 ST 段压低时应警惕后壁心肌梗死可能；需加做后壁导联心电图以明确是否存在后壁导联 ST 段抬高。超声心动图显示后壁运动减低也有助于诊断后壁心肌梗死。右冠状动脉闭塞可以导致急性下壁心肌梗死，如果右冠状动脉的分支血管锐缘支受到影响，则可以出现右室心肌梗死。右室心肌梗死给治疗带来一定的挑战，右侧胸壁导联 ST 段抬高有助于右室心肌梗死的诊断。

左束支传导阻滞（LBBB）或心室起搏可能掩盖由急性心肌梗死引起的 ST 段抬高。如果患者具有急性心肌梗死的临床特征且伴有 LBBB（尤其是新发生的 LBBB），应当怀疑存在 STEMI 并采取适当治疗措施。右束支传导阻滞（RBBB）不会掩盖 STEMI 引起的 ST 段抬高。

鉴别诊断

根据典型的临床症状和心电图表现，STEMI 一般不难诊断。但其他疾病有时也可以引起 ST 段抬高而使情况复杂化，如早复极、Takotsubo 综合征、急性心肌炎和急性心包炎等，其心电图表现很难与 STEMI 鉴别，从而干扰 STEMI 的诊断。对于有胸部不适症状且 ST 段抬高的患者，有时需要行冠状动脉造影以避免漏诊这一致命性疾病，尽管部分冠状动脉造影患者最终确诊为其他疾病。

诊断性检查 肌钙蛋白（cTnI 和 cTnT）是心肌细胞的肌节蛋白，血液中肌钙蛋白升高是心肌损伤的特异性标志物。肌钙蛋白在心肌损伤 2～4 h 后开始升高，可持续 2 周。CK-MB 在诊断心肌损伤方面特异性不如肌钙蛋白，但仍可用于急性心肌梗的辅助诊断。CK-MB 在急性心肌梗死发生 4 h 内开始升高，但是持续时间短于肌钙蛋白。在肌钙蛋白持续升高的情况下，CK-MB 再次升高可以提示再发心肌梗死。慢性肾功能不全可以导致肌钙蛋白假性升高，cTnT 较 cTnI 更为明显。除心肌损伤标志物外，急性心肌梗死患者还需要进行血常规、血生化、血脂、凝血酶原时间（PT）和部分凝血活酶时间（PTT）等检查。急性心肌梗死患者常出现白细胞升高，反映了心肌坏死的炎症性。

患者入院后应行 X 线胸片检查以评估肺水肿的情况，或观察有无主动脉夹层引起的纵隔增宽。超声心

suspicious for dissection. Echocardiography is important in delineating the extent of MI and assessing EF. In cases of diagnostic ambiguity, early use of echocardiography can demonstrate the presence of regional wall motion abnormalities consistent with acute MI. Echocardiography with color Doppler is also helpful in diagnosing complications of acute MI such as infarct-related mitral regurgitation or ventricular septal defect (VSD), pericardial effusion, or evidence of pseudoaneurysm as a result of myocardial rupture. Follow-up echocardiography in the months after acute MI can also reveal recovery of LV function. Radionuclide tracer studies are not useful in diagnosing acute MI. CT, cardiac MRI, and transesophageal echocardiography are all useful in diagnosing aortic dissection when there is an increased index of suspicion. Cardiac MRI can also distinguish myopericarditis.

Treatment

Acute STEMI is caused by occlusion of the epicardial coronary artery by thrombus after rupture of a vulnerable plaque. The process of myocardial necrosis is time dependent, so diagnosis and treatment of STEMI to preserve myocardium must occur as quickly as possible. More than half of deaths occur within 1 hour after onset of symptoms, before the patient can be reached for emergency care. Patients often delay seeking care for symptoms of acute MI despite efforts to alert the public to the risk of ignoring symptoms of chest discomfort. Emergency medical personnel who respond to patients with possible MI begin to institute initial therapy in the field. Patients are monitored with ECG for rhythm disturbances such as ventricular tachycardia (VT) or ventricular fibrillation (VF) that require prompt cardioversion or defibrillation. Oxygen is administered via nasal cannula, and intravenous access is established. Aspirin (162 to 325 mg) is administered to the patient, and sublingual nitroglycerin may also be given in an attempt to relieve chest discomfort. Some emergency response systems perform 12-lead ECGs and telemeter the results to the emergency department, allowing for early diagnosis of STEMI and early decision making regarding revascularization strategies.

Once the patient arrives in the emergency department, an ECG, if not already available, will be performed within 5 minutes. If the ECG is nondiagnostic, a second study is obtained no more than 20 minutes after presentation. A diagnosis of STEMI triggers decision making regarding reperfusion strategies that are used by the particular institution (see Chapter 64, "ST Elevation Acute Myocardial Infarction and Complications of Myocardial Infarction," in *Goldman-Cecil Medicine*, ❖ 26th Edition). Hospitals that are capable of performing emergency cardiac catheterization for the purpose of reperfusion therapy have an established rapid response system to activate the catheterization laboratory for this urgent therapy. There is evidence that primary PCI therapy for STEMI is superior to fibrinolytic therapy, but its use depends on the timely availability of a well-trained catheterization team. The quality of primary PCI is signified by a so-called door-to-balloon time of less than 90 minutes. Likewise, the standard for fibrinolytic therapy is a door-to-needle time of less than 30 minutes. Regardless of the means of reperfusion, it is important for the hospital treating patients with STEMI to have a structured protocol for timely diagnosis, decision making, and initiation of therapy.

In addition to aspirin, the patient should be given a loading dose of a P2Y12 inhibitor (ticagrelor 180 mg, clopidogrel 600 mg or prasugrel 60 mg), assuming he or she will be treated with primary PCI. Unfractionated heparin in a dose of 60 IU/kg should be administered (no more than 4000 IU bolus) with a drip rate of 12 IU/kg/hour (maximum dose, 1000 IU/hour). LMW heparin may also be used (enoxaparin 30 mg IV bolus with 1 mg/kg subcutaneously every 12 hours for patients younger than 75 years of age who have normal renal function). Other agents such as glycoprotein IIb/IIIa inhibitors or bivalirudin are administered depending on the protocols of the catheterization laboratory.

Patients are commonly given sublingual nitroglycerin 0.4 mg (repeat every 5 minutes for no more than three total doses), which often helps to diminish chest discomfort. Intravenous nitroglycerin may be helpful for control of both persistent pain and hypertension if present. Intravenous morphine (2 to 4 mg, repeated every 5 to 15 minutes as needed) is also frequently used for pain control. Although there has been no consensus statement on the use of morphine in ACS, recently there have been several studies that have suggested an increased risk of in-hospital mortality associated with its use presumed secondary to reduced antiplatelet activity of P2Y12 inhibitors. Intravenous β-blockers such as metoprolol (5-mg bolus every 10 minutes for a total dose of 15 mg) are indicated in the treatment of STEMI but should be avoided in the face of heart failure, severe COPD, hypotension, or bradycardia. β-Blockers (metoprolol, propranolol, atenolol, timolol, and carvedilol) have been shown to significantly reduce the risk of future MI and cardiovascular mortality. Statin therapy, as mentioned for NSTEMI, is recommended for all patients with STEMI as a presenting symptom regardless of their history of hypercholesterolemia. Other adjunctive measures include bedrest for the first 12 hours, ongoing oxygen by nasal cannula with pulse oximeter monitoring, continuous rhythm monitoring, anxiolytic agents as needed, and stool softeners. Atropine is kept in reserve for the treatment of hemodynamically significant bradycardia, which may occur with inferior MI.

ACE-inhibitor therapy also plays an important role in the long-term survival of patients after STEMI. ACE-inhibitor therapy has been shown to reduce the incidence of heart failure, recurrent MI, and long-term mortality after STEMI. ACE inhibitors commonly used for this purpose include lisinopril, captopril, enalapril, and ramipril. The decision to initiate ACE-inhibitor therapy is directed by the patient's tolerance. Care is warranted early after STEMI, because the patient may be prone to hypotension related to ACE-inhibitor therapy. A low dose should be administered first, with gradual upward titration.

Aldosterone receptor blockade with eplerenone (25 to 50 mg/day) reduces cardiovascular mortality after MI in patients with heart failure and a reduced EF of less than 40% or diabetes. Spironolactone also reduces mortality in patients with heart failure and a history of remote MI.

Reperfusion therapy. Timely reperfusion therapy, either thrombolytic therapy or primary PCI, is critical to limiting the extent of MI and reducing the risks of future morbidity and mortality. Primary PCI has been shown to have advantages over thrombolytic therapy, with higher immediate and long-term vessel patency. Primary PCI depends on the availability of cardiac catheterization facilities and staff to conduct the reperfusion procedure quickly (see earlier discussion). If the patient has not had access to a catheterization facility for longer than 2 hours after presentation, thrombolytic therapy is a reasonable alternative.

In the randomized, placebo-controlled Gruppo Italiano per lo Studio della Streptochinasi nell'Infarto (GISSI) study, thrombolytic therapy with intravenous streptokinase was shown to reduce the risk of mortality in patients with STEMI if it was administered early after presentation. The time-dependent nature of therapy was also demonstrated, in that patients treated more than 12 hours after the onset of symptoms had no measurable benefit from thrombolysis. The next generation of thrombolytic agents, recombinant tissue-type plasminogen activators (rt-PA), improved on mortality reduction when compared with streptokinase (30-day mortality rate, 7.3% with streptokinase vs. 6.3% with rt-PA). The advantage of rt-PA appeared to be related to enhanced vessel patency at 90 minutes after administration (80% with rt-PA vs. 53% to 60% with streptokinase). Subsequent forms of rt-PA,

动图对于评估心肌梗死范围和射血分数十分重要。在早期诊断不明确时，超声心动图发现的节段性室壁运动异常有助于急性心肌梗死的诊断。彩色多普勒超声检查有助于发现急性心肌梗死的机械并发症，如梗死相关的二尖瓣关闭不全、室间隔穿孔、心包积液或心肌破裂引起的假性室壁瘤等。急性心肌梗死后数月随访复查超声心动图可以评估左心功能恢复情况。放射性核素检查一般不用于诊断急性心肌梗死。对于高度怀疑主动脉夹层的患者可行心血管CT、心脏MRI或经食管超声心动图等检查；心脏MRI还可用于鉴别心肌心包炎。

治疗

易损斑块破裂诱发血栓形成，从而阻塞心外膜冠状动脉是STEMI的病理基础。"时间就是心肌"，STEMI患者应尽快得到诊断和治疗，才能更有效地挽救存活心肌。STEMI所致死亡中，超过一半发生于发病后1 h内，这些患者往往来不及急诊救治。尽管健康教育呼吁公众重视胸部不适症状，但仍有很多出现症状的急性心肌梗死患者不能及时就诊。急救医疗人员应在现场就开始对疑诊急性心肌梗死患者进行初始治疗，包括监测心电图以识别室性心动过速（室速，VT）或心室颤动（室颤，VF）等心律失常，一旦发生应立即电转复或电除颤；通过经鼻导管吸氧给予氧疗；建立静脉通路；予口服阿司匹林162～325 mg，舌下含服硝酸甘油可能缓解胸部不适症状。有些应急反应系统在完成12导联心电图后，远程传输回急诊科，有助于STEMI的早期诊断及血运重建策略的制定。

患者到达急诊室后，如无院外心电图则应在5 min内采集第一份心电图；如这份心电图不能明确诊断，应在20 min内再次复查心电图。一旦确诊STEMI，应制订再灌注治疗策略并由特定医疗中心执行（见 *Goldman-Cecil Medicine* 第26版第64章，"急性ST段抬高型心肌梗死和心肌梗死并发症"）。可实施心脏导管检查和血运重建治疗的医院应有完备的应急响应系统，能够及时启动导管室并完成急诊介入手术。证据显示，对于STEMI患者急诊PCI优于溶栓治疗，但这有赖于训练有素的介入团队，并能够快速响应。急诊PCI要求"门球（door-to-balloon）"时间小于90 min，溶栓治疗则要求"门-针（door-to-needle）"时间小于30 min。无论采取哪种再灌注治疗方案，治疗STEMI的医院都应该制订完善的流程体系，才能够快速诊断、制订治疗方案，并尽早启动治疗。

对于要接受急诊PCI的患者，应该给予负荷剂量的阿司匹林和P2Y12抑制剂（替格瑞洛180 mg、氯吡格雷600 mg或普拉格雷60 mg）。普通肝素应按照60 IU/kg剂量给药（最大剂量不超过4000 IU），静脉滴注速度为12 IU/（kg·h）（最大剂量不超过1000 IU/h）。也可使用低分子量肝素（对于年龄小于75岁、肾功能正常患者，可予依诺肝素30 mg静脉推注，随后1 mg/kg每12 h皮下注射）抗凝。其他药物，如糖蛋白Ⅱb/Ⅲa抑制剂和比伐卢定，也可以按照导管室的方案使用。

舌下含服硝酸甘油（每次0.4 mg，每5 min重复给药，一般不超过3次）有助于缓解心前区不适症状。持续胸痛合并高血压时可静脉使用硝酸甘油。静脉推注吗啡（每次2～4 mg，必要时可每5～15 min重复给药）用于镇痛治疗。吗啡用于治疗急性冠脉综合征尚无共识，最近几项研究也表明吗啡可能增加心肌梗死患者的住院死亡风险，可能与吗啡导致P2Y12抑制剂的抗血小板活性降低有关。静脉应用β受体阻滞剂（如美托洛尔 5 mg 弹丸式静脉推注，每10 min重复给药，最大量15 mg）推荐用于治疗STEMI，但在急性心力衰竭、严重COPD、低血压或心动过缓等情况下应避免使用。β受体阻滞剂（美托洛尔、普萘洛尔、阿替洛尔、噻吗洛尔、卡维地洛）还可以显著降低远期再发心肌梗死和心血管死亡风险。同NSTEMI一样，推荐所有STEMI患者，无论有无高胆固醇血症病史，均应使用他汀类药物治疗。其他辅助治疗措施包括心肌梗死后的头12 h卧床休息，鼻导管吸氧并监测脉搏血氧饱和度，持续心电监测，根据需要使用抗焦虑药物，以及使用通便药保持排便通畅。应常备阿托品，以用于治疗引起血流动力学障碍的严重心动过缓，下壁心肌梗死时常出现这种情况。

ACE抑制剂（ACEI）已被证实能够降低STEMI患者心力衰竭、再发心肌梗死及远期死亡风险，因此在STEMI患者的长期生存中起着重要作用。常见的ACEI包括赖诺普利、卡托普利、依那普利和雷米普利。能否加用ACEI取决于患者对药物的耐受性，比如在STEMI早期，患者就容易出现与ACEI相关的低血压。因此，ACEI应小剂量起始，根据患者临床情况逐渐加量。

醛固酮受体拮抗剂依普利酮（25～50 mg/d）能够降低心肌梗死后射血分数<40%的心力衰竭或糖尿病患者的心血管死亡风险。螺内酯也能降低陈旧性心肌梗死和心力衰竭患者的死亡率。

再灌注治疗 及时进行再灌注治疗（溶栓治疗或急诊PCI）可以限制心肌梗死的范围，对于降低远期再发心肌梗死和死亡的风险至关重要。急诊PCI较溶栓治疗具有更高的近期和远期血管通畅率，因而在治疗STEMI方面更具优势。但急诊PCI需要医院具备必要的心导管检查设备和能够快速实施再灌注治疗的医疗团队。如果预估患者不能在发病2 h内到达具备急诊介入条件的医院，溶栓治疗是合理的替代治疗策略。

一项随机、安慰剂对照临床试验GISSI（Gruppo Italiano per lo Studio della Streptochinasi nell'Infarto）结果显示，早期溶栓治疗（静脉注射链激酶）可显著降低STEMI患者死亡风险。该研究还表明，溶栓治疗具有明显的时效性，如果患者发病12 h后行溶栓治疗则几乎没有获益。新一代溶栓药，重组组织型纤溶酶原激活剂（rt-PA）在降低死亡率方面优于链激酶（30天死亡率rt-PA为6.3%，链激酶为7.3%），这种优势主要与rt-PA给药后90 min血管通畅率更高有关（rt-PA为80%，链激酶为53%～60%）。而更新型的rt-PA

although easier to administer, did not further reduce mortality. The major attribute of thrombolytic therapy is its ease of administration, but there is a significant risk (0.5% to 1%) of catastrophic bleeding complications in the form of intracerebral hemorrhage. Age older than 75 years, female gender, hypertension, and concomitant use of heparin increase the risk of this complication. In the case of failed thrombolytic therapy, rescue PCI may be pursued.

Primary PCI has been shown to be superior to thrombolytic therapy based on lower overall mortality rates and reduced risk of recurrent nonfatal MI. It is also associated with higher vessel patency rates and a low risk of intracranial hemorrhage. Primary PCI is frequently performed by mechanical aspiration of thrombus and placement of a coronary stent. Balloon angioplasty may or may not be needed during this procedure. Patients should receive preprocedure P2Y12 inhibitor (ticagrelor 180 mg, clopidogrel 600 mg or prasugrel 60 mg). For patients who are not able to take oral medications, whose platelet inhibition may not be at therapeutic levels at the time of stent placement, or who are at high risk for life-threatening bleeding requiring cessation of antiplatelet therapy, cangrelor (an intravenous P2Y12 inhibitor given at 30 mcg/kg bolus followed by infusion of 4 mcg/kg/minute) may be considered given its rapid onset and offset of platelet inhibition.

Bivalirudin was shown in a clinical trial of primary PCI to be superior to both heparin- and glycoprotein IIb/IIIa–based anticoagulation with lower post-MI mortality and fewer bleeding complications. Centers that are dedicated to primary PCI as the preferred therapy are likely to have the best outcomes when operators are sufficiently skilled and the institution cares for this patient population on a regular basis. Primary PCI is the best option for patients in cardiogenic shock (within 18 hours after onset of shock), for patients with prior CABG (graft occlusion is not amenable to thrombolysis), and for patients older than 70 years of age (conferring a reduced risk of intracerebral hemorrhage compared with thrombolysis).

Complications of Myocardial Infarction
Recurrent Chest Pain

MI is associated with a number of possible problems related to the extent of injury (Table 7.6). Patients can experience post-infarction angina that may reflect re-occlusion of the infarct related vessel. This can occur either in patients who underwent primary PCI with stent placement (stent thrombosis) or thrombolysis. Post-infarction angina usually requires cardiac catheterization for appropriate diagnosis and treatment. Patients with transmural MI are also subject to pericarditis 2 to 4 days after the event. This diagnosis is usually established by the symptom nature and pattern (worse with inspiration or supine position, improved with sitting), which is different from their initial presentation with acute MI. A less common event is the development of pericarditis due to Dressler syndrome up to 10 weeks after acute MI. This is likely an immune-mediated phenomenon. Pericarditis is treated with aspirin or nonsteroidal anti-inflammatory drugs.

Arrhythmias

The highest risk of life-threatening arrhythmias is during the first 24 to 48 hours after the onset of acute MI. Ischemic myocardium is susceptible to arrhythmia generation, probably based on micro-reentry associated with ischemic myocardium. The significant mortality risk in the early hours of acute MI is largely attributed to arrhythmias such as VF or VT. The risk of VF is about 3% to 5% in the early hours of MI and diminishes over 24 to 48 hours. One of the benefits of rhythm monitoring during the first 48 hours after presentation is prompt recognition and treatment of life-threatening ventricular arrhythmias.

TABLE 7.6 Complications of Acute Myocardial Infarction

Functional
Left ventricular failure
Right ventricular failure
Cardiogenic shock

Mechanical
Free-wall rupture
Ventricular septal defect
Papillary muscle rupture with acute mitral regurgitation

Electrical
Bradyarrhythmias (first-, second-, and third-degree atrioventricular blocks)
Tachyarrhythmias (supraventricular, ventricular)
Conduction abnormalities (bundle branch and fascicular blocks)

Accelerated idioventricular rhythm occurs early in the course of MI and may be associated with reperfusion. This arrhythmia is well tolerated and does not require specific therapy.

Ventricular arrhythmias occurring late (>48 hours) after acute MI usually are associated with large underlying MIs and heart failure. Late episodes of VF or VT portend a poor prognosis. Immediate therapy for VF is electrical defibrillation. VT that causes hemodynamic embarrassment is treated with synchronized electrical cardioversion. β-Blocker therapy may help to suppress arrhythmias in patients who are prone to them, as may the use of amiodarone. Correction of residual ischemia may also play a role in controlling VF or VT events. Patients with late VF or hemodynamically significant VT are candidates for an implantable cardioverter defibrillator device (ICD). An ICD can also improve survival in asymptomatic patients with a persistently reduced EF less than 30% at 40 days after their acute MI. ICD therapy is also indicated if the EF is less than 35% at 40 days after MI in a patient with symptomatic heart failure.

Atrial fibrillation (AF) occurs in 10% to 15% of patients after MI. Those more prone to AF include patients with older age, large MI, hypokalemia, hypomagnesemia, hypoxia, or increased sympathetic activity. Rate control with β-blockers (e.g., metoprolol), digoxin, calcium-channel blockers (e.g., diltiazem) or some combination of these agents is warranted, as is the use of intravenous heparin to reduce the risk of systemic embolization. Cardioversion is warranted in the face of rapid rates that cause ischemia, heart failure, or hypotension. Amiodarone is sometimes used to help maintain sinus rhythm for the first few months after MI-related AF.

Sinus bradycardia or AV block due to increased vagal tone is common in cases of inferior MI (30% to 40%). Reperfusion of the right coronary artery may be associated with significant bradycardia (Bezold-Jarisch reflex). Atropine (0.5 to 1.5 mg IV) can resolve severe inferior MI–related bradycardia. In contrast, heart block and wide-complex escape rhythms associated with anterior MI suggest an infra–AV node block. This may be worsened by the use of atropine.

Advanced degrees of heart block may require the placement of a permanent pacemaker. Intermittent second-degree or third-degree AV block associated with bundle branch block or symptomatic AV block are indications for a permanent pacemaker. Type I AV block (Wenckebach) is usually not persistent and rarely causes symptoms that warrant a permanent pacemaker.

Heart Failure and Low-Output States

MI involving 20% to 25% of the left ventricle can result in significant heart failure manifesting with dyspnea due to pulmonary congestion

给药方法更加方便，但未能进一步降低死亡风险。溶栓治疗易于实施，但发生致命性出血并发症风险较高（0.5%～1%），主要表现为颅内出血。年龄大于75岁、女性、高血压、同时应用肝素等因素会增加出血风险。此外，如果溶栓治疗失败，则应尽早行补救性PCI。

急诊PCI疗效优于溶栓治疗，体现在急诊PCI相关总死亡率、再发非致死性心肌梗死风险和颅内出血风险更低，同时具有更高的血管通畅率。急诊PCI包括机械性血栓抽吸和冠状动脉支架置入；而球囊血管成形术并非必要的操作。（译者注：除阿司匹林之外，）术前患者应该服用负荷剂量的P2Y12抑制剂（替格瑞洛180 mg，氯吡格雷600 mg或普拉格雷60 mg）。如果患者无法口服抗血小板药物，或在进行支架手术时抗血小板药物的抑制作用尚未达到治疗水平，或有致命性出血高风险而必须停用抗血小板药物的患者，可以使用起效迅速、半衰期较短的坎格瑞洛［一种P2Y12抑制剂的静脉制剂，先予30 μg/kg弹丸式静脉推注，后以4 μg/（kg·min）持续静脉泵入］。

临床研究显示，与肝素联用糖蛋白Ⅱb/Ⅲa抑制剂的抗凝方案相比，围手术期使用比伐卢定抗凝可以降低心肌梗死后死亡率和出血发生率。将急诊PCI作为优选治疗方案的医疗中心往往能给STEMI患者带来更好的预后，尤其是拥有技术娴熟的手术医师和术后照护经验丰富的医护团队。心源性休克（休克发病18 h内）、既往CABG（桥血管闭塞不适宜溶栓）及70岁以上（溶栓治疗相关颅内出血风险高）的患者应首选急诊PCI。

心肌梗死并发症

复发性胸痛

心肌梗死可以产生多种并发症，这些并发症都与心肌损伤密切相关（表7.6）。梗死后心绞痛可以由于梗死相关血管的再次闭塞而导致，急诊PCI行支架置入术后（支架内血栓形成）和溶栓治疗后均可出现这种情况。梗死后心绞痛往往需行心脏导管检查以明确诊断和及时治疗。心包炎可发生于透壁性心肌梗死后2～4天，其诊断通常根据患者的症状性质和特点（胸痛症状在吸气或仰卧位加重，坐位减轻），这和急性心肌梗死所致的胸痛性质不同。另一种更少见情况是由Dressler综合征引起的心包炎，可在心肌梗死发病长达10周内出现，这种心包炎可能是免疫介导的现象。可使用阿司匹林或非甾体抗炎药治疗心包炎。

心律失常

致命性心律失常多发生于急性心肌梗死后24～48 h内。缺血状态的心肌更容易发生心律失常，主要与缺血心肌细胞间的微折返有关。室速或室颤等心律失常是急性心肌梗死早期最主要的死亡原因。室颤在急性心肌梗死后数小时内的发生率为3%～5%，24～48 h后的发生风险逐渐下降。因此，推荐在急性心肌梗死发病48 h内进行心电监护，以及时发现并处理致命性心律失常。

加速性室性自主心律常发生于心肌梗死早期，多与再灌注相关。患者对这种心律失常耐受性较好，无须特殊干预。

表7.6　急性心肌梗死并发症
功能性 左心衰竭 右心衰竭 心源性休克
机械性 游离壁破裂 室间隔穿孔 乳头肌断裂伴急性二尖瓣反流
心律失常 缓慢性心律失常（一、二、三度房室传导阻滞） 快速性心律失常（室上性、室性心动过速） 传导异常（束支和分支阻滞）

急性心肌梗死后迟发性室性心律失常（48 h后）多与大面积心肌梗死和心力衰竭相关。迟发的室速和室颤提示患者预后不佳。室颤一旦发生应立即行电除颤；影响血流动力学的室速也应给予同步电转复。β受体阻滞剂或胺碘酮可以降低高危人群致命性心律失常的发生风险；另外，纠正残存的缺血状态也有助于控制室速和室颤的发生。发生迟发性室颤和影响血流动力学的室速患者需评估植入式心脏复律除颤器（ICD）的必要性。对于心肌梗死40天后，射血分数≤30%的无心力衰竭症状患者，ICD可以有效改善这些患者的生存率。射血分数≤35%的有心力衰竭症状患者也有ICD植入指征。

心肌梗死后心房颤动（房颤，AF）发生率约为10%～15%，尤其是高龄、大面积心肌梗死、低钾血症、低镁血症、低氧血症和交感神经张力升高的患者更易发生。β受体阻滞剂（如美托洛尔）、地高辛、钙通道阻滞剂（如地尔硫䓬）或上述药物的联用，可用于控制房颤的心室率；静脉应用肝素可以降低房颤相关体循环栓塞风险。当心室率过快引起心肌缺血、急性心力衰竭或低血压时，应予以转复。有时，可在发生心肌梗死相关房颤的最初几个月，应用胺碘酮以维持窦性心律。

约30%～40%的下壁心肌梗死患者可出现迷走神经张力升高相关的窦性心动过缓和房室传导阻滞；开通右冠状动脉时可出现显著的心动过缓（Bezold-Jarisch反射）。阿托品（0.5～1.5 mg静脉推注）可改善严重的下壁心肌梗死相关的心动过缓。需要注意的是，前壁心肌梗死相关的心脏传导阻滞和宽QRS波逸搏心律往往提示房室结以下部位的传导阻滞，使用阿托品可能会恶化。

高度传导阻滞患者可能需要植入永久起搏器。对于伴有束支传导阻滞的间歇二度或三度房室传导阻滞及有症状的房室传导阻滞患者，具有植入永久起搏器的指征。二度Ⅰ型房室传导阻滞（文氏现象，wenckebach）多为暂时性的，很少引起心动过缓相关症状，一般不需要植入永久起搏器。

心力衰竭和低心排状态

心肌梗死累及20%～25%的左心室心肌时，可导致明显的心力衰竭，临床表现为肺淤血相关的呼吸困难症状和左心功能不全相关的第三、第四心音等体征。心肌梗死范围超过40%时，则可导致心源性休克，死

and findings of LV dysfunction such as an S_3 or S_4. Cardiogenic shock is associated with loss of 40% of the myocardium. This condition carries a very high risk of mortality. In the era of widespread use of reperfusion therapy, the incidence of post-MI heart failure or cardiogenic shock has declined. Early use of reperfusion therapies limits infarct size and the risk of complications related to heart failure. When acute heart failure occurs with MI, therapeutic interventions including oxygen, intravenous morphine, and diuretics can help stabilize the patient. Nitroglycerin can also help by reducing the elevated preload. Long-term therapy for heart failure related to reduced EF after acute MI includes the use of ACE inhibitors (or ARBs), appropriate β-blockers, aldosterone receptor antagonists such as eplerenone or spironolactone, and diuretics as needed.

The acutely infarcted ventricle requires an increased filling pressure and volume to optimize its performance. Patients with acute MI may become relatively fluid depleted due to nausea, vomiting, or decreased fluid intake, leading to reduced LV volume and a fall in cardiac output. This can translate into hypotension that is best treated by judicious administration of fluids.

Acute inferior MI is usually associated with a low mortality risk once the early arrhythmia-prone hours have passed. Occlusion of the right coronary artery and a significant acute marginal branch can lead to right ventricular infarction. Approximately 10% to 15% of patients with inferior MI have associated right ventricular infarction. This condition produces a significant increase in mortality risk (in-hospital mortality, 25% to 30% vs. <6%). Hallmarks of right ventricular infarction include elevated jugular venous pressure with Kussmaul sign and hypotension. Right ventricular function frequently recovers, but it may be necessary to administer sufficient volume to maintain right heart output. Short-term inotropic support with dobutamine is sometimes needed, and venodilators and diuretics should be avoided. High-degree AV block, usually transient with inferior MI, may worsen hemodynamics and necessitate temporary AV sequential pacing. AF may not be tolerated and may require cardioversion.

Cardiogenic Shock

Cardiogenic shock is a clinical syndrome associated with extensive loss of myocardium, which leads to a reduced cardiac index (<1.8 L/min/m^2) in the face of elevated LV filling pressures (pulmonary capillary wedge pressure >18 mm Hg), resulting in systemic hypotension and reduced organ perfusion. This shock state is associated with mortality rates in the range of 70% to 80%. Aggressive diagnosis with hemodynamic monitoring and appropriate support with an inotropic agent and invasive mechanical support as indicated can help to stabilize the patient. Mechanical circulatory support includes the intra-aortic balloon pump (IABP), Impella ventricular assist device (VAD), and extracorporeal membrane oxygenation (ECMO). One benefit of the IABP is that it can quickly be placed in the cath lab to both augment cardiac output as well as diastolic filling of the coronary arteries. IABP therapy is at best temporizing, and the patient's survival depends on the presence of reversible factors such as ischemia that respond to revascularization or correction of a mechanical complication of MI (e.g., mitral regurgitation or VSD). IABP therapy cannot be used in the face of significant aortic insufficiency and may not be feasible in the presence of significant peripheral vascular disease. Despite the hemodynamic support it provides, the IABP has never been proven in a randomized trial to improve mortality, and thus its use is based on clinician decision making rather than routine use. Some centers now are opting for more advanced levels of support in particularly ill patients including the Impella or ECMO as a bridge to recovery or long-term VAD/transplant.

In patients with cardiogenic shock secondary to acute MI it is key to reestablish perfusion to affected areas of the heart as able. More recent theories have suggested that rather than the "door to balloon time" emphasized in STEMI, the emphasis in patients in shock should be to achieve early improvement in perfusion with mechanical support as needed and then address revascularization. If multivessel disease is discovered in a patient in shock, the culprit lesion should be addressed, and other high-grade diseases can be addressed at a later time.

Mechanical Complications

Mechanical complications of acute MI include mitral regurgitation (due to ischemic papillary muscle dysfunction or rupture), VSD, free wall rupture, and LV aneurysm formation. These problems usually occur during the first week after MI, and they account for as much as 15% of MI-related mortality. A new murmur, sudden onset of heart failure, or hemodynamic collapse should also raise suspicion of a mechanical complication of MI. Patients who either were not reperfused or were reperfused late after onset of MI are most at risk for these problems. Echocardiography usually identifies the mechanical problem, and hemodynamic assessment with right heart catheterization can aid the diagnosis. Surgical correction of the defect is usually required.

Papillary muscle rupture or dysfunction leading to acute severe mitral regurgitation results in severe heart failure and up to 75% mortality within 24 hours after onset. Afterload reduction with intravenous nitroprusside and the use of IABP can help to stabilize the patient, but surgical valve repair or replacement will be needed to provide some chance of survival. Surgery is associated with a 25% to 50% mortality risk, but that still is better than the risk with medical or IABP therapy only.

Elderly patients, particularly those with hypertension, are more prone to MI-related VSD. Thrombolytic therapy may also place patients at risk for this complication. Acute VSD with resultant left-to-right shunting can produce severe hemodynamic instability. As with acute mitral regurgitation, afterload reduction and IABP may help to stabilize the patient, but ultimately surgical repair will be required. Moderate to large VSDs are not well tolerated and are associated with significant mortality risk. VSDs related to anterior MI may offer a better opportunity for surgical repair than those resulting from inferior MI. Some patients have been helped by the use of percutaneous closure devices, which can afford an opportunity to delay surgery until there is better tissue healing in the infarct area.

LV free wall rupture is similar to VSD in terms of risk for occurrence and underlying myocardial pathology. Free wall rupture is usually associated with sudden death due to cardiac tamponade. On occasion, a pseudoaneurysm forms and the patient can be treated surgically.

Thromboembolic Complications

In earlier years, thromboembolism in the form of either cardioembolic stroke or pulmonary embolism contributed to 25% of post-MI in-hospital mortality, and clinical events were diagnosed in 10% of patients. The risk of thromboembolism is linked to the presence of LV mural clot, which is more likely to be found in anterior MI with associated apical akinesis and deep venous thrombosis due to prolonged bedrest. Contemporary methods of care for acute MI have greatly reduced the risk of post-MI thromboembolism.

Reperfusion therapy, when applied in a timely fashion, results in less extensive MI and less impairment of LV function. Patients with anterior MI treated with reperfusion therapy are less likely to have extensive apical akinesis, which is the breeding ground for mural thrombus. It is advised that patients treated for acute MI have an echocardiogram to assess for overall LV function; in the case of anterior MI, the presence of apical mural thrombus can be detected by echocardiography.

亡风险显著增加。随着再灌注治疗的广泛应用，心肌梗死后心力衰竭和心源性休克发生率已显著降低，主要得益于早期再灌注治疗可减少心肌梗死面积，降低心力衰竭相关并发症的发生风险。当发生心肌梗死后急性心力衰竭时，应予以氧疗、吗啡和利尿剂静脉推注；硝酸甘油通过降低心脏前负荷也可发挥作用。对于心肌梗死后射血分数减低的心力衰竭，长期治疗方案应包括 ACEI/ARB、β 受体阻滞剂、醛固酮受体拮抗剂（如依普利酮或螺内酯），必要时可加用利尿剂等。

发生急性心肌梗死后，心室需要一定的充盈压和容量来维持心输出量。但急性心肌梗死患者往往由于恶心、呕吐、摄入量减少等原因而处于低血容量状态，进而导致左心室前负荷和输出量降低，临床可表现出低血压状态；可通过适当补液纠正这种状态，但补液需慎重。

在渡过早期容易出现心律失常的时间段后，单纯急性下壁心肌梗死患者的死亡风险一般很低（住院死亡率约 6%）。但约有 10%~15% 的下壁心肌梗死患者可合并右冠状动脉及其较大锐缘支动脉闭塞引起的右心室梗死，此时患者死亡风险显著升高（住院期间死亡率高达 25%~30%）。右心室梗死的临床表现包括颈静脉压升高导致的 Kussmaul 征和低血压状态。尽管右心室功能多能快速恢复，但仍需补充足够的容量以维持右心输出量；有时需短期使用多巴胺等正性肌力药以维持血流动力学稳定；同时避免使用血管扩张剂和利尿剂。此外，下壁心肌梗死可伴发一过性高度房室传导阻滞，常导致患者血流动力学不稳定，此时可考虑植入临时起搏器。下壁心肌梗死患者对快心室率的房颤往往耐受性较差，需及时转复。

心源性休克

心源性休克是由大面积心肌梗死导致心输出量显著降低［心脏指数 < 1.8 L/(min·m²)］、左心室充盈压明显升高（肺毛细血管楔压 > 18 mmHg），临床表现为低血压、外周器官低灌注的一种临床综合征。心源性休克死亡率高达 70%~80%。有创血流动力学监测，并使用正性肌力药物和必要的机械循环辅助装置有助于稳定患者的血流动力学状态。机械循环辅助装置包括主动脉内球囊反搏（IABP）、Impella 心室辅助装置（VAD）和体外膜肺氧合（ECMO）。IABP 可在导管室快速置入，增加心输出量并改善冠脉舒张期灌注。但 IABP 作用有限，仅起到短期辅助作用，患者的预后主要取决于其他可逆因素，包括血运重建能否有效改善心肌缺血，心肌梗死相关机械并发症（如二尖瓣关闭不全或室间隔穿孔）是否得到纠正。IABP 的绝对禁忌证是主动脉瓣重度反流，相对禁忌证是严重周围动脉疾病。尽管 IABP 能提供一定的血流动力学支持，但临床随机对照试验显示 IABP 未能有效降低心源性休克患者的死亡率，因此 IABP 不作为心源性休克的常规治疗手段，主要由临床医师根据患者具体病情决定是否使用。目前一些医院可为病情危重的心源性休克患者提供更高级的循环支持系统（包括 Impella 和 ECMO），为患者心功能恢复或植入长期心室辅助装置（译者注：如人工心脏）或心脏移植争取治疗时间。

急性心肌梗死相关心源性休克治疗的关键是尽可能恢复心脏缺血区域的血液灌注。最新理论建议，与"门球时间"是影响 STEMI 预后的首要因素不同，心源性休克应更强调先通过机械循环支持，以尽早改善重要器官灌注，然后再行血运重建。如心源性休克患者合并多支冠脉病变，建议急诊 PCI 只处理罪犯病变，其他狭窄病变可择期再处理。

机械并发症

急性心肌梗死的机械并发症包括：乳头肌功能障碍或断裂引起的二尖瓣关闭不全、室间隔穿孔、心室游离壁破裂和左心室假性室壁瘤形成。这些情况通常发生于心肌梗死后 1 周内，所导致的死亡约占心肌梗死总死亡的 15%。当出现新发心脏杂音、突发心力衰竭及血流动力学迅速恶化时，需警惕机械并发症发生。未进行再灌注治疗或未及时行再灌注治疗的患者，更容易发生机械并发症。超声心动图通常可以发现这些机械并发症，右心导管检查进行血流动力学评估可协助诊断。机械并发症大多需要进行外科手术治疗。

乳头肌断裂或功能异常引起的急性重度二尖瓣关闭不全可导致严重心力衰竭，75% 的患者会在 24 h 内死亡。静脉使用硝普钠和置入 IABP 可降低心脏后负荷，有助于稳定患者血流动力学状态；但往往需要外科手术行瓣膜修补或置换才可增加患者存活机会。尽管外科手术死亡风险高达 25%~50%，但单纯药物或 IABP 治疗的死亡风险更高。

老年患者，尤其是合并高血压的患者更容易出现心肌梗死相关的室间隔穿孔。溶栓治疗也可以增加室间隔穿孔风险。急性室间隔穿孔引起的左向右分流可导致严重的血流动力学不稳定。与二尖瓣关闭不全类似，降低心脏后负荷和 IABP 治疗有助于稳定患者的血流动力学状态，但外科手术修补仍是必需的。患者往往无法耐受中等或大的室间隔穿孔导致的血流动力学障碍，死亡风险极高。前壁心肌梗死相关的室间隔缺损可能比下壁心肌梗死相关的室间隔缺损更适合进行外科修补。一些患者也可考虑行经皮介入封堵，从而可能推迟外科手术直到室间隔梗死部位组织愈合良好。

左心室游离壁破裂的发病风险和病理学特点与室间隔穿孔类似。游离壁破裂通常会因心脏压塞而发生猝死。偶有患者形成左心室假性室壁瘤，需行外科手术治疗。

血栓栓塞并发症

在早些年，血栓栓塞（包括心源性卒中和肺栓塞）事件发生率约 10%，死亡率占心肌梗死后住院死亡率的 25%。血栓栓塞的风险与左心室附壁血栓和深静脉血栓形成有关，前者更容易出现在伴有心尖运动消失的前壁心肌梗死患者，后者与长期卧床有关。现代急性心肌梗死后护理方法已大大降低了心肌梗死后血栓栓塞事件发生的风险。

及时的再灌注治疗可减少心肌梗死面积，并降低左心功能受损程度。目前对于及时接受再灌注治疗的前壁心肌梗死患者已很少出现大面积心尖部运动丧失，从而显著减

If LV mural thrombus is present, the patient should receive therapeutic anticoagulation with unfractionated or LMW heparin while oral anticoagulation with warfarin is initiated. Warfarin therapy should be continued for 6 months after MI when LV apical mural thrombus is detected. Early ambulation after MI, along with the use of compression stockings and subcutaneous heparin prophylaxis (unfractionated or LMW) for deep venous thrombosis, has greatly diminished the threat of pulmonary embolism.

PROGNOSIS

Risk Stratification After Myocardial Infarction

Key to understanding an individual patient's risk for future coronary events or mortality related to MI is a thorough assessment of drivers for those risks: status of LV function and its impact on clinical functional status, residual myocardial ischemia, and spontaneous or exercise-induced arrhythmias. Appropriate predischarge assessments provide a comprehensive picture of the patient's risk status and prognosis.

Electrocardiographic Monitoring

Patients are routinely monitored by telemetry systems that capture arrhythmic events in the first 48 hours after MI. Late ventricular arrhythmias such as VF or sustained VT identify patients who are likely to benefit from ICD therapy. This is particularly true if EF is reduced to less than 40%. ICD implantation is also indicated for patients with persistently reduced EF (<30%).

Cardiac Catheterization and Noninvasive Testing

Predischarge risk stratification may involve cardiac catheterization, submaximal predischarge exercise stress testing (on days 4 to 6), or maximal exercise stress testing after discharge (at 2 to 6 weeks). The presence or absence of high-risk coronary anatomy is demonstrated for patients who have undergone primary PCI at the time of presentation. Many patients who have been treated with thrombolytic therapy undergo coronary angiography before discharge to determine the extent and severity of underlying CAD as well as the status of the culprit lesion. If coronary angiography is not performed, predischarge submaximal exercise testing (up to 70% of maximal predicted heart rate) is done to identify those who are at increased risk for postdischarge coronary ischemic events. Patients who undergo submaximal exercise stress testing in lieu of coronary angiography frequently have a follow-up maximal exercise stress test within 2 to 6 weeks after discharge. During stress testing, positive results that suggest the need for coronary angiography include exercise-induced angina, ST changes of ischemia (ST depression), exercise-induced hypotension, exercise-induced ventricular arrhythmias, and low functional capacity. The sensitivity and specificity of stress testing after MI is enhanced by the use of imaging modalities such as stress echocardiography or nuclear perfusion imaging. All patients should have their EF assessed, typically by echocardiography, before discharge.

Secondary Prevention, Patient Education, and Rehabilitation

The goal of secondary prevention is to reduce the risk of recurrent MI and cardiovascular mortality. Risk factor modification is key to the secondary prevention strategy. All patients should have their lipid status assessed at the time of admission, but statin therapy is warranted in patients with acute MI at presentation. The target LDL level is less than 100 mg/dL, preferably closer to 70 mg/dL. Smoking cessation is of critical importance because it can reduce the risk of reinfarction, and ongoing smoking can double the risk of recurrent MI or mortality in the first year after MI. Structured smoking cessation programs and the use of pharmacologic aids (e.g., nicotine patches or gum, bupropion, varenicline) can increase the success of smoking cessation efforts.

Antiplatelet therapy with aspirin (75 to 162 mg/day) is given indefinitely to all patients after MI. Regardless of whether primary PCI has been performed, patients will benefit from the additional use of a P2Y12 inhibitor for the first year after MI. Those patients who have received a stent during primary PCI should continue clopidogrel 75 mg/day, ticagrelor 90 mg twice daily, or prasugrel 10 mg/day for one year. There are some data suggesting that if the patient is tolerating dual-antiplatelet therapy (DAPT) well and has a low bleeding risk, there may be additional benefit to continuing DAPT even for up to three years.

The use of anticoagulation is indicated for patients with systemic or pulmonary thromboembolism, as well as persistent or paroxysmal AF, guided by their CHADS-2 score (congestive heart failure, hypertension, age ≥75 years, diabetes mellitus, and stroke). Patients who are at high risk for thromboembolism after acute MI, such as those with low EF related to anterior MI, can also be considered for prophylactic anticoagulation; however, there is no strong randomized data for this indication.

The high prevalence of patients who have both AF and the need for stent placement creates a conundrum involving the need for both anticoagulation and antiplatelet agents leading to a significantly increased risk of bleeding. Warfarin (target international normalized ratio [INR], 2.0 to 3.0) has been the historical choice for anticoagulation. Its use in conjunction with patients having undergone stenting was evaluated in several clinical trials that suggested that therapy with warfarin and clopidogrel had similar outcomes for ischemic or embolic events compared to "triple therapy" (warfarin, clopidogrel, and aspirin) but afforded a lower risk of bleeding. Since then, newer anticoagulant medications have been developed for nonvalvular AF that have merited their own series of trials, including the thrombin inhibitor dabigatran and the direct factor Xa inhibitors apixaban, edoxaban, and rivaroxaban. These drugs were also demonstrated to be effective when paired with clopidogrel with a lower bleeding risk compared to triple therapy. None of the trials referenced above utilized any other P2Y12 inhibitors aside from clopidogrel. Ultimately the decision regarding antithrombotic therapy length and composition will be provider dependent but should be based upon an assessment of the patient's bleeding and ischemic risk.

Acute anterior MI that has resulted in significant injury to the ventricle with an EF of less than 40% places the patient at risk for future negative remodeling of the left ventricle and potential heart failure. ACE-inhibitor therapy has been shown to reduce the risk of negative remodeling and the occurrence of heart failure in such patients. This group of patients also experiences a reduction in future recurrent MI risk with the use of ACE-inhibitor therapy. This observation does not appear to carry over to patients with stable CAD. ACE-inhibitor therapy (captopril, ramipril, lisinopril) is indicated for all patients after MI. The use of ARBs (e.g., valsartan, losartan) is reasonable for patients who are intolerant of ACE-inhibitor therapy. The aldosterone receptor antagonist eplerenone (25 mg/day, titrated to 50 mg/day) is indicated as additive therapy to ACE or ARB in MI patients who have reduced EF (<40%) or diabetes. Careful monitoring of serum potassium is required after initiation of eplerenone together with ACE or ARB.

β-Blocker therapy reduces mortality risk in patients who have reduced EF post-MI. This therapy should be avoided in patients with uncompensated heart failure early after MI or the presence of other contraindications. Metoprolol succinate (25 mg/day titrated up to 200 mg/day) or carvedilol (3.125-6.25 mg titrated to 25 mg twice each day) should be initiated at low doses and titrated upward as tolerated. The role of β-blockers in patients with no residual myocardial ischemia, arrhythmias, or normal EF is not clear.

少了附壁血栓发生风险。推荐所有急性心肌梗死患者行超声心动图检查以评估左心功能，对于前壁心肌梗死患者还可以及时发现心尖部附壁血栓。如果发生左心室附壁血栓应予普通肝素或低分子量肝素抗凝，同时开始口服华法林抗凝；华法林应持续应用至心肌梗死后 6 个月。鼓励心肌梗死后早期下床活动，使用弹力袜及预防性皮下注射肝素（普通肝素或低分子量肝素）抗凝以减少下肢深静脉血栓形成，以上措施可显著降低肺栓塞风险。

预后

心肌梗死后风险分层

了解心肌梗死患者远期发生冠状动脉缺血事件及死亡风险的关键在于全面评估以下危险因素：左心功能及其对临床功能状态的影响、残余的心肌缺血情况及有无自发或活动诱发的心律失常。心肌梗死患者出院前进行上述评估可以全面了解患者的事件发生风险和预后。

心电监测

建议在心肌梗死后 48 h 内常规进行心电监测，以及时发现心律失常事件。发生晚期室性心律失常（包括室颤或持续性室速）的患者植入 ICD 可能获益，尤其是射血分数 < 40% 的患者。射血分数持续减低（< 30%）的患者也建议植入 ICD。

心导管和无创性检查

心导管检查、出院前亚极量运动负荷试验（可在心肌梗死后第 4～6 天进行）和出院后极量运动负荷试验（可在出院后第 2～6 周完成）等检查可辅助评估心肌梗死患者出院后再发事件风险。行急诊 PCI 的患者可以通过同期冠脉造影评估有无高危冠脉病变；而对于接受溶栓治疗的患者，建议出院前行冠脉造影检查，以明确罪犯病变状况，并评估冠脉病变的范围及严重程度。若无法行冠脉造影检查，建议行亚极量运动负荷试验（达到最大预测心率的 70%），以识别出院后再发冠状动脉缺血事件的高危人群；同时建议以亚极量运动负荷试验替代冠状动脉造影检查的患者在出院后 2～6 周内行极量运动负荷试验。运动负荷试验阳性（包括运动诱发的心绞痛、缺血性 ST 段改变如 ST 段压低、运动导致的低血压、运动导致的室性心律失常发作或运动耐量降低）的患者应考虑行冠脉造影。也可以考虑行敏感性和特异性更高的负荷超声心动图或运动心肌核素显像等影像学检查。所有患者在出院前评估左心室射血分数，一般通过超声心动图检查进行。

冠心病二级预防、患者教育和康复治疗

冠心病二级预防的目标是减少再发心肌梗死和心血管死亡，其核心是冠心病危险因素的控制。所有患者住院期间均应检测血脂水平，但对于急性心肌梗死患者，无论血脂水平高低，在就诊时就应接受他汀类药物治疗。LDL 的目标值应 < 100 mg/dl，最好控制接近 70 mg/dl。戒烟可减少再发梗死风险，因此戒烟非常重要；而继续吸烟则可以使 1 年内再发心肌梗死和死亡风险增加 1 倍。系统制订戒烟方案并使用辅助药物（如尼古丁贴片或尼古丁口香糖、安非他酮和伐尼克兰）可提高戒烟成功率。

所有心肌梗死患者均应长期服用阿司匹林（75～162 mg 1 次 / 日）行抗血小板治疗；无论是否行急诊 PCI，加用 P2Y12 抑制剂使用 12 个月可带来明确获益。对于急诊 PCI 行冠状动脉支架置入的患者，应继续使用氯吡格雷 75 mg 1 次 / 日、替格瑞洛 90 mg 2 次 / 日或普拉格雷 10 mg 1 次 / 日至少 12 个月。有研究显示如患者能耐受双联抗血小板治疗（DAPT）且出血风险较低，可考虑延长双联抗血小板治疗至 36 个月，可能会带来额外获益。

存在体循环栓塞或肺栓塞的患者应接受抗凝治疗；对于持续性或阵发性房颤患者，可根据 CHADS-2 评分（允血性心力衰竭、高血压、年龄 ≥ 75 岁、糖尿病、卒中）来评估是否需要抗凝治疗。对于血栓栓塞高危（如前壁心肌梗死合并射血分数明显减低）患者，可考虑预防性抗凝治疗，但目前尚缺乏随机对照研究等明确证据支持这种治疗策略。

房颤患者需行冠状动脉支架置入术的情况并不少见，这类患者面临既需抗凝又需抗血小板治疗的难题，因为抗凝联合抗血小板治疗会显著增加出血风险。华法林 [目标国际标准化比值（INR）2.0～3.0] 是最早使用的抗凝药物。临床试验显示，华法林联合氯吡格雷与三联抗栓治疗（华法林 + 氯吡格雷 + 阿司匹林）相比，两组在缺血或栓塞事件发生率方面的结果相似，但出血风险更低。此后，一些新型抗凝药物被开发出来，并经过临床研究检验后，主要用于非瓣膜性房颤的抗凝治疗，包括直接凝血酶抑制剂达比加群酯及直接 Xa 因子抑制剂阿哌沙班、艾多沙班和利伐沙班。这些新型抗凝药物联合氯吡格雷较三联抗栓治疗相比仍然具有相似的抗栓疗效和更低的出血风险。需注意，上述临床试验均采用抗凝药物联合氯吡格雷而非其他 P2Y12 抑制剂。最终的抗栓治疗方案和时长只能由临床医师在充分权衡患者出血和缺血风险后决定。

急性前壁心肌梗死导致左心功能严重受损、射血分数下降 < 40% 的患者具有较高的远期左心室病理性重构和心力衰竭的发病风险。ACEI 不仅可以有效降低此类患者左心室病理性重构和心力衰竭的发病风险，还可降低再发心肌梗死风险；而对于稳定性 CAD 患者，使用 ACEI 似乎并不能带来上述获益。因此，所有心肌梗死患者均应接受 ACEI（如卡托普利、雷米普利、赖诺普利）治疗；对于不耐受 ACEI 的患者应予 ARB（如缬沙坦、氯沙坦等）。心肌梗死合并射血分数减低（< 40%）或者糖尿病的患者可考虑在 ACEI/ARB 基础上加用醛固酮受体拮抗剂依普利酮（起始 25 mg/d，可逐渐加量至最大剂量 50 mg/d），但上述药物联用需严密监测血钾水平。

β 受体阻滞剂可以降低心肌梗死后射血分数减低患者的死亡风险，但应避免用于心肌梗死后早期失代偿性心力衰竭或存在其他禁忌证的患者。琥珀酸美托洛尔（起始 25 mg/d，最大剂量 200 mg/d）或卡维地洛（起始 3.125～6.25 mg 2 次 / 日，最大剂量 25 mg 2 次 / 日）应从小剂量开始，逐渐加量至患者可耐受的最大剂量。

Nitrates, either short-acting sublingual nitroglycerin or long-acting versions, may be useful in the treatment of stable angina. Calcium-channel blocking drugs should be avoided in patients with reduced EF (<40%). In patients with normal EF, either diltiazem or verapamil may useful as a substitute in patients who are intolerant of β-blockers when either antianginal therapy or rate control for AF is needed. The dihydropyridine, amlodipine, may be a useful adjunct for control of hypertension or treatment of angina. It should be used with caution in the face of reduced EF.

After acute MI, women should refrain from initiating hormone therapy with estrogen or estrogen/progesterone preparations; these agents do not decrease the risk of recurrent MI but do increase the risk of thromboembolic events. The ongoing use of hormone therapy in women already receiving treatment should be individualized, with a bias toward discontinuing therapy. Diabetic patients need attention to their degree of glycemic control, with a target of hemoglobin A_{1c} less than 7%. Vitamin supplements have no clear role in therapy for MI patients. Fish oil supplements do not appear to benefit patients who have experienced acute MI.

Patient Education and Cardiac Rehabilitation

It is important to begin the education of patients early after acute MI so that they understand the value of their various prescribed medical therapies and the need for risk factor modification. Cardiac rehabilitation programs are very useful in the ongoing education of patients; they reinforce positive lifestyle changes and provide exercise training in the post-MI period. Such programs not only educate patients but also help them to regain confidence in their ability to perform the tasks of daily living and other activities they enjoy. Early follow-up with the physician after discharge is also important to ensure clinical stability and tolerance of medical therapy and to monitor the progress of lifestyle changes.

SUGGESTED READINGS

Amsterdam EA, Wenger NK, Brindis RG, et al: 2014 AHA/ACC Guideline for the Management of Patients with Non–ST-Elevation Acute Coronary Syndromes, J Am Coll Cardiol 64(24):e139–e228, 2014.

Arnett DK, Blumenthal RS, Albert MA, et al.: 2019 ACC/AHA Guideline on the primary prevention of cardiovascular disease: A Report of the American College of Cardiology/American Heart Association Task Force on Clinical Practice Guidelines, Circulation 140:e596–e646, 2019.

Fihn SD, Gardin JM, Abrams J, et al.: 2012 ACCF/AHA/ACP/AATS/PCNA/SCAI/STS Guideline for the diagnosis and management of patients with stable ischemic heart disease: a report of the American College of Cardiology Foundation/American Heart Association Task Force on Practice Guidelines, and the American College of Physicians, American Association for Thoracic Surgery, Preventive Cardiovascular Nurses Association, Society for Cardiovascular Angiography And Interventions, and Society of Thoracic Surgeons, J Am Coll Cardiol 60:e44–e164, 2012.

Hillis LD, Smith PK, Anderson JL, et al.: 2011 ACCF/AHA Guideline for coronary artery bypass graft surgery: A report of the American College of Cardiology Foundation/American Heart Association Task Force on Practice Guidelines. Developed in collaboration with the American Association for Thoracic Surgery, Society of Cardiovascular Anesthesiologists, and Society of Thoracic Surgeons, J Am Coll Cardiol 58:e123–e210, 2011.

Levine GN, Bates ER, Bittl JA, et al.: 2016 ACC/AHA Guideline focused update on duration of dual antiplatelet therapy in patients with coronary artery disease, J Am Coll Cardiol 68(10):1082–1115, 2016.

Levine GN, Bates ER, Blankenship JC, et al.: 2011 ACCF/AHA/SCAI guideline for percutaneous coronary intervention: a report of the American College of Cardiology Foundation/American Heart Association Task Force on Practice Guidelines and the Society for Cardiovascular Angiography and Interventions, J Am Coll Cardiol 58:e44–e122, 2011.

Levine GN, Bates ER, Blankenship JC, et al.: 2015 ACC/AHA/SCAI focused update on primary percutaneous coronary intervention for patients with ST-elevation myocardial infarction, J Am Coll Cardiol 67(10):1235–1250, 2016.

O'Gara PT, Kushner FG, Ascheim DD, et al.: 2013 ACCF/AHA Guideline for the management of ST-elevation myocardial infarction: a report of the American College of Cardiology Foundation/American Heart Association Task Force on Practice Guidelines, J Am Coll Cardiol 61(4):e78–e140, 2013.

对于没有残余心肌缺血、心律失常及射血分数正常的患者，β受体阻滞剂是否获益仍不清楚。

硝酸酯类药物（包括舌下含服的短效硝酸甘油和长效口服制剂）可用于治疗稳定型心绞痛患者；钙通道阻滞剂应避免用于射血分数＜40%的患者；对于不耐受β受体阻滞剂且射血分数正常的患者，可考虑使用地尔硫䓬或维拉帕米以控制心绞痛发作或房颤的快心室率；二氢吡啶类钙通道阻滞剂（如氨氯地平）可用于控制高血压和心绞痛发作，同样慎用于射血分数减低患者。

女性心肌梗死患者应避免使用雌激素或雌/孕激素复合制剂，这类药物不仅不能降低再发心肌梗死风险，反而可明确增加血栓栓塞风险。而对于已经接受激素治疗的患者，能否继续使用激素需个体化评价，尽量暂停激素治疗；糖尿病患者应注意监测血糖，糖化血红蛋白应控制＜7%；补充维生素对于治疗心肌梗死效果并不确切；目前也没有证据表明鱼油可以使急性心肌梗死患者获益。

患者教育和心脏康复治疗

在急性心肌梗死早期就应开展患者教育，使患者充分了解所使用药物的作用及控制冠心病危险因素的重要性。制订心脏康复方案在患者教育中非常重要，它可以督促患者改善生活方式，并指导心肌梗死后恢复期的运动康复训练；此外，心脏康复方案还能帮助心肌梗死患者重新恢复正常生活、甚至继续从事自己所热爱的体育运动的信心。心肌梗死患者出院后也应及时复诊，评估病情稳定性、服药依从性，并监督生活方式改善情况。

推荐阅读

Amsterdam EA, Wenger NK, Brindis RG, et al: 2014 AHA/ACC Guideline for the Management of Patients with Non–ST-Elevation Acute Coronary Syndromes, J Am Coll Cardiol 64(24):e139–e228, 2014.

Arnett DK, Blumenthal RS, Albert MA, et al.: 2019 ACC/AHA Guideline on the primary prevention of cardiovascular disease: A Report of the American College of Cardiology/American Heart Association Task Force on Clinical Practice Guidelines, Circulation 140:e596–e646, 2019.

Fihn SD, Gardin JM, Abrams J, et al.: 2012 ACCF/AHA/ACP/AATS/PCNA/SCAI/STS Guideline for the diagnosis and management of patients with stable ischemic heart disease: a report of the American College of Cardiology Foundation/American Heart Association Task Force on Practice Guidelines, and the American College of Physicians, American Association for Thoracic Surgery, Preventive Cardiovascular Nurses Association, Society for Cardiovascular Angiography And Interventions, and Society of Thoracic Surgeons, J Am Coll Cardiol 60:e44–e164, 2012.

Hillis LD, Smith PK, Anderson JL, et al.: 2011 ACCF/AHA Guideline for coronary artery bypass graft surgery: A report of the American College of Cardiology Foundation/American Heart Association Task Force on Practice Guidelines. Developed in collaboration with the American Association for Thoracic Surgery, Society of Cardiovascular Anesthesiologists, and Society of Thoracic Surgeons, J Am Coll Cardiol 58:e123–e210, 2011.

Levine GN, Bates ER, Bittl JA, et al.: 2016 ACC/AHA Guideline focused update on duration of dual antiplatelet therapy in patients with coronary artery disease, J Am Coll Cardiol 68(10):1082–1115, 2016.

Levine GN, Bates ER, Blankenship JC, et al.: 2011 ACCF/AHA/SCAI guideline for percutaneous coronary intervention: a report of the American College of Cardiology Foundation/American Heart Association Task Force on Practice Guidelines and the Society for Cardiovascular Angiography and Interventions, J Am Coll Cardiol 58:e44–e122, 2011.

Levine GN, Bates ER, Blankenship JC, et al.: 2015 ACC/AHA/SCAI focused update on primary percutaneous coronary intervention for patients with ST-elevation myocardial infarction, J Am Coll Cardiol 67(10):1235–1250, 2016.

O'Gara PT, Kushner FG, Ascheim DD, et al.: 2013 ACCF/AHA Guideline for the management of ST-elevation myocardial infarction: a report of the American College of Cardiology Foundation/American Heart Association Task Force on Practice Guidelines, J Am Coll Cardiol 61(4):e78–e140, 2013.

8

Cardiac Arrhythmias

Marcie G. Berger, Jason C. Rubenstein, James A. Roth

BASIC CELLULAR ELECTROPHYSIOLOGY

Cardiac myocytes actively maintain a negative resting membrane potential (E_m) through the differential distribution of ions between intracellular and extracellular compartments, which is an energy-dependent process that relies on ion channels, pumps, and exchangers. Transmembrane differences in voltage and ionic concentration create electrical and chemical forces that drive charged ions in and out of cells.

The resting E_m of cardiac myocytes is controlled by potassium ions (K^+). Active K^+ transport by the sodium-potassium adenosine triphosphatase pump (Na^+, K^+-ATPase) produces a transmembrane ionic gradient, with the intracellular concentration of K^+ exceeding the extracellular concentration. This favors the net efflux of K^+ from cells, down the chemical concentration gradient, yielding a resting negative charge within the cardiac myocytes. K^+ continues to flow from the intracellular to the extracellular compartment until the negative intracellular charge counterbalances the transmembrane K^+ concentration gradient at a potential called the *equilibrium potential* for K^+. This potential, at which the net K^+ current is zero, is close to the resting E_m of nonpacemaker cardiac myocytes. Pacemaker cells (i.e., sinoatrial and atrioventricular [AV] nodal cells) are characterized by a resting E_m of −50 to −60 mV. The resting E_m of atrial and ventricular myocytes is typically −80 to −90 mV.

The depolarization of a cardiac myocyte to threshold potential triggers a sequence of ionic movements resulting in a cardiac action potential (Fig. 8.1). The action potential is divided into five phases. Phase 0 is the rapid depolarization of nonpacemaker myocytes resulting from rapid sodium ion (Na^+) entry through fast Na^+ channels. These channels have three conformational states: closed (resting state), open (conducting Na^+ current), and inactivated, from which recovery is voltage dependent. Phase 1 is early, rapid, partial repolarization of the cell mediated by K^+ efflux. During phase 2, the plateau phase, there is a small net current flow, with inward calcium ion (Ca^{2+}) flow balanced by outward K^+ flow.

During phase 3, repolarization is mediated by an increase in K^+ efflux and a decline in Ca^{2+} influx. The dominant repolarizing current is I_{Kr}, the rapidly activating delayed rectifier K^+ current, a channel encoded by the *KCNE2* gene (also called *HERG*). The I_{Ks} current, or slowly activating delayed rectifier K^+ current, also contributes to repolarization. Phase 3 determines to a large degree the cellular refractory period. Importantly, I_{Kr} is inhibited by a large number of drugs that prolong the action potential duration.

Phase 4 is particularly significant in cardiac pacemaker cells because slow depolarization occurs from the resting membrane potential to the threshold potential. The resting E_m, rate of spontaneous phase 4 depolarization, and rate of phase 0 depolarization differentiate slow-response from fast-response cardiac myocytes. Slow-response cells, located in the sinoatrial node and AV node, normally display automaticity or spontaneous depolarization during phase 4. Resting E_m in slow-response cells is less negative, and Ca^{2+} current mediates phase 0 depolarization. Conduction in these pacemaker cells is slow, and recovery from inactivation is time dependent. The fast-response cells found in atrial myocytes, ventricular myocytes, and the His-Purkinje system display slow phase 4 depolarization and do not typically display automaticity. Their resting E_m is more negative, and the fast Na^+ current drives rapid phase 0 depolarization and rapid conduction. Recovery from inactivation in these cells is voltage dependent.

The sinus node typically displays the fastest phase 4 depolarization. Other cardiac tissues have the capacity to depolarize spontaneously, and subsidiary pacemakers may take over when sinus rates slow and under conditions of increased automaticity. Typically, the AV node, located above the AV ring, serves as the heart's secondary pacemaker, with a spontaneous rate of depolarization of 40 to 50 beats per minute. Automaticity of cardiac myocytes is increased when the slope of phase 4 depolarization increases, with a shift of threshold potentials to more negative values, or in the presence of more positive maximal diastolic potentials.

The sinus node is the primary intrinsic pacemaker, and spontaneous depolarization leads to action potential generation, with normal resting rates of 60 to 100 beats per minute. Depolarization then spreads through the atria to the AV node, where conduction slows, introducing a delay between atrial and ventricular activation, and then to the His-Purkinje system fibers, which originate at the AV node with the bundle of His and split to form the left bundle branch and the right bundle branch, rapidly conducting depolarization to the ventricular myocardium. Cardiac myocytes are joined by electrical synapses called *gap junctions*, which permit the flow of intracellular current from cell to cell.

Classification of Arrhythmias

Mechanistically, cardiac arrhythmias can be broadly divided into disorders of action potential formation and disorders of impulse conduction. Clinically, arrhythmias are classified as bradycardias and tachycardias, with further categorization according to arrhythmia origin. This information is used to guide evaluation and management strategies.

Electrophysiologic Mechanisms of Arrhythmias

Automaticity is a normal function of pacemaker cells, occurring during phase 4 depolarization. *Enhanced automaticity* occurs when pacemaker cells depolarize at a faster rate due to an increased slope of phase 4 depolarization, a shift of threshold potential to a more negative value,

心律失常

周晶亮　刘芃　译　李学斌　周益锋　审校　郑金刚　通审

基础细胞电生理学

心肌细胞通过细胞内外离子浓度差主动维持"外正内负"的静息膜电位（E_m），这一过程依赖于离子通道、离子泵和转运载体，并且需要消耗能量。跨膜电压差和离子浓度差产生电化学力，驱动带电离子进出细胞。

心肌细胞的静息膜电位由钾离子（K^+）控制。通过钠-钾三磷酸腺苷酶（Na^+, K^+-ATP 酶）对 K^+ 的主动跨膜转运产生钾离子浓度梯度，即细胞膜内 K^+ 浓度高于细胞膜外。这促使 K^+ 沿着化学浓度梯度通过细胞膜外流，使心肌细胞膜内电荷为负值。K^+ 继续从细胞膜内向膜外移动，直到膜内外电位差阻碍 K^+ 外流的力量与浓度差促使 K^+ 外流的力量平衡时，这时的膜电位称作 K^+ 平衡电位。此电位下，K^+ 跨膜净电流为零，接近非自律细胞的静息电位。自律细胞[如窦房结和房室结（AV）细胞]的静息电位为 -50 至 -60 mV。心房和心室肌细胞的静息电位通常为 -80 至 -90 mV。

心肌细胞去极化到阈电位会触发一系列离子跨膜运动，产生动作电位（图 8.1）。动作电位可分为五期。0 期是非自律细胞快速去极化，由快速 Na^+ 通道开放，钠离子（Na^+）快速内流引起。这些离子通道具有三种构象状态：关闭（静息状态）、开放（Na^+ 快速内流）和失活。离子通道失活后的恢复依赖于电压。1 期是细胞早期、快速和部分复极，通过 K^+ 外流介导。2 期称为平台期，跨膜净电流小，此期钙离子（Ca^{2+}）内流与 K^+ 外流互相抵消。

3 期，K^+ 外流增加和 Ca^{2+} 内流减少介导细胞复极。主导细胞复极的电流是 I_{Kr}，即快速激活的延迟整流 K^+ 电流，是由 KCNE2 基因编码的离子通道（也称为 HERG）。I_{Ks} 电流或称慢速激活的延迟整流 K^+ 电流，也参与了细胞复极。3 期在很大程度上决定了细胞的不应期。重要的是，I_{Kr} 可被许多延长动作电位持续时间的药物所抑制。

4 期对于自律细胞尤其重要，因为从静息电位到阈电位的缓慢去极化发生在这一期。根据静息电位、4 期自动去极化速率和 0 期去极化速率区分慢反应和快反应心肌细胞。位于窦房结和房室结的慢反应细胞通常在 4 期表现出自律性或出现自动去极化。慢反应细胞的静息电位负值较小，Ca^{2+} 内流介导 0 期去极化。这些自律细胞传导慢，从失活状态恢复活性具有时间依赖性。在心房肌细胞、心室肌细胞和希浦（His-Purkinje）系统中发现的快反应细胞显示 4 期缓慢地去极化，通常不显示自律性。它们的静息电位负值更大，0 期通过快速 Na^+ 电流迅速去极化，传导速度快。这些细胞从失活状态恢复活性呈现电压依赖性。

通常情况下窦房结 4 期自动去极化速率最快，其他心肌组织也具备自动去极化的能力，当窦房结自律性降低，并且其他心肌组织自律性增加的情况下，潜在起搏点可能取代窦房结成为异位起搏点。通常，位于房室环上方的房室结作为心脏的潜在起搏点，自动去极化速率为 40～50 次/分。当 4 期去极化速率增加，阈电位负值增大，或最大舒张电位数值减小时，心肌细胞自律性增加。

窦房结是最主要的心脏起搏点，自动去极化产生动作电位，静息时正常心率为 60～100 次/分。然后心肌细胞去极化通过心房传导至房室结，由于房室结存在传导延缓，引起心房和心室之间的激动延迟。然后心肌细胞去极化传导至希浦系统。希浦系统起源于房室结的希氏束，并分为左右束支，将心肌细胞去极化迅速传至心室。心肌细胞通过电突触相连接，称为缝隙连接。心肌细胞间细胞内电流通过缝隙连接流动。

心律失常的分类

从机制上讲，心律失常大致可分为动作电位形成障碍和冲动传导异常。临床上，心律失常通常分为心动过缓和心动过速，并根据心律失常的起源部位进一步分类。这些信息主要用来指导病情评估和治疗策略。

心律失常的电生理机制

自律性是起搏细胞的正常功能，发生在 4 期自动去极化。当起搏细胞 4 期自动去极化的斜率增加、阈电位下移（负值更大），或最大舒张电位数值减小时，去极化速率更快，自律性增加。上述变化可发生于交感神经兴奋的情况下。自律性增加可能是正常的（如适当的窦

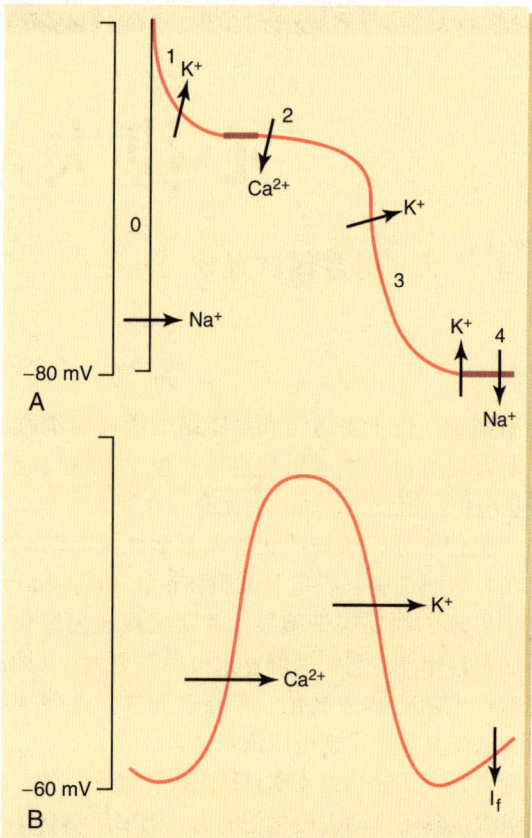

Fig. 8.1 Electrophysiologic basis of the cardiac cellular action potential. (A) Fast-response cells found in working myocardium and the specialized infranodal conduction system maintain a strongly negative resting membrane potential and a brisk phase 0 upstroke mediated by rapid sodium influx at the start of the action potential. (B) In contrast, slow-response cells found in the sinus node and atrioventricular nodal tissue exhibit less-negative resting membrane potentials, slower calcium-channel–dependent action potential upstrokes, and phase 4 depolarization.

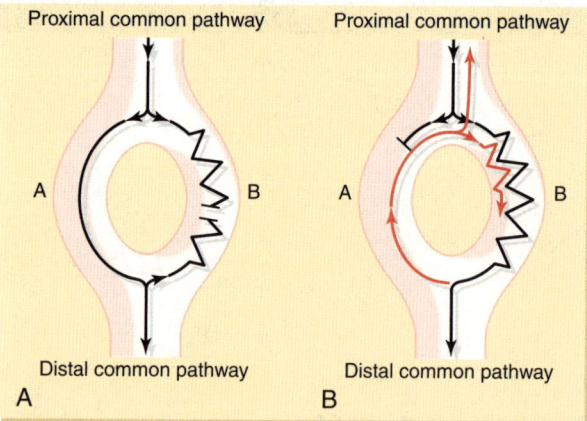

Fig. 8.2 Mechanism of reentry. Reentry requires two distinct pathways with different refractoriness and a region of slowed conduction. One pathway (A) has normal rapid conduction but a long refractory period. The second pathway (B) has slowed conduction but a relatively shorter refractory period. To initiate reentry, conduction must fail down one pathway in the antegrade direction but then permit later retrograde reactivation of this pathway. This is referred to as a *unidirectional block*. A fixed or functional obstacle must maintain separation of the two pathways. Although drawn schematically as a circular loop, the anatomy of circuits is often complex and circuitous and is different in different arrhythmia mechanisms. (A) In normal rhythm, the circuit is activated in an antegrade direction down both pathways. However, because of slowed conduction in the B limb, distal activation is mediated by the faster A pathway, which arrives first and may activate the slowly conducting pathway in a retrograde direction. This retrograde conduction is electrocardiographically concealed (invisible), collides with the antegrade wave front, and is extinguished, and no tachycardia results. (B) Reentry is usually initiated by a premature beat originating independently of the circuit. The premature beat fails to propagate down the rapidly conducting A limb due to differential refractoriness of the two limbs, but it is able to propagate down the slowly conducting B pathway, where it may encounter substantial delay due to increased conduction time with prematurity (i.e., decremental conduction), allowing recovery of the previously blocked rapidly conducting A limb. This permits the rapidly conducting A limb to act as a return path and for ultimate reentrant reactivation of the slowly conducting B pathway, initiating sustained reentrant tachycardia in the circuit.

or a shift of the maximal diastolic potential to a more positive value. These changes may occur with sympathetic stimulation. Enhanced automaticity may be normal (e.g., appropriate sinus tachycardia) or abnormal (e.g., inappropriate sinus tachycardia). Spontaneous depolarization occurring in nonpacemaker cardiac myocytes is called *abnormal automaticity*. Conditions such as ischemia, electrolyte abnormalities, and sympathetic stimulation may produce abnormal automaticity. Premature atrial and ventricular depolarizations, atrial tachycardia, and ventricular tachycardia (VT) may result.

Triggered activity occurs when secondary cardiac depolarizations are initiated by prior depolarizations. If these secondary depolarizations reach threshold potential, they may generate action potentials during or immediately after phase 3 of the action potential. *Early afterdepolarizations* (EADs) are observed when triggered depolarization occurs during phase 3 of the action potential. Inciters of EADs include QT-prolonging drugs, hypokalemia, and bradycardia. Patients with congenital long QT syndrome (LQTS) are prone to develop EADS, resulting in *torsades de pointes* (TdP).

When triggered activity occurs during phase 4, *delayed afterdepolarizations* (DADs) result. DADs are exaggerated at rapid heart rates and observed with digoxin toxicity and high-level catecholamine states, conditions that are associated with intracellular calcium overload. DADs are thought to be the chief arrhythmic mechanism underlying catecholaminergic polymorphic VT (CPVT).

Reentry is the dominant mechanism underlying clinical tachyarrhythmias. Reentry describes the reexcitation of a localized region of cardiac tissue by the same impulse, requiring bifurcating conduction pathways with different velocities and refractory periods. To permit reentry, unidirectional block in one pathway and slowed conduction in the other are required. Reentry is further categorized as anatomic, circling around a fixed anatomic obstacle, or functional, in which the unexcitable center of a reentrant circuit is not fixed but functionally refractory. Fig. 8.2 illustrates reentry as an arrhythmic mechanism. The two pathways join proximally and distally. Pathway A conducts rapidly but has a long refractory period. Pathway B is slowly conducting but has a shorter refractory period. A normally timed impulse enters the two pathways through the proximal common pathway, conducting rapidly down A and slowly down B. As the impulse from pathway A reaches the distal common pathway, while continuing distally, it may also turn around to activate B retrogradely. This impulse collides with the slowly conducting antegrade impulse in pathway B, extinguishing the impulse. However, a sufficiently premature stimulus

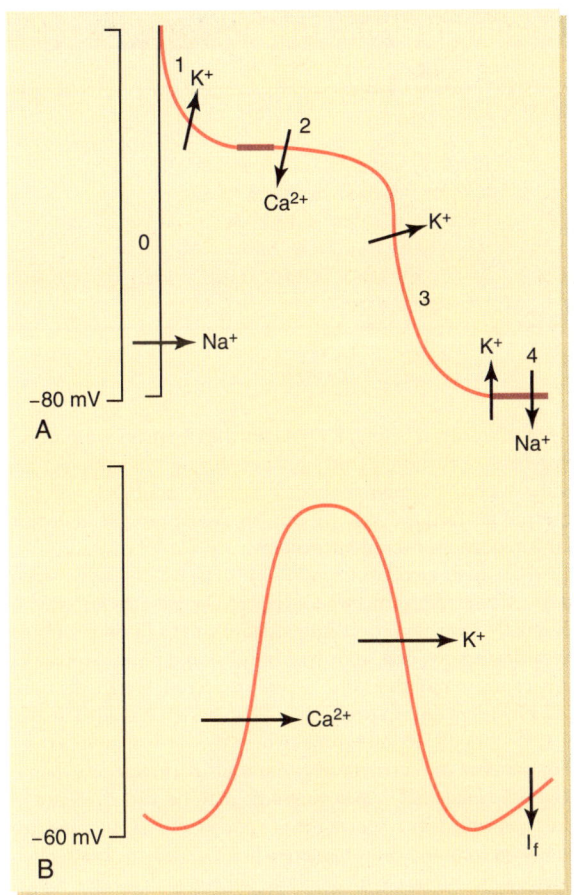

图 8.1 心肌细胞动作电位的电生理基础。(A) 心肌工作细胞和房室结下特殊传导系统中的快反应细胞维持极大的静息膜电位负值,而动作电位开始时钠离子快速内流引起 0 期快速上升。(B) 相比之下,窦房结和房室结组织中的慢反应细胞静息膜电位负值较小,动作电位上升较慢,依赖慢钙通道,并存在 4 期自动去极化

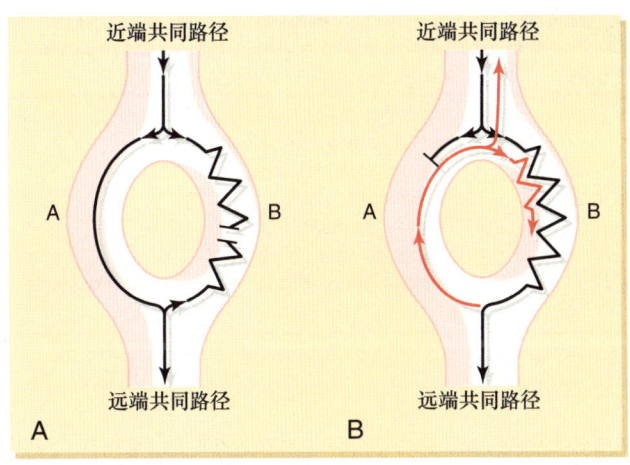

图 8.2 折返机制。折返需要两条不应期不同的路径和一个传导缓慢的区域。一条路径(A)传导正常,但不应期长。第二条路径(B)传导缓慢,但不应期相对较短。要启动折返环路,冲动必须在一条路径上出现无法前传,但随后允许该路径逆传的再激活,这称为单向阻滞。必须有一个固定的或功能性障碍维持两条路径的分离。尽管折返环路在示意图中被画成一个圆形环路,但其解剖结构通常复杂而曲折,并且在不同的心律失常机制中是不同的。(A) 在正常节律下,折返环路的两条路径在前传方向上同时被激活。但由于路径 B 传导缓慢,经路径 A 传导的激动首先到达,远端激活由传导更快的路径 A 介导,并可逆传激活传导缓慢的路径。这种逆向传导在心电图上看不见,逆传冲动与前传冲动相互碰撞并消除,不引发心动过速。(B) 折返性心律失常通常由一个起源于折返环路之外的期前刺激(早搏)诱发。由于两条路径的不应期差异,早搏未能沿着快速传导的路径 A 下传,但能够沿着缓慢传导的路径 B 下传,在那里它可能会因为早搏导致的传导时间增加(即递减传导)而遇到显著的延迟,先前前传被阻断的快速传导路径 A 脱离不应期,从而允许快速传导路径 A 作为逆传路径,最终导致缓慢传导路径 B 折返性再激活,启动折返环路中持续的折返性心动过速

性心动过速),也可能是异常的(如不适当的窦性心动过速)。在非起搏心脏肌细胞中发生的自发去极化称为异常自律性。缺血、电解质异常和交感神经刺激等情况可能导致自律性异常,结果导致心房期前收缩、心室期前收缩、房性心动过速和室性心动过速(室速,VT)的发生。

触发活动为心脏去极化之后继发的再次去极化。如果继发的去极化达到阈电位,可能在动作电位 3 期或紧接其后产生动作电位。早期后除极(EAD)见于动作电位 3 期触发去极化时。早期后除极的诱因包括药物导致 QT 间期延长、低钾血症和心动过速。先天性长 QT 综合征(LQTS)患者容易发生早期后除极,从而导致尖端扭转型室性心动过速(TdP)。

当触发活动发生在 4 期时,会产生延迟后除极(DAD)。延迟后除极于心率增快时加剧,可在洋地黄中毒、高水平儿茶酚胺等状态下观察到,与细胞内钙超载有关。延迟后除极是儿茶酚胺敏感性多形性室性心动过速(CPVT)的主要心律失常机制。

折返是临床快速性心律失常的主要机制。折返描述为心脏组织的局部区域被同一冲动再次激动,需要具有不同传导速度和不应期的分支传导路径。折返的产生需要一条路径存在单向阻滞,另一路径存在传导延缓。折返可进一步分为解剖性的、围绕固定的解剖障碍环绕,或者功能性的,其折返环路的非兴奋性中心并不固定,而是处于功能性不应期。图 8.2 展示了折返作为心律失常的机制。两条路径在近端和远端汇合。路径 A 传导速度快但不应期较长。路径 B 传导速度慢但不应期较短。一个正常冲动通过近端共同路径进入两条路径,沿路径 A 快速传导,沿路径 B 缓慢传导。当来自路径 A 的冲动到达远端共同路径时,继续向远端传导,同时也可能逆传激动路径 B。这个冲动与路径 B 中缓慢传导的顺行冲动相碰撞,阻止了冲动的下传。然而,当足够早的期前刺激进

TABLE 8.1 Singh–Vaughan Williams Classification of Antiarrhythmic Drugs

Class	Physiologic Effect[a]	Examples
I	Blocks sodium channels; predominantly reduces the maximum velocity of the upstroke of the action potential (phase 0)	
IA	Intermediate-potency blockade	Quinidine, procainamide, disopyramide
IB	Least-potent blockade	Lidocaine, tocainide, mexiletine, phenytoin
IC	Most-potent blockade	Flecainide, propafenone, moricizine
II	β-Adrenergic receptor blockade	Propranolol, metoprolol, atenolol
III	Potassium-channel blockade: predominantly prolongs action potential duration	Amiodarone, sotalol, bretylium, ibutilide, dofetilide, dronedarone
IV	Calcium-channel blockade	Verapamil, diltiazem

[a]Several agents have physiologic effects characteristic of more than one class.

may enter the proximal common pathway, finding pathway A with its long refractory period unexcitable, traveling slowly down pathway B, and finally reaching the distal common pathway. Due to the slow conduction velocity in pathway B, pathway A may no longer be refractory, and the impulse may successfully travel retrograde up pathway A, potentially repeatedly activating the circuit. Reentry is the most common mechanism producing supraventricular tachycardia (SVT) and VT.

❖ For a deeper discussion on this topic, please see Chapter 55, "Principles of Electrophysiology," in *Goldman-Cecil Medicine*, 26th Edition.

GENERAL APPROACH TO MANAGEMENT
Diagnostic Procedures
Electrocardiography

The baseline 12-lead electrocardiogram (ECG) is essential for the initial evaluation of patients with arrhythmic symptoms. The baseline ECG may indicate underlying structural heart disease, with Q waves or fractionated QRS complexes suggesting prior myocardial infarction (MI). Slow sinus rates or AV conduction abnormalities may point to susceptibility to symptomatic bradycardia. Delta waves confirm an accessory pathway and direct the evaluation of arrhythmic symptoms toward the diagnosis of Wolff-Parkinson-White (WPW) syndrome while localizing the accessory pathway.

Evidence for hereditary cardiomyopathies and cardiac ion channel disorders that predispose to sudden death may be detected on a baseline ECG. Patients with arrhythmogenic right ventricular (RV) dysplasia may have epsilon waves and inverted T waves in the right precordial leads. QT interval prolongation or shortening may indicate congenital or acquired long QT or short QT syndrome, respectively. Brugada syndrome can be diagnosed based on coved ST-segment elevation in leads V_1 and V_2.

A 12-lead ECG obtained during arrhythmic symptoms can establish the cause of a patient's symptoms. The specific mechanism underlying bradycardia and tachycardia can often be inferred from the ECG. Documentation of QRS morphology during VT or accessory pathway–mediated tachycardia on a 12-lead ECG aids in localizing the site of origin and guiding catheter ablation.

Ambulatory Monitoring

Although a 12-lead ECG obtained during arrhythmic symptoms is ideal, it is difficult to obtain in practice because of the transient and intermittent nature of these symptoms. Ambulatory recording devices permit electrocardiographic monitoring over longer periods to establish symptom-rhythm correlations.

Three types of monitoring devices are available. *Holter monitors* typically provide continuous electrogram storage for 24 to 48 hours. Holter monitoring is helpful for patients with frequent symptoms. The comprehensive rhythm record obtained during this sampling period provides useful information about heart rate variability, rate control with atrial fibrillation (AF), AF burden, asymptomatic arrhythmias, and the frequency of ventricular ectopy.

External event monitors or loop recorders, which can be worn for 30 days, store electrograms when triggered by patients for symptoms. Additionally, loop monitors employ algorithms to automatically detect tachycardia, bradycardia, and atrial fibrillation. Episode storage varies from seconds to minutes. After events are recorded, patients transmit the data by telephone. External loop recorders are intended to identify cardiac rhythm disturbances underlying infrequent symptoms.

For patients with arrhythmia symptoms occurring less than once per month, *implantable loop recorders* may be useful. These small devices implanted in a subcutaneous pocket in the left chest record patient-triggered and auto-triggered ECGs based on heart rate and AF detection criteria. With a 3-year anticipated battery longevity, implantable loop recorders are valuable in establishing the cause of recurrent infrequent syncope and arrhythmic symptoms. Implantable loop recorders, with a reported 98% sensitivity for AF detection, are useful both for AF management and AF surveillance in the setting of cryptogenic stroke, resulting in higher utilization of appropriate oral anticoagulation following stroke.

Electrophysiologic Testing

To perform electrophysiologic studies, temporary transvenous pacing catheters are positioned in multiple locations in the heart, permitting pacing and recording of intracardiac electrograms. Catheters are typically placed in the right atrium, the right ventricle, close to the bundle of His, and in the coronary sinus for left atrial recording and pacing. Electrophysiologic studies can define the mechanism of tachyarrhythmias and guide therapy. In patients with prior MI, induction of VT may assist in determining patient susceptibility to life-threatening arrhythmias and inform decisions regarding defibrillator implantation. Electrophysiologic testing also can evaluate sinus node function and AV conduction.

Pharmacologic Therapy

Antiarrhythmic drugs are traditionally divided according to the Singh–Vaughan Williams classification, which categorizes agents based on their primary physiologic effect (Table 8.1). When this classification system was first proposed, knowledge of electrophysiologic mechanisms was limited. Although the simplicity of categorizing antiarrhythmic drugs according to Singh–Vaughan Williams classes I through IV is appealing, the system has many limitations. A hybrid classification system, class I and III agents block ion channels, and class II and IV drugs block receptors. Some drugs cross classes and have several

表 8.1　Singh–Vaughan Williams 抗心律失常药物分类

分类		生理作用 [a]	举例
I		阻断钠通道；主要降低动作电位上升（0 期）的最大速率	
	IA	中效阻滞剂	奎尼丁、普鲁卡因胺、丙吡胺
	IB	弱效阻滞剂	利多卡因、托卡因、美西律、苯妥英钠
	IC	强效阻滞剂	氟卡尼、普罗帕酮、莫雷西嗪
II		β 受体阻滞剂	普萘洛尔、美托洛尔、阿替洛尔
III		钾通道阻滞剂：主要延长动作电位时程	胺碘酮、索他洛尔、溴苄乙胺、伊布利特、多非利特、决奈达隆
IV		钙通道阻滞剂	维拉帕米、地尔硫䓬

[a] 有的药物具有一类以上的生理作用特性。

入近端共同路径时，发现路径 A 由于不应期长而不能激活，从而沿路径 B 缓慢下传，到达远端共同路径。由于路径 B 中传导速度慢，此时路径 A 不再处于不应期，冲动可能成功地通过路径 A 逆传，从而反复激活回路。折返是产生室上性心动过速（室上速，SVT）和室速的最常见机制。

◆　有关此专题的深入讨论，请参阅 Goldman-Cecil Medicine 第 26 版第 55 章 "电生理学原理"。

处理原则

诊断流程

心电图（ECG）

基线 12 导联 ECG 对于心律失常症状患者的初始评估必不可少。基线心电图可能揭示潜在的结构性心脏病，异常 Q 波或碎裂 QRS 波群提示既往心肌梗死（MI）。窦性心动过缓或房室传导异常提示症状性心动过缓。Delta 波确认旁路存在，提示心律失常症状的评估方向为 Wolff-Parkinson-White（WPW）综合征的诊断，同时可对旁路进行定位。

基线 ECG 可提供导致猝死的遗传性心肌病和心脏离子通道疾病的证据。致心律失常型右室发育不良患者的右胸导联心电图可能存在 epsilon 波和 T 波倒置。QT 间期延长或缩短可能分别提示先天性或获得性长 QT 或短 QT 综合征。Brugada 综合征可以根据 V_1 和 V_2 导联的穹窿样 ST 段抬高进行诊断。

心律失常症状期间获得的 12 导联 ECG 有助于评估患者症状的原因。通常可以从 ECG 推断出心动过缓和心动过速的特定机制。VT 发作时或旁路介导的心动过速期间的 12 导联 ECG 上的 QRS 形态有助于定位起源部位并指导导管消融。

动态监测

尽管理想状态是在心律失常症状发作期间获得 12 导联 ECG，但由于这些症状通常为一过性和间歇性，在实践中较难实现。动态记录设备允许进行更长时间的心电图监测，以获得症状-心律相关性。

目前有三种类型的监测设备可供选择。Holter 监测器通常提供 24～48 h 的连续心电图存储。Holter 监测对于症状发作频繁的患者很有帮助。在这段时间内获得的综合性心律记录可提供心率变异性、心房颤动（房颤，AF）的心率控制、房颤负荷、无症状心律失常和室性异位搏动的发作频率等有用信息。

外部事件监测器或循环记录器可佩戴 30 天，出现症状时由患者触发心电图存储。此外，循环记录器的算法可自动检测心动过速、心动过缓和心房颤动。事件存储时间从几秒到几分钟不等。事件记录后，患者可通过电话传输数据。外部循环记录器有助于确认发作不频繁的与症状相关的心律异常。

对于心律失常症状发作频率低于每月 1 次的患者，植入式循环记录器可能有用。将这些小型设备植入患者左胸的皮下囊袋中，由患者触发或根据心率和房颤检测标准自动触发记录心电图。植入式循环记录器预期电池寿命为 3 年，对发作不频繁的复发性晕厥和心律失常症状的病因确认非常有价值。植入式循环记录器对房颤检测敏感性有报道达 98%，对房颤管理和隐源性卒中的房颤病因检测非常有用，可显著提高卒中后抗凝治疗的规范使用率。

电生理检查

为进行电生理研究，经静脉将临时起搏导管放置于心脏的多个位置，进行起搏和记录心内电图。导管通常放置在右心房、右心室、希氏束附近以及冠状窦以用于左心房的记录和起搏。电生理研究可以确认心动过速的机制和指导治疗。对既往心肌梗死患者的室速的诱发可能有助于确定患者的致命性心律失常易感性和指导除颤器植入的决定。电生理检查还可以评估窦房结功能和房室传导。

药物治疗

抗心律失常药物传统上按照 Singh-Vaughan Williams 分类，根据药物的主要生理效应进行归类（表 8.1）。该分类系统首次提出时，对电生理机制的了解尚有限。尽管根据 Singh-Vaughan Williams Ⅰ至Ⅳ类对抗心律失常药物进行分类简便易行，但该系统存在许多局限性。各类之间存在混杂，Ⅰ类和Ⅲ类药物阻断离子通道，Ⅱ类和Ⅳ类药物阻断受体。有些药物跨越类别并具有

TABLE 8.2 Selected Characteristics of Antiarrhythmic Drugs

Drug	Effect on Surface ECG	Effect on LV Function	Important Drug Interactions	Effect on Pacing and Defibrillation Thresholds	Major Route of Elimination
Quinidine	Prolongs QRS and QT	Negative inotrope	Increases digoxin level and warfarin effect Cimetidine increases quinidine level Phenobarbital, phenytoin, and rifampin decrease quinidine level	Increases PT and DT at high doses	Liver (CYP3A4) and kidney
Procainamide	Prolongs PR, QRS, and QT	Negative inotrope	Cimetidine, alcohol, and amiodarone increase procainamide level	Increases PT at high doses	Liver and kidney
Disopyramide	Prolongs QRS and QT	Negative inotrope	Phenobarbital, phenytoin, and rifampin decrease disopyramide level	Increases PT at high doses	Liver (CYP3A4) and kidney
Lidocaine	Shortens QT	None	Propranolol, metoprolol, and cimetidine increase lidocaine level	Increases DT	Liver (CYP2D6)
Mexiletine	Shortens QT	None	Increases theophylline level Phenobarbital, phenytoin, and rifampin decrease mexiletine level	Various effects	Liver (CYP2D6)
Flecainide	Prolongs PR and QRS	Negative inotrope	Increases digoxin level	Increases PT; variable effect on DT	Liver (CYP2D6) and kidney
Propafenone	Prolongs PR and QRS	Negative inotrope	Increases digoxin, theophylline, and cyclosporine levels; increases warfarin effect Phenobarbital, phenytoin, and rifampin decrease propafenone level Cimetidine and quinidine increase propafenone level	Increases PT; variable effect on DT	Liver (CYP2D6)
Dronedarone	Prolongs PR and QT; slows sinus rate	Negative inotrope	CYP3A4 inhibitors (ketoconazole, clarithromycin, calcium-channel blockers) increase dronedarone levels; additive effect with drugs that prolong QT (macrolides, class I and III antiarrhythmics) increasing risk of TdP; increases dabigatran levels	Little effect	Liver (CYP3A4)
Amiodarone	Prolongs PR and QT; slows sinus rate	None	Increases digoxin and cyclosporine levels; increases warfarin effect	Increases DT	Liver (CYP3A4)
Sotalol	Prolongs PR and QT; slows sinus rate	Negative inotrope	Additive effects with other β-blockers	Decreases DT	Kidney
Ibutilide	Prolongs PR and QT	None	Additive effect on QT prolongation with class IA and other class III antiarrhythmic agents	Decreases DT	Liver
Dofetilide	Prolongs QT	None	Verapamil, diltiazem, Cimetidine, and ketoconazole increase dofetilide level	Decreases DT	Liver and kidney

DT, Defibrillation threshold; *ECG*, electrocardiogram; *LV*, left ventricle; *PT*, pacing threshold; *TdP*, torsades de pointes.

mechanisms of action. There are drugs with antiarrhythmic action that are excluded from the classification, such as digitalis and adenosine. The system categorizes drugs based on their in vitro electrophysiologic effects in normal cardiac tissues.

Available antiarrhythmic drugs have limited efficacy and carry the risk of adverse events, including proarrhythmic potential. Knowledge of drug metabolism, interactions, electrophysiologic effects, and side effects is essential. Certain antiarrhythmics may suppress left ventricular systolic function and may impact pacing and defibrillation thresholds. Excepting β-blockers, none of the antiarrhythmics has been demonstrated to reduce mortality rates. In fact, the use of antiarrhythmic agents may confer an increased risk of cardiovascular mortality, particularly in heart failure patients. Tables 8.2 and 8.3 summarize major characteristics and side effects of commonly used antiarrhythmic drugs.

Class I Antiarrhythmic Agents

Class I antiarrhythmic drugs include sodium-channel blockers that bind fast sodium channels in their open and inactivated states and dissociate from sodium channels during their resting state. Blocking voltage-gated fast sodium channels slows phase 0 depolarization and conduction velocity. Class I agents demonstrate use-dependent blockade, and their effect is potentiated at faster heart rates. The drug dissociation rate from sodium channels during phase 4 of the action potential determines the degree to which these agents depress cardiac conduction velocity.

Class IA agents have a slow rate of drug dissociation from sodium channels, conferring moderate potency. In addition to blocking voltage-gated fast sodium channels, class IA drugs block delayed rectifier potassium channels. Slowing of conduction velocity and action potential prolongation are observed. All are antimuscarinic, especially

表 8.2 抗心律失常药物的特点

药物	对心电图的影响	对左心室（LV）功能的影响	重要的药物相互作用	对起搏和除颤阈值的影响	主要清除途径
奎尼丁	延长 QRS 和 QT	负性肌力	增加地高辛水平和华法林效应 西咪替丁增加奎尼丁水平 苯巴比妥、苯妥英钠和利福平降低奎尼丁水平	高剂量时增加 PT 和 DT	肝（CYP3A4）和肾
普鲁卡因胺	延长 PR、QRS 和 QT	负性肌力	西咪替丁、酒精和胺碘酮增加普鲁卡因胺水平	高剂量时增加 PT	肝和肾
丙吡胺	延长 QRS 和 QT	负性肌力	苯巴比妥、苯妥英钠和利福平降低丙吡胺水平	高剂量时增加 PT	肝（CYP3A4）和肾
利多卡因	缩短 QT	无	普萘洛尔、美托洛尔和西咪替丁增加利多卡因水平	增加 DT	肝（CYP2D6）
美西律	缩短 QT	无	增加茶碱水平 苯巴比妥、苯妥英、利福平降低美西律水平	多种效应	肝（CYP2D6）
氟卡尼	延长 PR 和 QRS	负性肌力	增加地高辛水平	增加 PT；改变 DT	肝（CYP2D6）和肾
普罗帕酮	延长 PR 和 QRS	负性肌力	增加地高辛、茶碱和环孢素水平；增加华法林效应 苯巴比妥、苯妥英钠和利福平降低普罗帕酮水平 西咪替丁和奎尼丁增加普罗帕酮水平	增加 PT；改变对 DT	肝（CYP2D6）
决奈达隆	延长 PR 和 QT；减慢窦性心率	负性肌力	CYP3A4 抑制剂（酮康唑、克拉霉素、钙通道阻滞剂）增加决奈达隆水平；与延长 QT 间期（大环内酯类、Ⅰ类和Ⅲ类抗心律失常药物）的药物叠加作用可增加 TdP 风险；增加达比加群酯水平	影响较小	肝（CYP3A4）
胺碘酮	延长 PR 和 QT；减慢窦性心率	无	增加地高辛和环孢素水平；增加华法林效应	增加 DT	肝（CYP3A4）
索他洛尔	延长 PR 和 QT；减慢窦性心率	负性肌力	与其他 β 受体阻滞剂有叠加作用	降低 DT	肾
伊布利特	延长 PR 和 QT	无	ⅠA 类和其他Ⅲ类抗心律失常药物对 QT 间期延长有叠加作用	降低 DT	肝
多非利特	延长 QT	无	维拉帕米、地尔硫䓬、西咪替丁和酮康唑增加多非利特水平	降低 DT	肝和肾

DT，除颤阈值；PT，起搏阈值；TdP，尖端扭转室速。

几种作用机制。有些具有抗心律失常作用的药物被排除在了分类之外，如洋地黄和腺苷。该分类依据的基础是药物对正常心脏组织的体外电生理效应。

现有的抗心律失常药物疗效有限，同时具有致不良事件风险，包括致心律失常的潜在不良反应。了解药物代谢、相互作用、电生理效应以及副作用至关重要。某些抗心律失常药物可能抑制左心室收缩，可能影响起搏和除颤阈值。除了 β 受体阻滞剂外，没有任何抗心律失常药物被证明可以降低死亡率。实际上，抗心律失常药物的使用可能会增加心血管死亡风险，特别是对心力衰竭患者。表 8.2 和表 8.3 总结了常用抗心律失常药物的主要特性和副作用。

Ⅰ类抗心律失常药物

Ⅰ类抗心律失常药物包括钠通道阻滞剂，它们在快钠离子通道的开放和失活状态下与其结合，在静息状态下与其解离，阻断电压门控快钠通道、减慢 0 期去极化和传导速度。Ⅰ类药物表现出使用依赖性阻滞，其效果在心率快时更明显。药物在动作电位 4 期与钠离子通道的解离速率决定了其对心脏传导速度的抑制程度。

ⅠA 类药物与钠通道解离的速率慢，具有中等效力。除了阻断电压门控快钠通道外，ⅠA 类药物还阻断延迟整流钾通道。可以观察到传导速度减慢和动作电位时程延长。这些药物都具有抗胆碱能作用，尤其是

TABLE 8.3 Common Side Effects of Select Antiarrhythmic Drugs

Drug	Major Side Effects
Quinidine	Nausea, diarrhea, abdominal cramping
	Cinchonism: decreased hearing, tinnitus, blurred vision, delirium
	Rash, thrombocytopenia, hemolytic anemia
	Hypotension, torsades de pointes (quinidine syncope)
Procainamide	Drug-induced lupus syndrome
	Nausea, vomiting
	Rash, fever, hypotension, psychosis, agranulocytosis
	Torsades de pointes
Disopyramide	Anticholinergic: dry mouth, blurred vision, constipation, urinary retention, closed angle glaucoma
	Hypotension, worsening heart failure
Lidocaine	CNS: dizziness, perioral numbness, paresthesias, altered consciousness, coma, seizures
Mexiletine	Nausea, vomiting
	CNS: dizziness, tremor, paresthesias, ataxia, confusion
Flecainide	CNS: blurred vision, headache, ataxia, tremor
	Congestive heart failure, ventricular proarrhythmia
Propafenone	Nausea, vomiting, constipation, metallic taste to food
	Dizziness, headache, exacerbation of asthma, ventricular proarrhythmia
β-Blockers	Bronchospasm, bradycardia, fatigue, depression, impotence
	Congestive heart failure
Calcium-channel blockers	Congestive heart failure, bradycardia, heart block, constipation
Amiodarone	Agranulocytosis, pulmonary fibrosis, hepatopathy, hyperthyroidism or hypothyroidism, corneal microdeposits, bluish discoloration of the skin, nausea, constipation, bradycardia, tremor, ataxia
Sotalol	Same as β-blockers, torsades de pointes
Dronedarone	Diarrhea, QT prolongation and torsades de pointes, death, bradycardia, congestive heart failure, hepatocellular injury, interstitial lung disease
Ibutilide	Torsades de pointes
Dofetilide	Torsades de pointes, headache, dizziness, diarrhea

CNS, Central nervous system.

disopyramide. Clinical applications include SVT, AF, atrial flutter, and VT. In the setting of atrial flutter and AF, class IA drugs are vagolytic. They may improve AV nodal conduction and should be used in conjunction with a β-blocker or calcium-channel blocker to avoid uncontrolled ventricular response rates. Quinidine is infrequently used due to its side effect profile, including diarrhea, thrombocytopenia, and QT prolongation, triggering polymorphic VT. Clinical studies highlight the proarrhythmic risk and increased mortality associated with quinidine therapy. Procainamide, available as an intravenous formulation, has an active metabolite N-acetylprocainamide (NAPA) and may induce a reversible lupus-like syndrome. Disopyramide, with its potent negative inotropic and antimuscarinic activity, has been used to treat vagally mediated AF.

Class IB agents rapidly dissociate from sodium channels during phase 4, providing weak sodium-channel blockade. Their therapeutic role is restricted to ventricular arrhythmias due to a lack of effect on the sinoatrial node, AV node, and atrial tissue. Lidocaine, which is available parentally, undergoes extensive first-pass hepatic inactivation. Lidocaine is more effective in relatively depolarized ventricular tissue due to preferential affinity for inactivated sodium channels; the drug is more potent in ischemic tissue. Mexiletine, which is available orally, has slower hepatic metabolism and a longer half-life than lidocaine.

Class IC drugs are potent fast sodium-channel blockers with little effect on K+ current. These agents have a role in the therapy of SVTs and VTs. Their use is relegated to patients without coronary disease or significant structural heart disease. The Cardiac Arrhythmia Suppression Trial proved that the use of flecainide and moricizine to suppress ventricular arrhythmias after MI increased mortality rates. These agents may convert AF to atrial flutter and slow atrial conduction sufficiently to permit 1:1 AV conduction during atrial flutter, necessitating the simultaneous use of AV nodal–blocking therapies in patients with atrial arrhythmias. Flecainide is associated with bronchospasm, leukopenia, thrombocytopenia, and neurologic side effects. Flecainide, which inhibits Ca^{2+} release from the sarcoplasmic reticulum cardiac ryanodine receptor, may be useful in the therapy for CPVT. Propafenone has β-blocking effects and can cause agranulocytosis, anemia, and thrombocytopenia.

Class II and IV Antiarrhythmic Agents

β-Adrenoceptor antagonists, the class II agents, inhibit sympathetic activation of cardiac automaticity and conduction, resulting in slowing of the heart rate, decreased AV node conduction velocity, and prolongation of the AV node refractory period. Side effects include bradycardia, hypotension, exacerbation of reactive airway disease, fatigue, worsening symptoms of peripheral vascular disease, and depression. β-Blockers have different half-lives, lipid solubilities, elimination routes, and specificities for $β_1$ and $β_2$ receptors.

Class IV agents include the nondihydropyridine calcium-channel blockers. Blockade of voltage-gated L-type calcium channels decreases AV nodal conduction velocity, increases AV nodal refractory period, slows sinus node automaticity, and decreases myocardial contractility. Calcium-channel blockers may cause hypotension, bradycardia, and heart failure. Clinical applications for these agents include rate control for atrial tachyarrhythmias, termination and suppression of SVT, and normal heart VT. In the setting of atrial arrhythmias with underlying WPW, they can potentiate accessory pathway conduction and should be avoided.

Class III Antiarrhythmic Agents

Class III antiarrhythmic agents are a heterogeneous group of drugs that block the potassium delayed rectifier currents responsible for phase 3 cardiac repolarization, prolonging the cardiac action potential duration and refractory period. These agents demonstrate reverse-use dependence, with more potent potassium-channel blockade at slower heart rates. Prolonging the action potential duration can be therapeutic or proarrhythmic (e.g., TdP). This class represents the dominant category of antiarrhythmic agents in use.

Amiodarone is an iodinated compound available orally and parentally. With oral administration, it is slowly absorbed. Because it concentrates in fat tissues, amiodarone has a large volume of distribution. This characteristic prolongs the time to reach steady-state levels and produces a long elimination half-life, approximately 35 to 100 days. Amiodarone's pharmacology is complex, with class I through IV activity, although its primary therapeutic mechanism is prolongation of the action potential duration. It is effective in treating SVTs and VTs. It is hepatically metabolized and proven safe to use in the setting of congestive heart failure. Amiodarone is commonly used to treat atrial and ventricular arrhythmias in patients with structural heart disease and renal failure. Amiodarone is the only antiarrhythmic agent to demonstrate improved survival to hospital admission after cardiac arrest. This finding led to amiodarone prioritization within the ACLS pulseless

表 8.3　抗心律失常药物的主要副作用

药物	主要副作用
奎尼丁	恶心、腹泻、腹部绞痛 奎宁中毒：听力下降、耳鸣、视物模糊、谵妄 皮疹、血小板减少、溶血性贫血 低血压、尖端扭转型室性心动过速（奎尼丁晕厥）
普鲁卡因胺	药源性狼疮综合征 恶心、呕吐 皮疹、发热、低血压、精神异常、粒细胞缺乏症、尖端扭转型室性心动过速
丙吡胺	抗胆碱能：口干、视物模糊、便秘、尿潴留、闭角型青光眼； 低血压、心力衰竭加重
利多卡因	CNS：头晕、口周麻木、感觉异常、意识改变、昏迷、癫痫发作
美西律	恶心、呕吐 CNS：头晕、震颤、感觉异常、共济失调、意识模糊
氟卡尼	CNS：视物模糊、头痛、共济失调、震颤 充血性心力衰竭、致室性心律失常
普罗帕酮	恶心、呕吐、便秘、食物金属异味 头晕、头痛、哮喘急性发作、药物性室性心律失常
β受体阻滞剂	支气管痉挛、心动过缓、疲劳、抑郁、阳痿 充血性心力衰竭
钙通道阻滞剂	充血性心力衰竭、心动过缓、心脏传导阻滞、便秘
胺碘酮	粒细胞缺乏症、肺纤维化、肝病、甲状腺功能亢进或甲状腺功能减退、角膜微沉淀、皮肤青紫变色、恶心、便秘、心动过缓、震颤、共济失调
索他洛尔	与β受体阻滞剂相同、尖端扭转型室性心动过速
决奈达隆	腹泻、QT间期延长和尖端扭转型室性心动过速、死亡、心动过缓、充血性心力衰竭、肝细胞损伤、间质性肺病
伊布利特	尖端扭转型室性心动过速
多非利特	尖端扭转型室性心动过速、头痛、头晕、腹泻

CNS，中枢神经系统。

丙吡胺。临床应用包括室上速、心房颤动、心房扑动和室速。心房扑动和心房颤动的情况下，ⅠA类药物具有抑制迷走神经兴奋的作用。它们能改善房室结传导，应与β受体阻滞剂或钙通道阻滞剂联合使用，以避免心室率失控。奎尼丁由于其副作用（包括腹泻、血小板减少和QT延长，诱发多形性VT）而很少使用。临床研究发现奎尼丁治疗相关的致心律失常风险和死亡率增加。普鲁卡因胺可静脉给药，具有活性代谢物N-乙酰普鲁卡因胺（NAPA），可诱发可逆性类狼疮综合征。丙吡胺由于其强效的负性肌力和抗胆碱能活性，已用于治疗迷走神经介导的心房颤动。

ⅠB类药物在4期与钠离子通道迅速解离，钠通道阻断作用弱。由于对窦房结、房室结和心房组织没有影响，它们的治疗作用仅限于室性心律失常。利多卡因可注射用药，主要经由首过肝脏代谢灭活。利多卡因对失活的钠离子通道亲和力更强，在相对去极化的室性组织中更有效；该药物在缺血组织中效果更强。美西律可口服给药，肝脏代谢较慢，半衰期比利多卡因长。

ⅠC类药物是强效的快速钠离子通道阻断剂，对钾离子（K^+）影响很小。这些药物对室上速和室速具有治疗作用。它们的使用限于没有冠状动脉疾病或明显结构性心脏病的患者。心脏心律失常抑制试验（The Cardiac Arrhythmia Suppression Trial）证明，使用氟卡尼和莫雷西嗪抑制心肌梗死后的室性心律失常增加死亡率。此类药物可能将心房颤动（AF）转化为心房扑动，并因显著减慢心房传导，导致心房扑动时1∶1室传导，故治疗房性心律失常时需联用房室结阻滞治疗。氟卡尼与支气管痉挛、白细胞减少、血小板减少和神经系统副作用有关。氟卡尼抑制肌浆网兰尼碱受体的Ca^{2+}释放，在CPVT治疗中可能有效。普罗帕酮具有β受体阻断作用，并可导致粒细胞缺乏症、贫血和血小板减少。

Ⅱ类和Ⅳ类抗心律失常药物

β肾上腺素受体阻滞剂，即Ⅱ类药物，通过抑制心脏自律性和传导性的交感神经激活，减缓心率、降低房室结传导速度，并延长房室结的不应期。副作用包括心动过缓、低血压、加重气道反应性疾病、疲劳、外周血管疾病症状恶化和抑郁。β受体阻滞剂具有不同的半衰期、脂溶性、排泄途径和对β1及β2受体的特异性。

Ⅳ类药物包括非二氢吡啶类钙通道阻滞剂。阻断电压门控L型钙离子通道减慢房室结传导速度，增加房室结不应期，降低窦房结自律性，并降低心肌收缩力。钙通道阻滞剂可导致低血压、心动过缓和心力衰竭。这些药物的临床应用包括控制快速性房性心律失常的心室率、终止和抑制室上速，以及正常心脏的室速。在房性心律失常合并预激综合征（WPW）的情况下，此类药物可增强旁路的传导，应避免使用。

Ⅲ类抗心律失常药物

Ⅲ类抗心律失常药物为一类异质性药物，阻断心肌细胞复极化3期的延迟整流钾电流，延长心脏动作电位的持续时间和不应期。这些药物表现出反向使用依赖性，在心率较慢时钾离子通道阻断作用更强。延长动作电位持续时间既可以是治疗性的，也可以致心律失常（如TdP）。这一类药物是当前临床使用的主要的抗心律失常药物。

胺碘酮是一种碘化合物，可口服和静脉给药，口服时吸收缓慢。由于胺碘酮在脂肪组织中蓄积，因此具有较大的分布容积。这一特性延长了达到稳态水平的时间，并产生较长的半衰期，大约为35～100天。胺碘酮药理作用复杂，其主要治疗机制是延长动作电位时程，但还同时具有Ⅰ至Ⅳ类药物的活性。它对室上速和室速治疗有效。经肝脏代谢，已证明在充血性心力衰竭情况下使用安全。胺碘酮通常用于治疗结构性心脏病和肾衰竭患者的房性和室性心律失常。胺碘酮是唯一证实能改善心搏骤停后入院存活率的抗心律失常药物。这一发现

VT/VF algorithm. Widespread chronic use of amiodarone has been limited by significant side effects necessitating drug discontinuation in up to 20% of patients. Serious adverse effects include potentially irreversible pulmonary fibrosis, optic neuropathy producing visual impairment, hyperthyroidism, and severe hepatic toxicity. Less serious adverse effects include hypothyroidism, neurologic toxicity, sun sensitivity, QT prolongation, and bradycardia.

Sotalol blocks β-adrenoreceptors and delayed rectifier K+ channels, decreasing sinoatrial node automaticity, slowing AV conduction velocity, and prolonging repolarization. It effectively treats a large number of ventricular and supraventricular arrhythmias.

Dofetilide, a selective class III agent used primarily to treat atrial arrhythmias, blocks delayed rectifier K+ channels to prolong action potential duration and QT intervals. The risk of TdP is about 1% among patients without structural heart disease but as high as 4.8% among patients with congestive heart failure.

Ibutilide, an intravenous class III agent, is used for the acute termination of recent-onset AF and atrial flutter. The risk of polymorphic VT with administration of ibutilide is 8.3%.

Dronedarone is an orally available class III drug demonstrated to reduce the risk of first hospitalization due to cardiovascular events or death from any cause for patients in sinus rhythm with a history of paroxysmal or persistent AF. Dronedarone may not be used in the setting of permanent AF or in patients with New York Heart Association (NYHA) class IV heart failure or symptomatic heart failure with recent decompensation because the drug increases the risk of cardiovascular death in these populations. Other major side effects of dronedarone are severe hepatotoxicity, interstitial lung disease, bradycardia, and QT prolongation.

Other Antiarrhythmic Agents

The Singh–Vaughan Williams classification scheme does not describe several agents commonly used in cardiac arrhythmia management. *Adenosine* is a parenteral agent with an elimination half-life of 1 to 6 seconds. The drug binds to A1 receptors to activate K+ channels, decreasing the action potential duration and hyperpolarizing membrane potentials in the atria, sinoatrial node, and AV node. Indirectly, adenosine blocks catecholamine-stimulated adenylate cyclase activation, decreasing cAMP and consequently decreasing Ca^{2+} influx. Used clinically for its ability to produce transient AV block, adenosine can terminate SVT when the AV node contributes to the reentrant circuit. By slowing atrial-ventricular conduction, adenosine can also establish the presence of underlying atrial tachycardia or atrial flutter when the arrhythmia mechanism is unclear.

Digoxin inhibits Na^+, K^+-ATPase, increasing intracellular Na^+ concentrations and stimulating the Na^+-Ca^{2+} exchanger to increase intracellular Ca^{2+}, accounting for its positive inotropic effect. Digoxin also acts through the autonomic nervous system to enhance vagal tone, slowing sinus rates, shortening the atrial refractory period, and prolonging AV conduction. Digoxin is therefore used for rate control in patients with atrial arrhythmias. Renally excreted, digoxin has a narrow therapeutic range. Digoxin toxicity may lead to high-grade AV block, tachyarrhythmias, blurred vision, nausea, dizziness, and severe hyperkalemia.

Cardioversion and Defibrillation

Direct current cardioversion and defibrillation represent the cornerstone of acute therapy for unstable tachyarrhythmias and play an important role in the termination of medication-refractory stable tachyarrhythmias. Organized VTs and SVTs may be terminated by synchronized cardioversion—shock delivery synchronized to the QRS complex—to restore normal rhythm. Synchronization is critical to avoid induction of VF by delivering energy during the relative refractory period of the cardiac cycle. Defibrillation entails the asynchronous delivery of electrical current to depolarize a critical mass of myocardium and terminate VF. Successful defibrillation is time dependent, with the likelihood of success declining by approximately 10% per minute from the onset of VF.

Defibrillation may be delivered internally through an implantable cardioverter-defibrillator (ICD) or externally through an automatic external defibrillator (AED). Current-generation AEDs use biphasic waveforms, achieving greater first-shock efficacy compared with older devices delivering monophasic waveforms. ICDs, implanted in patients for primary and secondary prevention of sudden cardiac death (SCD), deliver defibrillation shocks directly to the endocardium through an RV lead. With direct delivery of energy, relatively lower energy levels (<40 J) are typically effective.

Ablation

Catheter ablation plays an important role in the therapy of a broad range of arrhythmias, such as SVT, atrial arrhythmias, and VT. The ascendance of catheter ablation derives in part from the poor efficacy and side effect profiles of available antiarrhythmic drugs. Radiofrequency ablation (i.e., applying radiofrequency-range energy) and cryoablation (i.e., administering freezing temperatures, to produce localized cellular and tissue injury) are commonly used.

Focal and reentrant arrhythmias are defined and localized, permitting targeted delivery of ablation energy to eliminate the tachyarrhythmia. Ablation is associated with varied success and complication rates, depending on the mechanism and location of the arrhythmogenic focus. Cure rates for typical tricuspid-caval isthmus–dependent atrial flutter, AV nodal reentry tachycardia (AVNRT), and accessory pathway–mediated tachycardias exceed 95%, with low complication rates of about 2%. Although an important therapeutic option in the treatment of AF and VT, success rates are lower and procedural risks are higher.

For a deeper discussion on this topic, please see Chapter 56, ❖ "Approach to the Patient with Suspected Arrhythmia," in *Goldman-Cecil Medicine*, 26th Edition.

BRADYCARDIA

Bradycardia, defined as a heart rate of less than 60 beats per minute, may occur as a consequence of physiologic adaptations or pathology. Bradycardia always results from failure of sinus node function or AV conduction disturbances, or both processes. Clinically significant bradycardia or pauses may result from autonomic disturbances, drugs, chronic intrinsic conduction system disease, or acute cardiac damage as occurs with endocarditis or infarction.

Normal Conduction System: Anatomy and Physiology

Because of the normal gradient of intrinsic automaticity, heart rate usually is determined by intrinsic automaticity of the sinus node. The sinus node is a complex of cells that extends from the superior vena cava and along the upper right atrial free wall in the sulcus terminalis. Blood supply is derived from the sinus node artery, which arises from the right coronary in 66% or left coronary in 34% of patients.

Activation proceeds through the right atrium to the AV node, which is located in the low interatrial septum adjacent to the tricuspid annulus. The AV node is a complex structure with at least three preferential atrial insertions. The anterior atrial insertion has a short conduction time and usually determines the normal AV conduction time in sinus rhythm. The posterior right and left atrial insertions have long conduction times. Because they do not normally mediate

提示在ACLS无脉VT/VF诊疗流程中优先使用胺碘酮。由于高达20%的患者因明显副作用而需要停药，限制了胺碘酮的长期广泛使用。严重的不良反应包括可能不可逆的肺纤维化、导致视力损害的视神经病变、甲状腺功能亢进和严重的肝毒性。相对较轻的不良反应包括甲状腺功能减退、神经毒性、日光敏感、QT间期延长和心动过缓。

索他洛尔阻断β肾上腺素受体和延迟整流K^+通道，降低窦房结自律性，减缓房室传导速度，并延长复极化，可有效地治疗多种室性和室上性心律失常。

多非利特，一种主要用于治疗房性心律失常的选择性Ⅲ类药物，通过阻断延迟整流K^+通道来延长动作电位时程和QT间期。在非结构性心脏病患者中，尖端扭转型室性心动过速（TdP）的风险约为1%，但在充血性心力衰竭患者中高达4.8%。

伊布利特，一种静脉给药的Ⅲ类药物，用于急性终止新近发作的心房颤动和心房扑动。伊布利特给药时发生多形性室速的风险为8.3%。

决奈达隆是一种口服Ⅲ类药物，其对于既往阵发性或持续性心房颤动病史且目前为窦性心律的患者，已证实可减少因心血管事件首次住院或全因死亡的风险。决奈达隆不应用于永久性心房颤动或纽约心脏协会（NYHA）Ⅳ级心力衰竭或近期失代偿性症状性心力衰竭患者，因为该药可增加上述人群的心血管死亡风险。决奈达隆的其他主要副作用为严重的肝毒性、间质性肺病、心动过缓和QT间期延长。

其他抗心律失常药物

Singh-Vaughan Williams 分类方案并未包含心律失常治疗的一些其他常用药物。腺苷是一种静脉药物，清除半衰期为1～6 s。该药物结合A1受体激活K^+通道，减少心房、窦房结和房室结的动作电位时程和降低超极化膜电位。腺苷间接地阻断儿茶酚胺对腺苷酸环化酶的激活，减少cAMP，从而减少Ca^{2+}内流。在临床上，腺苷由于能够导致一过性房室传导阻滞，可以终止房室结参与折返环路的室上速。通过减缓心房-心室传导，腺苷还可以在心律失常机制不明时确定潜在的房性心动过缓或心房扑动。

地高辛抑制Na^+-K^+-ATP酶，增加细胞内钠离子浓度，并刺激Na^+-Ca^{2+}交换体增加细胞内钙离子浓度，产生正性肌力作用。地高辛还通过自主神经系统发挥作用，增强迷走神经张力，减缓窦性节律，缩短心房不应期，延长房室传导。因此地高辛可用于控制房性心律失常患者的心室率。地高辛经肾排泄，治疗窗窄。地高辛中毒可能导致高度房室传导阻滞、快速性心律失常、视物模糊、恶心、头晕以及严重的高钾血症。

心脏复律和除颤

直流电复律和电除颤是治疗血流动力学不稳定的快速性心律失常的急救基石，在终止药物难治性快速性心律失常中也发挥重要作用。规整的室速和室上速可通过同步电复律终止——与QRS波群同步的电击——以恢复正常心律。同步至关重要，可以避免在心动周期的相对不应期发放电击而诱发心室颤动。除颤通过非同步电击使超过临界量心肌去极化而终止心室颤动。除颤的成功呈时间依赖性，从心室颤动发作开始，每过1 min成功率下降约10%。

可以通过植入式心脏复律除颤器（ICD）从体内发放电击进行除颤，也可以通过自动体外除颤器（AED）从体外电击。现今一代AED使用双相波，与旧设备单相波相比，首次电击效果更好。ICD植入患者体内用于心源性猝死（SCD）的一级和二级预防，通过右室电极导线直接向心内膜发放电击除颤。由于直接发放电击，相对较低的能量水平（<40 J）即通常有效。

导管消融

导管消融在很多种心律失常治疗中发挥重要作用，如室上速、房性心律失常和室速。导管消融的兴起部分源于现有抗心律失常药物疗效较差及其副作用。射频消融（即应用射频能量）和冷冻消融（即施加低温，产生局部细胞和组织损伤）是常用的方法。

局灶性和折返性心律失常可标测和定位，允许针对性地发放消融能量以消除快速性心律失常。消融具有不同的成功率和并发症发生率，取决于心律失常的机制和起源灶位置。典型三尖瓣-腔静脉峡部依赖性心房扑动、房室结折返性心动过速（AVNRT）和旁路介导的心动过速的治愈率超过95%，并发症发生率低，约为2%。导管消融虽然也是治疗心房颤动和室速的重要选择，但成功率相对较低，手术风险较高。

有关此专题的深入讨论，请参阅 *Goldman-Cecil Medicine* 第26版第56章"怀疑心律失常患者的处理方法"。

心动过缓

心动过缓定义为每分钟心跳少于60次，可能是生理性适应的结果，也可能是病理状况。心动过缓通常是由于窦房结功能障碍或房室传导紊乱，或两者皆有。临床上显著的心动过缓或停搏可能源于自主神经紊乱、药物、慢性自身传导系统疾病，或者如发生于心内膜炎或心肌梗死时的急性心脏损伤。

正常传导系统：解剖学和生理学

出于自律性的正常梯度，心率通常由窦房结的自律性所决定。窦房结为一细胞群，位于右心房上部，从上腔静脉延伸至右心房游离壁的界沟内。血供来自窦房结动脉，该动脉在66%的患者中起源于右冠状动脉，在34%的患者中起源于左冠状动脉。

激动通过右心房传递至房室结，其位于低位房间隔，靠近三尖瓣环。房室结结构复杂，至少有三个房性插入点。心房前部插入点传导时间短，通常决定正常窦性心律中的正常房室传导时间。右房后部和左房插入点传导时间长。人类中它们通常不介导房室传导，所以功

AV conduction in humans, they are functionally vestigial. However, the posterior slowly conducting insertions become important in mediating paroxysmal supraventricular tachycardia (PSVT). The AV node derives its blood supply from the AV nodal artery, which is supplied by the right coronary artery in 73% or the left coronary artery in 27% of patients.

After entry into the AV node, conduction proceeds to the His bundle through the fibrous annulus and along the membranous septum before splitting into a leftward Purkinje branch, the left bundle, which ramifies over the left ventricular endocardium, and a rightward branch, the right bundle, which similarly ramifies over the RV endocardium. The leftward branch may be damaged proximally, resulting in full left bundle branch block, or damaged more distally in its anterior or posterior divisions, resulting in fascicular hemiblock patterns.

Normal Autonomic Regulation of Heart Rate

Normal heart rate is a consequence of tonic and phasic autonomic modulation of intrinsic sinus node automaticity. The intrinsic heart rate in the absence of autonomic modulation ranges from 85 to 110 beats per minute and is somewhat faster than normal resting heart rates. That the normal heart rate is slower than the intrinsic rate is a consequence of the dominance of parasympathetic tone over adrenergic tone in the resting state.

Based on a review of Holter recordings in a normal population, the normal resting heart rate is 46 to 93 beats per minute in men and 51 to 95 beats per minute in women. It has been proposed that 50 to 90 is a clinically more accurate working definition of normal heart rate for adults than the traditional 60 to 100 beats per minute commonly used by consensus. However, heart rates well below these estimates may be seen in normal people, especially during hours of sleep. For these reasons, defining a cutoff value for pathologic bradycardia in the absence of symptoms is problematic for an otherwise healthy patient.

The maximal stress-induced heart rate (HR_{max}) is related to maximal sympathetic stimulation, accompanied by withdrawal of parasympathetic tone. This is commonly estimated as $HR_{max} = (220 - age)$.

Sinus Node Dysfunction

Sick sinus syndrome, also called *sinus node dysfunction,* is a common clinical syndrome that increases in prevalence with age. The estimated prevalence is 1 case per 600 patients older than 65 years of age, and it accounts for about one half of all pacemaker implantations. Sinus node dysfunction is a consequence of two distinct processes: failure of intrinsic automaticity and failure of propagation of sinus node impulses to the surrounding atrial tissue, also referred to a *sinus node exit block.*

Sinus node dysfunction manifests clinically as one of several patterns: persistent or episodic sinus bradycardia, inability to appropriately augment rate with exercise (i.e., chronotropic incompetence), sinus pauses, or commonly a combination of these patterns. The sinus node is at the top of a cascade of automaticity and is normally backed up by a competent AV junctional escape mechanism. Severe bradycardia and associated symptoms due to sinus node dysfunction always imply sinus node dysfunction and simultaneous failure of normal subsidiary escape mechanisms. In the setting of a competent escape mechanism, even severe sinus node dysfunction may be completely asymptomatic, clinically well tolerated, and require no specific therapy.

Resting Sinus Bradycardia

Sinus bradycardia is frequently observed during routine clinical practice. Modest sinus bradycardia in the high 40s in men and 50s in women is normal and called *bradycardia* only because of the conventional choice of 60 beats per minute as the lower limit of normal rates. Because there is no set rate at which sinus bradycardia can be labeled as pathologic, pathologic sinus node dysfunction is best defined as significant bradycardia associated with symptoms plausibly attributable to bradycardia.

Modest persistent bradycardia is often asymptomatic. When symptoms occur, they are commonly nonspecific, such as fatigue, listlessness, or dyspnea, making the attribution of symptoms to resting bradycardia difficult. Sinus bradycardia may also exacerbate congestive heart failure and limit effective use of β-blocker therapy, a cornerstone of therapy for heart failure, coronary disease, and tachyarrhythmias. When inappropriate sinus bradycardia is persistent, especially when severe, plausible symptoms are present, and alternative causes of symptoms have been excluded, pacemaker implantation is reasonable. Asymptomatic sinus bradycardia should rarely be treated with pacing unless a need for medical therapy is expected to further exacerbate bradycardia.

Chronotropic Incompetence

Cardiac output during exercise is increased by augmentation in stroke volume and an increase in heart rate. If heart rate rise with exercise is inadequate, exertional symptoms such as fatigue or dyspnea may ensue. As in the case of resting sinus bradycardia, unless severe, attribution of symptoms to chronotropic incompetence is difficult. Various criteria for this condition have been proposed that rely on the inability to achieve a set fraction of age-predicted heart rate or heart rate reserve. As for resting sinus bradycardia, the decision to implant a pacemaker for chronotropic incompetence is a matter of judgment more than criteria.

Sinus Pauses or Arrest

An abrupt failure of sinus node automaticity or failure of propagation from the sinus node to the atrium can result in a pause in atrial activity. P waves are absent, and if of adequate duration and not accompanied by a competent subsidiary escape mechanism, it can result in abrupt symptoms of lightheadedness, presyncope or true syncope. Sinus pauses of less than 3 seconds are commonly seen for normal subjects, who are rarely symptomatic. Sinus pauses exceeding 3 seconds and not occurring during sleep are often pathologic and may result in symptoms. Sinus pauses associated with simultaneous symptoms and documentation of pauses lasting 3 seconds or longer in patients with a history of symptoms plausibly related to bradycardia are indications for pacemaker therapy.

Sinoatrial Exit Block

Sinus node dysfunction is often accompanied by significant atrial fibrosis, which may lead to a block in the tissues surrounding the sinus node complex and impede propagation to the atrial tissue. Bradycardia due to sinus node dysfunction may result, not from a failure of automaticity, but from failure of propagation from the sinus node complex to the atrium. Because sinus node activity is not directly apparent from the surface ECG, the diagnosis is made indirectly by the observation of abrupt halving in the sinus P-wave rate, followed by an abrupt return to the baseline sinus rate (Fig. 8.3C and D). Although other patterns may be observed, 2:1 exit block is the most common. Therapy for sinoatrial exit block is identical to that for intermittent sinus bradycardia (discussed earlier).

Bradycardia-Tachycardia Syndrome as a Consequence of Sinus Node Dysfunction

Bradycardia-tachycardia ("brady-tachy") syndrome refers to a clinically significant tachyarrhythmia sometimes accompanied by clinically significant bradycardia. The term may be confusing because the mechanism of tachycardia is often unrelated to the mechanism of bradycardia.

能上退化。但是，后部缓慢传导的插入点在介导阵发性室上性心动过速（PSVT）时变得很重要。房室结的血液供应来自房室结动脉，该动脉在 73% 的患者中由右冠状动脉供应，在 27% 的患者中由左冠状动脉供应。

进入房室结后，传导通过纤维环下行至希氏束，穿过室间隔膜部并分成向左的浦肯野分支即左束支，其于左心室心内膜面分布，以及向右的分支即右束支，于右心室心内膜面分布。左侧分支可能在近端受损，导致完全性左束支传导阻滞，或在其较远端的前或后分支受损，导致分支阻滞。

自主神经系统正常心率调节

正常心率是自主神经系统对窦房结内在自律性的张力性和时相性调节的结果。在没有自主神经系统调节的情况下，固有心率范围为每分钟 85～110 次，比正常的静息心率稍快。正常心率比固有心率慢是因为在静息状态下，副交感神经张力占主导地位。

根据对正常人群 Holter 记录回顾，男性正常静息心率为每分钟 46～93 次，女性为每分钟 51～95 次。有提议对于成年人将 50～90 次/分界定为临床更准确的正常心率，而不是传统共识使用的 60～100 次/分。然而，正常人的心率可能远低于上述值，尤其是睡眠期间。因此，对于没有症状的健康患者，定义病理性心动过缓的界值是存在困难的。

最大应激性心率（HR_{max}）与最大程度的交感神经刺激，伴有副交感神经张力的减弱有关。通常预测为 $HR_{max} = (220 - 年龄)$。

窦房结功能障碍

病态窦房结综合征，也称为窦房结功能障碍，是一种常见的临床综合征，发病率随年龄的增长而增加。估算 65 岁以上人群患病率为每 600 人中 1 例，且占所有起搏器植入病因的大约一半。窦房结功能障碍是两个不同病理过程的结果：自律性受损和窦房结冲动传递到周围心房组织的障碍，也称为窦房结传出阻滞。

窦房结功能障碍在临床上表现为以下几种形式：持续或间歇性窦性心动过缓、运动时心率无法适宜增加（即变时功能不全）、窦性停搏，或通常是这些形式的组合。窦房结位于自律性级联的顶端，良好的房室结逸搏功能通常为其做好了后备支持。由窦房结功能障碍而引起严重心动过缓和相关症状通常意味着窦房结功能障碍和次级起搏点正常逸搏机制的同时异常。在逸搏机制功能正常的情况下，即使出现严重的窦房结功能障碍也可能完全无症状，临床上耐受良好并且不需要特定治疗。

静息窦性心动过缓

窦性心动过缓在常规临床实践中比较常见。男性心率在每分钟 40 多次，女性在每分钟 50 多次的轻度窦性心动过缓是正常的，之所以称为心动过缓，仅仅是因为通常选择每分钟 60 次作为正常心率下限。由于没有固定的心率可以将窦性心动过缓标记为病理性，病理性窦房结功能障碍的最好定义为明显心动过缓、伴有可合理归因于心动过缓的症状。

轻度持续性心动过缓通常无症状。当出现症状时，它们通常是非特异性的，如疲劳、倦怠或呼吸困难，将上述症状归因于静息心动过缓较为困难。窦性心动过缓可能加剧充血性心力衰竭，并限制 β 受体阻滞剂的有效使用，而 β 受体阻滞剂是心力衰竭、冠状动脉疾病和快速性心律失常治疗的基石。当不恰当的窦性心动过缓持续存在，特别是伴有严重相关症状，同时排除其他可能导致症状的病因，植入起搏器是合理的。无症状的窦性心动过缓很少需要起搏治疗，除非其他医学治疗会进一步加剧心动过缓。

变时功能不全

运动时，心输出量的增加是通过每搏输出量增加和心率增加来实现的。如果运动时心率增加不足，可能会出现疲劳或呼吸困难等运动症状。与静息窦性心动过缓的情况一样，除非相对严重，将症状归因于变时功能不全较为困难。对此，已经提出的各种标准，依赖于无法达到根据年龄预估的心率或心率储备。与静息窦性心动过缓一样，治疗变时功能不全的植入起搏器决策更多的是一种判断而不是标准。

窦性停搏

窦房结自律性的突发障碍或窦房结到心房的传导阻滞可导致心房活动暂停。P 波缺失，如果持续时间足够长且没有伴随有效的次级起搏点逸搏机制，可导致头晕、晕厥前兆或晕厥的突发症状。正常情况下少于 3 s 的窦性停搏常见，很少出现症状。非睡眠期间发生的超过 3 s 的窦性停搏通常是病理性的，可导致相关症状。存在窦性心动过缓相关症状史的患者记录到持续时间 3 s 或更长的窦性停搏，同时出现相关症状，是起搏器治疗的指征。

窦房传出阻滞

窦房结功能障碍通常伴随着心房显著纤维化，这可能导致窦房结复合体周围组织的阻滞，阻碍窦房结冲动向心房组织传导。由窦房结功能障碍引起的心动过缓的原因可能不是自律性受损，而是窦房结到心房的传导阻滞。由于窦房结活动在体表心电图上非直接可见，通过观察窦性 P 波节律突然减半，随后突然恢复到基线窦性节律（图 8.3C 和 D）而间接得出诊断。尽管还可能观察到其他模式，但 2∶1 传出阻滞是最常见的。窦房传出阻滞的治疗与间歇性窦性心动过缓的治疗相同（见前面讨论）。

窦房结功能障碍导致的窦性心动过缓-心动过速综合征

窦性心动过缓-心动过速（"慢-快"）综合征指的是临床显著心动过缓有时伴有临床显著快速性心律失常。这个术语可能令人困惑，因为心动过速的机制通常与心动过缓的机制无关。

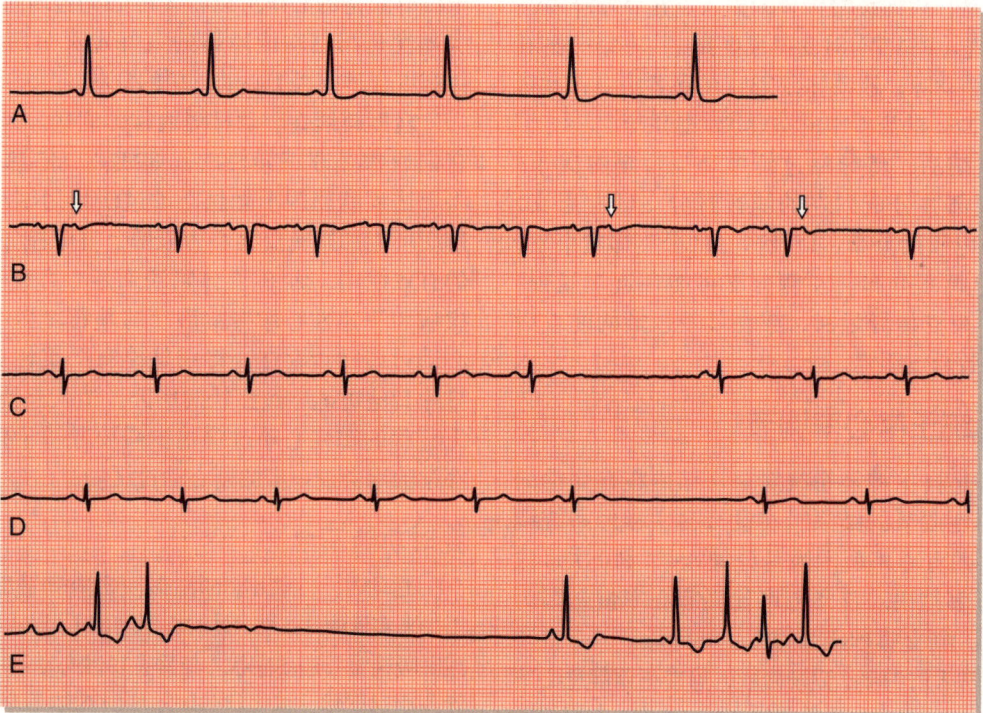

Fig. 8.3 Sinus node dysfunction. (A) Sinus bradycardia in a patient receiving metoprolol. This bradycardia results from diminished normal automaticity of the sinus node. (B) Pauses related to blocked premature atrial contractions (PACs). Blocked PACs are a common cause for apparent sinus pauses because the PAC may be early enough to be concealed by the T wave of the preceding beat *(arrows)*. The pauses are not a sign of sinus node dysfunction but rather a physiologic response to an early coupled PAC. (C) The sinus pause is an abnormal finding that suggests sinus node disease. The pause is exactly two sinus cycles and may represent sinoatrial exit block. (D) Sinoatrial Wenckebach type exit block. As is the case with the RR interval preceding atrioventricular nodal Wenckebach, progressive shortening of the PP interval preceding a doubling in sinus cycle length likely represents Wenckebach exit block from the sinus node tissue to the atrium. (E) Bradycardia-tachycardia syndrome due to sinus node dysfunction. An episode of rapidly conducted atrial fibrillation or flutter terminates and is followed for a protracted period of sinus arrest before recovery of sinus rhythm and ultimate relapse of rapidly conducted atrial fibrillation. These pauses may result in syncope or near-syncope.

This syndrome most commonly manifests as intermittent pathologic atrial arrhythmias, often intermittent AF with concomitant sinus node dysfunction resulting in long pauses or symptomatic sinus bradycardia when the patient is in sinus rhythm. A typical manifestation of this syndrome is a prolonged period of asystole after termination of AF (see Fig. 8.3E) due to slow recovery of sinus node automaticity with resultant presyncope or syncope.

The combination of two seemingly independent processes is in part a consequence of the high prevalence of AF and sinus node dysfunction in the elderly and the need to use potent drugs to decrease ventricular response during AF with resultant unintended secondary sinus node dysfunction between periods of atrial arrhythmias. This type of bradycardia-tachycardia syndrome represents an important form of clinical sinus node dysfunction and is a common indication for pacemaker implantation.

Sinus node dysfunction causing bradycardia-tachycardia should be distinguished from a common, unrelated form of bradycardia-tachycardia syndrome, which is characterized by chronic rather than intermittent AF with periods of rapid and slow ventricular responses. This condition is often incorrectly referred to as *sick sinus syndrome*. However, in this syndrome, the atrium is chronically fibrillating, and the sinus node therefore has no influence on heart rate. Bradycardia or protracted pauses in the setting of chronic AF is a consequence of impaired AV conduction and is unrelated to sinus node dysfunction.

Atrioventricular Conduction Disturbances

AV conduction disturbances include disorders in which the normal physiologic AV relationship is not maintained due to pathologic delay in AV conduction or to intermittent or complete loss of AV conduction. The PR interval includes three distinct phases of AV conduction. Although the individual components of AV conduction can be readily recorded by a His bundle catheter in an electrophysiology laboratory, the salient features of AV conduction disturbances can usually be elucidated by careful interpretation of the surface ECG without resorting to invasive recording techniques.

The right atrial conduction time from the area of the sinus node where the P wave begins to the region of the AV node occupies a short first portion of the PR interval and usually lasts no more than 30 milliseconds. Because the atrial conduction time is short and does not change much over time in a given patient, it can conveniently be ignored when assessing AV conduction. The second portion of the PR interval is the propagation time through the AV node, which is normally 50 to 120 milliseconds. The last component of the PR interval is the time for propagation through the His bundle and bundle branches, which is typically 30 to 55 milliseconds. Although this last portion, constituting His-Purkinje conduction, is short, it is the major prognostic component of AV conduction and therefore clinically important. Because the last portion of the PR interval is the time from the onset

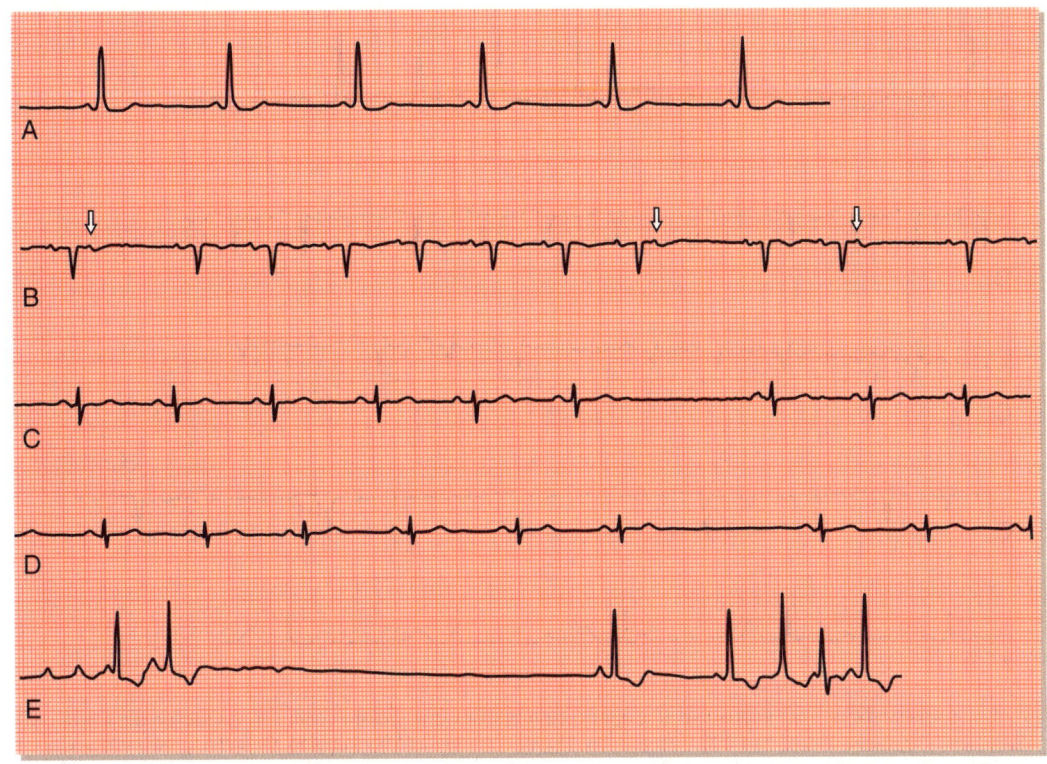

图8.3 窦房结功能异常。（A）接受美托洛尔治疗的患者出现窦性心动过缓。这种心动过缓是由于窦房结正常自律性减弱所致。（B）与房性期前收缩（PAC）阻滞相关的停搏。PAC阻滞被视为窦性停搏的常见原因，因为PAC可以早到被前一次心跳的T波掩盖（箭头）。这类停搏并非窦房结功能障碍，而是对短联律间期PAC的生理反应。（C）窦性停搏是一种异常表现，提示窦房结疾病。停搏时间恰好是两个窦性周期的长度，可能代表窦房传出阻滞。（D）窦房文氏（Wenckebach）传出阻滞。与房室结文氏（Wenckebach）阻滞前的RR间期类似，在窦性周期长度加倍之前PP间期逐渐缩短，代表窦房结组织至心房的文氏出口阻滞。（E）窦房结功能障碍引起的心动过缓-心动过速综合征。快速传导的心房颤动或心房扑动发作终止后，可能会出现一段长时间的窦性停搏，随后恢复窦性节律，最终再次发作快速传导的心房颤动。这些停搏可导致晕厥或近晕厥

该综合征最常见的表现为间歇性病理性房性心律失常，通常为阵发性心房颤动伴窦房结功能障碍，导致患者处于窦性心律时出现长间歇或症状性窦性心动过缓。该综合征的典型表现是在心房颤动终止后出现长时间停搏（见图8.3E），这是因为窦房结自律性恢复缓慢，可导致晕厥前兆或晕厥。

两种过程看似独立，部分关联原因是老年人心房颤动和窦房结功能障碍均有高患病率，心房颤动发作期间使用有效药物来控制心室率无意中导致房性心律失常间歇期间窦房结功能障碍。这种类型的心动过缓-心动过速综合征是临床窦房结功能障碍的重要形式，是起搏器植入的常见指征。

窦房结功能障碍引起的心动过缓-心动过速需要与一种常见但不相关的心动过缓-心动过速综合征区分开来，后者特点是慢性而非间歇性心房颤动，伴有间断性快速和缓慢的心室率。该情况通常被错误地称为病态窦房结综合征。但该综合征中心房是慢性颤动，此时心率并非窦性心律，因此窦房结对心率没有影响。在慢性心房颤动情况下，心动过缓或长间歇是由于房室传导受损所致，与窦房结功能障碍无关。

房室传导障碍

房室传导障碍包含由于房室传导的病理性延迟或房室传导的间歇性或完全丧失导致的无法维持正常生理性房室关系的一类疾病。PR间期包括三个不同的房室传导阶段。尽管房室传导的各个组成部分可以通过电生理实验室中的希氏束导管轻松记录，但通常可以通过仔细观察体表心电图来阐明房室传导障碍的显著特征，而无需求助于侵入性记录技术。

右心房传导时间为由P波起始的窦房结区域至房室结区域，占据PR间期的第一部分，相对较短，通常持续不超过30 ms。对于既定患者，由于心房传导时间短且大多数时候变化不大，因此在评估房室传导时可以将其简单忽略。PR间期的第二部分是房室结的传导时间，通常为50～120 ms。PR间期的最后一个组成部分是希氏束和束支的传导时间，通常为30～55 ms。尽管由希氏束-浦肯野系统传导的这最后一部分时间很短，但它是影响房室传导预后的主要组成部分，因此在临床上很重要。因为PR间期的最后一部分是从希氏束开始到心室激动的时间，所以通常称为HV间期。尽管

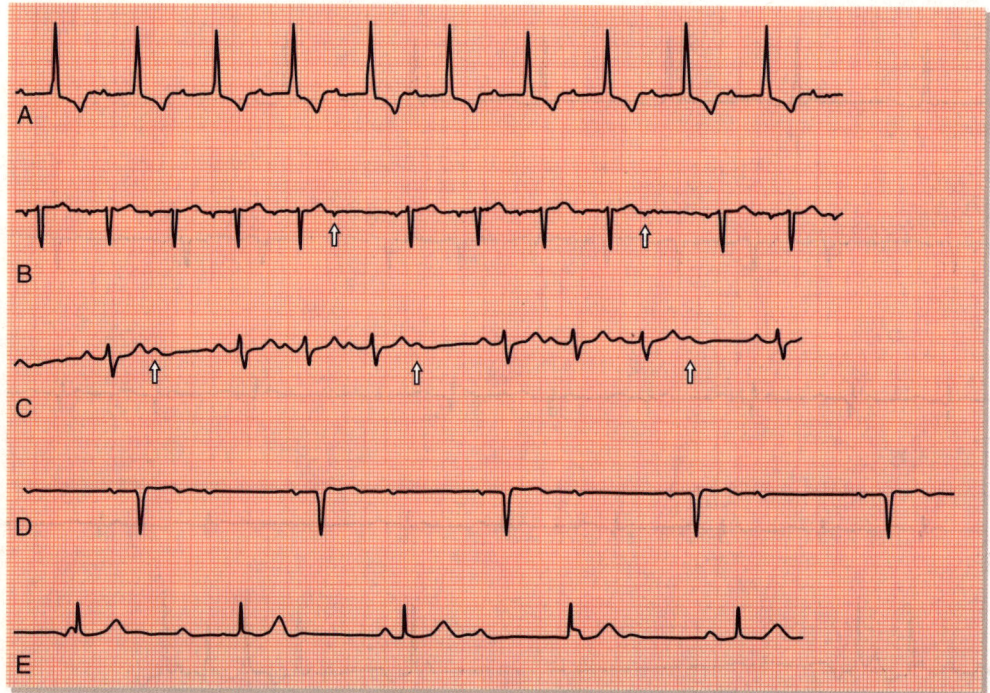

Fig. 8.4 Heart block. (A) First-degree atrioventricular (AV) block is associated with 1:1 conduction but a prolonged PR interval more than 200 milliseconds. (B) Mobitz type I (Wenckebach) second-degree AV block. Notice the progressive PR prolongation preceding the blocked P wave *(arrows)* followed by recovery of conduction with a shorter PR interval before repetition of the same pattern. (C) Mobitz type II second-degree AV block. Notice that the PR interval does not prolong in the beat preceding the blocked P wave *(arrows)*. (D) A 2:1 second-degree AV block. Notice that every other P wave fails to conduct. Because there are never two consecutively conducted P waves to assess for the presence or absence of progressive prolongation, this type of block is neither Mobitz I nor Mobitz II. (E) Complete heart block with a junctional escape rhythm. Notice that the atrial rate is faster than the ventricular rate and that there is AV dissociation. The narrow QRS escape rhythm implies a level of block high in the conduction system near the AV node.

of His bundle to the time of ventricular activation, it is commonly referred to as the HV interval. Although the HV interval cannot be measured directly from the surface ECG, a block in the His-Purkinje system can be inferred from the characteristic features that can be gleaned from review of the surface ECG.

First-Degree Atrioventricular Block

First-degree AV block is defined as a PR interval exceeding 0.2 seconds (200 milliseconds) in the setting of otherwise preserved AV conduction (Fig. 8.4A). First-degree block implies a conduction delay in one of the components of AV conduction, usually at the level of the AV node or His-Purkinje system (i.e., infranodal conduction system). First-degree AV block is usually asymptomatic, but it is a sign of AV conduction system disease and may be a diagnostic clue to the mechanism of intermittent electrocardiographically undocumented symptoms in a patient with unexplained syncope.

Second-Degree Atrioventricular Block

Second-degree AV block is defined as intermittent failure of AV conduction with interspersed periods of intact AV conduction. Second-degree AV block, like sinus bradycardia and pauses, may be seen normally during hours of sleep as well as in athletes with high parasympathetic tone. Alone, it is not an indication of AV conduction system disease.

Second-degree block may be asymptomatic, may be associated with mild symptoms such as palpitations, or if resulting in protracted pauses or persistent bradycardia, may result in hemodynamic symptoms, including lightheadedness, syncope, and fatigue. Second-degree AV block at the level of the AV node is usually indolent and gradually progressive. Because of stable junctional escape mechanisms associated with progression to complete heart block at the level of the AV node, second-degree AV block at this level tends to have a benign prognosis and, in the absence of symptoms, can be followed safely without intervention.

Second-degree block in the infranodal conduction system, which is composed of the His bundle and bundle branches, can be malignant with a tendency to progress abruptly and unpredictably to higher degrees of AV block accompanied by unstable or absent subsidiary escape mechanisms. After a patient becomes symptomatic, the infranodal block may progress to complete heart block and, in some cases, to sudden death. Despite its malignant nature, SCD is rarely attributable to complete heart block, suggesting that most patients have symptoms permitting intervention before progression to sudden death.

Because of the profound difference in natural history of second-degree AV block at the AV node and that at an infranodal level, the major clinical task in evaluating patients with second-degree AV block is to establish the probable level of the block. The surface ECG and pattern of block are quite useful.

Mobitz type I second-degree atrioventricular block. Also referred to a Wenckebach block, *Mobitz type I second-degree AV block* is a progressive prolongation in the PR interval before development of AV

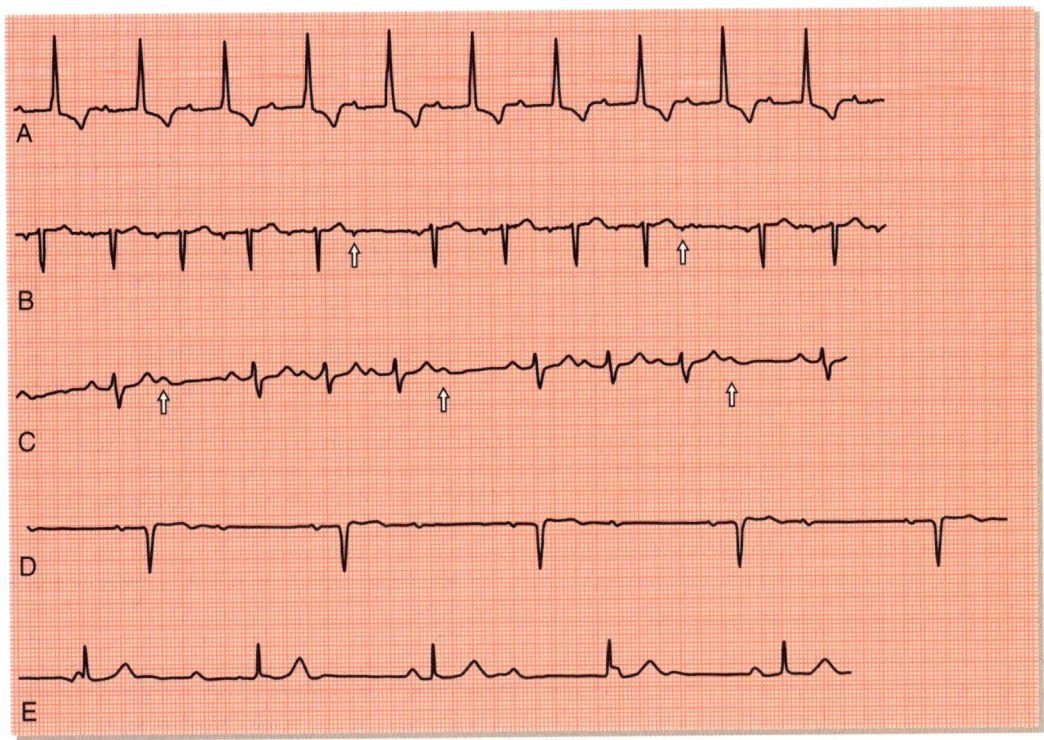

图 8.4 心脏阻滞。(A) 一度房室传导阻滞表现为 1:1 的传导比例,但 PR 间期延长至超过 200 ms。(B) 莫氏 I 型 (Wenckebach) 二度房室传导阻滞。注意 P 波被阻滞（箭头所示）前 PR 间期逐渐延长,随后传导恢复,PR 间期变短,然后重复同样的模式。(C) 莫氏 II 型二度房室传导阻滞。注意在被阻滞的 P 波（箭头所示）前一跳 PR 间期没有延长。(D) 2:1 型二度房室传导阻滞。注意每隔一个 P 波未能下传。因为没有两个连续下传的 P 波来评估 PR 间期是否存在逐渐延长,所以这种类型的阻滞既不属于莫氏 I 型也不属于莫氏 II 型。(E) 完全性心脏传导阻滞伴交界性逸搏心律。注意房率快于室率,存在房室分离。窄 QRS 波群逸搏心律提示阻滞位于传导系统的较高位置,靠近房室结

HV 间期不能直接从体表心电图上进行测量,但从体表心电图的典型特征中可以推断出希氏束-浦肯野系统的传导阻滞。

一度房室传导阻滞

一度房室传导阻滞定义为 PR 间期超过 0.2 s（200 ms）,除此之外房室传导仍然存在（图 8.4A）。一度传导阻滞意味着房室传导的某个组成部分出现传导延迟,通常位于房室结或希氏束-浦肯野系统（即房室结下传导系统）的水平。一度房室传导阻滞通常无症状,但它是房室传导系统疾病的一个标志,可能是未记录到心电图的间歇性不明原因晕厥患者的诊断线索。

二度房室传导阻滞

二度房室传导阻滞定义为房室传导的间歇性障碍,穿插有正常房室传导。像窦性心动过缓和窦性停搏一样,发生在睡眠期间或副交感神经张力高的运动员中的二度房室传导阻滞可能是正常的。单独来看,它并不是房室传导系统疾病的指标。

二度房室传导阻滞可以无症状,也可能伴有轻微症状如心悸,或者出现长时间的停搏或持续性心动过缓时导致血流动力学症状包括头晕、晕厥和疲乏。位于房室结水平的二度传导阻滞通常逐步且缓慢进展。即使房室结水平进展为完全性阻滞,由于存在稳定的结区逸搏机制,该水平的二度房室传导阻滞预后良好,在没有症状的情况下可以安全地随访,无需干预。

位于希氏束和束支的房室结下传导系统的二度传导阻滞,可能是恶性的,可突然和不可预测地进展到更高程度的房室传导阻滞,伴有次级逸搏机制的不稳定或缺失。患者出现症状后,房室结下阻滞可能进展为完全性阻滞,某些情况下可导致猝死。尽管其表现为恶性进展,但很少由于完全性阻滞发生猝死,提示大多数出现症状的患者在进展到猝死之前都具有干预时机。

位于房室结水平和位于房室结下水平的二度房室传导阻滞自然病程存在明显不同,因此评估二度房室传导阻滞患者的主要临床任务是判断可能存在的阻滞位置。此时体表心电图和阻滞类型非常有用。

莫氏（Mobitz）I 型二度房室传导阻滞 也被称为文氏（Wenckebach）阻滞,莫氏 I 型二度房室传导阻滞在房室阻滞发生之前 PR 间期逐渐延长,通常一个周期

block, usually for one cycle followed by recovery of conduction with a return to the baseline PR interval (see Fig. 8.4B). Because the degree of prolongation of the PR interval is less with each successive beat before the block, the RR intervals can paradoxically shorten in the final beats before the block.

Mobitz I AV block typically is associated with block at the level of the AV node. However, this pattern is rarely seen with advanced infranodal disease in the His bundle and bundle branches. Because Mobitz type I AV block usually occurs at the level of the AV node, infranodal conduction is commonly normal and associated with a narrow conducted QRS complex. In ambiguous cases, other clues may be helpful. Because AV node function is improved with exercise, Mobitz I block tends to normalize with activity and return at rest. Second-degree block at the level of the AV node is improved with atropine and exacerbated by carotid sinus massage. If associated with periods of complete heart block, a block at the level of the AV node is associated with a junctional escape with a QRS morphology similar to that in conducted sinus rhythm. In contrast, the observation of a wide complex escape that is different from the conducted QRS points to infranodal causes of block in the His-Purkinje system. The block may be malignant (discussed later) and require expeditious use of ventricular pacing to prevent catastrophic bradycardia.

Mobitz type II second-degree atrioventricular block. Mobitz type II second-degree AV block is intermittent failure of AV conduction during stable atrial rates without antecedent PR prolongation and followed by recovery of AV conduction (see Fig. 8.4C). Mobitz II AV block is believed to always be a sign of block in the infranodal tissues, including the His bundle and bundle branches. Whereas infranodal block may rarely display Mobitz I (Wenckebach) periodicity, AV block at the level of the AV node does not result in true Mobitz II AV block periodicity.

The finding of Mobitz II AV block is always reason for concern. Although it may result from block in the His bundle or subsidiary bundle branches, block within the His bundle accompanied by a narrow QRS complex is uncommon. In practice, Mobitz II AV block is usually preceded by the development of fixed bundle branch block. It has been believed that such bundle branch block patterns implied disease of the bundle branches themselves as they ramify within the ventricles. However, in many cases of left bundle branch block, the disease process may actually be within the His bundle affecting fibers that will ultimately extend to the left bundle branch. Regardless of the exact anatomic level of clinical bundle branch block, it remains a good clinical rule that most patients exhibiting Mobitz II AV block will also exhibit a full bundle branch block pattern during periods of conduction between episodes of second-degree AV block.

In ambiguous cases, other clues may be helpful. Because infranodal function improves relatively little with exercise, infranodal block tends to worsen with the increasing heart rates associated with exercise or stress. Atropine is not helpful for infranodal block, and because it may accelerate sinus rates, it may cause a patient to progress to higher degrees of AV block with a consequent decrease in the conducted ventricular rate. Exogenous catecholamines such as isoproterenol infusion may be helpful acutely but should not be relied on. Because of its malignant potential, hemodynamically significant Mobitz II AV block should be addressed with early temporary or permanent pacing.

2:1 and High-Grade Atrioventricular Blocks

2:1 AV block is a failure of conduction of every other P wave (see Fig. 8.4D). This pattern is most commonly seen with an infranodal block in the His bundle or bundle branches. However, 2:1 AV block may also be observed in advanced AV nodal disease. It can be distinguished from the more common infranodal form of 2:1 block by the typical Mobitz I periodicity accompanied by a usually narrow QRS complex at other times in the same patient. Because two consecutive conducted P waves are not available to assess the Mobitz pattern, a 2:1 AV block is neither truly Mobitz I nor Mobitz II, although it is common in clinical practice to describe 2:1 block as Mobitz II.

High-grade AV block is second-degree AV block with conduction failure of two or more consecutive P waves. High-grade AV block is neither Mobitz I nor Mobitz II. Although Mobitz periodicity cannot be assigned, like other forms of second-degree AV blocks, the level of block must be established to assess prognosis and guide therapy. In this case, the ancillary clues described for Mobitz blocks remain useful.

Third-Degree Atrioventricular Block

Third-degree AV block or equivalently complete heart block is a complete failure of AV conduction. In the setting of underlying sinus rhythm, this is an atrial rate faster than the ventricular rate associated with AV dissociation (see Fig. 8.4E). However, when the underlying rhythm is AF, the definition of complete heart block cannot rely on the demonstration of AV dissociation. Because conducted AF always results in an *irregular* ventricular response, the finding of a *regular and slow* ventricular response during AF implies an associated complete heart block.

As is the case for second-degree AV block, the level of the third-degree block determines the clinical behavior and prognosis of complete heart block. Complete heart block at the level of the AV node is associated with a generally stable junctional escape with rates between 40 and 50 beats per minute and usually with a narrow QRS complex. If the patient had a bundle branch block before the development of complete heart block, a block at the level of the AV node is associated with a wide QRS escape, identical to the conducted QRS before the development of a block.

Complete heart block at an infranodal level is associated with a wide and slow ventricular escape rhythm, which often is slower than 40 beats per minute with a QRS different from the antecedent conducted morphology. Unfortunately, infranodal escape rhythms may be absent entirely, leading to asystole and loss of consciousness. When infranodal complete heart block is suspected, regardless of tolerance of the ventricular escape rhythm, prompt institution of temporary or permanent ventricular pacing is appropriate.

TACHYCARDIAS

Overview and Classification

Tachyarrhythmias are categorized as supraventricular and ventricular arrhythmias. SVT relies mechanistically on the atrium, the AV node, or both. During SVT, normal depolarization of the ventricles by the His-Purkinje system typically produces a narrow complex tachycardia. SVT can manifest as a wide-complex tachycardia in the setting of aberrancy with left bundle branch block or right bundle branch block conduction, or antegrade conduction down an accessory pathway, producing an abnormal sequence of ventricular activation. Ventricular tachyarrhythmias do not depend on the atrium or AV node; they originate in the ventricles, generating a wide-complex tachycardia.

Supraventricular Tachycardias

SVTs can be categorized as paroxysmal supraventricular tachycardia (PSVT), focal atrial tachycardia, atrial flutter, and AF. This classification scheme, which addresses the underlying arrhythmic mechanism, clinical presentation, and prognosis, guides evaluation and therapy.

PSVT typically manifests in young patients without structural heart disease. The PSVT syndrome is characterized by recurrent tachypalpitations with abrupt onset and offset. Focal atrial tachycardia is more

之后传导恢复并回到基线 PR 间期（见图 8.4B）。由于在阻滞前每次心跳的 PR 间期延长程度逐渐减小，在阻滞前的最后几次心跳中可能出现 RR 间期反常地缩短。

莫氏 I 型房室传导阻滞通常与房室结水平阻滞相关。然而很少情况下亦可见该类型为位于希氏束和束支阻滞的房室结下病变。由于莫氏 I 型房室传导阻滞通常发生在房室结水平，房室结下传导通常是正常的，并伴有窄 QRS 波群。在不明确的情况下，寻找其他线索可能有帮助。由于房室结功能在运动中能得到改善，莫氏 I 型阻滞在活动时趋于正常并在休息时恢复阻滞。阿托品可改善房室结水平的二度阻滞，而颈动脉窦按摩可加剧。如果出现完全性阻滞，房室结水平的阻滞存在结区逸搏，QRS 波形态与窦性心律相似。相反，观察到异于下传 QRS 形态的逸搏 QRS 波群增宽提示阻滞位于房室结下水平的希氏束-浦肯野系统。这种阻滞可能是恶性的（后面讨论），需要迅速采取心室起搏以防止发生灾难性的心动过缓。

莫氏（Mobitz）II 型二度房室传导阻滞 莫氏 II 型二度房室传导阻滞是在房性心律稳定时房室传导的间歇性阻滞，没有 PR 间期逐渐延长，且随后恢复房室传导（见图 8.4C）。莫氏 II 型房室传导阻滞提示阻滞位于房室结下水平，包括希氏束和束支。虽然房室结下阻滞可能罕见地表现为莫氏 I 型（Wenckebach）阻滞，但位于房室结水平的阻滞不会导致真正的莫氏 II 型房室传导阻滞。

发现莫氏 II 型房室传导阻滞通常需引起重视。尽管它可能源于希氏束或束支阻滞，但伴有窄 QRS 波群的希氏束内阻滞并不常见。在临床实践中，莫氏 II 型房室传导阻滞通常先于固定的束支出现阻滞。人们曾认为该束支阻滞模式意味着束支本身及其心室内的分支存在病变。但是在许多左束支传导阻滞病例中，实际发病过程可能在希氏束内，病变最终延伸至左束支。无论临床束支阻滞的确切解剖水平如何，大多数表现为莫氏 II 型房室传导阻滞的患者也会在二度房室传导阻滞发作间期表现出完全性束支阻滞，这仍然是一个很有价值的临床规律。

在情况不明确时，其他线索可能提供帮助。因为运动对房室结下传导系统功能改善不大，运动或压力导致心率增加时，房室结下阻滞常加重。阿托品对房室结下阻滞无效。并且阿托品可使窦性心率加快，可能导致房室阻滞进展到更高程度，导致下传的心室率降低。诸如异丙肾上腺素输注之类的外源性儿茶酚胺在急救情况下可能有所帮助，但不应依赖于此。由于其潜在恶性性质，对于血流动力学上改变显著的莫氏 II 型房室传导阻滞应早期采取临时或永久起搏。

2：1 和高度房室传导阻滞

2：1 房室传导阻滞是每两个 P 波中有一个未能下传（见图 8.4D）。这种类型最常见于希氏束或束支的房室结下阻滞。然而，2：1 房室传导阻滞也可能在房室结病变进展时出现。如果同一患者其他时间常伴随窄 QRS 波群的典型莫氏 I 型周期性表现，可以以此与更常见的房室结下水平的 2：1 阻滞进行区分。由于缺乏两个连续传导的 P 波不足以评估莫氏类型，2：1 房室传导阻滞既不是真的莫氏 I 型也不是莫氏 II 型，尽管在临床实践中通常将 2：1 阻滞描述为莫氏 II 型。

高度房室传导阻滞是连续 2 个或更多 P 波未能下传的二度房室传导阻滞。高度房室传导阻滞既不是莫氏 I 型也不是莫氏 II 型。尽管不能区分莫氏类型，跟其他形式的二度房室传导阻滞一样，必须确定阻滞的水平以评估预后并指导治疗。在这种情况下，描述莫氏阻滞的辅助线索仍然有用。

三度房室传导阻滞

三度房室传导阻滞，等同于完全性阻滞，是房室传导的完全障碍。在潜在窦性心律下，房率快于室率，伴房室分离（见图 8.4E）。然而，当潜在心律为心房颤动时，完全性阻滞的判断不能依赖于房室分离。由于心房颤动下传的心室律常不规则，心房颤动期间出现规律而缓慢的心室律意味着完全性阻滞。

正如二度房室传导阻滞一样，三度阻滞所处的阻滞水平决定了心脏完全性阻滞的临床处理和预后。房室结水平的完全性阻滞通常存在稳定的结区逸搏，速率在 40～50 次 / 分之间，通常伴有窄 QRS 波群。如果患者在进展为完全性阻滞之前有束支阻滞，房室结水平的阻滞可出现宽 QRS 逸搏波，与进展为完全性阻滞之前的下传 QRS 波群形状相同。

房室结下水平的完全性阻滞，室性逸搏心律 QRS 波群宽而慢，通常小于 40 次 / 分，并且 QRS 波群形态与之前不同。不幸的是，房室结下水平的逸搏心律可能完全缺失，导致心室停搏和意识丧失。当怀疑房室结下水平的完全性阻滞时，无论对室性逸搏心律的耐受性如何，应及时采取临时或永久性心室起搏。

心动过速

概述和分类

心动过速分为室上性和室性心动过速两大类。室上性心动过速（室上速，SVT）在机制上依赖于心房、房室结或上述两者。室上速发作期间，激动通过希氏束-浦肯野系统传导，心室去极化产生窄 QRS 波群心动过速。存在左束支或右束支传导阻滞或激动通过旁路下传时，可导致心室激动顺序异常，室上速可表现为宽 QRS 波群心动过速。室性心动过速（室速，VT）不依赖于心房或房室结；它们起源于心室，为宽 QRS 波群心动过速。

室上性心动过速

室上性心动过速可以分为阵发性室上性心动过速（PSVT）、局灶性房性心动过速、心房扑动和心房颤动。这种分类方案针对潜在的心律失常机制、临床表现和预后，指导评估和治疗。

阵发性室上速通常见于没有结构性心脏病的年轻患者。其症状特点是阵发性心悸伴随突然发作和终止。局

often observed in patients with underlying atrial enlargement and valvular heart disease. AF and atrial flutter are associated with advancing age, hypertension, structural heart disease, diabetes, obstructive sleep apnea, and pulmonary disease. Unlike PSVT, AF carries an increased risk of stroke, heart failure, and death.

Paroxysmal Supraventricular Tachycardia

The incidence of PSVT is 35 cases per 100,000 person-years, with a prevalence of 2.25 per 1000 person-years. Patients report recurrent tachypalpitations. Associated symptoms may include shortness of breath, lightheadedness, chest pain, and syncope. Anginal chest pain and ischemic ST-segment depression are common and related to increased myocardial oxygen demand coupled with the loss of normal diastolic coronary perfusion time. These findings do not necessarily indicate underlying coronary artery disease and typically resolve with tachycardia termination.

PSVT typically occurs independent of structural heart disease and may manifest at any point from infancy to advanced age. PSVT relies on reentry, which is localized in the AV node in approximately 60% of cases and uses a concealed or manifest accessory pathway in 40%. Unless a delta wave indicative of WPW is identified, the underlying mechanism of PSVT may not be apparent on initial clinical presentation.

An ECG obtained during PSVT can provide useful clues to establish the diagnosis and guide management. The AV relationship should be assessed during tachycardia. By ascertaining the relationship of the P wave to the preceding QRS complex, it is possible to classify PSVT as a *short RP tachycardia* or a *long RP tachycardia*. Short RP tachycardias demonstrate a short RP pattern with P waves embedded within or occurring closely after the preceding QRS complex. Short RP tachycardias occur with reentrant SVT when the retrograde VA conduction time is shorter than the antegrade AV conduction time. This pattern is observed in the two most common forms of PSVT: typical AV nodal reentry tachycardia and reciprocating AV tachycardia related to an accessory pathway.

Long RP tachycardias are characterized by an RP interval that is longer than the next PR interval during tachycardia. This pattern occurs when the retrograde VA conduction time in reentrant arrhythmias is long due to a slowly conducting retrograde pathway during tachycardia. Atypical AV node reentry, in which retrograde conduction occurs over the slow AV nodal pathway, is the most common example of a long RP reentrant tachycardia.

Atrioventricular nodal reentry tachycardia. AVNRT is the most common form of PSVT. The arrhythmic mechanism depends on two distinct pathways in the AV node: a slowly conducting pathway with a short effective refractory period (i.e., slow pathway) and a rapidly conducting pathway with a longer refractory period (i.e., fast pathway). The fast pathway is located anteriorly near the bundle of His, and the slow pathway posteriorly near the coronary sinus ostium. Although dual pathways are a common feature of the AV node, patients with clinical tachycardia have more robust slow pathway conduction.

Tachycardia is most commonly triggered by a premature atrial contraction that blocks in the fast pathway due to its prolonged refractory period and conducts slowly antegrade down the slow pathway, producing a long PR interval on the ECG. On reaching the distal common pathway where the fast and slow AV nodal inputs meet, if the fast pathway is no longer refractory, the impulse may penetrate the fast pathway in a retrograde direction and rapidly activate the atrium, producing a short RP interval and reinitiating reentry down the slow pathway and up the fast pathway. In typical slow-fast AVNRT, the RP interval is so short that the P wave is often buried in the preceding QRS complex (Fig. 8.5A).

Atypical fast-slow AVNRT may occur with antegrade conduction over the fast pathway and retrograde conduction over the slow pathway. This form of AVNRT is uncommon and produces a long RP pattern on the ECG with characteristically deeply inverted retrograde P waves in leads II, III, and aVF.

Vagal maneuvers cause temporary AV nodal blockade and may terminate sustained AVNRT. Alternatively, intravenous adenosine is a highly effective acute therapy. The need for chronic or definitive therapy is determined by symptoms, arrhythmia frequency, and patient preference. Catheter ablation of the slow pathway at the posterior AV node is highly successful, eliminating AVNRT with a greater than 95% success rate and a low risk of complications. Drug therapy with β-blockers and calcium-channel blockers directed at the AV node may be helpful for chronic suppression. Occasionally, class IC and III antiarrhythmics may be required. AVNRT should be easily distinguished from automatic junctional tachycardia, with a narrow complex and rapid, irregular rhythm typically demonstrating AV dissociation (see Fig. 8.5B).

Reciprocating atrioventricular tachycardia and preexcitation syndromes. Congenital anomalous extranodal AV muscle fibers or accessory pathways may arise as a consequence of incomplete development of the AV annulus. These pathways are usually observed in patients with otherwise anatomically normal hearts, although right-sided accessory pathways are infrequently associated with Ebstein's anomaly and left-sided accessory pathways with hypertrophic cardiomyopathy.

Accessory pathways, or bypass tracts, may conduct antegrade, retrograde, or bidirectionally. They typically fail to demonstrate decremental conduction or the slowed conduction with increasingly frequent stimulation that characterizes the AV node. Accessory pathways capable of antegrade conduction produce early activation of the ventricle in sinus rhythm because conduction over the accessory pathway surpasses conduction over the AV node. The relatively rapid AV conduction produces a shortened PR interval, and eccentric ventricular activation over the pathway slurs the QRS onset, resulting in a delta wave (see Fig. 8.5C). If the accessory pathway is capable only of retrograde conduction, the baseline ECG in sinus rhythm does not show evidence of an accessory pathway, and the extranodal AV connection is called *concealed*.

Short PR intervals during sinus rhythm are also observed in patients with Lown-Ganong-Levine syndrome. These patients have a normal-appearing QRS complex without a delta wave because ventricular activation occurs through the His-Purkinje system (see Fig. 8.5D).

Whether accessory pathways are concealed or manifest, the most common associated arrhythmia is *orthodromic AV reentrant tachycardia* (AVRT). Tachycardia is mediated by antegrade conduction down the AV node to the ventricle and subsequent retrograde conduction up the accessory pathway to activate the atrium, then antegrade again down the AV node. Because the ventricles are activated during tachycardia exclusively over the AV node, the resulting tachycardia is typically a narrow complex unless aberrancy occurs (see Fig. 8.5E). A short RP pattern is observed on the ECG, although the RP is slightly longer than commonly observed in a typical AVNRT. Because the atria and ventricles constitute portions of the reentrant circuit, tachycardia depends on 1:1 AV conduction.

Less frequently, *antidromic AV reentrant tachycardia* is seen in patients with accessory pathways capable of antegrade conduction. The accessory pathway provides the antegrade limb of the reentrant circuit, and the AV node serves as the retrograde pathway, resulting in a wide QRS tachycardia due to complete preexcitation of the ventricles, or activation of the ventricles entirely over the accessory pathway.

Special considerations for patients with supraventricular tachycardia and delta waves in sinus rhythm. Asymptomatic patients may have delta waves on the ECG, which is called a *WPW pattern*. Prevalence

灶性房性心动过速更常见于潜在心房扩大和瓣膜性心脏病的患者。心房颤动（AF）和心房扑动与年龄增长、高血压、结构性心脏病、糖尿病、阻塞性睡眠呼吸暂停和肺部疾病相关。与阵发性室上速不同，心房颤动增加卒中、心力衰竭和死亡的风险。

阵发性室上性心动过速

阵发性室上速的发病率为35例/10万人年，患病率为2.25例/1000人年。患者描述为反复快速性心悸。相关症状可能包括呼吸急促、头晕、胸痛和晕厥。心绞痛性胸痛和缺血性ST段降低常见，这与心肌需氧量增加和舒张期冠状动脉正常灌注时间无法保证相关。这些发现并不一定提示潜在冠状动脉疾病，通常在心动过速终止后缓解。

阵发性室上速通常与结构性心脏病无关，可在婴儿到老年任何一个时间点表现出来。阵发性室上速依赖于折返机制，约60%的病例病变局限于房室结，40%通过隐匿或显性旁路。除非识别出预激综合征（WPW）的delta波，否则阵发性室上速（PSVT）的潜在机制在最初临床表现中可能不明显。

在阵发性室上速发作期间获得的心电图可以提供有用的线索，以确立诊断并指导管理。在心动过速期间应评估房室关系。通过确定P波与前一个QRS波群的关系，可以将阵发性室上速分类为短RP间期心动过速或长RP间期心动过速。短RP间期心动过速显示RP间期缩短，P波嵌入在前一个QRS波群内或紧随其后。短RP间期心动过速发生在逆传室房（VA）传导时间比顺行房室（AV）传导时间短的折返性室上速中。这在两种最常见的阵发性室上速中均可见到：典型房室折返性心动过速和与旁路相关的房室折返性心动过速。

长RP间期心动过速的特征是心动过速发作期间的RP间期比下一个PR间期长。当心动过速期间逆传室房（VA）传导时间由于逆传路径传导缓慢而较长时，便会出现该模式。非典型房室结折返，逆传发生在房室结慢径上，是长RP折返性心动过速最常见的例子。

房室结折返性心动过速（AVNRT） 房室结折返性心动过速是阵发性室上速的最常见形式。心律失常机制依赖于房室结中的两个不同路径：一个缓慢传导路径，有效不应期短（即慢径）和一个快速传导路径，不应期较长（即快径）。快径位于靠近希氏束的前部，慢径位于冠状窦口附近的后部。尽管双径是房室结的常见特征，但患有临床心动过速的患者具有更稳健的慢径传导。

心动过速通常由房性早搏触发，由于快径不应期长，快径传导受阻，从而沿慢径缓慢顺行下传，产生心电图上的长PR间期。在达到房室结快慢径汇合的远端共同途径时，如果快径已脱离不应期，冲动可能通过快径逆传，迅速激活心房，产生短RP间期，并沿慢径下传和快径逆传发作折返。在典型的慢-快型房室结折返性心动过速中，RP间期非常短以至于P波通常埋在前一个QRS波群中（图8.5A）。

非典型的快-慢型房室结折返性心动过速可能发生于经快径顺传和慢径逆传。这种形式的房室结折返性心动过速不常见，在心电图上表现为长RP间期，在Ⅱ、Ⅲ和aVF导联中出现特征性的深倒置逆传P波。

迷走神经刺激可导致房室结暂时阻滞，可终止持续的房室结折返性心动过速。此外，静脉注射腺苷也是一种高效的紧急治疗措施。根据症状、心律失常频率和患者意愿确定长期控制或根治的需求。在房室结后部慢径的导管消融可以非常成功，根治房室结折返性心动过速的成功率超过95%，且并发症风险低。应用β受体阻滞剂和钙通道阻滞剂针对房室结进行药物治疗可能有助于长期控制。偶尔可能需要使用ⅠC类和Ⅲ类抗心律失常药物。房室结折返性心动过速易与交界性心动过速区分，后者具有窄QRS波群和快速而不规则的节律，通常显示房室分离（见图8.5B）。

房室折返性心动过速和预激综合征 先天性异常的房室结之外的肌纤维或附加径路可能是房室环发育不完全而产生的结果。这些径路通常见于解剖结构正常的患者，尽管右侧附加径路可罕见地与Ebstein畸形相关，左侧附加径路与肥厚型心肌病相关。

附加径路，或称旁路，可以顺传、逆传或双向传导。它们通常不表现出房室结特有的递减传导或随着刺激频率增加而出现传导减慢。因为旁路的传导快于房室结的传导，能够顺传的旁路在窦性心律中可引起心室的提前激动。相对快速的房室传导导致PR间期缩短，通过旁路传导的心室激动导致QRS波起始变钝，形成delta波（见图8.5C）。如果旁路只能逆传，窦性心律的基线心电图不显示旁路的证据，此类额外的房室连接被称为隐匿性旁路。

Lown-Ganong-Levine综合征患者在窦性节律下也可观察到短PR间期。这些患者有一个看似正常的QRS波群，没有delta波，原因是心室激活为通过希氏束-浦肯野（His-Purkinje）系统传导的（见图8.5D）。

无论旁路是隐匿的还是显性的，最常见的心律失常是顺向型房室折返性心动过速（AVRT）。心动过速通过房室结顺向传导至心室，随后通过旁路逆传激活心房，然后再次通过房室结顺传。因为心动过速期间心室的激动完全通过房室结传导，所以呈现窄QRS波群心动过速，除非发生差异性传导（见图8.5E）。尽管RP间期比典型房室结折返性心动过速中所见到的略长，但在心电图上仍观察到短RP间期。因为心房和心室构成了折返环的一部分，心动过速依赖于1∶1的房室传导。

较少见的是，可在旁路能够顺行传导的患者中观察到逆向型房室折返性心动过速。旁路提供折返环路的顺传路径，房室结作为逆传路径，心室完全预激或完全通过旁路激活产生宽QRS波群心动过速。

窦性心律下delta波的室上性心动过速患者的特殊情况 无症状患者可在心电图上出现delta波，称为WPW（Wolff-Parkinson-White）现象。WPW现象在一

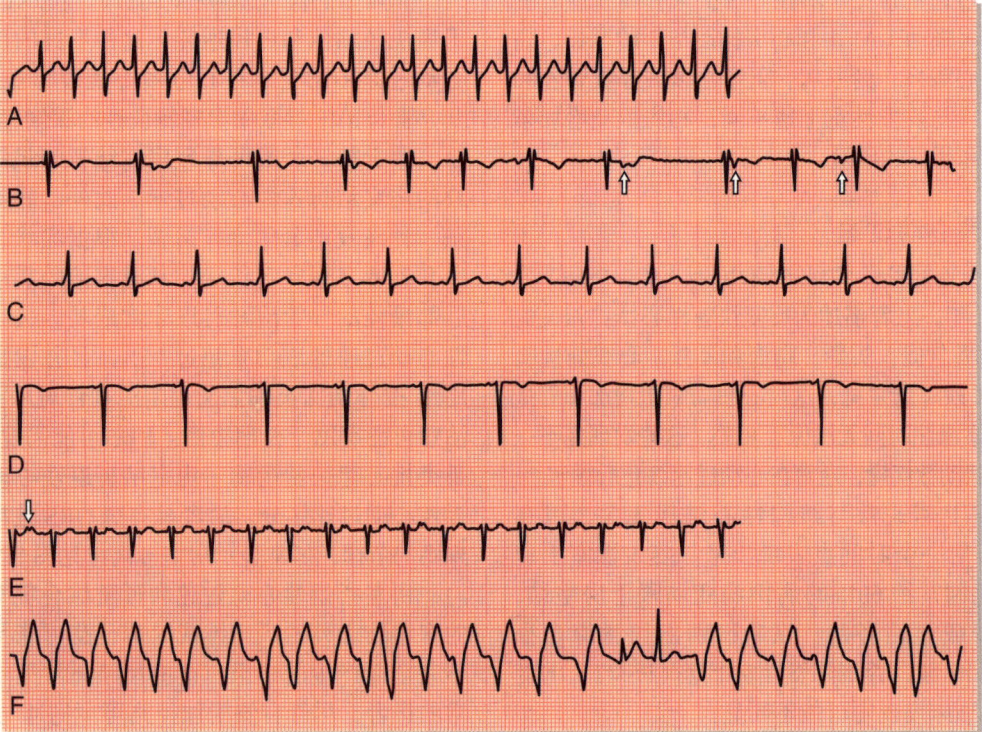

Fig. 8.5 Atrioventricular (AV) nodal (junctional) rhythm disturbances. (A) Supraventricular tachycardia. The lack of visible P waves during tachycardia suggests that they are concealed within the QRS complex, a pattern indicative of underlying AV nodal reentrant tachycardia. (B) Automatic junctional tachycardia. Notice the AV dissociation during tachycardia. The P waves *(arrows)* are dissociated from the QRS complexes. (C) Sinus rhythm with a short PR interval due to the presence of delta waves in a patient with Wolff-Parkinson-White (WPW) syndrome. The slurred QRS upstroke of the delta wave results from early activation of the ventricle by the extranodal bypass tract, followed by fusion with rapid conduction down the normal conduction system and resulting in narrowing of the terminal QRS. (D) Sinus rhythm with a short PR interval but no delta waves. Despite the short PR, the P wave is normally vectored, excluding a junctional rhythm that appears similar but with an inverted P wave. A short PR interval in sinus rhythm without delta waves is caused by an abnormally rapid AV nodal conduction and is described as a Lown-Ganong-Levine pattern. (E) Supraventricular tachycardia. Unlike tracing A, there is a clear P wave *(arrow)* inscribed immediately after each QRS in the ST segment. This pattern is seen most commonly with orthodromic AV reciprocating tachycardia in a patient with WPW syndrome. The early P wave in WPW is caused by retrograde conduction up the accessory pathway after ventricular activation during tachycardia. (F) Preexcited atrial fibrillation (AF) in a patient with WPW syndrome. Notice the rapid and irregular ventricular response with widening of the QRS due to preexcitation. This pattern results from rapid conduction of the AF down the accessory pathway, bypassing the normal conduction system. As in this arrhythmia, occasional conduction down the AV node may occur during ongoing tachycardia, resulting in periods with a narrow QRS complex.

of the WPW pattern in the general population is approximately 1 case per 1000 people. Accessory pathways may be poorly conducting and less likely to promote tachycardia, accounting for the absence of symptoms. These patients have a favorable prognosis, particularly if spontaneous and abrupt cessation of ECG preexcitation (delta wave) occurs with exercise or during ambulatory monitoring. In many cases, no specific therapy is required for asymptomatic patients.

Asymptomatic young patients participating in high-risk activities with WPW pattern may be subjected to invasive electrophysiologic testing for risk stratification. Patients with delta waves demonstrating clinical SVT or suggestive arrhythmic symptoms are said to have WPW syndrome, and invasive electrophysiologic testing is ordinarily recommended in these patients. Invasive testing helps to stratify the risk of sudden cardiac death.

Curative ablation is highly effective, with a success rate of 95%, and poses a low risk of procedural complications. Chronic therapy with antiarrhythmic drugs that prolong the accessory pathway refractory period (i.e., class IA, IC, or III agents) may be effective, but the potential for adverse drug effects has made accessory pathway ablation the treatment of choice for symptomatic and high-risk patients.

The use of agents that slow AV nodal conduction in patients with WPW syndrome warrants special mention. Digoxin, β-blockers, and calcium-channel blockers should not be used in patients with WPW because they slow conduction through the AV node, resulting in preferential excitation of the ventricles over the accessory pathway. In the setting of AF or atrial flutter, this may cause rapid ventricular rates and hemodynamic instability.

Wolff-Parkinson-White syndrome and atrial fibrillation. WPW syndrome is associated with a 0.25% per year risk of sudden cardiac death (SCD), which is related to the development of AF with rapid antegrade conduction over the accessory pathway producing VF. This risk is greatest for patients demonstrating very short preexcited RR

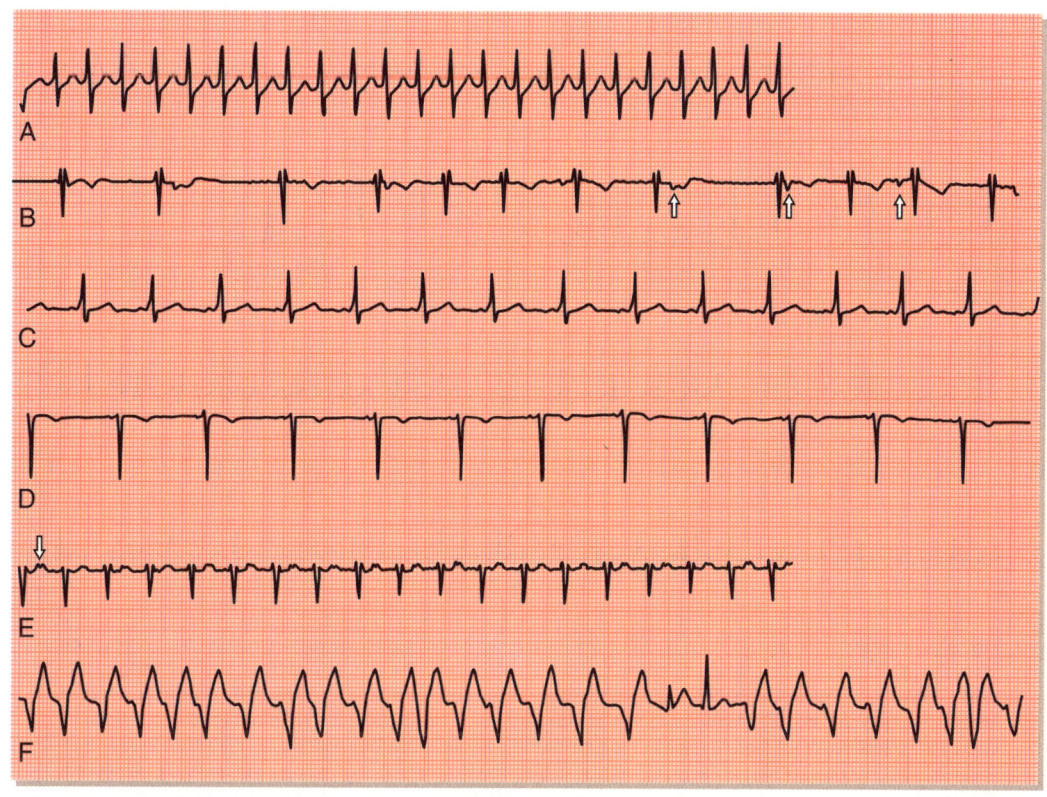

图8.5 房室（AV）结性（交界性）节律异常。（A）室上性心动过速。心动过速发作期间P波不可见提示它们可能隐藏在QRS波群中，这种模式提示潜在的房室结折返性心动过速。（B）自律性交界性心动过速。注意心动过速期间的房室分离。P波（箭头所示）与QRS波群分离。（C）Wolff-Parkinson-White（WPW）综合征患者由于存在delta波，窦性心律下PR间期缩短。含delta波的QRS上升支顿挫是由于心室被房室结外的旁路提前激活，随后与正常传导系统的快速传导融合，导致QRS末端变窄。（D）窦性心律伴短PR间期但无delta波。尽管PR间期缩短，但P波正向，排除了与窦性心律相似但P波倒置的交界性心律。窦性心律中没有delta波的短PR间期是由异常的快速房室结传导引起的，称为Lown-Ganong-Levine（LGL）综合征。（E）室上性心动过速。与A图不同，在每个QRS波群后的ST段上清晰地记录到P波（箭头所示）。这种模式最常见于WPW综合征患者的顺向房室折返性心动过速。WPW综合征中的早现的P波是在心动过速发作期间心室激动后通过旁路逆行传导形成的。（F）WPW综合征患者的预激性心房颤动（AF）。注意心室律快速且不规则，由于预激造成QRS波变宽。这种模式是由于心房颤动（AF）通过旁路快速传导，绕过了正常的传导系统。正如该心律失常心电图所示，在持续的心动过速期间偶尔可通过房室结传导出现窄QRS波群

般人群中的患病率大约为千分之一。旁路传导性有可能较差，此时诱发心动过速可能性较小，这解释了为什么没有症状。这类患者预后良好，特别是如果心电图预激波（delta波）在运动或动态监测期间出现自发和突然消失。许多情况下，无症状患者不需要特殊治疗。

参与高风险活动的无症状年轻患者，如果具有WPW现象，可能需要接受侵入性电生理检查进行危险分层。临床上表现为室上速或提示性心律失常症状的delta波患者称为WPW综合征。此类患者通常建议进行有创电生理检查。有创检查有助于对心源性猝死的风险进行分层。

治疗性消融非常有效，成功率为95%，手术并发症风险低。长期使用延长旁路不应期的抗心律失常药物（即IA、IC或III类药物）可能有效，但药物相关副作用的潜在风险使得旁路消融成为有症状和高风险患者的首选治疗。

WPW综合征患者使用减慢房室结传导药物时需要特别注意。洋地黄、β受体阻滞剂和钙通道阻滞剂不可用于WPW综合征患者，因为它们减慢房室结传导，导致旁路成为激动心室的首选路径。在心房颤动或心房扑动发作的情况下，可能导致心室率过快和血流动力学不稳定。

WPW综合征和心房颤动 WPW综合征与每年0.25%的心源性猝死（SCD）风险相关，这与心房颤动通过旁路快速下传导致心室颤动相关。对于心房颤动

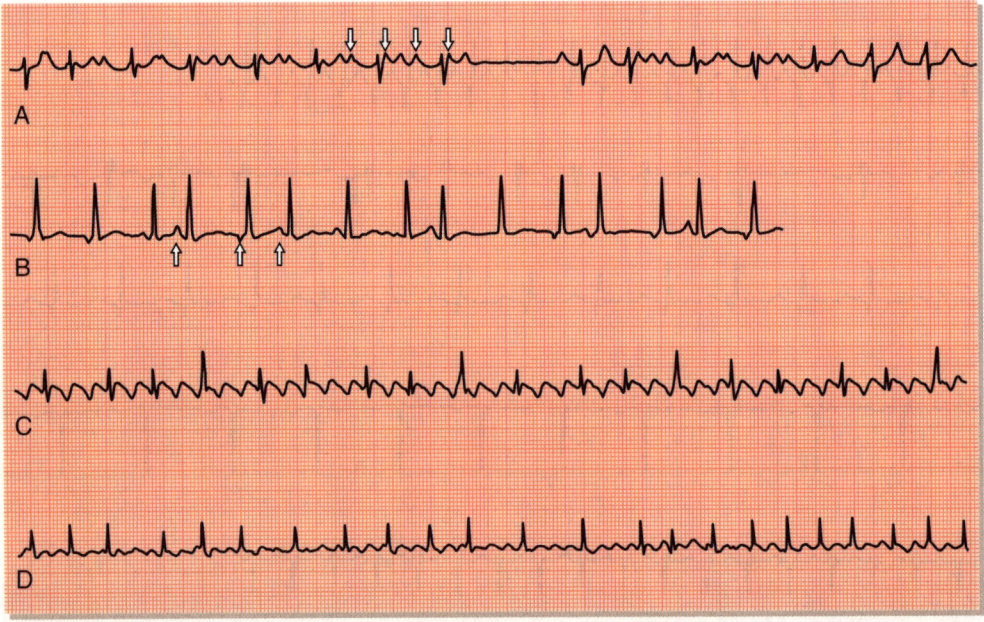

Fig. 8.6 Atrial arrhythmias. (A) Runs of focal atrial tachycardia with variable atrioventricular (AV) block. The tachycardia occurs in salvos with interspersed periods of sinus rhythm. The P waves *(arrows)* during tachycardia appear uniform although their cycle length varies, resulting in variable patterns of AV conduction and an irregular ventricular rate. (B) Multifocal atrial tachycardia. Notice the incessant atrial premature beats *(arrows)* with at least three distinct morphologies. Because of the irregularly irregular response, this arrhythmia can be easily misdiagnosed as atrial fibrillation (which lacks discrete P waves) if the tracing is not carefully reviewed. (C) Atrial flutter with rapid, variable conduction. Notice the continuous sawtooth atrial activity. Although commonly manifesting with stable 2:1 block and a regular response, the block varies in this patient, progressing through periods of 2:1 and 3:1 ratios and resulting in an irregular ventricular response. (D) Atrial fibrillation with a rapid ventricular response. Notice the wavering baseline without distinct P waves and an irregularly irregular response.

intervals during AF. For some WPW patients, SCD may be the initial presentation. Successful catheter ablation of the accessory pathway eliminates this possibility.

Patients with WPW and rapidly conducted AF have the characteristic electrocardiographic findings of a rapid, irregularly irregular, wide QRS rhythm with various degrees of QRS widening or preexcitation from beat to beat (see Fig. 8.5F). During AF in the setting of underlying WPW, activation of the ventricle over the AV node produces concealed retrograde activation of the accessory pathway, prolonging the refractory period of the pathway and moderating the rate of antegrade accessory pathway conduction.

Treating patients with AV nodal–blocking therapy decreases concealed retrograde activation of the pathway, facilitating antegrade accessory pathway conduction and potentiating hemodynamic instability. Appropriate acute therapy includes drugs that prolong the accessory pathway refractory period, such as intravenous procainamide, ibutilide, or amiodarone. In the event of hemodynamic instability, electrical cardioversion is preferred.

Role of catheter ablation in Wolff-Parkinson-White syndrome. Catheter ablation is highly effective for treating WPW, with success rates of approximately 95% and recurrence rates of only 5%. Procedural complications are uncommon, with major complications occurring in 2% to 4% of cases and deaths related to ablation occurring in 0.1%.

Although antiarrhythmic drug therapy may control symptoms, the expense and risks of pharmacologic therapy along with the safety and efficacy of ablation have made radiofrequency ablation the first-line therapy for symptomatic WPW. Because older patients with asymptomatic WPW patterns have a favorable prognosis, they should not routinely be subjected to ablation.

Atrial Arrhythmias
Overview and Classification

Atrial arrhythmias depend entirely on the atria but are mechanistically independent of AV conduction. As a consequence, intra-atrial arrhythmias persist despite the development of spontaneous or pharmacologically induced AV block. Tachycardias originating in the atria may be organized and repetitive, resulting from automaticity or intra-atrial reentry, or may be chaotic and disorganized, as is the case in AF. Therapy is directed at moderating the ventricular response during episodes of tachycardia or suppressing the underlying atrial arrhythmia.

Focal arrhythmias originate from a point source in one of the atria, and circumferential spread encompasses the remainder of the atrium. These arrhythmias display distinct P waves separated by a clear isoelectric segment. Focal arrhythmias commonly have an automatic mechanism, but in some cases, they may result from micro-reentry involving an anatomically small portion of the atrium (e.g., around a single pulmonary vein), followed by radial spread to the rest of the atrium. Although most commonly a single abnormal focus may be active, in the setting of severe physiologic stress, multiple foci may be active simultaneously, leading to a chaotic electrocardiographic appearance with multiple distinct P waves, referred to as *multifocal atrial tachycardia* (MAT) (Fig. 8.6B). Automatic arrhythmias tend to be episodic and nonsustained, sometimes recurring incessantly. Cycle length often varies within a run, between runs, and with changes in autonomic tone.

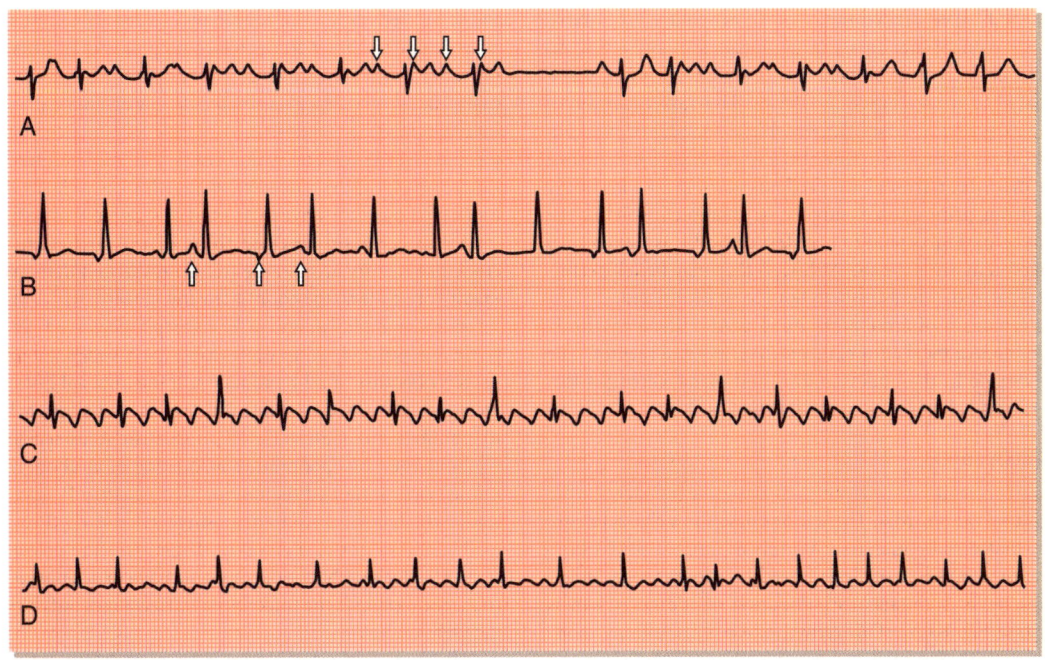

图 8.6　房性心律失常。（A）局灶性房性心动过速伴随不定的房室（AV）阻滞。一串心动过速发生在窦性心律之间。心动过速时的 P 波（箭头）看起来呈单形性，但它们的周长有所变化，导致房室传导模式变化和不规则的心室律。（B）多源性房性心动过速。注意连续的至少 3 个不同形态的房性早搏（箭头）。由于心室律绝对不规整，如果没有仔细回顾心电记录，这种心律失常很容易被误诊为心房颤动（心房颤动没有散在的 P 波）。（C）心房扑动伴快速、多变的心室下传。注意连续的锯齿状心房波。尽管通常表现为具有稳定的规律 2:1 阻滞和规整的心室律，但该患者阻滞比例有变化，间断以 2:1 和 3:1 比例下传，并导致心室律不规整。（D）心房颤动伴快心室率。注意基线波动、无明显 P 波且心室律绝对不规整

期间预激 RR 间期非常短的患者，上述猝死风险最大。对于部分 WPW 综合征患者，SCD 可能是最初的临床表现。成功消融旁路可避免这种可能性。

具有 WPW 综合征和旁路快速传导的心房颤动患者具有快速、不规则、宽 QRS 波的典型心电图节律表现，每跳 QRS 波群增宽或预激程度不同（见图 8.5F）。在 WPW 综合征基础上合并心房颤动发作期间，通过房室结下传的心室激动对旁路产生隐匿性逆传激活，延长旁路的不应期，调节顺行旁路的传导速率。

阻断房室结的治疗减少了旁路的隐匿性逆传激活，促进旁路顺向传导，并加剧血流动力学不稳定。恰当的急救治疗包括延长旁路不应期的药物，如静脉注射普鲁卡因胺、伊布利特或胺碘酮。在血流动力学不稳定的情况下，首选电复律。

导管消融在 WPW 综合征中的作用　导管消融治疗 WPW 综合征非常有效，成功率约为 95%，复发率仅为 5%。手术并发症不常见，严重并发症发生于 2%～4% 的病例中，与消融相关的死亡发生率为 0.1%。

尽管抗心律失常药物治疗可控制症状，但结合药物治疗的费用和风险以及消融的安全性和有效性，使得射频消融成为症状性 WPW 综合征的一线治疗。由于无症状 WPW 现象的老年患者预后良好，因此他们不进行常规消融。

房性心律失常

概述和分类

房性心律失常完全依赖于心房，但从机制上来说独立于房室传导。因此，即使出现了自发性或药物引起的房室阻滞，心房内心律失常仍会持续。起源于心房的心动过速，可能是自律性或心房内折返导致的规整的心动过速。在心房颤动发生时也可能是杂乱无序的。治疗房性心律失常的方法可以为在心动过速发作时通过减慢房室传导而治疗，也可以针对房性心律失常本身治疗。

局灶性心律失常起源于心房中某个点，呈同心圆样向心房其余部位扩布。大多数时候心房内仅有一个异常激动灶，但在明显生理应激的情况下，有可能触发多个激动灶，导致形态紊乱的心电图，伴有多种不同形态的 P 波，即多源性房性心动过速（MAT）（图 8.6B）。自律性心律失常倾向于发作性和非持续性，有时也会无休止反复发作。心动过速周长常常会随自主神经张力的改变，在同一次发作内以及不同发作之间变化。

Macro-reentrant atrial arrhythmias are a consequence of stable reentrant circuits, which encompass large portions of the atria. All such circuits require a central obstacle and a region of slowed atrial conduction related to atrial dilation or fibrosis. The most common of these arrhythmias is *typical atrial flutter,* which is mediated by right atrial reentry around normal anatomic obstacles. In addition to typical flutter, reentry may occur around acquired obstacles, most commonly scars resulting from prior cardiac surgery or ablation involving the atria. Reentrant arrhythmias tend to manifest clinically as paroxysmal sustained or persistent arrhythmias. Although they may be self-terminating and episodic, individual episodes tend to be protracted.

The final mechanism of atrial arrhythmia is AF. This arrhythmia involves components of focal automatic mechanisms and reentry. The major advances made in the understanding and management of this common arrhythmia are reviewed in the following sections.

Focal Atrial Tachycardia

Focal atrial tachycardia also is referred to as ectopic atrial tachycardia and automatic atrial tachycardia. These terms describe a characteristic clinical pattern that usually manifests as runs of unifocal PACs lasting for seconds or minutes, usually followed by spontaneous termination and subsequent spontaneous reinitiation of additional salvos of tachycardia (see Fig. 8.6A). This arrhythmia less commonly manifests as a paroxysmal sustained tachycardia. When mapped in the electrophysiologic laboratory, these arrhythmias have a focal origin, and although they are sometimes triggered by rapid pacing, suggesting triggered activity, they appear to be automatic rather than a reentrant mechanism.

The electrocardiographic features are characteristic and usually permit accurate diagnosis. Because the arrhythmia is focal and automatic, the morphology of the first PAC of the run is identical to the subsequent PACs. Cycle length tends to vary between and within runs, and tachycardia is unaffected by intermittent AV block, which may occur during the runs. The same focus often fires erratically between runs, resulting in frequent atrial ectopy that is morphologically similar to the P wave observed during the runs.

The arrhythmia appears to be caused by intracellular calcium overload and resultant triggered activity related to delayed afterdepolarizations, making it responsive to calcium-channel blockers and β-blockers. The paroxysmal sustained form of this arrhythmia is also adenosine responsive, giving the false impression of dependence on AV conduction. The use of digoxin may exacerbate triggered causes of atrial tachycardia. Class IC agents, such as flecainide and propafenone, may be useful in patients without structural heart disease or coronary artery disease. Amiodarone can also be used in these patients for rhythm control. The arrhythmia is readily amenable to catheter ablation if ectopy occurs frequently enough to permit mapping.

Typical Atrial Flutter

Atrial flutter is a persistent atrial arrhythmia with an atrial rate of at least 250 beats per minute (see Fig. 8.6C). Because the normal AV node cannot conduct 1:1 at these rates, this arrhythmia characteristically manifests with 2:1 conduction and a ventricular response of about 140 to 150 beats per minute. During 2:1 conduction, the difficulty in perceiving flutter waves may lead to diagnostic confusion. Typical atrial flutter is the most common form of this arrhythmia, and it is mediated by macro-reentry restricted to the right atrium. The central obstacles in this circuit consist of normal anatomic structures, accounting for its stereotyped pattern.

Typical atrial flutter is mediated by counterclockwise reentry around the tricuspid valve as viewed from the ventricle. The valve prevents anterior collapse of the circuit, and posteriorly a long ridge in the atrial wall (i.e., crista terminalis) forms a functional line of block, preventing the circuit from collapsing posteriorly. Because the normal obstacles already exist, flutter development results from the abnormally slowed conduction related to atrial enlargement, fibrosis, or edema, which sometimes is combined with shortened atrial refractory periods due to catecholamine stress. Typical counterclockwise atrial flutter demonstrates a deeply negative F wave in leads II, III, and aVF; a sharply positive F wave in V_1; and a negative F wave in V_6.

A less common reversed form of this arrhythmia is caused by clockwise reentry around the tricuspid valve. It demonstrates an ECG exactly opposite to the counterclockwise form, with a strongly positive F wave in leads II, III, and aVF; a sharply negative F wave in V_1; and a positive F wave in V_6. In both cases, the F waves are often difficult to perceive because of 2:1 conduction. If the unusual F-wave vector is not recognized, the ECG may be misinterpreted as sinus tachycardia. Clues to identification of atrial flutter are persistent, unexplained heart rates of about 150 beats per minute with a variation of only a few beats per minute over time and the finding of a negative P wave in the inferior leads, which is expected to be positive in sinus rhythm.

The most fruitful method of diagnosis is the provocation of transient AV block with carotid sinus massage or adenosine infusion. This transiently exposes the underlying flutter waves but does not terminate the arrhythmia.

Although acute therapy involves rate control or cardioversion if drugs are poorly tolerated, long-term rate control for this arrhythmia is difficult. Drug doses that result in acceptable block at rest often fail to control exercise rates, and doses that result in exercise rate control often provoke bradycardia at rest. Early restoration of sinus rhythm is preferred for this arrhythmia.

Atrial flutter is a common transient arrhythmia in acute care hospital settings. The right atrial wall is thin, and pericarditis resulting from cardiac or thoracic surgery results in atrial edema and inflammation that may permit adequate slowing and promote transient atrial flutter. Acute pulmonary decompensation may result in right heart failure and may promote transient atrial flutter. In all of these settings, endogenous or pharmacologic catecholamine stimulation exacerbates the arrhythmia. Transient therapy for up to a month is appropriate in these settings.

When atrial flutter occurs in the absence of an acute precipitant, long-term therapy is required. Given the difficulty of achieving rate control in atrial flutter and the need for antiarrhythmic agents with associated potential morbidity to maintain sinus rhythm, catheter ablation has become the primary means of treating this arrhythmia. Antiarrhythmic therapy for atrial flutter is similar to that for AF (discussed later). Antiarrhythmic drug therapy should be reserved for temporary treatment of likely transient flutter or for patients who are not suitable candidates for invasive management. Catheter ablation of typical atrial flutter is a low-risk procedure with a long-term success rate exceeding 90% in experienced centers.

Atypical Atrial Flutter and Macro-Reentrant Atrial Tachycardia

In addition to the typical atrial flutter circulating around normal anatomic obstacles, atrial disease with associated fibrosis or, more commonly, atrial scars created at the time of prior catheter or surgical ablation or cardiac surgery for valvular or congenital heart disease may create alternative substrates for intra-atrial reentry. Common to these arrhythmias is a significant region of scar with a channel of surviving myocardium bridging the scar or between the scar and a normal anatomic obstacle. Within the channel, conduction is slow and electrocardiographically silent, resulting in an isoelectric PP interval. Because the circuit is different from that of typical atrial flutter, the P-wave morphology is atypical.

稳定的折返环会导致大折返性房性心动过速。这些折返环都需要依赖中心屏障和心房内缓慢传导区，后者与心房扩大或纤维化相关。最常见的大折返性房性心律失常是典型性心房扑动，由围绕正常解剖屏障的右心房折返所介导。除了典型性心房扑动之外，折返可以围绕获得性屏障发生，既往心脏外科手术或消融所致的瘢痕最为常见。折返性心律失常可以表现为阵发性或持续性心律失常。虽然可以自行终止并呈发作性，但个别发作会有迁延倾向。

房性心律失常的最后一种机制是心房颤动。心房颤动涉及局灶性自律性机制和折返的成分。这种常见心律失常的认识和治疗方面所取得的主要进展将在下文中进行介绍。

局灶性房性心动过速

局灶性房性心动过速也称异位性房性心动过速和自律性房性心动过速。这些名词描述了一个特征性的临床现象，通常表现为持续数秒至数分钟的单源性房性期前收缩，通常会自行终止，随后出现反复发作的心动过速（见图8.6A）。这种心律失常较少出现突发的持续性心动过速，在电生理检查标测时，这些心律失常为局灶性起源，尽管它们有时由快速起搏触发，提示可能为触发活动所致，但它们似乎是自律而非折返机制所致。

由于其心电图特征明显，通常易于做出正确诊断。因为这种心律失常是局灶性、自律性的，所以发作时第一个房性期前收缩的形态与随后的期前收缩形态相同。发作时或发作间，心动过速周长倾向于改变，心动过速不受发作时可能出现的间歇性的房室传导阻滞影响。同一个起源点也常在发作的间期不规律激动，导致频繁出现房性异位搏动，其P波形态类似于心动过速发作时的P波。

细胞内钙超载和延迟后除极引发的触发活动导致了此类心律失常，故可应用钙通道阻滞剂和β受体阻滞剂进行治疗。腺苷同样可治疗此类心律失常，产生其依赖房室传导的错误印象。地高辛可加剧房性心动过速。IC类药物，如氟卡尼和普罗帕酮，可用于没有结构性心脏病或冠状动脉疾病的患者。胺碘酮也可用于这类患者的节律控制。若异位搏动发作频繁，能完成标测，则易于进行导管消融治疗。

典型心房扑动

心房扑动（房扑）是持续性房性心律失常，心房率为每分钟至少250次（见图8.6C）。由于这种快的心房率不能经正常房室结1∶1下传，心电图特征性地表现为2∶1传导和140～150次/分的心室率。2∶1传导时，难以辨识的扑动波可能导致误诊。典型心房扑动是这种心律失常最常见的形式，由右心房内的大折返环所致。折返环中心的屏障由正常的解剖结构组成，因此形成固定的发作模式。

从右心室方向观察典型心房扑动，可见围绕三尖瓣逆时针方向折返。瓣膜维持折返环的前半部分，而在后面，心房的界嵴（脊）提供功能性阻滞线，维持折返环的后半部分。由于正常屏障已经存在，心房增大、纤维化或水肿所致的异常缓慢传导，有时还可伴儿茶酚胺应激所致的心房不应期缩短，均可诱发心房扑动。典型的逆时针方向心房扑动在Ⅱ、Ⅲ和aVF导联表现为深的负向F波，V_1导联中锐利的正向F波，V_6导联中的负向F波。

与上述心律失常方向相反的心房扑动，是由围绕三尖瓣环的顺时针折返所致，这类心房扑动较为少见。心电图表现为与逆时针形态完全相反：在Ⅱ、Ⅲ和aVF导联中F波明显正向，V_1导联出现锐利的负向F波，V_6导联F波正向。以上两种心房扑动，如果出现2∶1传导，则F波经常难以辨识。如果未能识别异常的F波向量，则心电图可能被误认为窦性心动过速。心房扑动的识别线索包括持续的、不可解释的约150次/分的心室率，较长时间内每分钟心率仅有数次的差别，并且在下壁导联中出现负向P波，而窦性心律下壁导联为正向P波。

心房扑动最有效的诊断方法是激发出短暂的房室传导阻滞，方法包括按摩颈动脉窦和推注腺苷。这会使潜在的心房扑动波短暂显现，但不终止心房扑动。

急性期治疗虽涉及心率控制和药物难以耐受时的复律治疗，但长期心率控制较为困难。静息时使房室传导阻滞、心率达标的药物剂量，通常难以控制活动时心率，而活动时心率达标，可能引起静息时心动过缓。早期恢复窦性心律是此类心律失常的首选治疗。

心房扑动是重症监护病房常见的短暂性心律失常。右心房壁薄，心脏或胸外科手术所致的心包炎导致心房水肿和炎症，可产生足够的阻滞并诱发短暂性心房扑动。急性肺失代偿可能导致右心衰竭，并可能诱发短暂心房扑动。在所有这些情况下，内源性或药源性儿茶酚胺刺激可加剧心房扑动。在这些情况下可使用最长1个月的短期治疗方案。

若出现心房扑动却没有急性起因，则需长期治疗。鉴于抗心律失常药物难以实现心房扑动时的心率控制，以及维持窦性心律所需抗心律失常药潜在的副作用，导管消融已成为治疗这种心律失常的主要手段。心房扑动的抗心律失常治疗与心房颤动相似（将在下文讨论）。抗心律失常药物治疗可作为短暂性心房扑动的短期治疗方案或患者不适合介入治疗时的备选方法。导管消融典型心房扑动是一种低风险操作，在经验丰富的医学中心，远期成功率超过90%。

非典型心房扑动与大折返性房性心动过速

除围绕正常解剖学屏障的典型心房扑动折返之外，心房内折返的另一种基质会由以下情况导致，包括伴有心房纤维化的心房疾病，更常见的是既往导管或外科消融史，以及心脏瓣膜手术或先天性心脏病手术导致的心房瘢痕。此类心律失常的共同之处是存在一块关键瘢痕区，由存活心肌形成的通路对瘢痕，或对瘢痕和正常解剖屏障之间进行桥接。通路内传导缓慢且为心电静默状态，导致PP间期为等电位线。该折返环不同于典型心房扑动，故出现非典型的P波形态。

When the rate is 250 beats per minute or greater, the arrhythmia is arbitrarily classified as atypical atrial flutter, and when the rate is less than 250 beats per minute, it is arbitrarily classified as atrial tachycardia. Like typical atrial flutter, these arrhythmias are paroxysmal sustained or persistent arrhythmias, and when manifesting with 2:1 conduction, they may be misdiagnosed as sinus tachycardia if the abnormal P-wave vector and fixed heart rate over time are not recognized. Therapy and prognosis are otherwise similar to those for typical atrial flutter.

Atrial Fibrillation
Overview and Classification
AF is a chaotic atrial rhythm related to continuous and variable activation of the atria. There are no distinct P waves or periods of atrial quiescence. It is characterized electrocardiographically by a wavering baseline associated with an irregular ventricular response (see Fig. 8.6D).

AF is the most common clinically significant arrhythmia. It affects 2.2 million people in the United States. Its prevalence is between 0.4% and 1% in the general population, and it increases with age, reaching 8% in those older than 80 years. Patients with AF have a higher risk of stroke, heart failure, and mortality. However, the role of AF as an independent determinant of mortality is uncertain because it commonly coexists with other important conditions. Patients with lone AF do not have an increased mortality rate, and carefully designed trials exploring the benefit of maintenance of sinus rhythm over rate control show, in most populations, no survival benefit for sinus rhythm. One exception may be in patients with systolic heart failure in addition to AF where ablation of AF may have a survival advantage. The recently completed CASTLE-AF (Catheter Ablation vs. Standard Conventional Treatment in Patients with LV Dysfunction and AF) showed a significant reduction in mortality with catheter ablation of AF in this select population. AF is often classified by its clinical presentation and pattern. When AF is first detected, it is called *new onset*, and its ultimate pattern is initially undetermined. When AF relapses during follow-up, it is called *recurrent* and classified by its clinical pattern. If AF terminates spontaneously, it is called *paroxysmal* AF. Although episodes lasting up to 7 days are defined as paroxysmal, most episodes of paroxysmal AF terminate within the first 24 hours and many terminate within minutes or hours of onset. When AF lasts longer than 7 days, it is designated as *persistent*. AF that persists for a long interval, typically more than a year, without return of an interim period of sinus rhythm (spontaneously or as a result of medical intervention such as cardioversion) is termed long-standing persistent AF. Finally, when a clinical decision is made to no longer try to maintain sinus rhythm, the term *permanent* AF is used.

Mechanisms of Atrial Fibrillation
Because of its chaotic nature, it has been difficult to study AF, and its mechanisms remain incompletely understood. The initiation of spontaneous AF is a consequence of rapid electrical firing from preferential focal sites of origin. The most common site of focal origin is from left atrial muscle sleeves extending along the outer surface of the pulmonary veins. When firing does not originate from a pulmonary vein, it is commonly from the left atrial tissue immediately adjacent to one of the veins or occasionally from one of the other thoracic veins such as the ostium of the superior vena cava or the ostium of the coronary sinus. Atrial rates recorded in and around the pulmonary veins are significantly higher than at other atrial sites, suggesting that activity in the region of the veins is important in perpetuating AF after initiation.

These insights have produced highly effective techniques for the cure of AF. Ablation techniques designed to isolate these trigger sites from the atrium have success rates of 70% to 80% for the cure of paroxysmal AF and somewhat lower rates for the cure of persistent AF. Ablation restricted to the region of the pulmonary veins and adjacent left atrium is curative in most patients with AF, implying that most cases of AF are arrhythmias entirely contained within and maintained by the left atrium and connecting veins. In the same way that typical atrial flutter is the characteristic arrhythmia of the right atrium, AF is the characteristic arrhythmia of the left atrium.

Anticoagulation and Atrial Fibrillation
During AF (and to some extent, atrial flutter), the atria have incomplete and ineffective contractions. Blood stasis occurs and may result in the formation of intracardiac thrombus, which may lead to thromboembolism and stroke. The overall risk of stroke in patients with AF is 5% per year. Certain risk factors may adjust this risk, including age, gender, rheumatic heart disease, prior stroke, left ventricular dysfunction, vascular disease, hypertrophic cardiomyopathy, left atrial enlargement, hypertension, and diabetes.

Scoring systems have been developed to estimate a patient's AF-related stroke risk based on his or her constellation of risk factors. Formerly, the most used system was the $CHADS_2$ score (*c*ardiac failure, *h*ypertension, *a*ge ≥75 years, *d*iabetes mellitus, and prior *s*troke). This system has been well validated in assessing the stroke risk of patients with AF. It assigns a single point for age of 75 years or older, diabetes, history of heart failure, and hypertension. It assigns two points for a history of stroke or transient ischemic attack. A score of 0 correlates with a relatively low risk of stroke at 1.9% per year, a score of 1 has a stroke risk of 2.8% per year, a score of 2 has a risk of 4.0% per year, and a score of 3 or higher has a stroke risk of more than 5.9% per year.

The $CHADS_2$ underwent further refinement to increase the granularity of stroke risk stratification with the creation of the CHA_2DS_2-VASc (*v*ascular disease, *a*ge, and *s*ex) scoring system, currently the primary score for thromboembolic risk stratification. In this system, congestive heart failure, hypertension, diabetes mellitus, vascular disease, age between 65 and 74 years, and female gender are assigned 1 point, and age of 75 years or older and prior stroke are assigned 2 points. A CHA_2DS_2-VASc score of 0 was associated with a 0% stroke rate, a score of 1 with a 0.6% per year risk, a score of 2 with a 1.6% risk, and a score of 3 with a risk of 3.9%. This system may be most useful for identifying truly low-risk patients.

After a patient's individualized stroke risk is determined, it can be balanced against the risk of anticoagulation to determine what would be appropriate for stroke prevention. A useful tool for estimating bleeding risk due to oral anticoagulation is the HAS-BLED (*h*ypertension, *a*bnormal renal/liver function, *s*troke, *b*leeding history or predisposition, *l*abile international normalized ratio, *e*lderly, *d*rugs/alcohol) score. Patients with a HAS-BLED score of 0 had a risk of 0.59 severe bleeds per 100 patient-years, those with a score of 1 had a risk of 1.51, those with a score of 2 had a risk of 3.20, and those with a score of 3 had a risk of 19.51.

In patients with an acceptable bleeding risk, and with a CHA_2DS_2-VASc score of 2 or greater in men or 3 or greater in women, the 2019 AHA guidelines recommend oral anticoagulation to help prevent embolic stroke. Recommended agents include warfarin, dabigatran, rivaroxaban, apixaban or edoxaban. For patients with low CHA_2DS_2-VASc scores, aspirin is no longer recommended. Oral anticoagulants might be reasonable for intermediate CHA_2DS_2-VASc scores (1 in men and 2 for women), but this has less evidence.

Warfarin is the longest-studied antithrombotic used for reducing the rate of AF-related stroke and reduces the risk by 50%. Warfarin can be difficult to administer; the level of blood-thinning effect must be constantly monitored with international normalized ratio (INR) blood testing. An INR less than 2.0 is associated with higher rates of ischemic

当频率≥250次/分时，此类心律失常可归类为非典型心房扑动，当频率<250次/分时，则可归类为房性心动过速，这种分类具有随意性。同典型心房扑动类似，这种心律失常为阵发性或持续性，当表现为2:1传导时，如未能识别出异常P波形态和固定不变的心率，也可被误认为窦性心动过速。治疗和预后类似于典型心房扑动。

心房颤动

概述和分类

心房颤动（房颤）是心房激动持续和变化的混乱性心房节律。其无明显的P波或有一段时间的心房静止。心房颤动的心电图特征为基线摆动伴心室律不规整（图8.6D）。

心房颤动是最常见的有临床意义的心律失常。美国患病人数约为220万。一般人群的患病率为0.4%～1%，并且随年龄增长而增加，80岁以上的人群中患病率达8%。心房颤动患者的卒中、心力衰竭和死亡风险更高。然而，由于经常合并其他严重疾病，心房颤动是否为死亡率增加的独立决定因素仍不明确。孤立性心房颤动患者死亡率并不增加，且精细设计的探索维持窦性心律和心室率控制的试验也显示，在绝大多数人群中，维持窦性心律并没有生存率获益。一个例外是心房颤动合并收缩性心力衰竭患者，心房颤动消融可能有生存率的优势。近期完成的导管消融对比标准传统治疗左心室功能障碍合并心房颤动患者（CASTLE-AF）研究显示对这部分人群，导管消融心房颤动可显著降低死亡率。心房颤动通常根据其临床表现和模式进行分类。当首次检查到心房颤动时，称为新发心房颤动，其最终形式在初期无法确定。当心房颤动在随访期间复发时，其被称为复发性心房颤动，并通过其临床模式分类。如果心房颤动自发终止，则称为阵发性心房颤动。不超过7天的心房颤动均为阵发性心房颤动，大多数阵发性心房颤动发作会在24h内终止，很多在几分钟或几小时内终止。当心房颤动持续超过7天时，定义为持续性心房颤动。持续很长的时间，通常超过1年，且从未暂时恢复窦性心律（自发或医学干预，如心脏复律）的心房颤动称为长程持续性心房颤动，最终，如果做出临床决策，不再试图维持窦性心律，即为永久性心房颤动。

心房颤动的机制

由于心房颤动混乱的特点，使得对其研究一直很困难，心房颤动的机制仍然没有被完全理解。心房颤动是由于优势局灶起源点快速发放电冲动而出现的。局部起源灶大多来自于沿着肺静脉外表面延伸的左心房肌袖。当电活动不是源自肺静脉时，其通常来自紧邻一条肺静脉的左心房组织，或偶尔来自其他心脏静脉，如上腔静脉口或冠状窦口。肺静脉内及周围记录到的心房率显著高于心房其他位置，这表明静脉区域中的激动对于心房颤动初发后的维持十分重要。

这些重要发现衍生出了高效的心房颤动治疗技术。消融技术意在将这些触发部位与心房隔离，对于治愈阵发性心房颤动有着70%～80%的成功率，而对持续性心房颤动治愈率较低。局限于肺静脉及相邻的左心房区域的消融可治疗大多数心房颤动，这意味着大多数心房颤动病灶完全包含于左心房及其连接的静脉内，并由其维持。同理，心房扑动为右心房的特征性心律失常，而心房颤动为左心房特征性心律失常。

抗凝治疗与心房颤动

心房颤动（包括心房扑动）时，心房不完全或无效收缩。产生血流淤滞，可形成心内血栓，导致血栓栓塞和脑卒中。心房颤动患者的脑卒中总体风险为每年5%。以下危险因素会影响风险水平。包括年龄、性别、风湿性心脏病、既往卒中史、左心室功能障碍、肥厚型心肌病、左心房增大、高血压和糖尿病。

评分系统汇总患者危险因素以评估其心房颤动相关卒中风险。过去最常用的评分系统是$CHADS_2$评分（心力衰竭，高血压，年龄≥75岁，糖尿病和既往卒中史）。在评估心房颤动患者的脑卒中风险方面，该系统已得到很好的验证。它将75岁或以上、糖尿病、心力衰竭史和高血压均计为1分，卒中或短暂性脑缺血发作史为2分。0分与相对低的每年1.9%的卒中风险相关，1分的脑卒中风险为每年2.8%，2分的风险为每年4.0%，≥3分的患者每年卒中风险超过5.9%。

对$CHADS_2$评分进一步改进，细化了卒中风险分层，制定了CHA_2DS_2-VASc（血管疾病、年龄和性别）评分系统，是目前进行血栓栓塞风险分层的主要评分。

在该评分系统中，充血性心力衰竭、高血压、糖尿病、血管疾病、65～74岁和女性分别计1分，≥75岁和既往卒中史计2分。CHA_2DS_2-VASc评分为0提示年卒中风险为0%，1分为每年脑卒中风险为0.6%，2分为1.6%，3分为3.9%。该系统对于识别真正低危的患者最为有用。

在确定患者的个体化卒中风险后，可以将其与抗凝的风险进行权衡，以确定恰当的卒中预防治疗。评估口服抗凝出血风险的实用工具是HAS-BLED（高血压、肝肾功能异常、卒中、出血史或出血倾向、国际标准化比值不稳定、老年人、药物/酒精滥用）评分。HAS-BLED评分为0的患者具有每100患者-年中0.59次严重出血风险，1分为1.51，2分为3.20，3分为19.51。

对于出血风险可接受，CHA_2DS_2-VASc评分男性≥2分、女性≥3分的患者，2019年美国心脏协会（AHA）指南推荐口服抗凝药以预防栓塞性卒中。推荐的药物包括华法林、达比加群、利伐沙班、阿哌沙班，对于CHA_2DS_2-VASc评分低的患者，不再推荐阿司匹林。对于CHA_2DS_2-VASc评分中危的患者（男性1分、女性2分），口服抗凝药可能也是合理的，但证据较少。

在降低心房颤动相关卒中发生率的抗栓药物中，华法林的研究时间最长，可将风险降低50%。华法林可能难以管理，必须使用国际标准化比值（INR）来持续监测抗凝效果。INR<2.0发生缺血性卒中的概率较高；INR

stroke; a level greater than 3.0 is associated with increased intracranial bleeding. On average, a therapeutic INR (between 2.0 and 3.0) is maintained in only two thirds of cases, and there are many drug and dietary interactions with warfarin.

Several newer oral anticoagulants (NOACs) have effectiveness and bleeding risk rates similar to warfarin, but they do not require drug level monitoring. They include dabigatran, rivaroxaban, apixaban, and edoxaban. These drugs have been studied in large patient groups and found to be noninferior to warfarin, and some may be superior in certain aspects. NOACs are preferred in eligible patients over warfarin except in cases of moderate-to-severe mitral stenosis or the presence of a mechanical heart valve.

Percutaneous occlusion of the left atrial appendage with the Watchman device has been compared to Coumadin in patients with nonvalvular atrial fibrillation and found generally to offer similar protection against stroke. Oral anticoagulation remains the preferred therapy for stroke prevention in most patients; however, in those who are poor candidates for long-term anticoagulation (because of the propensity for bleeding or poor drug tolerance or adherence), the Watchman device provides an alternative.

The highest risk of stroke related to AF occurs at time of conversion to sinus rhythm achieved spontaneously or by chemical or electrical cardioversion. If thrombus has formed within the left atrium or left atrial appendage, it may not leave the atria during AF due to ineffective atrial mechanics. However, after sinus rhythm is restored, the improved atrial function may eject the thrombus and cause embolic stroke or other systemic embolic sequelae. Even with restoration of electrical atrial systole, the recovery of normal atrial mechanics may be delayed several days to weeks (i.e., atrial stunning). To reduce the risk of pericardioversion stroke, it is important to reduce the risk of preexisting thrombus and to prevent formation in the time period immediately after cardioversion.

The risk of preexisting thrombus can be reduced by 3 weeks of oral anticoagulation or Doppler transesophageal echocardiography (TEE) before cardioversion. These steps are recommended for any patient who has been in AF for an unknown period or has been documented to be in AF more than 48 hours. Although thrombi have been identified in patients with AF for shorter periods, current clinical practice presumes that most thrombus formation requires at least 48 hours. Thrombus related to AF occurs most commonly in the left atrial appendage, which cannot be well visualized by transthoracic echocardiography; TEE is often recommended before cardioversion for optimal imaging of the left atrial appendage. After cardioversion, at least 4 weeks of oral anticoagulation is recommended for everyone, with the exception of low CHA_2DS_2-VASc score patients (0 in men or 1 in women) who had AF less than 48 hours prior to the cardioversion, in whom postconversion anticoagulation may be omitted.

Acute Management of Atrial Fibrillation: Rate Control

The acute management of AF centers on the control of the ventricular response, timely restoration of sinus rhythm, and identification of potentially reversible factors that might have precipitated the arrhythmia. AF with rapid ventricular response results in acute deterioration in stroke volume and cardiac output and an increase in myocardial oxygen demand with the potential for coronary ischemia. Patients who are symptomatic must be controlled promptly. When pursuing rate control for acute AF of recent onset, the fastest way to achieve rate control is the restoration of sinus rhythm. If rate control in ongoing rapidly conducted AF proves difficult or is not well tolerated, cardioversion should be undertaken early.

For the acute control of rapidly conducted AF, intravenous administration of a β-blocker (i.e., esmolol, metoprolol, or propranolol) or a nondihydropyridine calcium-channel blocker (i.e., diltiazem or verapamil) is preferred. In the setting of decompensated heart failure, the use of a calcium-channel blocker may exacerbate heart failure and should be avoided. In this setting, digoxin is a useful agent for resting rate control. Digoxin is also a useful second-line drug in addition to a calcium-channel or β-blocker for resting rate control. If this therapy is ineffective or not tolerated, intravenous amiodarone is a useful rate control agent, especially in the setting of congestive heart failure, and it may facilitate restoration of sinus rhythm.

Long-term targets for rate control of permanent AF have been a matter of debate. The Rate Control Efficacy in Permanent Atrial Fibrillation II (RACE II) study showed no advantage to strict rate control. Targeting a resting rate of less than 80 beats per minute showed no advantage over a target of less than 110 and was much harder to achieve. For long-term management, the results suggest that achieving a resting heart rate of less than 110 beats per minute may be sufficient and safe.

Acute Management of Atrial Fibrillation: Restoration of Sinus Rhythm

When sinus rhythm is restored in the first 48 hours of acute AF, the thromboembolic risk is low, and anticoagulation is not required. New-onset AF should be managed with a plan to restore sinus rhythm during this period if possible. At least one half of new-onset AF episodes terminate spontaneously in the first 24 to 48 hours.

Pharmacologic conversion of atrial fibrillation. Pharmacologic conversion of AF can be undertaken when restoration of sinus rhythm is not urgent. Several antiarrhythmic drugs have been effective in increasing the rate of early conversion of AF. Pharmacologic conversion usually is more successful with AF of recent onset than with chronic AF.

Oral agents with efficacy in the early conversion of AF include flecainide, propafenone, and dofetilide. Oral amiodarone and sotalol have been associated with a 27% and 24% conversion rate, respectively, occurring after 28 days of therapy. However, due to low early conversion rates, these oral drugs are not recommended for conversion. Intravenous agents with efficacy for early conversion include ibutilide and amiodarone. Ibutilide is limited by a relatively high 4% rate of drug-induced QT prolongation and TdP VT. This risk is even higher in the setting of LV dysfunction, electrolyte disturbances, or heart failure. Ibutilide should be reserved for the pharmacologic conversion of stable patients with a baseline normal QT interval. In contrast, intravenous amiodarone is well tolerated by unstable patients and is the preferred pharmacologic agent for conversion in the critically ill.

Electrical cardioversion of atrial fibrillation. Electrical cardioversion should be performed urgently in the case of severe compromise related to acute AF, including angina, heart failure, hypotension, and shock. Cardioversion should also be attempted at least once electively in most cases of new-onset AF regardless of tolerance. When performing electrical cardioversion, an anterior-posterior patch or paddle position is more effective than the conventional anterior-to-lateral patch or paddle position used for ventricular defibrillation. Although low-output discharges may be effective in some patients, a strategy of starting at higher outputs decreases the number of shocks required and the average cumulative energy delivered. An initial shock energy of 200 J is recommended. After a failed initial shock, full output should be used for the next attempt.

Long-Term Maintenance of Sinus Rhythm

Antiarrhythmic therapy. Despite the association of AF with an increase in stroke-related and all-cause mortality, no study has established a benefit for pharmacologic maintenance of sinus rhythm in terms of stroke risk or survival. This may be because AF is

＞ 3.0 与颅内出血增加有关。平均而言，仅有 2/3 的病例能够维持治疗性 INR（2.0 ～ 3.0），华法林与许多药物和食物存在相互作用。

一些新型口服抗凝药（NOAC）的有效性和出血风险与华法林类似，但无需监测药物水平；包括达比加群、利伐沙班、阿哌沙班和艾多沙班，在大型患者群体中的研究发现这些药物不劣于华法林，并在某些方面可能优于华法林。除了合并中到重度二尖瓣狭窄和有机械瓣的病例之外，对于符合条件的患者，NOAC 相较于华法林应作为首选。

对于非瓣膜性心房颤动，使用 Watchman 封堵器行经皮左心耳封堵术和香豆素类药物（华法林）相比总体上具有相似的预防卒中效果。口服抗凝药仍然是绝大多数患者首选的卒中预防治疗；然而，在不适合长期抗凝的患者中（由于出血倾向、药物不耐受或依从性差），Watchman 封堵器提供了替代方案。

心房颤动在自发、通过药物或电复律转复为窦性心律时发生卒中的风险最高。如果在心房颤动期间，左心房或左心耳已形成血栓，心房颤动时心房没有有效机械运动，血栓可能不会从心房脱落。而在恢复窦性心律后，心房功能改善可导致血栓脱落，引起栓塞性卒中或其他体循环栓塞并发症。即使心房电活动恢复，心房正常机械收缩也可能要延迟几天到几周才能恢复正常（如心房顿抑）。降低转复期间的卒中风险，重点在于减小已经形成血栓的风险，且在心律转复后应立即预防血栓形成。

口服抗凝药 3 周或转复前进行经食管超声心动图（TEE）检查，可以减小已形成血栓的风险。所有心房颤动持续时间不明或记录到心房颤动超过 48 h 的患者，均推荐以上流程。尽管已证实有的心房颤动患者在更短时间内出现血栓，但目前的临床实践仍假定大多数血栓需要至少 48 h 才能形成。与心房颤动相关的血栓最常发生于左心耳中，经胸超声心动图（TTE）不能良好显示；通常建议心脏复律前行 TEE 获取左心耳的最佳成像。心脏复律后，除了 CHA_2DS_2-VASc 评分低（男性 0 分，女性 1 分）且复律前心房颤动持续不到 48h 的患者可能无需抗凝外，其他所有患者推荐至少口服 4 周的抗凝药物。

心房颤动的急性期治疗：心室率控制

心房颤动的急性期治疗核心是心室率控制、及时恢复窦性心律和识别可能导致心律失常的潜在可逆因素。心房颤动伴快速心室率导致每搏输出量、心输出量的急性下降和心肌氧耗量增加，并可能诱发冠状动脉缺血，因此必须迅速治疗有症状的患者。对新发的急性心房颤动进行心室率控制时，最快方法是恢复窦性心律。对于持续快速下传心室的心房颤动，如果心率控制被证实很困难或无法耐受，应尽早进行心脏复律。

心房颤动伴快速心室率的急性期治疗，首选静脉内使用 β 受体阻滞剂（如艾司洛尔、美托洛尔或普萘洛尔）或非二氢吡啶类钙通道阻滞剂（如地尔硫草或维拉帕米）。在存在失代偿性心力衰竭的情况下，使用钙通道阻滞剂可能加重心力衰竭，应予避免。在这种情况下，地高辛可有效控制静息心率。除钙通道阻滞剂或 β 受体阻滞剂可用于控制静息心率外，地高辛是一种有效的二线药物。如果这种治疗无效或不能耐受，静脉内给予胺碘酮也可用于心室率控制，特别是在充血性心力衰竭的情况下，而且胺碘酮可促进恢复窦性心律。

永久性心房颤动的长期心率控制目标已经成为一个有争议的话题。永久性心房颤动的心率控制有效性（RACE Ⅱ）研究显示严格控制心室率并没有获益。静息心率＜ 80 次 / 分与＜ 110 次 / 分相比，并无优势且更难实现。长期治疗的结果表明，静息心率小于每分钟 110 次可能已足够且安全。

心房颤动的急性期治疗：恢复窦性心律

在急性心房颤动 48 h 内恢复窦性心律，血栓栓塞风险低且不需要抗凝。如果可能的话，新发心房颤动的治疗计划应为在这一期间恢复窦性心律。至少一半的新发心房颤动在最初 24 ～ 48 h 内自行终止。

心房颤动的药物复律 当不急于恢复窦性心律时，可进行药物复律。数种抗心律失常药物能有效地提高心房颤动的早期转复率。相比慢性心房颤动，近期新发的心房颤动药物转复通常更容易成功。

心房颤动早期复律的有效口服药物包括氟卡尼、普罗帕酮和多非利特。口服胺碘酮或索他洛尔 28 天后，分别有 27% 和 24% 的心房颤动转复为窦性心律。然而，由于早期转复率低，不推荐应用这些口服药物转复。可早期复律的静脉制剂包括伊布利特和胺碘酮。伊布利特有相对较高的概率（4%）发生药物诱导的 QT 间期延长和尖端扭转型室性心动过速，故使用受限。这种风险在左心室功能障碍、电解质紊乱和心力衰竭的状态下发生率更高。伊布利特仅用于基础 QT 间期正常的稳定患者的药物复律。不稳定的患者对静脉内给予胺碘酮耐受良好，使其成为危重疾病时首选的转复用药。

心房颤动的电复律 急性心房颤动在出现包括心绞痛、心力衰竭、低血压和休克等相关严重并发症的情况下，应紧急进行电复律。大多数新发心房颤动，也应该有选择地尝试至少一次心脏复律，而不考虑耐受性如何。当进行电复律时，前-后放置电极片/电极板比传统用于心室颤动的前-侧位置更有效。虽然较低输出能量对一些患者可能有效，但是从更高能量输出开始可减少电击次数，降低了平均累积能量。建议初始电击能量为双相 200 J。在初次放电失败后，应选择最高能量进行下一次尝试。

长期维持窦性心律

抗心律失常治疗 尽管心房颤动与卒中相关死亡和全因死亡率增加相关，但是没有研究证实药物维持窦性心律可降低脑卒中风险或改善生存率。这可能是因为心

merely a marker and not a mechanism of mortality. It may also be a consequence of the relative inefficacy of pharmacologic therapy in the maintenance of sinus rhythm and the difficulty of establishing whether patients thought to be in sinus rhythm are consistently in sinus rhythm at follow-up.

The largest and best designed trial addressing this issue was the Atrial Fibrillation Follow-up Investigation of Rhythm Management (AFFIRM) trial. The study included 4060 patients randomly assigned to rhythm control with antiarrhythmic drugs, most commonly amiodarone, or to rate control without attempts to maintain sinus rhythm. AFFIRM demonstrated no advantage in stroke or mortality rates using a strategy of sinus rhythm maintenance compared with rate control. Either strategy can be offered to patients with an expectation of similar outcomes with regard to hard end points. The decision to pursue sinus rhythm usually is determined by the management of symptoms that may be better addressed by maintaining sinus rhythm in selected patients.

In the absence of antiarrhythmic drugs, more than 80% of patients relapse during the first year after cardioversion of AF. Antiarrhythmic drugs remain the primary strategy for maintaining sinus rhythm after cardioversion and for preventing symptomatic episodes in patients with paroxysmal AF. However, antiarrhythmic therapy has many limitations, and alternative ablative therapies may over time overtake antiarrhythmic therapy in the management of AF.

All antiarrhythmic drugs have the potential for proarrhythmia, the unintended precipitation of a new arrhythmic problem caused by the drug. Adverse rhythm effects of drugs may include sinus node dysfunction, heart block, promotion of drug-slowed atrial flutter permitting rapid 1:1 conduction, and promotion of potentially lethal ventricular arrhythmias. Class I drugs such as flecainide, propafenone, and disopyramide may result in significant direct myocardial depression and consequent exacerbation of heart failure. The array of potential adverse effects of antiarrhythmic drugs is beyond the scope of this chapter, but certain essential concepts are important to recognize.

Class I drugs such as flecainide and propafenone, which work by slowing conduction, have a high risk of ventricular proarrhythmia and potential for sudden death in the setting of heart failure, LV dysfunction, and coronary artery disease. Use of these drugs is restricted to patients with preserved cardiac function and no evidence of obstructive coronary artery disease. However, in this selected group of patients with normal hearts, these drugs are exceedingly safe, well tolerated, and often effective.

Class III drugs, which prolong repolarization and refractoriness, include sotalol, dofetilide, dronedarone, and amiodarone. They are safe for patients with coronary artery disease, and in the case of dofetilide and amiodarone, they are safe for those with congestive heart failure. However, sotalol and dofetilide may provoke TdP, even in patients with normal cardiac function, and they must be used with caution. Amiodarone has greater long-term efficacy than other drugs and a lower risk of proarrhythmia, but long-term somatic toxicity consisting of thyroid dysfunction, pulmonary, and occasional hepatotoxicity limits the use of this drug in older patients or those with limited expected longevity or an inability to safely tolerate alternative agents due to advanced cardiac disease or proarrhythmia. Amiodarone is highly effective for the short-term, acute management of arrhythmias in critically ill patients when the potential risk of long-term toxicity is not an issue.

Dronedarone was derived by modification of the amiodarone molecule. Like amiodarone, the drug has a low risk of proarrhythmia and TdP VT. Unlike amiodarone, the drug does not cause thyroid toxicity. In common use, hepatotoxicity is also uncommon with dronedarone. However, rare cases of hepatic failure have been associated

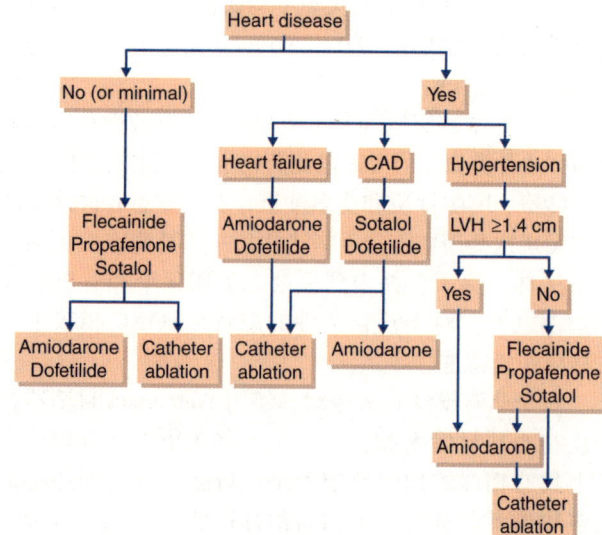

Fig. 8.7 A strategy for the selection of therapy to maintain sinus rhythm in patients with recurrent atrial fibrillation. Patients are stratified by the presence or absence of structural heart disease, and drugs expected to have the greatest efficacy and lowest therapeutic risk in each group are selected. Catheter ablation becomes a therapeutic option after failure of at least one antiarrhythmic drug. The class IC drugs flecainide and propafenone are not advised for patients with heart failure or coronary artery disease (CAD). Amiodarone is an acceptable first-line drug for those with heart failure and severe left ventricular hypertrophy. Because of its potential for somatic toxicity, amiodarone is otherwise reserved as a second-line agent that is used as an alternative to catheter ablation.

with dronedarone use. Dronedarone has increased mortality rates for patients with recently decompensated heart failure and when used as a simple rate control agent in patients with permanent AF. It is contraindicated in these settings.

In addition to being useful agents for the prevention of AF, sotalol, dronedarone, and amiodarone provide substantial rate control during relapses of AF. However, rate control with other antiarrhythmic agents may not be adequate to prevent rapid conduction with relapse, and class I drugs such as flecainide may accelerate response at the time of relapse. Antiarrhythmic drugs other than sotalol, dronedarone, or amiodarone should therefore be combined with a rate control agent such as a β-blocker or nondihydropyridine calcium-channel blocker during long-term therapy. Fig. 8.7 is a proposed strategy for antiarrhythmic drug selection for the long-term maintenance of sinus rhythm in patients with AF.

Surgical ablation of atrial fibrillation. The surgical treatment of AF was pioneered by Cox with the development of the atrial maze procedure. The procedure was predicated on the concept that AF was maintained by multiple interacting wave fronts of activity. By surgically dividing the atria into narrow channels, most with connection back to the sinus node, it was thought that AF could be abolished while preserving physiologic activation and contraction of the atrium. The circuitous path left for atrial activation and the multiple barriers created in the atrium intended to prevent AF gave rise to the term *maze procedure* to describe the technique. The initial procedure was thought to be highly successful but was associated with significant surgical risks and problems with sinus node dysfunction. Because of the surgical complexity of making and then closing multiple incisions in the atria and the complications associated with the procedure, the initial cut-and-sew maze procedure has fallen out of clinical use.

房颤动仅仅是一种标志事件而不是死亡机制；也可能是药物治疗维持窦性心律相对困难，并且难以确定在随访期间被认为是窦性心律的患者是否一直维持窦性心律。

心房颤动节律管理的随访研究（AFFIRM）试验是针对这个问题最大、设计最好的试验。该研究将 4060 例患者随机分为用抗心律失常药物（最常用的是胺碘酮）的节律控制组和心室率控制而不试图维持窦性心律组。AFFIRM 结果显示：相较于心室率控制，维持窦性心律未显示出脑卒中或死亡率的优势。因二者硬终点结果相似，予患者任一种治疗策略均有类似的预后。在经过选择的患者，维持窦性心律获得了更好的症状控制，故通常决定维持窦性心律。

在未应用抗心律失常药物的情况下，超过 80% 的患者在心房颤动复律后的第 1 年内复发。抗心律失常药物仍然是心脏复律后维持窦性心律和预防阵发性心房颤动患者症状性发作的主要治疗策略。但药物抗心律失常治疗有许多局限性，备选的消融治疗可能随着时间的推移取代心房颤动的抗心律失常药物治疗。

所有抗心律失常药物都有潜在的致心律失常作用，即药物所致的意外的心律失常问题。药物的致心律失常作用包括窦房结功能障碍、心脏传导阻滞、药物减慢心房扑动周长引发快速 1:1 房室传导和诱发潜在的致死性室性心律失常。Ⅰ类药物如氟卡尼、普罗帕酮和丙吡胺可产生显著的直接心肌抑制作用并导致心力衰竭加重。抗心律失常药物的一系列潜在不良反应内容超出了本章的范围，但对某些基本概念的认识十分重要。

通过减慢传导而作用的Ⅰ类药物如氟卡尼和普罗帕酮具有致室性心律失常作用和加重心力衰竭以及左心室功能障碍和冠状动脉疾病情况下发生猝死的可能性。这些药物仅限于心功能正常且没有阻塞性冠状动脉疾病证据的患者使用。在心功能正常患者组中，这些药物非常安全，耐受性良好，并且通常有效。

延长复极时间和不应期的Ⅲ类药物包括索他洛尔、多非利特、决奈达隆和胺碘酮，对冠状动脉疾病患者是安全的，而多非利特和胺碘酮对于充血性心力衰竭的患者也是安全的。但索他洛尔和多非利特可引起尖端扭转型室性心动过速，甚至在心功能正常的患者中也可发生，所以必须谨慎使用。胺碘酮具有比其他药物更好的长期疗效和较低的致心律失常风险，但长期的全身毒性，包括甲状腺功能障碍、肺和少见的肝毒性，使得该药物仅用于老年、预期寿命有限、由于严重心脏病不能应用其他药物或因其他药物的致心律失常作用而不能耐受的患者。对于危重患者的短期、急性心律失常治疗，长期毒性的潜在风险并不是问题，胺碘酮是非常有效的。

决奈达隆是胺碘酮分子修饰后的衍生药。与胺碘酮类似，该药致心律失常和致尖端扭转型室性心动过速的风险较低。与胺碘酮不同，该药无甲状腺毒性；常

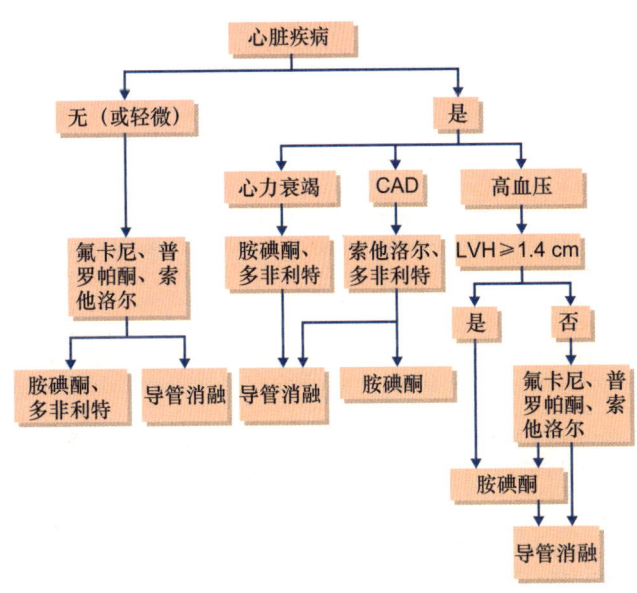

图 8.7　对于复发性心房颤动患者，维持窦性心律的治疗策略。根据患者是否存在结构性心脏病而进行分层，并在每组中选择最大预期效果和最低治疗风险的药物。在至少一种抗心律失常药物治疗无效后，可选择导管消融。IC 类药物氟卡尼和普罗帕酮不建议用于心力衰竭或冠状动脉疾病（CAD）患者。对于心力衰竭和严重左心室肥厚患者，胺碘酮是一种可接受的一线药物。胺碘酮具有潜在的全身毒性，可成为替代导管消融的二线用药。LVH，左心室厚度

规使用时肝毒性也不常见。但决奈达隆与罕见的肝衰竭有关。决奈达隆增加近期失代偿性心力衰竭患者死亡率，使用决奈达隆控制永久性心房颤动患者心室率会增加其死亡率，故在这些情况下禁用。

除了可预防心房颤动，索他洛尔、决奈达隆和胺碘酮在心房颤动复发期间可控制心室率。而其他抗心律失常药物不能充分地控制快速心室率，并且Ⅰ类抗心律失常药物如氟卡尼可提高复发时的心室率。长期治疗时，除了索他洛尔、决奈达隆和胺碘酮之外的抗心律失常药物应与控制心室率药物如 β 受体阻滞剂或非二氢吡啶类钙通道阻滞剂联用。图 8.7 是心房颤动患者长期维持窦性心律的最佳方案。

心房颤动的外科消融治疗　Cox 的心房迷宫手术是心房颤动外科治疗先驱。心房颤动由心房内多个相互作用的波面活动维持，是该操作的理论基础。通过手术将心房分割成狭窄通道，其大多与窦房结连接，进而消除心房颤动，同时维持心房的生理激动和收缩功能。在心房留下迂曲的激动途径并在心房中形成旨在预防心房颤动的多个屏障，故使用迷宫手术来描述该技术。此操作最初被认为非常成功，但伴随较高的手术风险及窦房结功能障碍问题。因在心房中制造并封闭多个切口的手术操作复杂，以及手术相关的并发症发生率较高，临床已不再使用原始的切割-缝合迷宫手术。

Although the original maze procedure is no longer used, many techniques have been developed to simplify the operation by substituting linear thermal ablation (by heating or cooling tissue) to create lines of conduction block in the atria without the need for extensive atrial dissection and reconstruction. Surgical ablation is commonly applied in patients with a history of AF who are undergoing concomitant heart operations for other indications such as valvular or coronary disease. Less frequently, surgical ablation has been applied as a standalone procedure for the sole management of AF. In that setting, various minimally invasive techniques have been developed. However, the techniques used vary widely from one center to another and long-term reporting of outcomes is inconsistent. In a large series that included 282 patients undergoing an open bi-atrial ablation procedure, 78% were in sinus rhythm without antiarrhythmic therapy at the 1-year follow-up evaluation.

Another important potential benefit of surgical ablation for AF is that it provides an opportunity to eliminate the left atrial appendage as a potential site of thrombus formation and source of thromboembolism. This can be accomplished by complete amputation of the appendage with oversewing of the appendage or clamping off the opening to the appendage with special devices designed for this purpose. This may be especially important in patients with absolute or relative contraindications to anticoagulation.

Catheter ablation of atrial fibrillation. Catheter ablation has become a common procedure for the management of AF after failure of initial attempts at medical therapy. Initial attempts to cure AF using catheter techniques were based on attempts in the early 1990s to emulate the linear lesion set of the Cox maze procedure with multiple endocardial lesions. High complication rates and limited efficacy led to abandonment of this approach.

In 1998, Haissaguerre reported the important role of rapid activity originating in the musculature of the pulmonary veins in initiation of paroxysmal AF. This led to the development of procedures designed to target the pulmonary veins and eventuated in the technique of electrical pulmonary vein isolation (PVI), which is currently the primary ablative approach to treatment of paroxysmal AF by catheter techniques. This technique has had acceptably high success rates (≈70%) at multiple centers for the treatment of paroxysmal AF without antiarrhythmic therapy.

Despite the high success rate of catheter PVI ablation for the treatment of paroxysmal AF, this technique has not proved reliably effective in the management of more persistent forms of AF, especially long-standing persistent AF. This likely reflects the importance of factors other than pulmonary vein activity in the initiation and maintenance of persistent AF that are not addressed by PVI ablation. Multiple ablative techniques are currently used in an attempt to increase the success rates for patients with persistent AF. They have included addition of linear lesions to block reentrant wave fronts, ablation of regions of unusually rapid atrial activity during ongoing AF, and interruption of stable rotors of atrial activity identified during multisite mapping of AF. Although these techniques have improved success rates in limited series, it is uncertain which, if any, of these methods represents the optimal approach to the ablation of long-standing persistent AF.

In summary, catheter ablation is the preferred secondary strategy for treatment of symptomatic AF after initial attempts at medical therapy have failed. Simple pulmonary vein isolation has a high success rate for the management of patients with paroxysmal AF. Success rates for all ablative techniques are lower for persistent AF, especially for long-term AF. As in the case of surgical ablation, multiple techniques are used at various centers, and the different strategies for follow-up and definitions of response have made it difficult to ascertain the relative efficacy of the various approaches in common use.

Catheter ablation of the atrioventricular node. Although less commonly used today than in the past, the older technique of catheter ablation of the AV node resulting in complete heart block followed by placement of a ventricular pacemaker to maintain physiologic heart rates remains an option for patients when rate control cannot be achieved medically. This technique continues to have an important role in the management of patients who are too infirm to safely undergo AF ablation or in patients for whom ablative techniques have failed to control the arrhythmia.

For a deeper discussion on this topic, please see Chapter 58, ❖ "Supraventricular Cardiac Arrhythmias," in *Goldman-Cecil Medicine*, 26th Edition.

SYNCOPE

Syncope is a sudden loss of consciousness that is transient. Syncope has cardiac causes (e.g., low cerebral blood pressure) and noncardiac causes. Common causes and categories of syncope are outlined in Table 8.4. Cerebrovascular disease or stroke uncommonly manifests as syncope unless a large cerebral territory is involved. Syncope is a common reason for emergency room or hospital admission.

The diagnostic approach to a patient with syncope is given in Fig. 8.8. Most causes can be identified by the medical history and physical examination alone. Conditions surrounding the syncopal episode often suggest a cause. For example, vasovagal episodes often occur during stress, pain, straining, coughing, or urination. Exercise-induced syncope may indicate obstructive coronary disease, channelopathies such as long QT or CPVT, obstructive cardiomyopathy, aortic stenosis, or arrhythmia. A history of palpitations or syncope with no warning may be related to cardiac arrhythmias. Very long episodes of syncope (>5 minutes) suggest noncardiac causes. A recent change in medications or dizziness with position changes suggests orthostatic hypotension. Witnessed limb movements or posturing is not specific for neurologic causes and can result from any type of cerebral hypoperfusion, even from cardiac causes.

Beyond the history, physical examination, and routine ECG, further testing has little diagnostic utility. Holter or loop recorders may be useful. Implantable loop recorders may have utility in cases of recurrent, infrequent syncope. Electrophysiologic testing may be useful in some patients with other abnormalities suggesting an arrhythmic cause.

Despite thorough evaluations, more than 30% of patients with syncope have no identifiable cause. Cardiac causes of syncope have the highest morbidity and mortality rates. Because patients with unknown causes of syncope have long-term outcomes similar to those with noncardiac syncope, the major goal of an evaluation is to identify cardiac causes of syncope.

VENTRICULAR ARRHYTHMIAS AND SUDDEN CARDIAC DEATH

Ventricular ectopy is defined as cardiac beats that originate from within the right or left ventricular muscle or conduction system. Premature ventricular contractions (PVCs) can occur singly or as ventricular couplets or triplets. VT is four or more consecutive beats that originate from the ventricle at a rate of at least 100 beats per minute. VT is classified as *sustained* if it lasts longer than 30 seconds or requires termination due to hemodynamic instability; otherwise, it is classified as *nonsustained* VT (NSVT).

Ventricular ectopy also may be classified based on maintenance of a similar electrocardiographic morphology. The beats of monomorphic VT (MMVT) appear to be identical and usually originate from

虽然原始迷宫手术已不再使用,但已有许多如替代性线性热消融(通过在心房中加热或冷却组织)从而产生心房内传导阻滞线等简化技术出现,不需要大量的切开和重建心房。手术消融通常用于有心房颤动病史,同时因其他适应证如瓣膜或冠状动脉疾病而接受心脏外科手术的患者。较少情况下,会单独就治疗心房颤动进行外科消融。在这种情况下,各种微创技术被开发出来。然而,不同中心所使用的技术差异很大,长期报告的结果不一致。在包括282例开放性双心房消融术的大型研究中,在没有抗心律失常治疗情况下,78%的患者在1年随访时仍维持窦性心律。

心房颤动的外科消融的另一个重要获益是提供了机会,以消除左心耳作为血栓形成的潜在位点和血栓栓塞来源的可能。这可以通过缝合完全阻断左心耳或使用特殊设计的装置封堵左心耳开口来完成。这对于抗凝存在绝对或相对禁忌证的患者尤为重要。

心房颤动的导管消融 导管消融已成为在心房颤动初始药物治疗失败后常见的操作。早期使用导管技术治愈心房颤动的尝试是模拟Cox在20世纪90年代早期开创的、造成一组线性损伤的迷宫手术,进行多处心内膜损伤。较高并发症发生率和有限的疗效使得这种术式已被废弃。

1998年,Haissaguerre报道了阵发性心房颤动起源于肺静脉肌肉组织中的快速电活动。促进了以肺静脉为治疗靶点的操作发展,最终促成了肺静脉电隔离(PVI)技术的产生,这也是目前导管治疗阵发性心房颤动的主要消融术式。在多个医学中心,这种技术对未予抗心律失常治疗的阵发性心房颤动有着较高的成功率(约70%)。

尽管导管PVI消融治疗阵发性心房颤动有着较高的成功率,这种技术还未证实对于持续时间更长的心房颤动疗效可靠,特别是长程持续性心房颤动。这可能提示持续性心房颤动的产生和维持中,肺静脉电活动以外因素的重要性,而PVI消融并未解决。目前有多种消融技术试图提高持续性心房颤动患者的消融成功率。包括添加线性消融阻滞折返波面,在心房颤动期间消融异常快速的心房活动区域,以及在行心房颤动多点标测时识别并阻断心房活动的稳定转子。尽管在某些研究中证实这些技术提高了成功率,但是仍不确定这些方法中的哪种(如果有的话)是长程持续性心房颤动消融治疗的最佳方法。

总之,在最初的药物治疗失败后,导管消融是治疗症状性心房颤动首选的次级治疗策略。单纯肺静脉隔离对于阵发性心房颤动患者有很高的治疗成功率。持续性心房颤动的所有消融技术成功率均较低,特别是长程持续性心房颤动。类似于手术消融,各个医学中心使用的心房颤动消融技术不尽相同,并且随访策略和有效治疗的定义不同使得难以确定常用的不同术式效果。

导管消融房室结 虽然和过去相比,导管消融房室结已不太常用,但在当患者无法应用药物控制心室率时,这种陈旧的、产生完全性心脏阻滞之后放置心室起搏器以维持生理性心率的房室结导管消融技术,仍是一种选择。这种技术对于治疗过于虚弱且不能安全地进行心房颤动消融的患者或消融术未能控制心律失常的患者仍然有着重要作用。

有关此专题的深入讨论,请参阅 *Goldman-Cecil Medicine* 第26版第58章"室上性心律失常"。 ❖

晕厥

晕厥是短暂的突发意识丧失。晕厥有心脏性原因(如低脑血压)和非心脏性原因。表8.4列出了晕厥的常见原因和分类。脑血管疾病或卒中通常不表现为晕厥,除非涉及脑区域较大。晕厥是急诊或住院的常见原因。

对晕厥的患者的诊断方法如图8.8所示。大多数病因通过问询病史和体格检查即可确定。晕厥发作前后的情况常常对病因有所提示。例如血管迷走性发作通常在应激、疼痛、紧张、咳嗽或排尿期间发生。运动诱发的晕厥可能提示阻塞性冠状动脉疾病、离子通道病变如长QT综合征或儿茶酚胺敏感性多形性室性心动过速、梗阻性心肌病、主动脉瓣狭窄或心律失常。没有先兆症状的心悸或晕厥可能与心律失常有关。非常长的晕厥发作(>5 min)提示非心脏性原因。近期更换药物或与体位变化相关的头晕提示直立性低血压。目击到的肢体运动或姿势不是神经系统病因所特有的,可以由任何原因甚至由心脏性原因所致的脑灌注不足引起。

除了病史、体格检查和常规心电图,进一步检查没有太大诊断意义。Holter或循环记录器可能有用。植入式循环记录器对偶发的复发性晕厥有用。如果患者存在一些其他提示心律失常病因的异常,电生理检查可能有用。

尽管进行了彻底的评估,仍有超过30%的晕厥患者没有明确原因。心脏性晕厥有着最高的致病性和死亡率。不明原因的晕厥患者与非心脏性晕厥患者长期预后相似,故评估的主要目的是鉴别晕厥的心脏性原因。

室性心律失常和心源性猝死

室性异位搏动是指源自右心室或左心室心肌或传导系统的心脏搏动。室性期前收缩(PVC)可以单独出现或呈现成对或连续3个出现。室性心动过速(室速,VT)是心室产生的≥4次连续搏动且频率≥100次/分。如持续时间超过30 s或因血流动力学不稳定而需终止,则归类为持续性室速,否则分类为非持续性室速(NSVT)。

此外,还可以基于是否维持单一的心电图形态对室性异位搏动进行分类。单形性室速(MMVT)每

TABLE 8.4 Causes of Syncope

Cause	Features
Peripheral Vascular or Circulatory	
Vasovagal syncope (neurally mediated)	Prodrome of pallor, yawning, nausea, diaphoresis; precipitated by stress or pain; occurs when patient is upright, aborted by recumbency; fall in blood pressure with or without a decrease in heart rate
Micturition syncope	Syncope with urination (probably vagal)
Post-tussive syncope	Syncope after paroxysm of coughing
Hypersensitive carotid sinus syndrome	Vasodepressor and/or cardioinhibitory responses with light carotid sinus massage
Drugs	Orthostasis; occurs with antihypertensive drugs, tricyclic antidepressants, phenothiazines
Volume depletion	Orthostasis; occurs with hemorrhage, excessive vomiting or diarrhea, Addison's disease
Autonomic dysfunction	Orthostasis; occurs in diabetes, alcoholism, Parkinson's disease, deconditioning after a prolonged illness
Central Nervous System	
Cerebrovascular	Transient ischemic attacks and strokes are unusual causes of syncope; associated neurologic abnormalities are usually identified
Seizures	Warning aura sometimes present, jerking of extremities, tongue biting, urinary incontinence, postictal confusion
Metabolic	
Hypoglycemia	Confusion, tachycardia, jitteriness before syncope; patient may be taking insulin
Cardiac	
Obstructive	Syncope is often exertional; physical findings consistent with aortic stenosis, hypertrophic obstructive cardiomyopathy, cardiac tamponade, atrial myxoma, prosthetic valve malfunction, Eisenmenger's syndrome, tetralogy of Fallot, primary pulmonary hypertension, pulmonic stenosis, massive pulmonary embolism
Arrhythmias	Syncope may be sudden and occurs in any position; episodes of dizziness or palpitations; may be history of heart disease; bradyarrhythmias or tachyarrhythmias may be responsible—check for hypersensitive carotid sinus

the same area of the heart. *Ventricular flutter* is a term that may be used to describe MMVT with rates of more than 300 beats per minute. Polymorphic VT (PMVT) has a more variable appearance on the ECG than MMVT. TdP is a special form of PMVT that has a repetitive, undulating periodicity and usually implies a long-QT triggered mechanism. VF is the most chaotic form of ventricular ectopy. It is associated with no meaningful cardiac output and usually leads to death unless rapidly treated. The other forms of VT may eventually degrade into VF.

Determining whether a patient has a rhythm of ventricular origin usually is done by 12-lead surface ECG. Ventricular ectopy typically has a wide QRS morphology (Fig. 8.9). Not all wide QRS morphologies are ventricular in origin, and there are criteria for determining whether a wide-complex tachycardia is supraventricular or ventricular. SVT may appear as a wide-complex tachycardia if it conducts to the ventricle with aberrancy (e.g., bundle branch block) or through an accessory pathway (e.g., WPW syndrome). Features that may help distinguish between SVT and VT include AV dissociation with capture beats and fusion beats and the QRS morphology and duration (Table 8.5). The Brugada algorithm is commonly used for determining the site of origin of wide-complex tachycardia. The tachycardia has a ventricular origin in more than 90% of patients with a history of ischemic heart disease.

VT may occur by the same mechanisms as other tachycardias, such as reentry, enhanced automaticity, or triggered activity. VT often occurs as a reentrant tachycardia around an area of prior MI scar in the left ventricle. VT in the chronic phase of ischemic heart disease is mediated by reentry through channels or sheets of surviving myocardium, especially in the partially spared border zone of a region of scar resulting from a prior MI. In these channels, conduction is abnormally slow due to poor coupling between sparse surviving myocytes. Susceptibility to sustained VT increases with worsening left ventricular dysfunction, likely due to the greater extent of ventricular scar.

VT can occur in the absence of ischemic heart disease in the form of idiopathic VT, nonischemic cardiomyopathies, hypertrophic cardiomyopathies, arrhythmogenic RV dysplasia, bundle branch reentry, cardiac ion channel disorders, or electrolyte disturbances. The right ventricular outflow tract (RVOT) is the most common origin of idiopathic VT, which is likely caused by triggered activity. This form of VT (or PVCs) is usually sensitive to catecholamines and may terminate with adenosine (i.e., adenosine-sensitive VT). Another common form of idiopathic VT originates from the left ventricular conduction system (i.e., fascicular VT) and may be verapamil sensitive. Idiopathic VTs are common targets for successful catheter ablation.

Nonsustained VT usually does not require specific therapy unless the patient is symptomatic. The Cardiac Arrhythmia Suppression Trial treated PVCs and NSVT after the acute phase of MI with class I antiarrhythmic drugs, and the trial demonstrated increased mortality rates when the arrhythmias were treated. If VT is attributed to reversible causes such as electrolyte disturbances or acute ischemia, the underlying mechanism should be treated. VT not due to reversible causes may be treated with β-blockers, antiarrhythmic drug therapy (e.g., amiodarone), or catheter ablation. If urgent treatment is required due to hemodynamic instability, direct current cardioversion is performed. It should be synchronized to the QRS complex if a regular morphology exists; otherwise, it should be nonsynchronized. Performing direct current cardioversion during the refractory period (T wave) of MMVT may degrade the rhythm to VF. An ICD often is used in patients who survive VT or VF to quickly treat recurrent episodes. Endocardial and epicardial catheter ablation has become an effective treatment for VT.

Prevention of Sudden Cardiac Death

SCD is defined as death within 1 hour of the onset of symptoms. It may result from a variety of cardiac or noncardiac conditions (Table 8.6). SCD is one of the most common causes of death, with 400,000 events occurring annually in the United States. The most common cause of SCD is VT

表 8.4 晕厥的原因

原因	机制
外周血管或循环系统	
血管迷走性晕厥（神经介导）	前兆：苍白、打呵欠、恶心、出汗，由于应激或疼痛诱发，发生在患者直立时，躺卧可终止，血压降低伴或不伴心率下降
排尿性晕厥	排尿时晕厥（可能与迷走神经有关）
咳嗽后晕厥	突发咳嗽后晕厥
颈动脉窦超敏综合征	轻度按摩颈动脉窦所致血管抑制和（或）心脏抑制
药物	直立性低血压；见于降压药、三环类抗抑郁药、噻嗪类利尿剂
容量不足	直立性低血压；见于出血、大量呕吐或腹泻、艾迪生病
自主神经功能障碍	直立性低血压；见于糖尿病、酒精中毒、帕金森病、长期患病后调节功能失调
中枢神经系统	
脑血管	短暂性缺血性发作和卒中不常导致晕厥，通常可发现神经系统相关异常
癫痫	有时会出现警告症状、四肢抽搐、咬舌、尿失禁、发作后意识障碍
代谢性	
低血糖	昏迷、心动过速、晕厥前颤抖，患者可能正在应用胰岛素
心脏性	
阻塞性	晕厥常为劳力性；体格检查结果符合主动脉瓣狭窄、梗阻性肥厚型心肌病、心脏压塞、心房黏液瘤、人工瓣膜功能异常、艾森门格综合征、法洛四联症、原发性肺动脉高压、肺动脉狭窄、大面积肺栓塞
心律失常	晕厥可能突然发生在任何体位；头晕或心悸发作；可能有心脏病史或由缓慢性或快速性心律失常所致，需检查颈动脉窦超敏综合征

搏形态一致，通常源自于心脏的同一区域。超过每分钟 300 次的单形性室速可称为心室扑动。多形性室速（PMVT）在心电图上有着比单形性室速更多的形态。尖端扭转型室性心动过速（TdP）是特殊类型的多形性室速，有重复性和周期波动性，常提示长 QT 间期的触发机制。心室颤动是心室异位搏动最混乱的形式。心室颤动时没有有效心输出量，如未能迅速治疗，多会导致死亡。其他形式的室速可最终发展为心室颤动。

通常用 12 导联体表心电图来判断患者是否为室性心律。室性异位搏动通常为宽 QRS 波群（图 8.9）。但并非所有的宽 QRS 波形都意味着源自心室，一些标准可用于区分宽 QRS 波群是室上性还是室性来源的。室上速如果伴室内差异性传导（如束支传导阻滞）或通过旁路（如 WPW 综合征）传导至心室，也可表现为宽 QRS 波心动过速。其他可以用于区分室上速和室速的特征包括通过心室夺获和室性融合波判断房室分离，以及 QRS 波群时程及形态（表 8.5）。Brugada 方法通常用于确定宽 QRS 波群心动过速的起源部位。缺血性心脏病史患者的心动过速 90% 为心室起源。

室速的发生机制与其他心动过速相同，如折返、自律性增强或触发活动。围绕左心室陈旧梗死瘢痕区域的折返常可导致室速。慢性缺血性心脏病患者的室速是由存活心肌的通路或层面中发生的折返介导的，尤其是在陈旧心肌梗死瘢痕边缘的部分存活心肌中。在这些通路中，稀疏的存活心肌细胞偶联较差，传导异常缓慢。持续性室速的易感性随着左心室功能障碍恶化而增加，可能与较大范围的心室瘢痕有关。

室速可以不伴有缺血性心脏病，其分类包括特发性室速、非缺血性心肌病、肥厚型心肌病、致心律失常型右心室发育不良、束支折返、心脏离子通道障碍或电解质紊乱。右心室流出道（RVOT）是特发性室速最常见的起源，其可能由触发活动所致。这种形式的室速（或室性早搏）通常对儿茶酚胺敏感，且可用腺苷终止（如腺苷敏感性室速）。另一种常见形式的特发性室速源自左心室传导系统（如分支型室速），可能对维拉帕米敏感。特发性室速是成功导管消融的常见治疗靶标。

除非患者有症状，非持续性室速通常不需要特殊治疗。心脏心律失常抑制试验（CAST）中，使用 I 类抗心律失常药物治疗梗死急性期后发生的室性早搏和非持续性室速，试验证实予抗心律失常治疗增加死亡率。如室速为可逆原因所致，如电解质紊乱或急性缺血，则应当对其潜在机制进行治疗，如为不可逆原因，则可用 β 受体阻滞剂、抗心律失常药物（如胺碘酮）或导管消融治疗。如因血流动力学不稳定需要紧急治疗，则行直流心脏电复律。如果 QRS 波群形态规则，则复律应与其同步，否则应选择非同步。在单形性室速的不应期（T 波）执行直流心脏电复律可能将节律恶化为心室颤动。植入式心脏复律除颤器（ICD）通常用于治疗室速或心室颤动的幸存者，用于快速治疗复发性发作。心内膜和心外膜导管消融已成为室速的有效治疗方式。

心源性猝死的预防

心源性猝死（SCD）定义为症状发作 1 h 内死亡。它可能由各种心脏或非心脏疾病引发（表 8.6）。心源性猝死是最常见的死因之一，在美国每年发生 400 000 次事件。心源性猝死的最常见原因是室速或心室颤动。

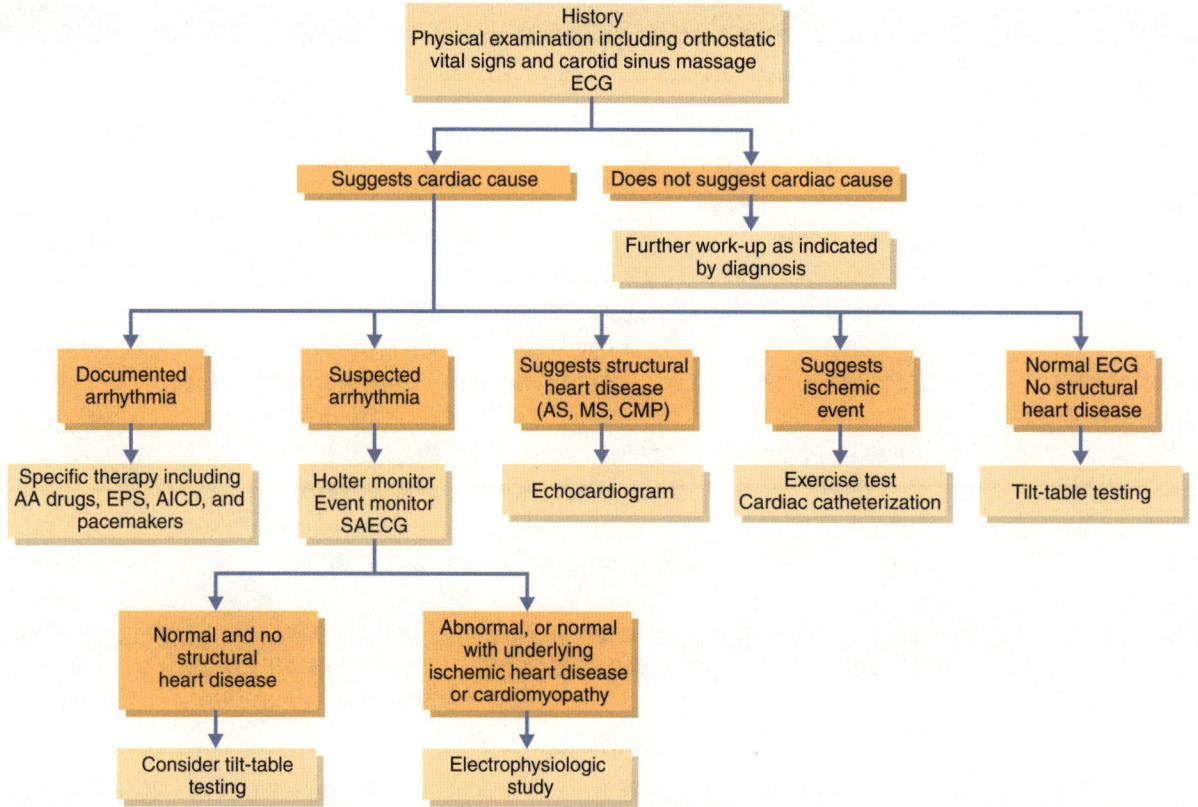

Fig. 8.8 Approach to the evaluation of syncope. *AA,* Antiarrhythmic; *AICD,* automatic implantable cardioverter-defibrillator; *AS,* aortic stenosis; *CMP,* cardiomyopathy; *ECG,* electrocardiogram; *EPS,* electrophysiologic study; *MS,* mitral stenosis; *SAECG,* signal-averaged ECG.

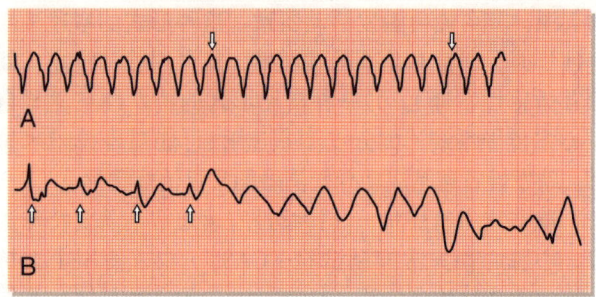

Fig. 8.9 Ventricular arrhythmias. (A) Monomorphic ventricular tachycardia (VT). Notice the wide QRS with a stable appearance with each beat. Detecting P waves during VT is difficult due to the overlying ventricular activity, but it is visible at several points on this tracing, some of which are marked by *arrows*. The AV dissociation is diagnostic of VT and excludes supraventricular tachycardia. (B) An initially organized agonal (preterminal) rhythm *(arrows)* degenerates into coarse ventricular fibrillation. Notice the irregular baseline and the absence of organized QRS complexes. During ventricular fibrillation, there is no forward cardiac output, and cardiac arrest immediately ensues.

TABLE 8.5 Differentiation of Ventricular Tachycardia From Supraventricular Tachycardia With Aberrancy

Helpful Features	Implications
Positive QRS concordance	Diagnostic of VT
AV dissociation, capture beats, or fusion beats	Diagnostic of VT
Atypical RBBB (monophasic R, QR, RS, or triphasic QRS in V_1; R:S ratio <1, QS or QR, monophasic R in V_6)	Suggests VT
Atypical LBBB (R >30 min or R to S [nadir or notch] >60 min in V_1 or V_2; R:S ratio <1, QS or QR in V_6)	Suggests VT
Shift of axis from baseline	Suggests VT
History of CAD	Suggests VT
QRS during tachycardia identical to QRS during sinus rhythm	Suggests SVT
Termination with adenosine	Suggests SVT

AV, Atrioventricular; *CAD,* coronary artery disease; *LBBB,* left bundle branch block; *RBBB,* right bundle branch block; *SVT,* supraventricular tachycardia; *VT,* ventricular tachycardia.

or VF. Cardiac conditions that increase the risk of SCD include LQTS, hypertrophic cardiomyopathy, Brugada syndrome, arrhythmogenic RV dysplasia, and nonischemic or ischemic cardiomyopathy. The most common cardiac condition that may lead to SCD is acute or distant MI.

The successful treatment of SCD due to VF usually requires rapid access to cardioversion; if treatment is delayed by more than 5 to 10 minutes, permanent brain injury is common. AEDs can reduce the time to defibrillation and improve survival when placed in public areas, although they have been less effective when installed in private residences, even for patients at risk for SCD.

ICDs used in the treatment of SCD have improved mortality rates. Patients who are at high risk for SCD are often offered an ICD to enable rapid defibrillation before the onset of anoxic brain injury. If a patient survives the first episode of SCD due to documented or presumed VT

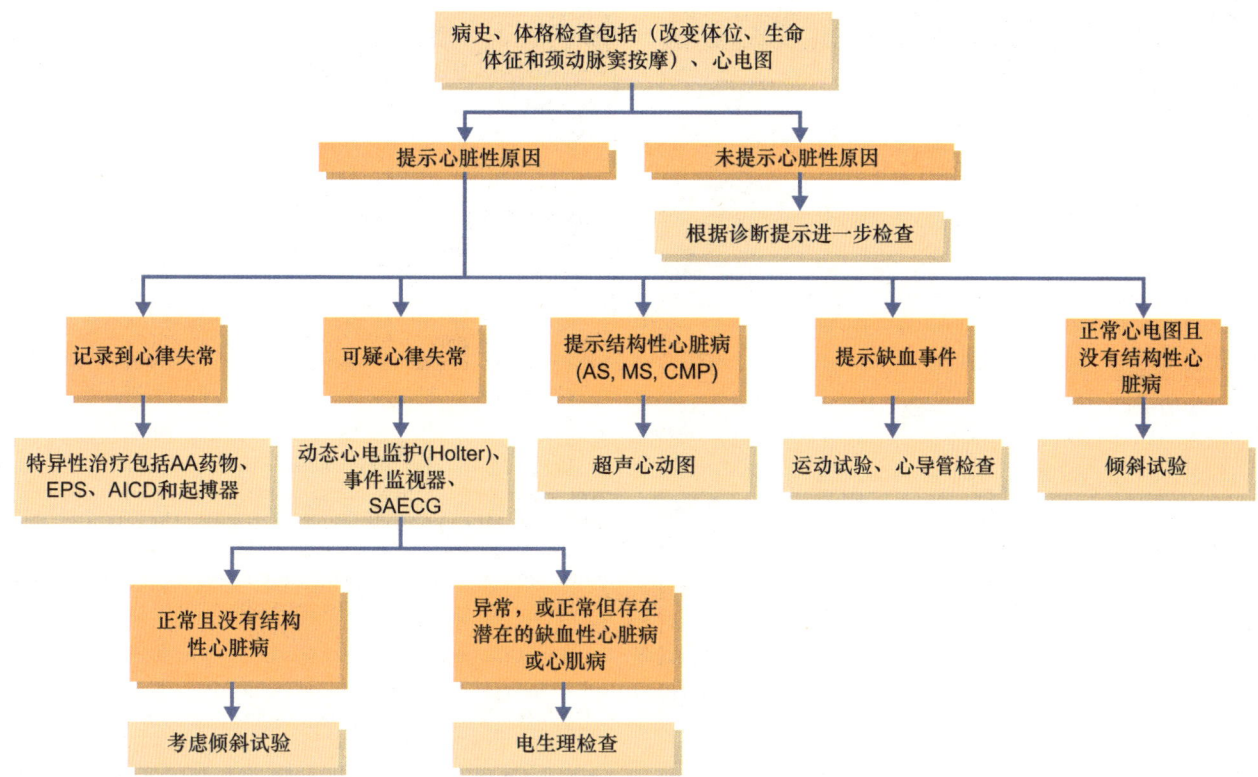

图 8.8 晕厥评估方法。AA，抗心律失常；AICD，自动植入式心脏复律除颤器；AS，主动脉瓣狭窄；CMP，心肌病；EPS，电生理检查；MS，二尖瓣狭窄；SAECG，信号平均心电图

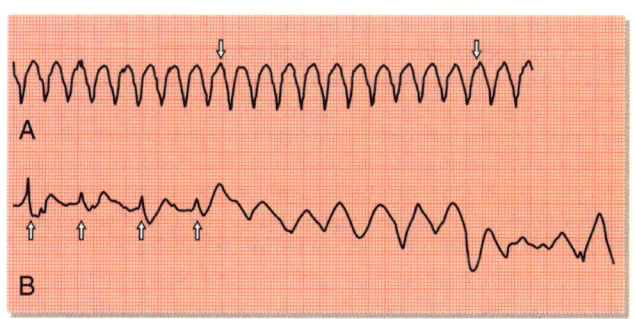

图 8.9 室性心律失常。（A）单形性室性心动过速（VT）。注意宽 QRS 波群，每搏为单一形态。室性心动过速期间，P 波被心室活动覆盖，故难以识别，但是在该记录上可见于数个点位，其中一些 P 波由箭头标记。房室分离支持室性心动过速的诊断，并可除外室上性心动过速。（B）初期的临终（死前）规整节律（箭头）恶化为粗大的心室颤动。注意不规则的基线及规整的 QRS 波群消失。在心室颤动期间，没有前向心输出量，因而出现心脏停搏

表 8.5 室上性心动过速伴差异性传导与室性心动过速的鉴别	
有助于鉴别的特性	意义
QRS 波群正向一致性	诊断 VT
房室分离、心室夺获或室性融合波	诊断 VT
非典型 RBBB［V_1 导联的呈 R、QR、RS 型或三相型 QRS 波群，V_6 导联 R∶S < 1，呈 QS、QR 或单相 R 波］	提示 VT
非典型 LBBB［V_1 或 V_2 导联中 R 波时限 > 30 ms 或 RS 时限（最低点或切迹）> 60 ms；V_6 导联 R∶S < 1，呈 QS 或 QR 型］	提示 VT
电轴偏移基线	提示 VT
冠状动脉疾病病史	提示 VT
心动过速时 QRS 波群与窦性心律时 QRS 波群相同	提示 SVT
可用腺苷终止	提示 SVT

LBBB，左束支传导阻滞；RBBB，右束支传导阻滞；SVT，室上性心动过速；VT，室性心动过速。

致心源性猝死风险增加的心脏疾病包括长 QT 间期综合征（LQTS）、肥厚型心肌病、Brugada 综合征、致心律失常型右心室发育不良和非缺血性/缺血性心肌病。导致心源性猝死的最常见心脏疾病是急性或陈旧性心肌梗死。

成功治疗心室颤动所致的心源性猝死需快速进行心脏复律，如果治疗延迟超过 5～10 min，常常出现永久性脑损伤。放置在公共区域的自动体外除颤器（AED）可以减少除颤的等待时间并提高生存率，但当安装在私人住所时效用较低，即使是对于存在心源性猝死风险的患者。

用于治疗心源性猝死的 ICD 可降低死亡率。心源性猝死高风险的患者常植入 ICD 以便在出现缺氧性脑损伤之前能够快速除颤。如果患者从第一次心源性猝死中幸存，猝死是由记录的或推测的室速或心室颤动

TABLE 8.6 Causes of Sudden Cardiac Death
Noncardiac Causes
Central nervous system hemorrhage
Massive pulmonary embolus
Drug overdose
Hypoxia secondary to lung disease
Aortic dissection or rupture
Cardiac Causes
Ventricular fibrillation
Myocardial ischemia or injury
Long QT syndrome
Short QT syndrome
Brugada syndrome
Arrhythmogenic right ventricular dysplasia
Ventricular tachycardia
Bradyarrhythmias, sick sinus syndrome
Aortic stenosis
Tetralogy of Fallot
Pericardial tamponade
Cardiac tumors
Complications of infective endocarditis
Hypertrophic cardiomyopathy (arrhythmia or obstruction)
Myocardial ischemia
Atherosclerosis
Prinzmetal angina
Kawasaki arteritis

TABLE 8.7 Predictors of Sudden Cardiac Death After Myocardial Infarction
Decreased left ventricular ejection fraction
Residual ischemia
Delayed enhancement on cardiac MRI
Late potentials on signal-averaged electrocardiography
Decreased heart rate variability
Prolonged QT on ECG
Induction of sustained MMVT with programmed electrical stimulation
Complex ventricular ectopy (e.g., NSVT) on ambulatory monitoring

ECG, Electrocardiogram; *MMVT,* monomorphic ventricular tachycardia; *MRI,* magnetic resonance imaging; *NSVT,* nonsustained ventricular tachycardia.

or VF from nonreversible or unknown causes, he or she is offered an ICD. ICDs are extremely successful in the detection and treatment of VT or VF. They do not always prevent loss of consciousness because it takes 15 to 20 seconds to treat the arrhythmia, and low cardiac output may cause syncope before restoration of normal rhythm, especially if several cardioversions are required.

The earliest ICD trials examined their use in the secondary prevention of SCD (i.e., treating patients who had already survived an episode of cardiac arrest). The largest study was the Antiarrhythmics Versus Implantable Defibrillators (AVID) trial, which randomized patients with a history of poorly tolerated sustained VT or cardiac arrest to empirical amiodarone or ICD implantation. In this trial and several others, ICD therapy was associated with a lower risk of arrhythmic and all-cause death compared with antiarrhythmic therapy.

Several trials have examined the use of ICDs for the primary prevention of SCDs (i.e., treating patients who are at risk for SCD). The first was the Multicenter Automatic Defibrillator Implantation Trial (MADIT), which enrolled patients with a prior MI and an ejection fraction of 35% or less who had frequent ventricular ectopy and inducible VT at electrophysiologic testing. The study demonstrated a substantial mortality reduction with ICD therapy. MADIT-II enrolled patients with a prior MI and an ejection fraction of 30% or less in the chronic phase, without requiring invasive testing. A significant mortality benefit was associated with ICD therapy.

The Sudden Cardiac Death in Heart Failure trial enrolled a broader population consisting of patients with ischemic and nonischemic cardiomyopathy, symptomatic heart failure, and an ejection fraction of 35% or less. A survival benefit was found for patients treated with an ICD compared with conventional therapy or empirical amiodarone therapy. The degree of benefit was similar for patients with ischemic or nonischemic cardiomyopathy, suggesting that primary prevention with ICDs for patients with prior MI or nonischemic cardiomyopathy and heart failure was appropriate.

The risk of SCD after MI is highest in the few months after the index event. However, ICDs have not been effective when implanted immediately after MI or revascularization procedures. The reason for this is unclear; it may reflect the large percentage of patients who have improved cardiac function early on, which decreases the risk of SCD and therefore the benefit of an ICD. Alternatively, the mechanism for SCD in the early period after an MI or revascularization procedure may be recurrent ischemia rather than reentrant tachycardia and therefore less amenable to ICD therapy. The Defibrillator in Acute Myocardial Infarction Trial (DINAMIT) randomized 675 patients with low ejection fractions immediately after MI to ICD or medical therapy; no difference in mortality rates was seen. The current recommendations are to avoid primary prevention with ICDs within 40 days of an MI or 3 months of revascularization.

A significant challenge in modern medicine is identifying patients who have an elevated risk of SCD to allow effective use of primary prevention interventions such as ICDs. Some known predictors of SCD after MI are shown in Table 8.7, but many are not specific or sensitive enough for practical use. Reduced ejection fraction has been the most successful noninvasive measure that can predict increased risk of SCD. An electrophysiologic study is a minimally invasive catheter procedure that with electrical stimulation can help to identify patients who are prone to VT. Electrophysiologic studies are most sensitive in patients with prior MI, but they may be less useful in other cardiac conditions. Cardiac magnetic resonance imaging (MRI), which can directly image cardiac function and cardiac scar or fibrosis, is showing great promise as a more sensitive and specific, noninvasive risk predictor of SCD.

Ventricular Tachycardia and Ventricular Fibrillation Without Evident Heart Disease

Ventricular arrhythmias occurring in the absence of structural heart disease usually carry a benign prognosis but can be associated with SCD in patients with genetic arrhythmic syndromes predisposing to life-threatening polymorphic VT. Genetic screening for these syndromes is important to identify at-risk family members.

Idiopathic Ventricular Tachycardia

Idiopathic VT most commonly originates from the outflow tracts, with approximately 80% localized to the RVOT and the remainder originating in the left ventricular outflow tract (LVOT), the aortic sinuses of Valsalva, and the region of the aortomitral continuity. Idiopathic RVOT VT manifests with the characteristic electrocardiographic findings of left bundle branch block and inferior axis VT QRS morphology. Triggered activity is the mechanism underlying outflow tract tachycardias. This calcium-dependent mechanism explains why an outflow tract VT often terminates with adenosine, β-blockers, and calcium-channel blockers.

表 8.6　心源性猝死的病因
非心源性病因
中枢神经系统出血
大面积肺栓塞
药物过量
肺部疾病继发的低氧血症
主动脉夹层或破裂
心源性病因
心室颤动
心肌缺血或损伤
长 QT 间期综合征
短 QT 间期综合征
Brugada 综合征
致心律失常型右心室发育不良
室性心动过速
缓慢性心律失常，病态窦房结综合征
主动脉瓣狭窄
法洛四联症
心脏压塞
心脏肿瘤
感染性心内膜炎的并发症
肥厚型心肌病（心律失常或梗阻）
心肌缺血
动脉粥样硬化
变异型心绞痛
川崎动脉炎

表 8.7　心肌梗死后心源性猝死的预测因子
左心室射血分数下降
残余心肌缺血
心脏 MRI 出现延迟强化
信号平均心电图出现晚电位
心率变异性降低
ECG 显示 QT 间期延长
程控电刺激诱导出持续性 MMVT
动态监测可见复杂室性早搏（如 NSVT）

ECG，心电图；MMVT，单形性室性心动过速；MRI，磁共振成像；NSVT，非持续性室性心动过速。

心肌梗死事件后的前几个月内心源性猝死的风险最高。然而，在心肌梗死或血运重建术后立即植入 ICD 的效果不佳。其原因尚不清楚，或许是因为大部分患者心功能在急性期有所改善，从而降低了心源性猝死的风险，并且因此降低了 ICD 的获益。另一种可能是在心肌梗死或血运重建术后的早期，心源性猝死的机制可能是复发性缺血而不是折返性心动过速，因此更不适于 ICD 治疗。除颤器用于急性心肌梗死试验（DINAMIT）中，将 675 例低射血分数的患者随机分为心肌梗死后立即进行 ICD 和药物治疗组，两组没有观察到死亡率的差异。当前的建议是在心肌梗死或血运重建 40 天到 3 个月内避免将 ICD 用于一级预防。

现代医学的一个重大挑战是识别心源性猝死高风险的患者，从而有效使用一级预防干预措施如 ICD。一些已知的心肌梗死后心源性猝死预测因素如表 8.7 所示，但许多因素对临床实际应用的特异性或敏感性不足。预测心源性猝死风险增加最有意义的无创检查是射血分数降低。电生理检查是微创导管操作，电刺激可以帮助识别易发室速的患者。电生理检查在陈旧性心肌梗死患者中最敏感，但在其他心脏疾病患者中不那么有用。心脏磁共振成像（MRI）可直接将心脏功能、心脏瘢痕和纤维化成像，作为一个更敏感和特异性更高的心源性猝死无创风险预测工具有着巨大的前景。

无心脏基础病的室性心动过速和心室颤动

在无结构性心脏病的情况下发生的室性心律失常通常预后良好，但对于遗传性心律失常综合征患者，也和易患威胁生命的多形性室速猝死相关。这些综合征的遗传筛查对于鉴别有风险的家庭成员具有重要意义。

特发性室性心动过速

特发性室速最常来自于心室流出道，约 80% 定位于右心室流出道，其余源于左心室流出道、主动脉窦和主动脉瓣二尖瓣连接区。特发性右心室流出道室速心电图表现为特征性的左束支传导阻滞和电轴向下的室速 QRS 波群形态。触发活动是流出道心动过速的机制。这种钙依赖机制解释了流出道室速通常可用腺苷、β 受体阻滞剂和钙通道阻滞剂终止的原因。

所致，其原因不可逆或不明，则应当植入 ICD。ICD 在室速或心室颤动的检测和治疗中极为成功。由于需要 15～20 s 来治疗心律失常，它们不总是能够防止意识丧失，在恢复正常节律之前的低心输出量可能引起晕厥，特别是如果需要数次心脏复律时。

最早的 ICD 试验探索了其在心源性猝死二级预防（即治疗心搏骤停幸存者）中的应用。最大规模的研究是抗心律失常药物对比植入式除颤器（AVID）试验，将难以耐受持续性室速或心搏骤停的患者随机分入经验性胺碘酮治疗组或 ICD 植入组。在这项试验和其他一些试验中，ICD 治疗与心律失常药物相比，心律失常死亡和全因死亡的风险明显降低。

数个实验研究探索了 ICD 在心源性猝死一级预防（即治疗心源性猝死风险患者）中的应用。第一项是多中心自动除颤器植入试验（MADIT），其招募了有心肌梗死病史且射血分数 ≤ 35%，伴频繁的室性异位搏动且电生理检查可诱发室速的患者。该研究表明 ICD 治疗可显著降低死亡率。MADIT-Ⅱ招募了有心肌梗死病史且在慢性期射血分数 ≤ 30%，不要求进行有创检查的患者。ICD 治疗组有着明显较低的死亡率。

心力衰竭中的心源性猝死试验招募了有心力衰竭症状且射血分数 ≤ 35% 的缺血性/非缺血性心肌病患者。与传统治疗或经验性胺碘酮治疗相比，ICD 治疗患者有生存率获益。缺血性和非缺血性心肌病患者的获益程度相似，提示对于陈旧性心肌梗死或非缺血性心肌病合并心力衰竭的患者，使用 ICD 一级预防是合适的。

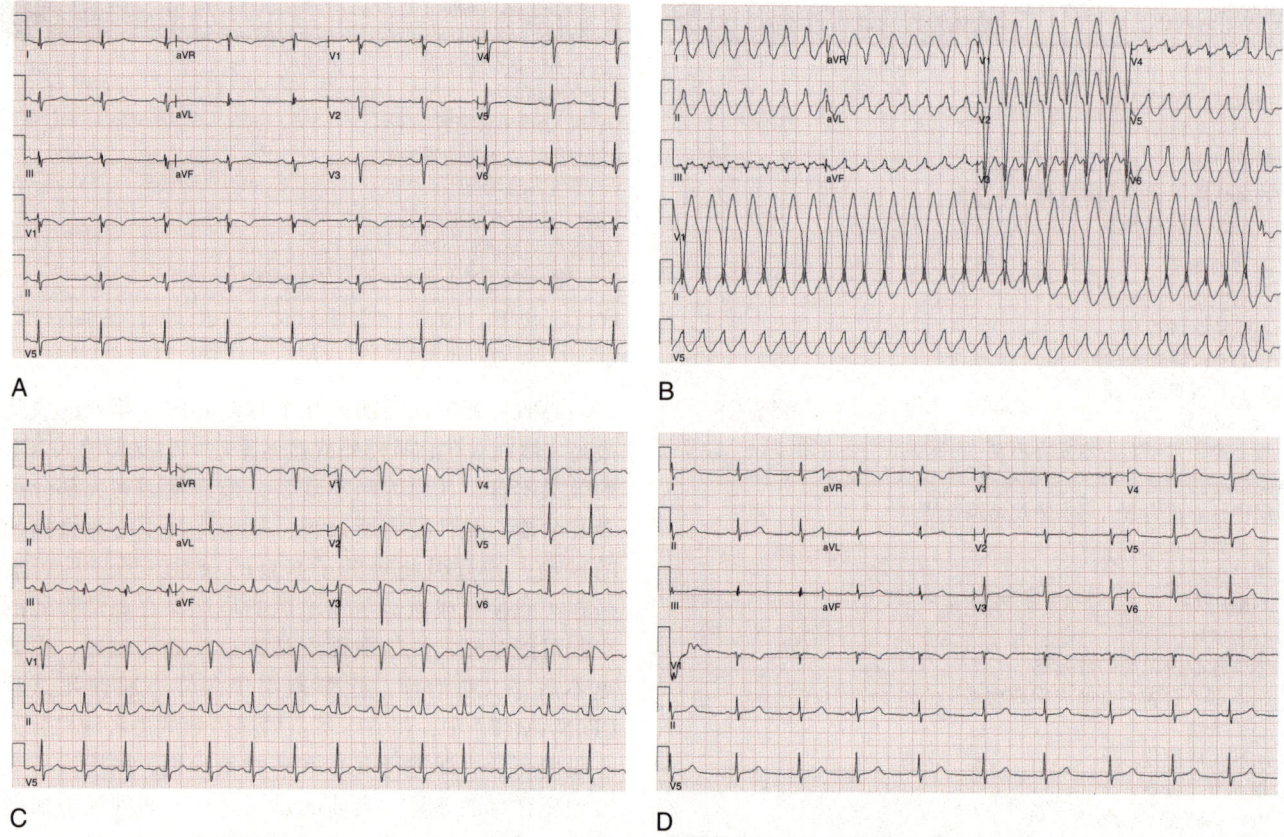

Fig. 8.10 Characteristic electrocardiograms associated with genetic disorders predisposing to SCD. (A) ARVC ECG demonstrating inverted T waves V_1-V_3 during sinus rhythm. (B) Monomorphic ventricular tachycardia with left bundle branch block morphology characteristic of ARVC. (C) Type I Brugada ECG pattern with coving ST elevation and T inversion in V_1-V_2. (D) ECG from patient with hereditary LQT1, with mutation KCNQ1.

Patients in their third or fourth decade typically have palpitations, shortness of breath, and lightheadedness at presentation. Reports of cardiac arrest are rare, and treatment is directed at controlling symptoms. β-Blockers and calcium-channel blockers are often used initially, although some patients require catheter ablation or antiarrhythmic drug therapy. A subset of asymptomatic patients may develop tachycardia-mediated cardiomyopathy due to frequent ventricular ectopy. The PVC burden posing the greatest risk for producing left ventricular dysfunction is likely more than 10,000 PVCs daily. Fortunately, PVC suppression with catheter ablation usually improves ventricular function.

Arrhythmogenic Right Ventricular Cardiomyopathy or Dysplasia

Arrhythmogenic right ventricular cardiomyopathy (ARVC) is an inherited cardiomyopathy with typically autosomal dominant transmission. It is associated with mutations affecting desmosomes, which are molecular complexes of cell adhesion proteins that bind cardiac myocytes. Although morphologic changes in the RV free wall predominate, biventricular or primary left ventricular variants occur. Due to myocyte death, large portions of the right ventricle are replaced with adipose tissue, leading to wall motion abnormalities, cardiac dysfunction, and aneurysm formation. Structural changes spread from the epicardium to the endocardium. RV imaging classically demonstrates RV enlargement with focal wall motion abnormalities and RV hypokinesis. The RV free wall is not well imaged by routine cardiac echocardiography, and MRI has become the gold standard for the diagnosis of ARVC.

ARVC patients develop ventricular arrhythmias with associated symptoms, including palpitations, lightheadedness, syncope, and SCD. Given the typical RV origin of arrhythmias in ARVC, the ventricular arrhythmias have a left bundle branch morphology (Fig. 8.10B). The surface ECG during sinus rhythm may demonstrate inverted T waves in the V_1 to V_3 leads or epsilon waves, which are low-amplitude deflections at the end of the QRS complex in the right precordial leads resulting from slowed RV conduction (Fig. 8.10A).

Distinguishing ARVC from idiopathic RVOT VT is essential because of the different prognostic and therapeutic implications of the two diagnoses. The diagnosis of ARVC is established by the ARVC Task Force Criteria. Risk factors for SCD of ARVC patients include prior aborted episodes of SCD, syncope, young age, LV dysfunction, and markedly diminished RV function.

Patients with documented ARVC typically receive ICDs. Adjunctive therapy with antiarrhythmic drugs or ablation, particularly strategies incorporating combined epicardial and endocardial ablation, may be useful in treating symptomatic VT.

Congenital Long QT Syndrome

Congenital LQTS is a genetic disorder characterized by abnormal cardiac repolarization producing QT prolongation on the ECG (corrected QT [QTc] >440 milliseconds in men and >460 milliseconds in women) (Fig. 8.10D). It is a leading cause of SCD in the young.

Mutations in 16 genes that participate in cardiac repolarization have been identified in patients with LQTS. Mutations of *KCNQ1* (encodes

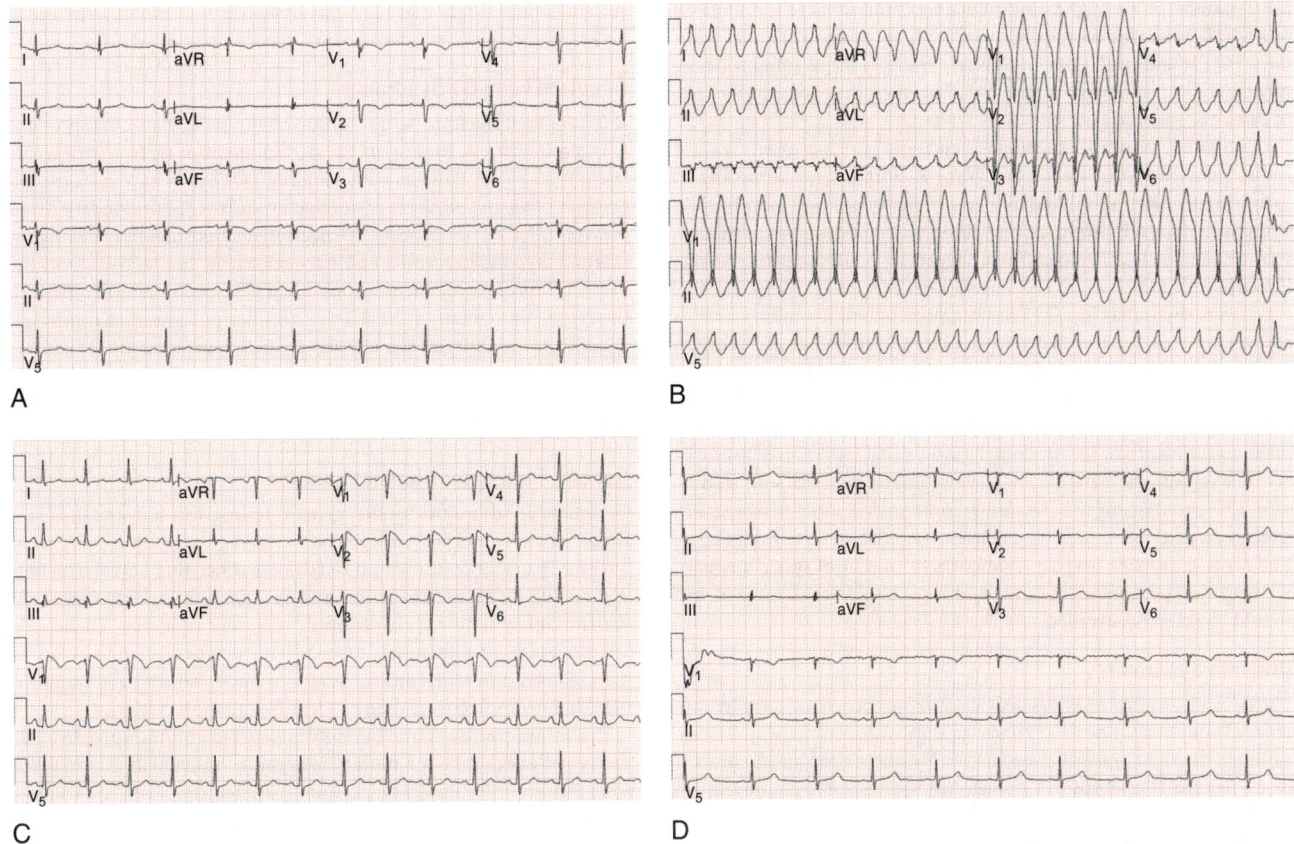

图 8.10 易发生心源性猝死的遗传性疾病的特征性心电图。（A）ARVC 心电图表现为窦性心律时 $V_1 \sim V_3$ 导联 T 波倒置。（B）ARVC 的典型单形性室性心动过速伴左束支传导阻滞形态。（C）Ⅰ型 Brugada 心电图形态，表现为 $V_1 \sim V_2$ 导联 ST 段穹顶样抬高和 T 波倒置。（D）遗传型 LQT1 伴 *KCNQ1* 突变患者心电图

患者 20～40 岁时通常表现为心悸、呼吸困难和头晕。心搏骤停很罕见，治疗针对于症状控制。β 受体阻滞剂和钙通道阻滞剂常为起始用药，尽管一些患者需要导管消融或其他抗心律失常药物治疗。一些无症状患者可能因频繁的室性异位搏动而发展为心动过速介导的心肌病。每日室性期前收缩（早搏）超过 10 000 个，期前收缩负荷导致左心室功能障碍的风险最高。幸运的是，导管消融抑制室性早搏通常可改善心室功能。

致心律失常型右心室心肌病或发育不良

致心律失常型右心室心肌病（ARVC）是一种典型的常染色体显性遗传性心肌病。与细胞桥粒的突变有关，而细胞桥粒是连接心肌细胞的细胞黏附性蛋白质分子复合物。ARVC 以右心室游离壁的形态学变化为主，但是也可出现双心室或主要是左心室改变。由于心肌细胞死亡，右心室的大部分被脂肪组织替代，导致室壁运动异常、心脏功能障碍和室壁瘤形成。结构改变从心外膜扩散到心内膜。右心室成像提示典型的右心室扩大、局灶性室壁运动异常和右心室低动力。右心室游离壁通过常规超声心动图成像欠佳，故 MRI 是 ARVC 诊断的金标准。

ARVC 患者可出现室性心律失常相关的症状，包括心悸、头晕、晕厥和心源性猝死。鉴于 ARVC 常为右心室起源，室性心律失常呈左束支传导阻滞形态（图 8.10B）。在窦性心律期间的体表心电图可以在 $V_1 \sim V_3$ 导联出现 T 波倒置或 epsilon 波，这是由于右心室传导减慢导致的右胸导联 QRS 波群末端处出现低振幅碎裂波（图 8.10A）。

区分 ARVC 及特发性右心室流出道室速很有必要，因为两种不同诊断的预后和治疗不同。ARVC 工作组制定了诊断 ARVC 的标准。ARVC 患者的心源性猝死的危险因素包括既往心源性猝死生还、晕厥、年轻、左心室功能障碍和显著的右心室功能低下。

确诊的 ARVC 患者通常应接受 ICD 治疗。辅助以使用抗心律失常药物或消融治疗，特别是心外膜和心内膜的联合消融，对症状性室速治疗或许有效。

先天性长 QT 间期综合征

先天性长 QT 间期综合征（LQTS）是一种遗传性疾病，其特征性表现为心脏复极异常，心电图上出现 QT 间期延长［男性校正 QT 间期（QTc）> 440 ms，女性 ≥ 460 ms］（图 8.10D）。它是年轻人心源性猝死的首位原因。

LQTS 患者中识别出参与心脏复极的 16 个基因突变。*KCNQ1* 突变（编码 I_{Ks} 钾通道的 α 亚基）产生 LQT1；

the α-subunit of the I_{Ks} potassium channel) produce LQT1; mutations of *KCNH2* (encodes the α-subunit of the I_{Kr} potassium channel) produce LQT2; and mutations of *SCN5A* (encodes the α-subunit of the cardiac sodium channel) cause LQT3. Together, they account for 75% of cases of congenital LQTS.

Decreased outward potassium currents or increased inward sodium currents prolong action potential duration, predisposing to early afterdepolarizations and TdP, a specific type of polymorphic VT. Symptoms typically begin during adolescence and include syncope, seizures, and SCD. The arrhythmia triggers in LQTS are gene specific. Patients with LQT1 are at risk during high adrenergic states, such as exercise; arrhythmias in LQT2 are triggered by sudden noises such as alarms; and LQT3 patients are more likely to experience arrhythmias during sleep. The autosomal dominant Romano-Ward variant has a prevalence of 1 case in 2000 live births.

Chronic treatment is directed at prevention of SCD. Initial therapy includes avoidance of QT-prolonging agents and initiation of β-blockers in symptomatic patients and asymptomatic patients with significant QT prolongation. ICDs are recommended after resuscitation from a cardiac arrest and for recurrent syncope despite β-blockade. The acute treatment of TdP is different from that of other forms of VT because many antiarrhythmic agents prolong the QT interval and should therefore be avoided.

Brugada Syndrome

The Brugada syndrome is a genetic disorder predisposing to polymorphic VT and SCD. The ECG characteristically displays coving ST elevation in the right precordial leads, V_1 to V_3, and a right bundle branch block pattern (Fig. 8.10C). These electrocardiographic abnormalities may be dynamic, and they are characteristically exacerbated by fever and therapy that blocks sodium channels.

The syndrome is linked to mutations in *SCN5A*, which encodes the cardiac sodium channel. Mutations result in a reduction in the sodium current. The mode of transmission is autosomal dominant. Patients typically have syncope or cardiac arrest, often occurring during sleep.

Although quinidine, by virtue of its ability to block transient outward potassium current (I_{to}), may have a therapeutic role, there are no established medical therapies to prevent VT in Brugada syndrome. Intravenous β-adrenergic stimulation with isoproterenol or a similar agent, by virtue of its ability to augment the sodium current, is potentially useful in the acute management of recurrent VT or VF in Brugada syndrome. Paradoxically, because of a protective effect of catecholamine stimulation, β-blockers are potentially harmful in patients with Brugada syndrome and should be avoided.

ICDs represent the only proven therapy for prevention of cardiac arrest. ICD therapy is recommended for secondary prevention of SCD. For high-risk patients with a spontaneous Brugada electrocardiographic pattern and syncope, primary prevention with an ICD is indicated.

Catecholaminergic Polymorphic Ventricular Tachycardia

CPVT is a genetic disorder that alters myocardial calcium handling, resulting in exercise-induced polymorphic or bidirectional VT. Exercise-triggered syncope or SCD during childhood is the common presenting symptom. About 50% to 60% of patients have an inherited or sporadic autosomal dominant mutation affecting the cardiac ryanodine receptor gene (*RYR2*), producing abnormal calcium-induced calcium release from the sarcoplasmic reticulum and intracellular calcium overload.

β-Blockers along with exercise restriction represent the primary therapy, although arrhythmia breakthrough is common. ICD therapy may be used for secondary prevention, although ICD shocks can produce catecholamine surges that may exacerbate the underlying arrhythmia. Left cardiac sympathetic denervation is useful in selected cases.

Acquired Long QT Syndrome

Environmental factors may prolong cardiac repolarization and produce QTc prolongation, leading to the development of early afterdepolarizations and TdP. Patients with acquired LQTS may have background genetics predisposing them to develop excessive QTc prolongation and polymorphic VT in response to electrolyte abnormalities (i.e., hypokalemia, hypomagnesemia, and hypocalcemia), bradycardia, and the use of QT-prolonging medications. Most QTc-prolonging drugs block the rapid component of the delayed rectifier potassium channel (I_{Kr}) encoded by the *KCNE2* gene. Drugs known to prolong the QTc interval are updated on an Internet registry. Therapy for acquired LQTS requires reversal of inciting physiologic factors and discontinuation of offending medications.

Genetic Testing for Channelopathies

Commercial laboratories offer genetic testing for congenital LQTS, Brugada syndrome, and CPVT. The yields of genetic testing vary from 25% for Brugada syndrome up to 80% for congenital LQTS. The limited sensitivity of current assays and the common finding of genetic variants of unknown significance represent ongoing challenges. Despite these considerations, cascade screening or screening of family members for a disease-causing mutation once characterized in a proband has been effectively used to identify mutation carriers.

Mutation-positive family members may benefit from prophylactic therapy. Reassurance for mutation-negative individuals is also valuable. Before ordering genetic testing, patients should be thoroughly informed of the risks, benefits, and limitations of testing. Genetic counselors ideally play an important advisory role.

For a deeper discussion on this topic, please see Chapter 59, "Ventricular Arrhythmias," in *Goldman-Cecil Medicine*, 26th Edition.

SUMMARY

Cardiac arrhythmias are caused by disorders of action potential formation or propagation and are broadly categorized as abnormally slow rhythms (i.e., bradycardias) or abnormally rapid rhythms (i.e., tachycardias). The cardiac cellular action potential is composed of five phases determined by the activity of multiple ion channels, including the rapid sodium channel, several potassium channels, and a calcium current. Disruptions of these currents may lead to abnormal automaticity and triggered activity, which may mediate pathologic tachyarrhythmias. Reentry is the dominant mechanism of clinically significant tachyarrhythmias and requires a functional or fixed obstacle to propagation, an area of slowed conduction, and differential refractoriness for initiation and perpetuation of the arrhythmia.

Antiarrhythmic drugs are commonly divided into four broad groups using the Singh–Vaughan Williams classification. Despite its clinical utility, many antiarrhythmic drugs have multiple effects and do not fit neatly into this framework. Some, such as adenosine and digoxin, fall completely outside of it. Class I drugs slow membrane conduction by blockade of the sodium channel. Class II drugs, or β-blockers, function by blockade of the cardiac β-receptor. Class III drugs prolong repolarization and the QT interval. Class IV drugs block the slow calcium channel and are primarily active in slow-response myocytes such as the sinus and AV node.

All bradycardia is a consequence of impairment of sinus node function or AV conduction, or both. Sinus and AV nodal function is strongly influenced by autonomic tone. Parasympathetic tone dominates at rest, and significant bradycardia and second-degree

KCNH2 突变（编码 I_{Kr} 钾通道的 α 亚基）产生 LQT2；*SCN5A* 的突变（编码心脏钠通道的 α 亚基）导致 LQT3。这三者共占先天性 LQTS 病例的 75%。

外向钾电流减少或内向钠电流增加延长了动作电位时程，促使早期后除极和尖端扭转型室速的发生，后者是一种特殊类型的多形性室速。症状通常在青春期开始，包括晕厥、抽搐和心源性猝死。LQTS 中的心律失常触发因素是基因特异性的。LQT1 患者在高肾上腺素状态如运动期间风险较高；LQT2 患者的心律失常由突然出现的噪声触发，如闹钟；LQT3 患者更可能在睡眠期间出现心律失常。常染色体显性遗传的 Romano-Ward 突变在活产新生儿中患病率为 1/2000。

长期治疗目标是预防心源性猝死。初始治疗包括避免应用延长 QT 间期的药物，有症状的患者和无症状但 QT 间期显著延长的患者使用 β 受体阻滞剂。使用 β 受体阻滞剂仍然出现心搏骤停复苏后的患者和反复晕厥的患者推荐植入 ICD。尖端扭转型室速的急性期治疗不同于其他形式的室速，许多抗心律失常药物可延长 QT 间期，应当避免应用。

Brugada 综合征

Brugada 综合征是一种易患多形性室速和心源性猝死的遗传性疾病。心电图特征性地显示右胸 $V_1 \sim V_3$ 导联的 ST 段穹顶样抬高和右束支传导阻滞形态（图 8.10C）。这些心电图异常可能是动态的，可因发热和钠通道阻滞剂的应用而特征性地显现。

该综合征与编码心脏钠通道的 *SCN5A* 突变相关。突变导致钠电流减小。此病呈常染色体显性遗传。患者常有晕厥或心搏骤停，通常在睡眠期间发生。

能够阻断瞬时外向钾电流（I_{to}）的奎尼丁，可能有一定治疗作用，但没有确切的药物治疗能预防 Brugada 综合征发生室速。使用异丙肾上腺素或类似的静脉 β 肾上腺素能激动剂，可增加钠电流，对于 Brugada 综合征的复发性室速或心室颤动的急性期治疗可能有效。与之相反的是，由于儿茶酚胺刺激的保护作用，β 受体阻滞剂对 Brugada 综合征患者有害，应避免使用。

ICD 是唯一被证实能预防心搏骤停的治疗方法。推荐使用 ICD 进行心源性猝死的二级预防。对于出现自发性 Brugada 心电图形态和晕厥的高危患者，应使用 ICD 进行一级预防。

儿茶酚胺敏感性多形性室性心动过速

儿茶酚胺敏感性多形性室性心动过速（CPVT）是一种影响心肌钙调节的遗传性疾病，会导致运动诱发的多形性或双向性室速。常见症状为儿童期的运动触发性晕厥或心源性猝死。约 50%～60% 的患者存在影响心脏雷诺丁受体基因（*RYR2*）的遗传或散发性常染色体显性突变，产生钙诱导的肌质网钙释放异常和细胞内钙超载。

首选治疗为 β 受体阻滞剂和限制运动，但仍常有心律失常发作。ICD 电击可使儿茶酚胺激增从而加剧潜在心律失常，但 ICD 治疗仍可用于二级预防。特定患者的左心交感神经去除术也有效果。

获得性长 QT 间期综合征

环境因素可致心脏复极延长并导致 QTc 延长，从而导致早期后除极和尖端扭转型室性心动过速。获得性长 QT 间期综合征的患者可能有遗传学背景，使得其易于受电解质异常（如低钾血症、低镁血症和低钙血症）、心动过缓和延长 QT 间期药物的影响，从而发生 QTc 过度延长和多形性室速。大多数延长 QTc 的药物会阻断由 *KCNE2* 基因编码的延迟整流钾通道（I_{Kr}）的快速部分。已知可延长 QTc 药物已在互联网注册并更新。获得性长 QT 间期综合征的治疗包括纠正生理易感因素和停用不恰当的药物。

离子通道病的基因检测

商业实验室可为先天性 LQTS、Brugada 综合征和 CPVT 提供基因检测。基因检出率从 Brugada 综合征的 25% 到先天性 LQTS 的 80% 不等。目前测定方法有限的敏感性和常见的意义不明的遗传变异仍是挑战。除这些顾虑外，级联筛查或家族成员筛查寻找先证者的致病突变，可有效地用于识别突变携带者。

突变阳性的家族成员可能从预防性治疗中受益。消除突变阴性个体的顾虑也有价值。在进行基因检测之前，应充分告知患者风险、收益和检测的局限性。遗传咨询师应当发挥重要的咨询作用。

有关此专题的深入讨论，请参阅 *Goldman-Cecil Medicine* 第 26 版第 59 章"室性心律失常"。

总结

动作电位形成或传导异常可导致心律失常，心律失常可大致分为缓慢性心律失常（即心动过缓）和快速性心律失常（即心动过速）。心脏细胞动作电位依离子通道的激活的不同（包括快速钠通道、数个钾通道和钙电流），可分为五期。这些电流的异常可致自律性异常和触发活动，并介导病理性快速性心律失常。有临床意义的快速性心律失常主要机制为折返，折返需要功能性或固定传导屏障、缓慢传导区和不同的不应期来启动和维持心律失常。

抗心律失常药物通常按照 Singh-Vaughan Williams 分类法分为四大类。尽管这个分类方法在临床应用，但许多抗心律失常药物具有多种作用，无法清晰分类。一些药物，如腺苷和地高辛，被完全排除在分类之外。Ⅰ类药物通过阻断钠通道使细胞膜传导减慢。Ⅱ类药物或称 β 受体阻滞剂，阻滞心脏 β 受体。Ⅲ类药物延长复极化和 QT 间期。Ⅳ类药物阻断慢钙通道，主要作用于慢反应心肌细胞，如窦房结和房室结。

所有心动过缓都是窦房结功能或房室传导障碍，或两者同时发生异常的结果。窦房结和房室结功能受自主神经张力的强烈影响。静息状态下副交感神经张力占优势，正常的患者在副交感神经张力增高时，尤

AV block may be observed in normal patients due to increased parasympathetic tone, especially during sleep or athletic training. Clinical sinus node dysfunction manifests as one of several syndromes, including sinus bradycardia, chronotropic incompetence, exit block, and bradycardia-tachycardia syndrome due to sinus pauses and bradycardia when concomitant atrial arrhythmias terminate to sinus rhythm.

AV conduction disturbances may occur at the AV nodal level or infranodal level. A block at the level of the AV node tends to be indolent, characterized by gradual progression and competent subsidiary escapes that usually protect the patient from catastrophic bradycardia. This permits asymptomatic patients to be followed clinically for the development of symptoms before intervention. In contrast, second- or third-degree infranodal block at the His bundle, or more commonly at the level of the bundle branches, is potentially malignant and is often not accompanied by stable escape mechanisms. If not managed appropriately, it can cause sudden death. Clues to an infranodal level of block are Mobitz II periodicity, associated bundle branch block, worsening heart block with tachycardia or exercise, and a wide QRS escape rhythm different from the conducted QRS in the setting of a high-degree or third-degree AV block.

Tachycardias are broadly categorized as SVTs, which depend on the atrium and AV conduction system, and ventricular arrhythmias, which depend on the ventricular myocardium. Supraventricular arrhythmias are further categorized as PSVTs, which depend on AV nodal conduction, and intra-atrial arrhythmias, which depend only on atrial tissue and not on AV conduction. The PSVTs include AVNRT and AV reciprocating tachycardia related to WPW syndrome. Intra-atrial arrhythmias include organized atrial arrhythmias, such as focal atrial tachycardia, atrial flutter, macro-reentrant atrial tachycardia, and AF, a common disorganized atrial arrhythmia. Recurrent atrial flutter and AF carry a risk of thromboembolism and, based on risk stratification, should be treated with antithrombotic therapy when appropriate. Catheter ablation has an important role in the management of all supraventricular arrhythmias but remains a second-line strategy for AF, for which success rates are lower and complication rates are higher than for other supraventricular arrhythmias.

Ventricular arrhythmias include isolated ventricular premature beats; short, nonsustained runs of tachycardia; and sustained ventricular arrhythmias. Sustained VT lasts more than 30 seconds or requires intervention before then. It is classified as monomorphic if beats all share a single electrocardiographic morphology, polymorphic if the electrocardiographic morphology is variable, TdP when the morphology is variable and the arrhythmia is associated with pathologic QT prolongation, and VF when the surface ECG continuously varies without distinct QRS complexes. VT is poorly tolerated and is the major cause of cardiac arrest. Although commonly seen in the setting of ischemic heart disease, idiopathic VT may be seen in the absence of structural heart disease.

Antiarrhythmic drugs have not been effective in reducing the risk of SCD after MI. In contrast, ICDs have been shown to improve mortality rates for patients with impaired LV function after an MI and patients with heart failure and impaired LV function with or without coronary disease.

In addition to advanced structural heart disease as a cause for VT, several syndromes may result in VT in the absence of evident structural heart disease. They include the syndrome of idiopathic VT, ARVC, arrhythmogenic RV dysplasia, congenital LQTS, Brugada syndrome, and CPVT. Several of these conditions are familial, and genetic testing and family screening have important roles in their management.

SUGGESTED READINGS

Al-Khatib SM, Stevenson WG, Ackerman MJ, et al.: 2017 AHA/ACC/HRS guideline for management of patients with ventricular arrhythmias and the prevention of sudden cardiac death, *Circulation* 138:e272–e391, 2018.

Calkins H, Hindricks G, Cappato R, et al.: 2017 HRS/EHRA/ECAS/APHRS/SOLAECE expert consensus statement on catheter and surgical ablation of atrial fibrillation, *Heart Rhythm* 14:e275–e444, 2017.

January CT, Wann LS, Calkins H, et al. AHA/ACC/HRS Focused Update of the 2014 AHA/ACC/HRS Guideline for the Management of Patients With Atrial Fibrillation. A Report of the American College of Cardiology/American Heart Association Task Force on Clinical Practice Guidelines and the Heart Rhythm Society 2019:25873.

Priori SG, Wilde AA, Horie M, et al.: Executive summary: HRS/EHRA/APHRS expert consensus statement on the diagnosis and management of patients with inherited primary arrhythmia syndromes, *Heart Rhythm* 10:e85–e108, 2013.

其是睡眠或运动员，也可出现明显的心动过缓和二度房室传导阻滞。窦房结功能障碍临床表现为几种综合征之一，包括窦性心动过缓、变时功能不全、传出阻滞和心动过缓-心动过速综合征。心动过缓-心动过速综合征指当房性心律失常终止恢复窦性心律时，伴随出现的窦性停搏和窦性心动过缓。

房室传导阻滞可发生于房室结水平或结下水平。房室结水平的阻滞倾向于无症状，逐步进展和有效的逸搏机制是其特征，可保护患者免于灾难性心动过缓。这使得无症状的患者可以临床随访直至发生症状进行干预。而在希氏束或更常见的束支水平处发生的二度或三度结下阻滞是潜在恶性的，通常没有稳定的逸搏机制。如果治疗不当，可能会导致猝死。阻滞位于结下水平的线索包括莫氏Ⅱ型阻滞，伴有束支传导阻滞，心动过速或运动时传导阻滞加剧，高度或三度房室传导阻滞时的宽大逸搏 QRS 波群异于房室正常传导时的 QRS 波群。

心动过速大致分类为室上性心动过速和室性心动过速。前者依赖于心房和房室传导系统，后者依赖于心室肌。室上性心律失常进一步分类为依赖于房室结传导的阵发性室上性心动过速（PSVT）和心房内心律失常，后者仅依赖于心房组织而非房室传导。阵发性室上性心动过速包括 AVNRT 和与 WPW 综合征相关的房室折返性心动过速。心房内心律失常包括：规律的房性心律失常，如局灶性房性心动过速、心房扑动、大折返性房性心动过速；常见的无规律的房性心律失常为心房颤动。复发性心房扑动和心房颤动有血栓栓塞的风险，应基于风险分层，在合适时进行抗栓治疗。导管消融在所有室上性心律失常的治疗中均具有重要作用，但相对于其他室上性心律失常，心房颤动导管消融成功率较低，并发症发生率较高，仍然是二线治疗策略（译者：现已成为一线治疗）。

室性心律失常包括单发室性早搏、短阵非持续性室性心动过速和持续性室性心律失常。持续性室性心动过速是指超过 30 s 或在 30 s 内需要干预的室性心动过速。心电图每搏形态一致则为单形性，心电图形态多变则为多形性，若形态多变且与病理性 QT 间期延长相关则为尖端扭转型室性心动过速，当体表心电图连续变化而没有明显的 QRS 波群时则为心室颤动。室性心动过速耐受性差，是心搏骤停的主要原因。虽然常见于缺血性心脏病，但特发性室性心动过速可见于无结构性心脏病的患者。

抗心律失常药物无法降低心肌梗死后心源性猝死风险。相比之下，ICD 已被证明可以降低心肌梗死后左心室功能受损、心力衰竭和左心室功能受损伴/不伴冠状动脉疾病患者的死亡率。

除严重结构性心脏病可导致室性心动过速之外，几种综合征可在无明显结构性心脏病的情况下导致室性心动过速。它们包括特发性室性心动过速、致心律失常型右心室心肌病、致心律失常型右心室发育不良、先天性长 QT 间期综合征、Brugada 综合征和儿茶酚胺敏感性多形性室性心动过速。其中数个疾病为家族性，基因监测和家族筛查在其治疗中具有重要作用。

推荐阅读

Al-Khatib SM, Stevenson WG, Ackerman MJ, et al.: 2017 AHA/ACC/HRS guideline for management of patients with ventricular arrhythmias and the prevention of sudden cardiac death, *Circulation* 138:e272–e391, 2018.

Calkins H, Hindricks G, Cappato R, et al.: 2017 HRS/EHRA/ECAS/APHRS/SOLAECE expert consensus statement on catheter and surgical ablation of atrial fibrillation, *Heart Rhythm* 14:e275–e444, 2017.

January CT, Wann LS, Calkins H, et al. AHA/ACC/HRS Focused Update of the 2014 AHA/ACC/HRS Guideline for the Management of Patients With Atrial Fibrillation. A Report of the American College of Cardiology/American Heart Association Task Force on Clinical Practice Guidelines and the Heart Rhythm Society 2019:25873.

Priori SG, Wilde AA, Horie M, et al.: Executive summary: HRS/EHRA/APHRS expert consensus statement on the diagnosis and management of patients with inherited primary arrhythmia syndromes, *Heart Rhythm* 10:e85–e108, 2013.

Pericardial and Myocardial Disease

Jennifer L. Strande, Panayotis Fasseas

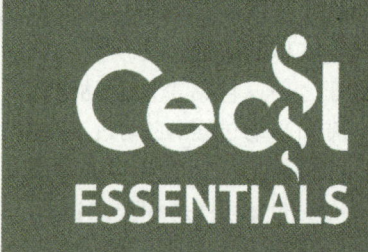

PERICARDIAL DISEASE

The pericardium is a thin, fibrous sac that envelops the heart and consists of two layers: visceral and parietal. The space between these two layers contains a small amount of fluid (15 to 50 mL), which is a plasma ultrafiltrate. The pericardium has mechanical, immunologic, and anatomic barrier functions.

Due to a paucity of randomized trial data and absence of practice guideline statements, the recommendations for assessment and treatment of pericardial disorders in this chapter are largely based on expert opinion and professional consensus.

Acute Pericarditis
Definition and Epidemiology
Acute pericarditis or inflammation of the pericardium has several causes. The exact incidence of acute pericarditis is unknown because a subclinical course is common.

Pathology
About 85% of cases are from idiopathic or viral causes. Less commonly, infection (other than viral), uremia, trauma, metabolic disorders, autoimmune disorders, and neoplastic involvement can also cause pericarditis. Causes of acute pericarditis are listed in Table 9.1.

Clinical Presentation
The classic manifestation of acute pericarditis is severe and sharp chest pain, which is often aggravated by a supine position, inspiration, and cough and relieved by sitting up and leaning forward. The pain is usually substernal and left precordial, and may radiate to the neck, shoulder, and scapular ridge, mimicking that of myocardial ischemia. Chest discomfort may be mild or absent in patients with connective tissue disorders, uremia, or neoplastic involvement. Patients may also have symptoms of low-grade fever, malaise, dyspnea, and less frequently, hiccups (i.e., phrenic nerve irritation).

In the absence of significant pericardial effusion, results of the inspection and palpation of the precordium are normal. A high-pitched, rasping pericardial friction rub is heard on cardiac auscultation in most patients with acute pericarditis. It may have three components corresponding to atrial contraction, ventricular systole, and early diastole, and it is best appreciated at end expiration with the patient leaning forward. It can be intermittent, and serial auscultation is recommended.

Diagnosis
The electrocardiographic (ECG) changes of acute pericarditis typically evolve over days to weeks. The early stage findings are characterized by diffuse ST segment elevation (i.e., concave upward) with upright T waves and PR depression. PR depression occasionally precedes the ST segment elevation. Resolution of the ST elevations is followed by diffuse T wave inversion. These ECG changes are not always seen and serial tracings should be obtained.

The laboratory findings of acute idiopathic pericarditis are not specific and consist of mild elevation of the white blood cell count, sedimentation rate, and C-reactive protein level. If indicated, specific testing for tuberculosis, human immunodeficiency virus (HIV), thyroid disease, or autoimmune disorders is recommended. However, routine performance of viral serologic testing has limited utility. Elevation of serum cardiac biomarkers (e.g., creatine kinase, troponin) reflects involvement of the adjacent myocardium. In uncomplicated acute pericarditis, the chest radiograph and echocardiographic findings are normal. Although not essential for the diagnosis of pericarditis, echocardiography is the diagnostic imaging modality of choice for the detection and determination of the hemodynamic significance of a pericardial effusion.

Treatment
Patients with uncomplicated idiopathic or viral pericarditis can be managed as outpatients. For patients with fever, large pericardial effusions, or elevated levels of cardiac biomarkers and for those with possible secondary causes or immunocompromised status, hospitalization for further investigation and treatment should be considered. Treatment consisting of high-dose nonsteroidal anti-inflammatory drugs (NSAIDs) is usually effective. Colchicine with NSAIDs or as monotherapy provides prompt resolution of symptoms and decreases the recurrence rate. The use of glucocorticoids results in rapid symptomatic improvement. However, glucocorticoids are associated with higher rates of symptomatic recurrence.

Prognosis
Most patients with idiopathic or viral pericarditis have an uneventful clinical course with complete recovery. Possible complications include recurrent pericarditis, cardiac tamponade, and constrictive pericarditis.

Pericardial Effusion and Cardiac Tamponade
Definition and Epidemiology
Pericardial effusion, an abnormal collection of fluid in the pericardial space, is a relatively common and incidental echocardiographic finding that is encountered in approximately 10% of studies. Cardiac tamponade occurs when fluid accumulation results in increased intrapericardial pressure, leading to cardiac compression, impaired ventricular filling, and reduced cardiac output. Accumulation of pericardial fluid can be caused by virtually any type of acute pericarditis. Pericardial effusions due to bacterial pericarditis (including tuberculosis), neoplastic involvement, uremic pericarditis, and trauma have a high incidence of progression to tamponade.

心包和心肌疾病

唐思琪 译 刘震宇 周强 审校 郑金刚 通审

心包疾病

心包是包裹心脏的纤维性薄囊袋状结构，由两层组成：脏层心包和壁层心包。两层之间的间隙内包含少量血浆超滤的液体（15～50 ml）。心包具有机械、免疫和解剖屏障功能。

由于缺少随机临床试验的数据和实践指南的推荐，本章中有关心包疾病评估和治疗的推荐主要基于专家意见和专业共识。

急性心包炎
定义和流行病学

急性心包炎或心包炎症有多种病因。由于亚临床病程的急性心包炎常见，故其确切发生率不详。

病理

约85%的心包炎病例为特发性或病毒性。感染（除病毒之外）、尿毒症、创伤、代谢性疾病、自身免疫性疾病、肿瘤侵犯也可导致心包炎，但较少见。急性心包炎的病因见表9.1。

临床表现

急性心包炎的典型表现为剧烈、尖锐的胸痛，常在仰卧位、吸气、咳嗽时加重，在坐位、身体前倾时缓解。疼痛部位通常位于胸骨后、左侧心前区，可放射至颈部、肩膀、肩胛脊，与心肌缺血性胸痛类似。结缔组织病、尿毒症或肿瘤侵犯所致心包炎可无症状，或仅表现为轻微心前区不适。患者可有低热、乏力、呼吸困难，少数患者可出现呃逆（即膈神经刺激症状）。

当无明显心包积液时，心前区视诊和触诊结果一般正常。大多数急性心包炎患者在心脏听诊时可闻及高频、抓刮样的心包摩擦音。心包摩擦音包括三个组成部分，分别对应心房收缩期、心室收缩期和心室舒张早期，在患者身体前倾、呼气末最易闻及。心包摩擦音可为间歇性，故推荐连续多次听诊。

诊断

急性心包炎的心电图通常在数天至数周内演变。早期表现为广泛ST段抬高（凹面向上），伴T波直立和PR段压低。PR段压低偶尔早于ST段抬高出现。在ST段抬高回落至基线后，可出现广泛T波倒置。上述心电图改变不一定总会出现，需多次复查心电图。

急性特发性心包炎的实验室检查结果缺乏特异性，可出现白细胞计数、红细胞沉降率、C反应蛋白水平轻度升高。如有指征，推荐进行结核、人类免疫缺陷病毒（HIV）、甲状腺疾病或自身免疫性疾病的特异性检查，但常规进行病毒血清学检查的作用有限。血清心脏标志物（如肌酸激酶、肌钙蛋白）升高反映邻近心肌受累。对于无并发症的急性心包炎，胸部X线检查、超声心动图多无异常。尽管超声心动图并非诊断心包炎所必需的影像学检查，但可明确心包积液的有无及其对血流动力学的影响。

治疗

对于无并发症的特发性或病毒性心包炎患者，可在门诊进行处理。对于伴有发热、大量心包积液、心脏标志物水平升高，以及可能存在继发性病因或免疫抑制状态的患者，应考虑住院进行进一步的检查和治疗。包含大剂量非甾体抗炎药（NSAID）的治疗通常有效。秋水仙碱单药或联合NSAID治疗可迅速缓解症状并减少复发。使用糖皮质激素可快速改善症状，但其与更高的症状复发率相关。

预后

多数特发性或病毒性心包炎患者的临床过程平稳，可完全缓解。可能出现的并发症包括复发性心包炎、心脏压塞和缩窄性心包炎。

心包积液和心脏压塞
定义和流行病学

心包积液指心包腔内的液体异常增多，是超声心动图检查时相对常见的附带发现，可见于约10%的超声心动图受检者。当心包腔内液体积聚导致心包腔内压力升高，引起心脏受压、心室充盈受限、心输出量下降时，可发生心脏压塞。所有类型的急性心包炎均可导致心包腔内液体的积聚。细菌性心包炎（包括结核）、肿瘤侵犯、尿毒症性心包炎和创伤所致心包积液进展为心脏压塞的比例较高。

TABLE 9.1	Causes of Pericarditis

Idiopathic
Infectious
  Viral (echovirus, coxsackievirus, adenovirus, cytomegalovirus, hepatitis B virus, Epstein-Barr virus, human immunodeficiency virus)
  Bacterial (*Staphylococcus, Streptococcus,* and *Mycoplasma* species; *Borrelia burgdorferi, Haemophilus influenzae, Neisseria meningitidis*)
  Mycobacterial (*Mycobacterium tuberculosis, Mycobacterium avium-intracellulare*)
  Fungal (*Histoplasma* and *Coccidioides* species)
  Protozoal
Immune or inflammatory
  Connective tissue disease (systemic lupus erythematosus, rheumatoid arthritis, scleroderma)
  Arteritis (polyarteritis nodosa, temporal arteritis)
  Late after myocardial infarction (Dressler syndrome), late postcardiotomy or thoracotomy
Drug induced
  Procainamide, hydralazine, isoniazid, cyclosporine
Trauma or damage to adjacent structures
  Penetrating trauma
  Acute myocardial infarction, cardiac surgery, coronary angioplasty, implantable defibrillators, pacemakers
  Pneumonia
Neoplastic disease
  Primary: mesothelioma, fibrosarcoma, lipoma
  Secondary (metastatic or direct extension): breast, lung, thyroid carcinoma, lymphoma, leukemia, melanoma
Radiation induced
Miscellaneous
  Uremia
  Hypothyroidism
  Gout

Pathology

The hemodynamic consequences of a pericardial effusion depend on the rate of accumulation. The normal pericardium has relatively limited reserve volume. The mechanical properties of the parietal pericardium are such that when stretched, it becomes rapidly inelastic and resistant to further expansion. As a result, rapidly accumulating effusions may result in significant hemodynamic compromise with only 100 to 200 mL of fluid. Conversely, when the accumulation of fluid is slow, the pericardium undergoes adaptive changes and can accommodate large (>1500 mL) effusions without the development of tamponade.

Clinical Presentation

The clinical manifestations of a pericardial effusion depend on the size and rate of fluid accumulation and may range from dyspnea, chest discomfort, and orthopnea to circulatory collapse, pulseless electrical activity, and death. Compression of adjacent structures such as the phrenic nerve and the recurrent laryngeal nerve can result in cough or hiccups and hoarseness, respectively. Compression of the esophagus may cause dysphasia.

A normal cardiac examination is not uncommon in patients with small effusions. With larger effusions, the apical impulse can be decreased or absent, and the cardiac sound may be muffled. In patients with acute pericarditis, disappearance of the pericardial friction rub may indicate development of an effusion. Compression of the left lung base can result in dullness to percussion, egophony, and bronchial breath sounds under the left scapula (i.e., Ewart sign).

Patients with tamponade usually appear to be in distress with tachypnea and tachycardia. The classic physical findings include hypotension, jugular venous distention with an absent *y* descent, and muffled or absent heart sounds. Pulsus paradoxus, a characteristic physical finding, is defined as a greater than 10 mm Hg of inspiratory decline of the systolic blood pressure. This results from the inspiratory decrease of the left ventricular stroke volume and systemic blood pressure. Under normal conditions, the intrathoracic pressure decreases during inspiration, resulting in enhanced right ventricular filling and enlargement. In cases of cardiac tamponade, the total heart volume is fixed, and the right ventricular expansion displaces the interventricular septum toward the left ventricle, with consequent reduction of the left ventricular stroke volume and systemic hypotension. Pulsus paradoxus is not pathognomonic of cardiac tamponade and can be detected in severe chronic obstructive airway disease, pulmonary embolism, bronchial asthma, constrictive pericarditis, and hypovolemic shock.

Diagnosis

The ECG findings of moderate to large pericardial effusions include low-voltage QRS complexes and occasionally electrical (QRS) alternans caused by the heart's swinging motion within the fluid-filled pericardium. The chest radiograph demonstrates an enlarged cardiac silhouette. Transthoracic echocardiography, the imaging modality of choice, provides information regarding the size, location (circumferential vs. loculated), and most importantly, the hemodynamic consequences of the pericardial effusion suggesting tamponade.

The two-dimensional findings of tamponade include right atrial and right ventricular collapse, distention of the inferior vena cava, and evidence of increased ventricular interdependence (Fig. 9.1). Doppler quantification of the mitral and tricuspid inflow velocity respiratory variation is more sensitive than two-dimensional echocardiography for determining the hemodynamic significance of pericardial effusions. Right heart catheterization demonstrates decreased cardiac output, elevated right atrial pressure with diminished or absent *y* descent, and equalization of the cardiac filling pressures (i.e., right atrial, pulmonary wedge, and diastolic pulmonary artery pressures).

Computed tomography (CT) and magnetic resonance imaging (MRI) can accurately identify pericardial effusions and may be used along with echocardiography to assess for loculated effusions, pericardial thickening, and extracardiac structures. A diagnostic pericardiocentesis should be performed for evaluating for bacterial, tuberculous, or malignant causes.

Treatment

Routine drainage of pericardial effusions is unnecessary in the absence of hemodynamic compromise. Cardiac tamponade is a life-threatening emergency requiring urgent drainage of the pericardial effusion. Fluid resuscitation should be initiated to increase preload and filling of the cardiac chambers. Inotropic and vasopressor support has limited utility. Surgical drainage is appropriate and therapeutic for loculated, purulent, and tuberculous effusions and for tissue biopsy.

Fluid should be analyzed for pH, cell count, glucose, protein, cholesterol, triglycerides, and acid-fast bacilli by Gram stain, culture, cytology, and laboratory tests. For patients with chronic, recurring effusions, the surgical creation of a pleuropericardial window provides a long-term solution.

Prognosis

The underlying cause of the pericardial effusion and the availability of effective treatment determine the prognosis.

表9.1 心包炎的病因
特发性
感染性
病毒（埃可病毒、柯萨奇病毒、腺病毒、巨细胞病毒、乙型肝炎病毒、EB 病毒、人类免疫缺陷病毒）
细菌（葡萄球菌、链球菌、支原体属；伯氏疏螺旋体、流感嗜血杆菌、脑膜炎双球菌）
分枝杆菌（结核分枝杆菌、鸟-胞内分枝杆菌）
真菌（组织胞浆菌、球孢子菌属）
原虫
免疫性或炎症性
结缔组织病（系统性红斑狼疮、类风湿关节炎、硬皮病）
动脉炎（结节性多动脉炎、颞动脉炎）
心肌梗死后综合征（Dressler 综合征），心脏切开术后，开胸术后
药物诱导
普鲁卡因胺，肼屈嗪，异烟肼，环孢素
创伤或邻近结构损伤
穿通伤
急性心肌梗死，心脏外科手术，冠状动脉成形术，植入型除颤器，起搏器
肺炎
肿瘤性疾病
原发性：间皮瘤，纤维肉瘤，脂肪瘤
继发性（转移或直接蔓延）：乳腺癌，肺癌，甲状腺癌，淋巴瘤，白血病，黑色素瘤
电离辐射诱导
其他
尿毒症
甲状腺功能减退
痛风

病理

心包积液的血流动力学结果取决于其积聚的速度。正常心包腔的储备容积相对有限。壁层心包的机械特性是，在被拉伸时会迅速失去弹性，从而使得进一步膨胀受限。因此，当心包积液迅速积聚时，仅 100～200 ml 积液即可对血流动力学产生严重影响。反之，当心包积液缓慢积聚时，心包可发生适应性变化，可容纳大量（>1500ml）积液而不发生心脏压塞。

临床表现

心包积液的临床表现取决于积液积聚的量和速度，可表现为呼吸困难、胸部不适、端坐呼吸、循环衰竭、无脉性电活动和死亡。若压迫邻近组织，如膈神经、喉返神经，分别会导致咳嗽或呃逆和声嘶。压迫食管可导致吞咽困难（译者注：原文为言语障碍 dysphasia，此处应为吞咽困难 dysphagia）。

仅有少量心包积液的患者，其心脏体格检查通常正常。当心包积液量大时，心尖搏动可减弱或不能被扪及，听诊心音低钝遥远。对于急性心包炎患者，心包摩擦音消失可能提示心包积液形成。当心包积液压迫左肺底组织时，在左肩胛骨下叩诊可呈浊音，听诊可闻及羊鸣音和支气管呼吸音（即 Ewart 征）。

发生心脏压塞的患者通常表现出痛苦状态伴呼吸急促和心动过速。经典体征包括低血压、颈静脉怒张伴 y 波消失、心音低钝遥远或消失。奇脉是心脏压塞的特征性体征，定义为吸气时收缩压下降超过 10 mmHg。这是因为吸气时左心室每搏输出量及收缩压下降所致。在正常情况下，吸气时胸腔内压下降，导致右心室充盈和扩大。在心脏压塞时，心脏总容量固定，右心室扩张导致室间隔向左心室方向移位，造成左心室每搏输出量下降和体循环低血压。奇脉并非心脏压塞的特异性体征，也可见于重度慢性阻塞性气道疾病、肺栓塞、支气管哮喘、缩窄性心包炎和低血容量性休克。

诊断

中到大量心包积液的心电图表现包括 QRS 波低电压，偶尔可见（QRS 波）电交替，后者为心脏在充满积液的心包腔中摆动所致。胸部 X 线检查可见心影扩大。经胸超声心动图是首选的影像学检查方式，可提供的信息包括心包积液的量、位置（环绕性/局灶性），最重要的是，可以了解其对血流动力学的影响是否引起了心脏压塞。

心脏压塞的二维超声心动图表现包括右心房和右心室塌陷、下腔静脉增宽，以及心室间相互依赖性增加的证据（图 9.1）。多普勒超声在定量测量二尖瓣瓣口和三尖瓣瓣口流入血流速度随呼吸的变化时，比二维超声心动图更为敏感，可以更好地判断心包积液的血流动力学影响。右心导管检查可见心输出量下降、右心房压升高、y 波减弱或消失，不同部位心脏充盈压（即右心房压、肺毛细血管楔压、肺动脉舒张末压）趋于同一水平。

计算机断层成像（CT）和磁共振成像（MRI）可准确识别心包积液，可与超声心动图联用，评价局灶性心包积液、心包增厚和心脏外结构。为了评估细菌性、结核性或恶性肿瘤心包积液病因，应进行诊断性心包穿刺。

治疗

在无血流动力学异常时，无需对心包积液进行常规引流。心脏压塞是危及生命的急症，应进行紧急心包积液引流。应启动液体复苏，以增加前负荷和心腔充盈。正性肌力药和血管加压药的作用有限。外科开窗引流是合理的引流方式，对局灶性、化脓性和结核性心包积液可起到治疗作用，可同时行组织活检。

对于引流出的心包积液，应进行以下分析，包括 pH 值、细胞计数、糖、蛋白质、胆固醇、甘油三酯、抗酸杆菌革兰氏染色、细菌培养、细胞学检查和化验检查。对于慢性、复发性心包积液患者，通过外科方式建立胸腔心包引流窗可行长期引流。

预后

心包积液患者的预后取决于心包积液的病因以及是否有有效的治疗。

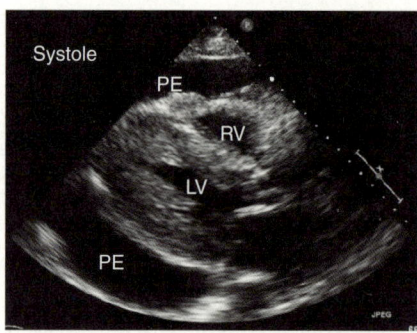 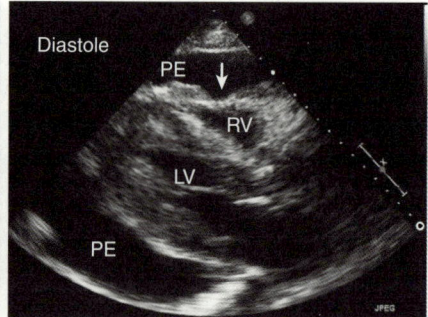

Fig. 9.1 Parasternal long axis echocardiographic views of the right ventricle in systole and diastole show right ventricular diastolic collapse *(arrow)* in a patient with a large, circumferential pericardial effusion. *LV*, Left ventricle; *PE*, pericardial effusion; *RV*, right ventricle.

Constrictive Pericarditis
Definition and Epidemiology
Pericardial constriction is caused by pericardial inflammation and is a condition characterized by a rigid, scarred pericardium that limits diastolic filling of the ventricles, resulting in increased intracardiac pressures. The most common causes are infection, prior cardiac surgery, trauma, and irradiation. Less common causes include connective tissue disorders, uremia, and neoplastic involvement of the pericardium. In developing countries, tuberculous pericarditis is a more common cause of pericardial constriction. Often a specific cause cannot be determined.

Pathology
Constriction is the end result of pericardial inflammation with scarring, fibrosis, calcification, and adhesion of the parietal and visceral layers of the pericardium. Although pericardial thickening is a usual pathologic finding, its absence does not exclude constriction.

Clinical Presentation
In the early stages, symptoms consist of dyspnea, fatigue, decreased exercise tolerance, and lower extremity edema. As the disease progresses, early signs and symptoms may be accompanied by ascites, anasarca, cachexia, and muscle wasting.

Physical examination reveals jugular venous distention with prominent *x* and *y* descents and an increase (or failure to decrease) of central venous pressure with inspiration (i.e., Kussmaul sign). The arterial blood pressure is usually normal, and pulsus paradoxus is absent in most patients. Ascites and hepatomegaly can be prominent with advanced disease. On cardiovascular examination, the apical impulse may be decreased, and the cardiac sounds muffled. An early diastolic sound (i.e., pericardial knock) corresponding to the abrupt cessation of early ventricular diastolic filling is pathognomonic of pericardial constriction, but it is not always detected.

Diagnosis
The diagnosis of pericardial constriction may be challenging and frequently requires the use of multiple imaging modalities. The electrocardiogram may display low QRS voltage, left atrial enlargement, and nonspecific T-wave changes. Atrial fibrillation occurs in one third of cases. The chest radiograph may reveal pleural effusions and pericardial calcification, which are best appreciated in the lateral projection.

Transthoracic echocardiography shows dilation of the inferior vena cava, abnormal interventricular septal motion, and pericardial thickening. Doppler echocardiography demonstrates abnormal respirophasic variations of the pulmonary and hepatic venous flow and mitral valve inflow. CT and MRI can accurately measure pericardial thickness.

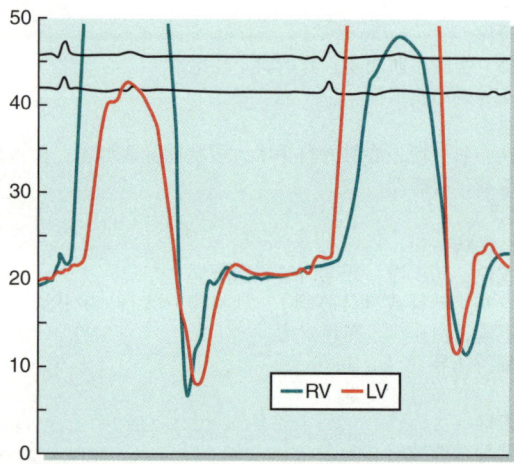

Fig. 9.2 Pressure recordings from a patient with constrictive pericarditis. Simultaneous right ventricular and left ventricular pressure tracings show equalization of diastolic pressure and dip-and-plateau morphology. *LV*, Left ventricle; *RV*, right ventricle.

Cardiac catheterization is essential in the diagnosis of pericardial constriction and differentiation from restrictive cardiomyopathy (RCM). The right atrial pressure tracing shows prominent *x* and *y* descents with equalization of the end-diastolic atrial and ventricular pressures. The ventricular pressure tracings show a rapid early diastolic filling of the ventricles, with abrupt cessation in middle and end diastole due to the finite volume of the rigid pericardium (i.e., dip-and-plateau morphology or the square root sign) (Fig. 9.2). Enhanced ventricular interdependence demonstrated by simultaneous measurement of right and left ventricular pressures during respiration is a more specific finding of pericardial constriction.

Treatment
Medical therapy with sodium restriction and diuretics is of limited efficacy and is only appropriate in patients who are not surgical candidates due to comorbidities. Pericardiectomy is the only definitive treatment for constrictive pericarditis.

Prognosis
Pericardiectomy is associated with substantial operative risk that depends on the extent of cardiac involvement and existence of comorbid conditions. Successful pericardial resection leads to resolution of the symptoms of constriction over a period of weeks to months. For patients who are not surgical candidates, the prognosis is poor.

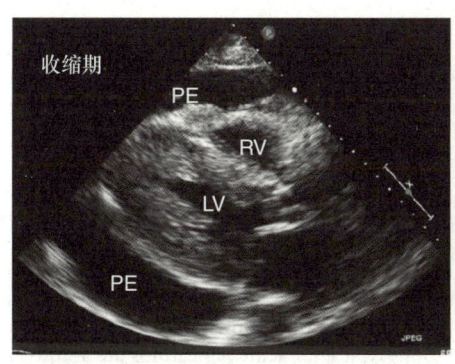
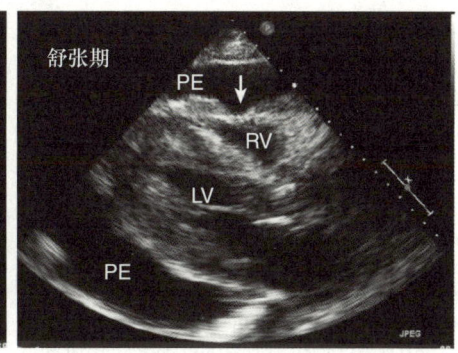

图 9.1 超声心动图胸骨旁长轴切面，对比一例大量环绕性心包积液患者的收缩期及舒张期右心室形态，显示右心室于舒张期塌陷（箭头）。LV，左心室；PE，心包积液；RV，右心室

缩窄性心包炎

定义和流行病学

心包缩窄由心包炎症所致，其特征性表现为心包僵硬、瘢痕化，限制心室充盈，进而导致心腔内压力升高。最常见的病因为感染、既往心脏手术、创伤和放射性损伤。少见的病因包括结缔组织病、尿毒症和肿瘤侵犯心包。在欠发达国家，结核性心包炎是缩窄性心包炎最常见的病因。在很多情况下，缩窄性心包炎的特定病因通常无法确定。

病理

心包缩窄是心包炎症的最终结果，表现为心包的瘢痕化、纤维化、钙化，以及壁层和脏层心包的粘连。尽管心包增厚是常见的病理表现，但无心包增厚并不能排除心包缩窄的存在。

临床表现

在早期阶段，症状包括呼吸困难、乏力、活动耐量下降和下肢水肿。随疾病进展，在早期症状和体征的基础上，可出现腹水、全身水肿、恶病质和肌肉萎缩。

体格检查可见颈静脉怒张伴明显加深的 x 波和 y 波，吸气时中心静脉压升高或无下降（即 Kussmaul 征）。动脉血压通常正常，多数患者无奇脉。在疾病晚期，患者可出现明显的腹水和肝脏肿大。在心脏查体方面，心尖搏动可以减弱、心音低钝遥远。舒张早期的额外心音（即心包叩击音）为心室充盈在舒张早期因心包缩窄而突然中止所致，是心包缩窄的特征性体征，但并非在所有患者中均可闻及。

诊断

心包缩窄的诊断难度大，通常需要借助多种影像学检查方法。心电图可见 QRS 波低电压、左心房扩大及非特异 T 波改变。1/3 的患者会出现心房颤动。胸部 X 线检查可见胸腔积液和心包钙化，后者在侧位投照时易见。

经胸超声心动图可见下腔静脉增宽、室间隔运动异常及心包增厚。多普勒超声心动图可见肺静脉和肝静脉血流以及二尖瓣流入血流随呼吸时相异常的变化。CT 和 MRI 可准确测量心包的厚度。

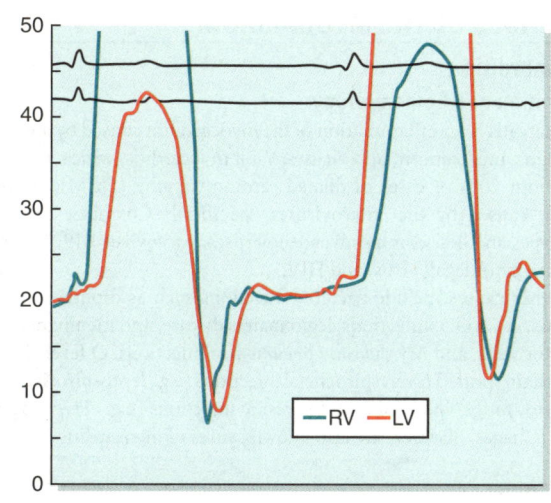

图 9.2 缩窄性心包炎患者的压力曲线记录。右心室和左心室的同步压力监测显示舒张期压力趋于同一水平和呈现下陷-高平形态。LV，左心室；RV，右心室

心导管检查对于诊断心包缩窄，并与限制型心肌病（RCM）进行鉴别至关重要。右心房压力监测显示加深的 x 波和 y 波，伴舒张末期心房和心室压力趋于同一水平。心室压力监测显示，在舒张早期，心室快速充盈，在舒张中、晚期，心室充盈受限于僵硬心包的有限容积而突然中止（即呈现下陷-高平形态或平方根征）（图 9.2）。通过同步测量右心室和左心室的压力，可见呼吸时心室间的相互依赖性增加，是心包缩窄更为特异性的表现。

治疗

包括限盐和利尿剂的内科治疗效果有限，且仅适用于因合并症而无法进行手术的患者。心包切除术是缩窄性心包炎唯一确定的治疗方法。

预后

心包切除术具有相当的手术风险，取决于心脏受累的范围和合并症情况。心包被成功切除后，心包缩窄的症状可在数周至数月内好转。对于无法进行手术的患者，其预后极差。

Effusive Constrictive Pericarditis

Effusive constrictive pericarditis is characterized by a pericardial effusion and a noncompliant or fibrotic parietal and visceral pericardium. Although it may result from any type of pericardial inflammation, it is usually seen after cardiac surgery or radiation injury. It likely represents a transition stage between acute pericarditis with effusion and pericardial constriction. It shares the clinical and hemodynamic features of both conditions.

Typically, drainage of the effusion does not result in resolution of symptoms, and the central venous and right atrial pressures remain elevated. In the early stage of the disease, patients may respond to prolonged treatment with NSAIDs. However, visceral and parietal pericardiectomy is often required. For a deeper discussion of this topic, please see Chapter 68, "Pericardial Diseases," in *Goldman-Cecil Medicine*, 26th Edition.

DISEASES OF THE MYOCARDIUM
Myocarditis
Definition and Epidemiology

Myocarditis is an inflammation of the myocardium caused by a variety of toxins, medications, and viruses. Viral myocarditis, which accounts for about 20% of cases of dilated cardiomyopathy (DCM), is commonly caused by the enteroviruses, specifically Coxsackie group B serotypes and, less commonly, adenoviruses, parvovirus B19, hepatitis C virus, cytomegalovirus, and HIV.

Other causes include bacterial infections such as diphtheria, brucellosis, clostridial infections, legionnaires disease, and meningococcal, streptococcal, and *Mycoplasma pneumoniae* infections. Q fever, Rocky Mountain spotted fever, spirochetal infections (e.g., leptospirosis, Lyme disease), fungal infections, and parasitic infections (e.g., *Trypanosoma cruzi* [Chagas' disease]) are also known causes of myocarditis.

Pathology

The pathogenesis of viral myocarditis is thought to begin with direct viral invasion of the myocardium and subsequent immunologic activation. Normal cellular and antibody-mediated immune responses lead to viral clearing and myocardial healing. However, a few patients go on to develop DCM and heart failure due to an abnormal immune response that furthers myocardial damage. The exact mechanisms are unknown, but they involve cytokines, autoantibodies, and possibly other processes associated with persistent, low-level viral replication in myocytes, leading to myocyte atrophy, myocyte apoptosis, and adverse remodeling of the ventricles. In nonviral infections, the damage is attributed to the bacterial toxins or abnormal immune responses, and in parasitic infections, it is largely immune mediated.

Multiple chemicals and drugs can lead to myocardial inflammation by direct effect or as part of a hypersensitivity reaction. Some of the common causes include cocaine, chemotherapeutics (e.g., daunorubicin, doxorubicin), and antibiotics.

Giant cell myocarditis is a rare disorder of uncertain origin, but it can be rapidly fatal. It is usually associated with ventricular arrhythmias and progressive, severe heart failure. Multinucleated giant cells seen on myocardial biopsy are pathognomonic.

Clinical Presentation

The clinical manifestations range from asymptomatic ECG abnormalities to cardiogenic shock. Patients report heart failure symptoms, including exercise intolerance, shortness of breath, fluid retention, and persistent fatigue. In the setting of viral myocarditis, they often report a viral prodrome, including fever, myalgia, fatigue, respiratory symptoms, or gastroenteritis that precedes the heart failure symptoms. Patients are often tachycardic and hypotensive. They may have an elevated jugular venous pressure, S_3 gallop, crackles, and peripheral edema. Myocarditis can masquerade as an acute coronary syndrome.

Diagnosis

Testing is performed to determine a possible infectious cause. Rising viral titers are often seen in cases of viral myocarditis. Serum cardiac enzymes (e.g., troponin, creatine kinase) are measured when myocarditis is suspected. Sinus tachycardia and nonspecific ST- and T-wave abnormalities are common ECG findings. When the pericardium is also involved by the inflammatory process, diffuse ST-segment elevations typical for acute pericarditis are also seen. Ventricular ectopy is common, and atrioventricular conduction defects are seen in myocarditis associated with Lyme disease.

Echocardiography is recommended in the initial diagnostic evaluation to identify ventricular remodeling, including increasing chamber size and ventricular systolic dysfunction. Cardiac MRI is a promising technique to detect myocardial inflammation and injury based on small, observational clinical studies.

Transvenous endomyocardial biopsy should be performed only when there is rapid deterioration of the clinical condition. Histopathologic abnormalities such as infiltrating white cells (i.e., macrophages, lymphocytes, and eosinophils), evidence of myocardial damage, and interstitial fibrosis help to establish acute myocarditis, but the determination is subject to significant intraobserver and interobserver variability. Often the biopsy does not provide a conclusive diagnosis. The endomyocardial biopsy is helpful in diagnosing giant cell myocarditis (i.e., multinucleated giant cells are seen) or hypersensitivity myocarditis (i.e., eosinophilic infiltrate is seen). Polymerase chain reaction testing can detect specific viral genomes in the myocardium.

Treatment

Supportive care is the mainstay of treatment. A few patients with fulminant or acute myocarditis require an intensive level of hemodynamic support and aggressive pharmacologic intervention similar to that for patients with advanced heart failure.

After initial hemodynamic stabilization, treatment should follow current American College of Cardiology and American Heart Association (ACC/AHA) recommendations for the management of left ventricular systolic dysfunction. Treatment includes β-adrenergic blockers, angiotensin-converting enzyme inhibitors, aldosterone receptor blockers, and diuretics.

No evidence-based guided therapy for viral myocarditis has been established. Clinical trials of various forms of antiviral or immunosuppressive therapy (e.g., prednisone, cyclosporine, azathioprine, intravenous immunoglobulin, interferon immunoadsorption) have not resulted in conclusive evidence of benefit. Treatment of nonviral myocarditis is aimed at eradication of the specific infectious agent. For Chagas' disease, treatment with antiprotozoal therapy, if initiated early in the course of infection, may be beneficial.

Hypersensitivity myocarditis and myocarditis associated with toxins respond to withdrawal of the offending agent. Immunosuppressive therapy has been effective in giant cell myocarditis.

Prognosis

The diverse clinical presentations and causes of myocarditis have limited the understanding of its natural history. It is thought that one third of the patients fully recover, one third of the patients have some sequelae in the form of left ventricular systolic dysfunction but are stable on medical therapy, and one third of patients progress to advanced heart failure. Patients who progress to chronic DCM have 5-year survival rates of less than 50%.

渗出性缩窄性心包炎

渗出性缩窄性心包炎的特征为同时存在心包积液和顺应性差或纤维化的壁层和脏层心包。尽管任何类型的心包炎症均可导致本病，但常出现于心脏手术后或放射性损伤后。渗出性缩窄性心包炎可能代表了急性心包炎伴心包积液和心包缩窄之间的过渡阶段。因此，其兼具两种疾病的临床和血流动力学特征。

对心包积液进行引流通常不能缓解症状，中心静脉压和右心房压仍旧升高。在疾病的早期阶段，患者可能对长期的 NSAID 治疗有反应。但患者大多需要接受脏层心包或壁层心包切开术治疗。关于此专题的更深入讨论，请参见 Goldman-Cecil Medicine 第 26 版第 68 章 "心包疾病"。

心肌疾病

心肌炎

定义和流行病学

心肌炎是由各种毒物、药物和病毒引起的心肌炎症。病毒性心肌炎占扩张型心肌病（DCM）病因的 20%，常由肠道病毒，尤其是柯萨奇病毒 B 组所致，少数由腺病毒、细小病毒 B19、丙型肝炎病毒、巨细胞病毒和 HIV 所致。

其他病因包括细菌感染，如白喉杆菌、布鲁氏菌、艰难梭菌、军团病、脑膜炎球菌、链球菌、肺炎支原体感染。Q 热、落基山斑点热、螺旋体（如钩端螺旋体病、莱姆病）感染、真菌感染、寄生虫［如美洲锥虫病（Chagas 病）］感染也是心肌炎的已知病因。

病理

病毒性心肌炎的发病机制被认为始于病毒直接侵犯心肌，随后激活免疫反应。正常由细胞及抗体介导的免疫反应可清除病毒和修复心肌。然而，一部分患者因为异常的免疫反应导致进一步的心肌损伤，进而发展为 DCM 和心力衰竭。其具体机制尚不明确，但细胞因子、自身抗体，以及与病毒在心肌细胞内持续低水平复制相关的其他过程可引起心肌细胞的萎缩、凋亡和心室的不良重构。在非病毒感染的患者中，心肌损伤与细菌毒素或异常的免疫反应有关，在寄生虫感染的患者中，心肌损伤多为免疫因素所介导。

多种化学品和药物可通过直接作用或参与超敏反应导致心肌炎症。常见原因包括可卡因、化疗药物（如柔红霉素、阿霉素）和抗生素。

巨细胞性心肌炎是一种病因不明的罕见疾病，可快速导致死亡。巨细胞性心肌炎常导致室性心律失常以及进行性加重的重度心力衰竭。在心肌活检标本中可见多核巨细胞是其特征性的表现。

临床表现

从无症状性心电图异常至心源性休克的各种临床表现均可出现。患者可有心力衰竭症状，包括活动耐量下降、气短、液体潴留和持续乏力。病毒性心肌炎患者在发病前常有前驱病毒感染症状，包括在心力衰竭症状前出现发热、肌肉酸痛、乏力、呼吸道症状或胃肠炎。患者常出现心动过速和低血压。查体可见颈静脉压升高、S_3 奔马律、湿啰音和外周水肿。心肌炎可出现类似急性冠脉综合征的表现。

诊断

需要完善检查以确定可能的感染原因。病毒滴度升高常见于病毒性心肌炎患者。当疑诊心肌炎时，需要进行血清心肌酶学检测（如肌钙蛋白、肌酸激酶）。窦性心动过速、非特异性 ST 段和 T 波异常是常见的心电图表现。当炎症过程累及心包时，可出现广泛 ST 段抬高，即急性心包炎的典型心电图表现。室性异位心律常见，房室传导阻滞可见于莱姆病相关的心肌炎。

推荐将超声心动图用于对心室重构的初步诊断性评估，包括心腔扩大和心室收缩功能异常。基于小样本量的观察性临床研究，心脏 MRI 是检查心肌炎症和损伤很有前景的技术。

当临床情况快速恶化时，应进行经静脉心内膜心肌活检。组织学异常，如白细胞（即巨噬细胞、淋巴细胞和嗜酸性粒细胞）浸润、心肌损伤相关表现，以及间质纤维化有助于确定急性心肌炎的诊断，但判读结果在观察者内部和观察者之间的变异性较大。活检结果经常无法提供明确的诊断。心内膜心肌活检对于诊断巨细胞性心肌炎（可见多核巨细胞）或过敏性心肌炎（可见嗜酸性粒细胞浸润）具有重要价值。聚合酶链反应可在心肌内检测到特定的病毒基因。

治疗

支持性治疗是心肌炎的主要治疗方法。一部分暴发性或急性心肌炎患者需要强力的血流动力学支持，及与晚期心力衰竭治疗相似的、积极的药物干预。

在血流动力学初步稳定后，应遵循目前美国心脏病学会（ACC）和美国心脏协会（AHA）针对左心室收缩功能障碍的推荐进行治疗。治疗包括 β 受体阻滞剂、血管紧张素转换酶抑制剂、醛固酮受体拮抗剂和利尿剂。

针对病毒性心肌炎，目前尚无基于循证医学证据的治疗方案。各种抗病毒治疗或免疫抑制治疗（如泼尼松、环孢素、硫唑嘌呤、静脉注射免疫球蛋白、干扰素免疫吸附治疗）的临床试验并未得出可使患者获益的明确证据。针对非病毒性心肌炎的治疗以清除特定病原体为主要目的。对于 Chagas 病，如果在感染早期启动抗原虫治疗，可能对患者有益。

过敏性心肌炎和毒物相关心肌炎在脱离致病物后可好转。免疫抑制治疗对于巨细胞性心肌炎有效。

预后

心肌炎的临床表现和病因的多样性限制了对其自然病程的认识。目前认为，1/3 患者可完全康复，1/3 患者可出现后遗症，表现为左心室收缩功能障碍，但在药物治疗后病情稳定，1/3 患者进展为晚期心力衰竭。进展为慢性 DCM 患者的 5 年生存率不足 50%。

TABLE 9.2 Cardiomyopathies

Disorder	Description and Cause
Dilated cardiomyopathy	Dilation and impaired systolic function of the left or both ventricles
Familial (genetic)	Known or unknown genetic mutations
Nonfamilial	Viral myocarditis, nonviral infective myocarditis, idiopathic (immune) myocarditis
	Toxins (drugs, alcohol)
	Pregnancy (peripartum cardiomyopathy)
	Nutritional (thiamine deficiency [beriberi], vitamin C deficiency [scurvy], selenium deficiency)
	Endocrine (diabetes mellitus, hyperthyroidism, hypothyroidism, hyperparathyroidism, pheochromocytoma, acromegaly)
	Autoimmune (rheumatoid arthritis, systemic lupus erythematosus, dermatomyositis)
	Tachycardia induced
Hypertrophic cardiomyopathy	Left and/or right ventricular hypertrophy, often asymmetrical (usually more prominent hypertrophy of the interventricular septum)
Familial (genetic)	Mutations of sarcoplasmic proteins (several hundred described)
	Metabolic storage diseases of the myocyte
Restrictive cardiomyopathy	Restrictive filling of the ventricles; ventricles are usually small, atria are markedly enlarged
Familial (genetic)	Mutations of sarcomeric proteins
	Familial amyloidosis (transthyretin, apolipoprotein)
	Hemochromatosis
	Desminopathy, pseudoxanthoma elasticum, glycogen storage diseases
	Unknown genetic mutations
Nonfamilial	Amyloidosis, sarcoidosis, carcinoid, scleroderma
	Endomyocardial fibrosis (hypereosinophilic syndrome, idiopathic, chromosomal defect, drugs)
	Radiation, metastatic cancer, anthracycline toxicity
Arrhythmogenic right ventricular	Progressive fibrofatty replacement of the right and, to a lesser degree, left ventricular cardiomyopathy
Familial	Unknown gene mutation
	Mutations of intercalated disk protein, cardiac ryanodine receptor, transforming growth factor-β3
Unclassified Cardiomyopathies	
Takotsubo (stress-induced) cardiomyopathy	Transient dilation and dysfunction of the distal parts of the left ventricle (apical ballooning) in the setting of a stressful situation; usually resolves within weeks
Left ventricular noncompaction	Characterized by prominent left ventricular trabeculae and deep intertrabecular recesses; familial in most cases, caused by arrest in the normal embryogenesis of the heart; apex and periapical regions of the left ventricle most affected; some patients remain asymptomatic, but others develop left ventricular dilation and systolic dysfunction
Cardiomyopathies associated with muscular dystrophies and neuromuscular disorders	Duchenne-Becker muscular dystrophy, Emery-Dreifuss muscular dystrophy, myotonic dystrophy, Friedreich's ataxia, neurofibromatosis, tuberous sclerosis
Ion channelopathies	Disorders caused by mutations in genes encoding ionic channel proteins; not considered cardiomyopathies because they are not associated with typical structural changes of the heart but rather manifest with electrical dysfunction; some classifications include these disorders as cardiomyopathies: long QT syndrome, short QT syndrome, Brugada syndrome, catecholaminergic polymorphic ventricular tachycardia

Cardiomyopathies

Cardiomyopathies are a heterogeneous group of diseases in which the major structural abnormality is limited to the myocardium. The four main cardiomyopathic groups are dilated, hypertrophic, restrictive, and arrhythmogenic right ventricular cardiomyopathy. Atrophic cardiomyopathy is a newer recognized group. Familial (genetic) and nonfamilial (acquired) forms of the diseases have been described.

Dilated Cardiomyopathy

Definition and epidemiology. Cardiac enlargement and systolic dysfunction in DCM result from a wide spectrum of genetic, inflammatory, toxic, and metabolic causes (Table 9.2), although most cases are idiopathic. Abnormal loading conditions such as hypertension, valvular disease, or coronary artery disease can lead to similar structural and functional changes; these conditions are not considered to be part of the DCM group and are discussed elsewhere.

Most cases are thought to result from acute viral myocarditis, a process described earlier. Exposures to cardiac toxins such as chemotherapeutic agents, alcohol, cocaine, and radiation, along with deficiency of nutrients such as thiamine (causes beriberi), vitamin C (causes scurvy), carnitine, selenium, phosphate, and calcium, can cause DCM. Peripartum cardiomyopathy is a rare cause of DCM that can develop during the last month of pregnancy and up to 6 months after delivery. The pathogenesis of this peripartum cardiomyopathy is not completely understood, and it is a diagnosis of exclusion. Risk factors include older maternal age, being African American, and having multiple pregnancies. Prolonged periods of supraventricular or ventricular tachycardia can lead to idiopathic DCM (i.e., tachycardia-induced cardiomyopathy). The structural and functional changes usually reverse after the rapid heart rhythm is controlled.

Familial forms of DCM may be responsible for 20% to 30% of cases. Specific mutations involve genes that encode proteins of the sarcomere, cytoskeleton, nuclear membrane, and mitochondria; many mutations remain unknown. The mode of inheritance is typically autosomal dominant, but it can be an X-linked or mitochondrial pattern.

Pathology. Marked enlargement of all four cardiac chambers is typical of DCM, although the disease sometimes is limited to the left

表 9.2　心肌病	
疾病	描述和病因
扩张型心肌病	左心室或双心室扩张及收缩功能障碍
家族性（遗传性）	已知或未知的基因突变
非家族性	病毒性心肌炎，非病毒感染性心肌炎，特发性（免疫性）心肌炎
	毒物（毒品、酒精）
	妊娠（围产期心肌病）
	营养性［维生素 B_1 缺乏（脚气病）、维生素 C 缺乏（坏血病）、硒缺乏］
	内分泌（糖尿病、甲状腺功能亢进、甲状腺功能减退、甲状旁腺功能亢进、嗜铬细胞瘤、肢端肥大症）
	自身免疫性（类风湿关节炎、系统性红斑狼疮、皮肌炎）
	心动过速诱导性
肥厚型心肌病	左心室和（或）右心室肥厚，常为非对称性（通常室间隔肥厚更为明显）
家族性（遗传性）	肌质蛋白的编码基因突变（已知数百种）
	心肌细胞代谢性贮积病
限制型心肌病	心室充盈受限；心室通常较小，心房明显扩大
家族性（遗传性）	肌节蛋白的编码基因突变
	家族性淀粉样变性（甲状腺素转运蛋白、载脂蛋白）
	血色病
	结蛋白病，弹性纤维假黄瘤，糖原贮积症
	未知的基因突变
非家族性	淀粉样变性，结节病，类癌，硬皮病
	心内膜心肌纤维化（嗜酸性粒细胞增多综合征、特发性、染色体缺陷、药物）
	放射性损伤，转移癌，蒽环类药物毒性
致心律失常型右心室心肌病	右心室和左心室（相对少见）心肌逐渐被纤维脂肪组织所替代
家族性	未知的基因突变
	闰盘蛋白、心脏雷诺定受体、转化生长因子 $β_3$ 的编码基因突变
未分类的心肌病	
Takotsubo（应激性）心肌病	在应激情况下，左心室远段短暂性扩张和功能障碍（心尖部呈球样）；通常在数周内缓解
左心室致密化不全	以左心室肌小梁增粗及肌小梁间隙加深为特征；多数病例为家族性，因胚胎期心肌致密化过程停滞所致；以左心室心尖和心尖周围受累为主；一部分患者可无症状，另一部分患者可出现左心室扩张和收缩功能障碍
与肌营养不良和神经肌肉疾病相关的心肌病	Duchenne-Becker 肌营养不良，Emery-Dreifuss 肌营养不良，强直性肌营养不良，Friedreich 共济失调，神经纤维瘤病，结节硬化症
离子通道病	由离子通道的编码基因突变导致；不考虑为心肌病，因为不伴有典型的心脏结构改变，而是表现为心脏电活动紊乱；有些分类标准将以下疾病纳入心肌病：长 QT 间期综合征，短 QT 间期综合征，Brugada 综合征，儿茶酚胺敏感性多形性室性心动过速

心肌病

心肌病是一组异质性疾病，其主要结构异常局限于心肌。心肌病主要分为 4 类：扩张型、肥厚型、限制型和致心律失常型右心室心肌病。萎缩性心肌病是一类新近被认识的心肌病。心肌病也可分为家族性（遗传性）和非家族性（获得性）。

扩张型心肌病

定义和流行病学　DCM 时的心脏扩大和收缩功能障碍源于广泛的病因，涵盖遗传性、炎症性、中毒性和代谢性因素（表 9.2），但多数病例为特发性。心脏负荷异常，如高血压、瓣膜病或冠状动脉疾病可导致相似的心脏结构和功能改变；但这些疾病不属于 DCM，将在其他章节进行讨论。

目前认为，多数 DCM 病例继发于前述的急性病毒性心肌炎。暴露于心脏毒性物质（如化疗药、酒精、可卡因）、电离辐射，以及营养物质缺乏［如维生素 B_1 缺乏（导致脚气病）、维生素 C 缺乏（导致坏血病）、肉毒碱缺乏、硒缺乏、磷缺乏、钙缺乏］，均可导致 DCM。围产期心肌病是 DCM 的罕见病因，可于妊娠最后 1 个月至分娩后 6 个月期间发病。围产期心肌病的发病机制尚未完全阐明，在排除其他疾病后才可诊断。其危险因素包括高龄产妇、非裔美国人、多胎妊娠。长期室上性或室性心动过速可导致特发性 DCM（即心动过速诱导的心肌病）。在快速心脏节律被控制后，心脏的结构及功能改变通常可逆转。

家族性 DCM 占所有病例的 20%～30%。特定突变涉及编码肌节、细胞骨架、核膜和线粒体蛋白的基因；很多突变尚未明确。遗传方式多为常染色体显性遗传，但也可以为 X 染色体连锁遗传或线粒体遗传。

病理　所有四个心腔均明显扩大是 DCM 的典型表现，尽管有时心腔扩大局限于左侧或右侧心腔。心腔

or right chambers. The dilation is out of proportion to the ventricular thickness. Histology reveals evidence of myocyte degeneration with irregular hypertrophy and atrophy of myofibers with often extensive interstitial and perivascular fibrosis.

Clinical presentation. DCM usually manifests with symptoms of heart failure such as fatigue, weakness, dyspnea, and edema. In some patients, the presenting episode is related to arrhythmia or an embolic event. On physical examination, signs of decreased cardiac output are often found, including cool extremities, narrow pulse pressure, and tachycardia. The cardiac examination reveals a laterally displaced apex. An S_3 gallop is common, along with murmurs of mitral and tricuspid regurgitation. Pulmonary edema manifests as auscultatory crackles over the lung fields, and breath sounds may be diminished if there are pleural effusions. In some patients, the clinical features of right ventricular heart failure may predominate, with jugular venous distention hepatomegaly, ascites, and peripheral edema.

Diagnosis. Standard diagnostic procedures include a chest radiograph, an electrocardiogram, serum markers, and echocardiography. The radiograph shows cardiomegaly, pulmonary venous congestion, and pleural effusions. The electrocardiogram may reveal enlargement of the heart chambers along with other nonspecific ST- and T-wave abnormalities. Serum B-type natriuretic peptide (BNP) levels are elevated.

Echocardiography provides a comprehensive evaluation of ventricular size and function and valvular function, and it can show a ventricular thrombus. Similar information can be obtained with MRI.

A complete work-up should rule out ischemic, valvular, and hypertensive heart disease as the cause of myocardial dysfunction, and it should include evaluation for potentially reversible causes of DCM (e.g., alcohol, nutritional deficiencies). Myocardial biopsy may be considered if the cause of DCM is in question. In patients with a strong family history, a referral for genetic testing should be considered.

Treatment. Potential reversible causes of DCM should be addressed (e.g., alcohol cessation, correction of nutritional deficiencies, removal of cardiotoxic agents). Treatment should follow current ACC/AHA recommendations for the management of left ventricular systolic dysfunction and include β-adrenergic blockers, angiotensin-converting enzyme inhibitors, aldosterone receptor blockers, and diuretics.

Patients with idiopathic DCM who have persistent, moderate to severe symptoms of heart failure and a QRS duration longer than 120 milliseconds may benefit from cardiac resynchronization therapy with a biventricular pacemaker. Survival of patients with a left ventricular ejection fraction less than 35% despite maximal medical management is improved with the use of implantable cardioverter-defibrillators (ICDs). Patients with limiting heart failure symptoms despite use of the previously described therapies may be considered for heart transplantation or support with a left ventricular assist device.

Prognosis. The prognosis of patients with DCM depends on the response to medical therapy. Some patients have a significant improvement in symptoms and cardiac function, but in others, the disease is progressive and associated with a high mortality rate.

Hypertrophic Cardiomyopathy

Definition and epidemiology. Hypertrophic cardiomyopathy (HCM) is a disease state characterized by left ventricular hypertrophy with nondilated ventricular chambers in the absence of an apparent cause for hypertrophy (e.g., hypertensive disease, aortic stenosis). This is a relatively common genetic disease (1 case in 500 people in the general population) with autosomal dominant inheritance, although spontaneous mutations have been described. More than 1400 mutations identified among at least eight genes encoding proteins of the cardiac sarcomere have been described, with mutations of the β-myosin heavy chain being the most common.

Pathology. The main pathophysiologic abnormalities seen in HCM are left ventricular outflow obstruction, diastolic dysfunction, mitral regurgitation, and arrhythmias. Obstruction of left ventricular outflow occurs in roughly one half of the patients. During systole, the hypertrophied septum bulges into the left ventricular outflow tract, creating a gradient between the lower part of the left ventricular cavity and the left ventricular outflow. This causes high-velocity turbulent flow through the narrowed path, which results in a suction force (i.e., Venturi effect) that pulls the anterior leaflet of the mitral valve into the outflow tract. This worsens the obstruction and causes mitral regurgitation. Diastolic dysfunction from impaired relaxation properties of the abnormal myocardium causes marked elevation of left ventricular filling and pulmonary venous pressures, pulmonary congestion, and limitation in cardiac output. Patients with HCM are also predisposed to supraventricular and ventricular arrhythmias.

Clinical presentation. HCM is a heterogeneous cardiac disease with a diverse course and clinical manifestations. Most patients probably do not suffer sequelae from this disease during their lifetimes. When the disease does result in complications, there are three relatively discrete but not mutually exclusive clinical manifestations: sudden cardiac death due to unpredictable ventricular tachyarrhythmia, most commonly in young asymptomatic patients (<35 years of age); heart failure characterized by exertional dyspnea (with or without chest pain) that may progress despite preserved systolic function and sinus rhythm; and atrial fibrillation that associates with various degrees of heart failure.

Heart failure symptoms result from the dynamic obstruction to left ventricular outflow and diastolic dysfunction. The most frequent symptom is dyspnea on exertion, followed by ischemic chest pain due to the increased oxygen demand by the hypertrophied ventricle and elevated wall tension that reduces blood flow to the subendocardium. Abnormalities of the structure of small myocardial arteries in HCM can contribute to myocardial ischemia. Presyncope or syncope can result from outflow tract obstruction and an inability to increase cardiac output during exertion or from arrhythmias that can be triggered by exertion. In some, sudden death caused by ventricular arrhythmia is the initial manifestation of the disease.

Physical examination findings include pulsus bisferiens, a brisk initial upstroke in pulse followed by a midsystolic dip corresponding to the development of left ventricular outflow tract obstruction, followed by another rise in late systole. Cardiac examination may reveal a forceful and sustained apical impulse, an audible S_4 gallop, and a harsh crescendo-decrescendo systolic murmur best heard along the left sternal border with radiation to the base of the heart.

Patients may also have an apical holosystolic murmur of mitral regurgitation. The intensity of the murmur of HCM varies with changing degrees of obstruction. This can be observed with physiologic or pharmacologic maneuvers that change preload (i.e., left ventricular filling) or contractility. The intensity of the murmur increases with a Valsalva maneuver, with assuming a standing position, and after administration of nitroglycerin or inotropic drugs. The intensity of the murmur decreases with squatting, volume loading, and administration of β-blockers.

Diagnosis. Clinical diagnosis is made most commonly with echocardiography and increasingly with cardiac MRI. The diagnosis is based on a maximal left ventricular wall thickness of 15 mm or more; a wall thickness of 13 to 14 mm is considered borderline. The diagnosis can be made in the setting of other compelling information (e.g., family history of HCM). Genetic testing is available to confirm the diagnosis and to screen family members.

Treatment. The ACC/AHA hypertrophic cardiomyopathy guideline recommends tailored therapy based on the individual patient. For

扩张与心室壁厚度不成比例。组织学表现为心肌细胞变性伴不规则肥大，以及肌纤维萎缩常伴广泛间质和血管周围纤维化。

临床表现 DCM通常表现为心力衰竭的症状，如乏力、虚弱、呼吸困难和水肿。一些患者的症状发作与心律失常或栓塞事件相关。体格检查时，常可见心输出量下降的体征，包括肢端凉、脉压小和心动过速。心脏查体可扪及心尖左移。听诊常可闻及S_3奔马律，以及二尖瓣和三尖瓣的反流性杂音。发生肺水肿时，肺野听诊可闻及湿啰音，如有胸腔积液，可有呼吸音减低。一些患者以右心衰竭的症状为突出表现，伴颈静脉怒张、肝脏肿大、腹水和外周水肿。

诊断 标准诊断流程包括胸部X线检查、心电图、血清标志物和超声心动图。胸部X线检查可见心脏扩大、肺静脉淤血和胸腔积液。心电图可提示心腔扩大，伴其他非特异性的ST段和T波异常。血清B型利钠肽（BNP）升高。

超声心动图可全面评估心室的大小、功能和瓣膜功能，可显示心室血栓。MRI亦可获取相同的信息。

完整的诊断流程应除外缺血性、瓣膜性和高血压性心脏疾病所导致的心肌功能障碍，并包括对潜在可逆性DCM病因（如酒精、营养缺乏）的评估。对于病因不明者，可考虑行心肌活检。对于有强烈家族史的患者，可考虑行基因检测。

治疗 应纠正DCM潜在的可逆性病因（如戒酒、纠正营养缺乏、停用心脏毒性药物）。应遵循目前ACC/AHA针对左心室收缩功能障碍的推荐进行治疗，包括β受体阻滞剂、血管紧张素转换酶抑制剂、醛固酮受体拮抗剂和利尿剂。

对于持续存在中重度心力衰竭症状、QRS波时限超过120 ms的特发性DCM患者，可能从植入双心室起搏器行心脏再同步化治疗中获益。对于虽经最大化药物治疗但左心室射血分数仍小于35%的患者，植入式心脏复律除颤器（ICD）可提高生存率。对于虽经上述治疗但仍存在限制性心力衰竭症状的患者，可考虑行心脏移植或左心室辅助装置支持治疗。

预后 DCM患者的预后取决于其对药物治疗的反应。一部分患者的症状及心功能可明显改善，但其他患者的病情呈进行性恶化，死亡率高。

肥厚型心肌病

定义和流行病学 肥厚型心肌病（HCM）是以左心室肥厚、不伴心室腔扩张、无明显导致心室肥厚的病因（如高血压、主动脉瓣狭窄）为特征的心肌病。HCM是一种相对常见的遗传病（一般人群的患病率为1/500），为常染色体显性遗传，也有自发突变的报道。目前已发现至少8个编码心脏肌节蛋白基因超过1400余种突变，以编码β-肌球蛋白重链基因最为常见。

病理 HCM主要病理生理异常为左心室流出道梗阻、舒张功能障碍、二尖瓣反流和心律失常。左心室流出道梗阻可见于约1/2的患者。在收缩期，肥厚的室间隔凸入流出道，使左心室腔较低部位与左心室流出道之间产生压力阶差。血流经过狭窄通道时形成高速湍流，产生吸力（即Venturi效应）将二尖瓣前叶吸入流出道，从而加重梗阻并造成二尖瓣反流。病变心肌的松弛能力下降可导致舒张功能障碍，进而造成左心室充盈压及肺静脉压升高、肺水肿和心输出量下降。HCM患者也易出现室上性和室性心律失常。

临床表现 HCM是一种异质性疾病，临床表现和疾病过程多种多样。多数患者可能终生不受其影响。当HCM出现并发症时，可出现三类相对独立但不互相排斥的临床表现：由难以预测的室性心动过速所导致的心源性猝死，最常见于年轻的无症状患者（年龄<35岁）；以劳力性呼吸困难（伴或不伴胸痛）为特征的心力衰竭，即使收缩功能正常且为窦性心律，病情仍可进行性加重；心房颤动，伴不同程度的心力衰竭。

心力衰竭的症状与左心室流出道的动态梗阻和舒张功能障碍有关。最常见的症状为劳力性呼吸困难，其次为缺血性胸痛（其机制为心室肥厚导致心肌需氧量增加，以及室壁张力增高造成心内膜下心肌血流量减少）。HCM心肌内小动脉的结构异常可参与心肌缺血的发病机制。先兆晕厥或晕厥的原因包括流出道梗阻、运动中心输出量无法增加或运动诱发的心律失常。在一些患者中，室性心律失常所导致的猝死是HCM的首发表现。

体格检查时可扪及双峰脉，即脉搏的初始波形曲线迅速上升，随后因左心室流出道梗阻导致波形曲线在收缩中期回落，随后波形曲线在收缩晚期再次上升。心脏查体可见有力的、持续性的、抬举样心尖搏动，听诊可闻及S_4奔马律，以及胸骨左缘粗糙、递增-递减型、向心底部放射的收缩期杂音。

患者可出现因二尖瓣反流所导致的心尖部全收缩期杂音。HCM杂音的强度随梗阻程度的变化而不同。此点可通过生理性或药理性因素改变前负荷（即左心室充盈）或收缩力来观察。Valsalva动作、站立位、应用硝酸甘油或强心药可使杂音增强。下蹲位、扩充血容量，以及应用β受体阻滞剂可使杂音减弱。

诊断 HCM的临床诊断多基于超声心动图，基于心脏MRI者逐渐增多。诊断依据为最大左心室室壁厚度≥15mm；左心室室壁厚度13～14 mm可考虑为临界增厚。如存在其他具有说服力的证据，也可做出诊断（如HCM家族史）。基因检测可用于明确诊断和进行家系筛查。

治疗 ACC/AHA肥厚型心肌病指南推荐针对每个患者进行个体化治疗。对于无症状患者，可考虑应用

Fig. 9.3 (A to C) Schematic diagrams of a septal myectomy. (From Nishimura RA, Holmes DR Jr: Clinical practice: hypertrophic obstructive cardiomyopathy, N Engl J Med 350:1320-1327, 2004.)

asymptomatic patients, the usefulness of β-blockade and verapamil may be considered. For patients symptomatic with dyspnea or angina, β-blockers and verapamil are recommended. If patients remain symptomatic, it is reasonable to add disopyramide to a β-blocker or verapamil.

Nonpharmacologic therapies should be considered in patients with considerable symptoms despite medical management. Septal reduction therapy is recommended only for patients with severe drug-refractory symptoms and left ventricular outflow tract obstruction (Fig. 9.3). Use of ICD therapy for prevention of sudden death is guided by the perceived risk for ventricular arrhythmias in individual patients. Some of the characteristics that have been associated with this risk are prior cardiac arrest or sustained ventricular tachycardia; great (>30 mm) ventricular wall thickness; syncope, especially if exertional or recurrent; and a first-degree relative with sudden cardiac death. Certain genotypes appear to convey an increased risk of sudden cardiac death. Patients with HCM should be excluded from most competitive sports and should avoid strenuous exercise.

Prognosis. The clinical course of HCM varies. Sudden cardiac death is the leading cause of mortality. Heart failure symptoms may gradually progress and patients who are unresponsive to conventional therapy may require heart transplantation.

Restrictive Cardiomyopathies

Definition and epidemiology. RCM is an uncommon form of cardiomyopathy characterized by impaired ventricular filling of nondilated ventricles. RCM can be genetic or acquired. Causes include infiltrative disorders (e.g., amyloidosis, sarcoidosis, Gaucher's disease, Hurler's syndrome, fatty infiltration), storage diseases (e.g., hemochromatosis, Fabry's disease, glycogen storage disease), other disorders (e.g., hypereosinophilic syndrome, carcinoid heart disease), drugs (e.g., serotonin, methysergide, ergotamine), and cancer treatment (e.g., irradiation, chemotherapy).

Pathology. In the purest form of the disease, the atria are disproportionately dilated compared with the normal ventricular size, and the left ventricle has normal or near-normal systolic function in the absence of hypertrophy. Histology is normally nondistinctive and can reveal normal findings or nonspecific degenerative changes, including myocyte hypertrophy, disarray, and degrees of interstitial fibrosis.

Clinical presentation. Patients often have symptoms and signs of pulmonary and systemic congestion. The most common symptoms include dyspnea, palpitations, fatigue, weakness, and exercise intolerance due to poor cardiac output. As central venous pressure continues to increase in advanced cases, there may be hepatosplenomegaly, ascites, and anasarca. The chest radiograph shows atrial enlargement, pulmonary venous congestion, and pleural effusions.

Diagnosis. The diagnosis of RCM should be considered for patients with predominantly right ventricular heart failure without evidence of cardiomegaly or systolic dysfunction. The correct diagnosis often is not made until months or years after symptom onset. Constrictive pericarditis can mimic RCM and establishing the correct diagnosis can be challenging. Distinctive features of the two disorders are described in Table 9.3.

Treatment. Treatment of RCM focuses on alleviating the symptoms of heart failure. Diuretics are used for decongestion, but intravascular depletion may compromise ventricular filling and lead to reduced cardiac output and hypotension. Supraventricular tachyarrhythmias are poorly tolerated. In patients with conduction system disease such as advanced atrioventricular block, a permanent pacemaker may be indicated. Specific therapies for underlying disorders include chemotherapy in amyloidosis, phlebotomy and iron chelation therapy in hemochromatosis, and steroids in sarcoidosis and endomyocardial fibrosis.

Prognosis. The course of RCM depends on the pathology, and treatment is often unsatisfactory. In the adult population, the prognosis usually is poor, with progressive deterioration and death due to low-output heart failure.

Arrhythmogenic Right Ventricular Cardiomyopathy

Definition and epidemiology. Arrhythmogenic right ventricular cardiomyopathy (ARVC) is an autosomal dominant disease characterized by specific myocardial pathology. The estimated prevalence of ARVC is about 1 case in 2000 to 5000 people, and it has a male predominance.

Pathology. The myocardium of the right ventricular free wall is progressively replaced by fibrous and adipose tissue. Right ventricular function is abnormal, with regional akinesis or dyskinesis or global right ventricular dilation and dysfunction.

Clinical presentation. The disease typically manifests in young adults as palpitations, dizziness or syncope, or sudden cardiac death. Symptoms of right ventricular failure are rare, despite evidence of right ventricular dysfunction on imaging studies.

Diagnosis. The clinical diagnosis of ARVC is suggested by integration of the information from the clinical presentation (e.g., arrhythmias), electrocardiogram, family history, and imaging studies. When available, histologic examination of the right ventricle confirms the diagnosis. The resting electrocardiogram may be normal, but common abnormalities include incomplete or complete right bundle branch block, the so-called epsilon waves that follow the QRS complex, and inverted T waves in the precordial leads. Right ventricular dilation and systolic dysfunction can be seen with echocardiography and MRI. The latter modality can also show myocardial fat.

Treatment. Treatment consists of ICD therapy to prevent sudden cardiac death, but the indications for implantation are not well defined. Antiarrhythmics and radiofrequency ablation of ventricular tachycardia are used in patients with frequent arrhythmias, but they have not been shown to reduce the risk of sudden cardiac death.

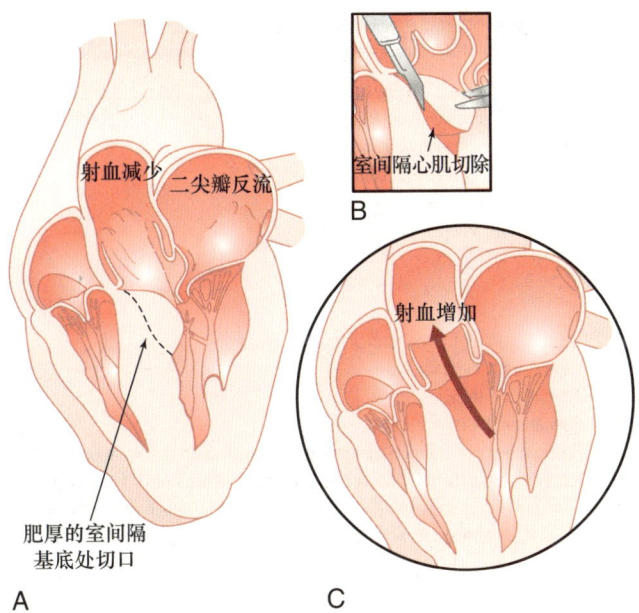

图 9.3 （A 至 C）室间隔心肌切除术示意图（引自 Nishimura RA, Holmes DR Jr: Clinical practice: hypertrophic obstructive cardiomyopathy, N Engl J Med 350: 1320-1327, 2004.）

β 受体阻滞剂和维拉帕米。对于出现呼吸困难或心绞痛症状的患者，推荐应用 β 受体阻滞剂和维拉帕米。如患者仍有症状，在 β 受体阻滞剂或维拉帕米的基础上加用丙吡胺是合理的治疗策略。

对于接受药物治疗后仍有明显症状的患者，应考虑非药物治疗。室间隔减容治疗仅推荐用于存在药物难以控制的严重症状且存在左心室流出道梗阻的患者（图 9.3）。应用 ICD 预防猝死需要基于每个患者发生室性心律失常的风险来决策。与猝死风险相关的因素包括：既往发生过心脏停搏或持续性室性心动过速；严重的左心室肥厚（> 30 mm）；晕厥，尤其是劳力诱发或反复发作的晕厥；一级亲属发生心源性猝死。某些基因型似乎与心源性猝死风险的增加有关。HCM 患者应禁忌参加大多数竞技体育运动，避免剧烈运动。

预后　HCM 的病程各不相同。心源性猝死是第一位的死亡原因。心力衰竭的症状可进行性加重，接受传统治疗后效果不佳的患者可能需要接受心脏移植。

限制型心肌病

定义和流行病学　限制型心肌病（RCM）是一种少见类型的心肌病，以心室舒张功能障碍、无心室扩张为特征。RCM 可分为遗传性和获得性。RCM 的病因包括浸润性疾病［如淀粉样变性、结节病、戈谢（Gaucher）病、赫尔勒（Hurler）综合征、脂肪浸润］，贮积病（如血色病、法布里病、糖原贮积症），其他疾病（如嗜酸性粒细胞增多综合征、类癌性心脏病），药物（如 5-羟色胺、二甲基麦角新碱、麦角胺）和癌症治疗（如放疗、化疗）。

病理　最典型的病例表现如下：与正常大小的心室相比，心房不成比例地扩大，左心室收缩功能正常或接近正常，且无心肌肥厚。组织学表现无特异性，可表现为正常或非特异性的退行性改变，包括心肌细胞肥大、排列紊乱和不同程度的间质纤维化。

临床表现　患者常出现肺循环和体循环淤血的症状和体征。最常见的症状包括呼吸困难、心悸、乏力、衰弱和因心输出量下降所导致的活动耐量减低。在晚期病例，由于中心静脉压持续升高，可出现肝脾肿大、腹水和全身性水肿。胸部 X 线检查可见心房扩大、肺静脉淤血和胸腔积液。

诊断　对于以右室心力衰竭为主要表现，但无心脏扩大或收缩功能障碍证据的患者，应考虑 RCM 的诊断。患者通常在症状出现数月至数年后，才得以确诊。缩窄性心包炎可与 RCM 的临床表现相似，二者常难以鉴别。两者的鉴别特征见表 9.3。

治疗　RCM 治疗的重点在于缓解心力衰竭症状。利尿剂被用于改善充血症状，但血管内容量不足又可使心室充盈减少，导致心输出量下降和低血压。患者对室上性快速性心律失常的耐受性差。对于合并传导系统异常，如高度房室传导阻滞的患者，可能需要植入永久起搏器。针对病因的特异性治疗包括针对淀粉样变性的化疗、针对血色病的放血治疗和铁螯合治疗，以及针对结节病和心内膜心肌纤维化的糖皮质激素治疗。

预后　RCM 的病程取决于病理类型，治疗效果多不满意。由于低输出量性心力衰竭导致的病情进行性恶化和死亡，成年患者的预后通常很差。

致心律失常型右心室心肌病

定义和流行病学　致心律失常型右心室心肌病（ARVC）是一种常染色体显性遗传病，以特异性病理改变为特征。ARVC 的患病率估计为 1/(2000 ~ 5000)，多见于男性。

病理　右心室游离壁的心肌逐渐被纤维或脂肪组织所替代。右心室功能异常，可见节段性无运动或运动减低，或整个右心室扩张和功能障碍。

临床表现　ARVC 通常在年轻成年人中发病，表现为心悸、头晕或晕厥，或心源性猝死。尽管影像学检查可见右心室功能障碍的证据，但出现右心室心力衰竭的症状少见。

诊断　整合来自于临床表现（如心律失常）、心电图、家族史和影像学检查的信息，有助于提示 ARVC 的临床诊断。如果具备条件，右心室的心肌组织学检查可确定诊断。静息心电图可能正常，常见的异常包括不完全性或完全性右束支传导阻滞、QRS 波后出现 epsilon 波，以及胸前导联 T 波倒置。超声心动图和 MRI 可见右心室扩张和收缩功能障碍。MRI 可同时显示心肌脂肪。

治疗　包括植入 ICD 以预防心源性猝死，但植入的指征尚未明确。抗心律失常药和针对室性心动过速的射频消融被用于心律失常频繁发作的患者，但无证据显示其可降低心源性猝死的风险。疑诊或确诊 ARVC

TABLE 9.3 Differentiation of Restrictive Cardiomyopathy From Constrictive Pericarditis

Type of Evaluation	Restrictive Cardiomyopathy	Constrictive Pericarditis
Physical examination	Kussmaul sign present Apical impulse may be prominent Regurgitant murmurs are common	Kussmaul sign may be present Apical impulse usually not palpable Pericardial knock may be present
Electrocardiography	Low QRS voltage (especially in amyloidosis) Pseudoinfarction pattern Bundle branch blocks AV conduction disturbances Atrial fibrillation	Low QRS voltage Repolarization abnormalities
Chest radiography		Calcification of the pericardium may be present
Echocardiography	Marked enlargement of the atria Increased wall thickness (especially in amyloidosis)	Atria usually of normal size Normal wall thickness Pericardial thickening may be seen
Doppler echocardiography	Restrictive mitral inflow (dominant E wave with short deceleration time) No significant variation (<10%) of transvalvular velocities with respiration Reversal of forward flow in hepatic veins during inspiration	Restrictive mitral inflow (dominant E wave with short deceleration time) Increased velocity of RV filling and decreased velocity of LV filling with inspiration; opposite with expiration; variation in velocity exceeds 15% Reversal of forward flow in hepatic veins during expiration
Cardiac catheterization	Prominent atrial *x* and *y* descents (w sign) Dip-and-plateau appearance of ventricular diastolic pressure Diastolic pressures increased but not equalized; LV diastolic pressure higher than RV diastolic pressure	Prominent atrial *x* and *y* descents (w sign) Dip-and-plateau appearance of ventricular diastolic pressure Increase and equalization of diastolic pressures Discordance of RV and LV peak systolic pressures (with inspiration, RV systolic pressure increases and LV systolic pressure decreases)
Endomyocardial biopsy	May reveal specific cause of restrictive cardiomyopathy	No specific findings on endomyocardial biopsy Pericardial biopsy may reveal abnormality
Computed tomography, magnetic resonance imaging		Pericardial thickening

AV, Atrioventricular; *LV,* left ventricular; *RV,* right ventricular.

Patients with a probable or definite diagnosis of ARVC should be excluded from competitive sports.

Prognosis. The prognosis for these patients remains uncertain.

Unclassified Cardiomyopathies

Some cardiomyopathies that do not fit the current categories are described in Table 9.2.

For a deeper discussion of this topic, please see Chapter 54, "Diseases of the Myocardium and Endocardium," in Goldman-Cecil Medicine, 26th Edition.

SUGGESTED READINGS

Elliott P, Andersson B, Arbustini E, et al: Classification of the cardiomyopathies: a position statement from the European Society of Cardiology Working Group on Myocardial and Pericardial Diseases, Eur Heart J 29:270–276, 2008.

Gersh BJ, Maron BJ, Bonow RO, et al: 2011 ACCF/AHA guideline for the diagnosis and treatment of hypertrophic cardiomyopathy: a report of the American College of Cardiology Foundation/American Heart Association Task Force on Practice Guidelines. Developed in collaboration with the American Association for Thoracic Surgery, American Society of Echocardiography, American Society of Nuclear Cardiology, Heart Failure Society of America, Heart Rhythm Society, Society for Cardiovascular Angiography and Interventions, and Society of Thoracic Surgeons, J Am Coll Cardiol 58:e212–e260, 2011.

Kindermann I, Barth C, Mahfoud F, et al: Update on myocarditis, J Am Coll Cardiol 59:779–792, 2012.

Maron BJ, Ackerman MJ, Nishimura RA, et al: Task Force 4: HCM and other cardiomyopathies, mitral valve prolapse, myocarditis, and Marfan syndrome, J Am Coll Cardiol 45:1340–1345, 2005.

Maron BJ, Towbin JA, Thiene G, et al: Contemporary definitions and classification of the cardiomyopathies: an American Heart Association scientific statement from the Council on Clinical Cardiology, Heart Failure and Transplantation Committee; Quality of Care and Outcomes Research and Functional Genomics and Translational Biology Interdisciplinary Working Groups; and Council on Epidemiology and Prevention, Circulation 113:1807–1816, 2006.

Yancy CW, Jessup M, Bozkurt B, et al: 2013 ACCF/AHA guideline for the management of heart failure: a report of the American College of Cardiology Foundation/American Heart Association Task Force on Practice Guidelines, Circulation 128:1810–1852, 2013.

表 9.3 限制型心肌病与缩窄性心包炎的鉴别

评估方法	限制型心肌病	缩窄性心包炎
体格检查	存在 Kussmaul 征 心尖搏动可能被明显扪及 常可闻及反流性杂音	可能存在 Kussmaul 征 心尖搏动通常不能被扪及 可能闻及心包叩击音
心电图	QRS 波低电压（尤其见于淀粉样变性） 假性心肌梗死改变 束支传导阻滞 房室传导阻滞 心房颤动	QRS 波低电压 复极异常
胸部 X 线		可能存在心包钙化
超声心动图	心房明显扩大 室壁增厚（尤其见于淀粉样变性）	心房通常大小正常 室壁厚度正常 可能存在心包增厚
多普勒超声心动图	跨二尖瓣血流受限（E 峰增高伴 E 峰减速时间缩短） 跨瓣血流速度不随呼吸出现明显变化（< 10%） 吸气时肝静脉前向血流呈反向流动	跨二尖瓣血流受限（E 峰增高伴 E 峰减速时间缩短） 吸气时右心室充盈加快、左心室充盈减慢；呼气时情况相反；血流速度的变化率超过 15% 呼气时肝静脉前向血流呈反向流动
心导管检查	心房 x 波和 y 波加深（w 征） 心室舒张压呈下陷-高平形态 舒张压增加但不趋于一致；左心室舒张压高于右心室舒张压	心房 x 波和 y 波加深（w 征） 心室舒张压呈下陷-高平形态 舒张压增加且趋于一致 右心室和左心室峰值收缩压不一致（吸气时右心室收缩压增加，左心室收缩压下降）
心内膜心肌活检	可发现限制型心肌病的特异性病因	心内膜心肌活检无特异性发现 心包活检可发现异常
计算机断层成像，磁共振成像		心包增厚

的患者应禁忌参加竞技体育运动。

预后 此类患者的预后尚不明确。

未分类的心肌病

不符合现有分类标准的一些心肌病列于表 9.2。

❖ 有关此专题的深入讨论，请参阅 *Goldman-Cecil Medicine* 第 26 版第 54 章，"心肌和心内膜疾病"。

推荐阅读

Elliott P, Andersson B, Arbustini E, et al: Classification of the cardiomyopathies: a position statement from the European Society of Cardiology Working Group on Myocardial and Pericardial Diseases, Eur Heart J 29:270–276, 2008.

Gersh BJ, Maron BJ, Bonow RO, et al: 2011 ACCF/AHA guideline for the diagnosis and treatment of hypertrophic cardiomyopathy: a report of the American College of Cardiology Foundation/American Heart Association Task Force on Practice Guidelines. Developed in collaboration with the American Association for Thoracic Surgery, American Society of Echocardiography, American Society of Nuclear Cardiology, Heart Failure Society of America, Heart Rhythm Society, Society for Cardiovascular Angiography and Interventions, and Society of Thoracic Surgeons, J Am Coll Cardiol 58:e212–e260, 2011.

Kindermann I, Barth C, Mahfoud F, et al: Update on myocarditis, J Am Coll Cardiol 59:779–792, 2012.

Maron BJ, Ackerman MJ, Nishimura RA, et al: Task Force 4: HCM and other cardiomyopathies, mitral valve prolapse, myocarditis, and Marfan syndrome, J Am Coll Cardiol 45:1340–1345, 2005.

Maron BJ, Towbin JA, Thiene G, et al: Contemporary definitions and classification of the cardiomyopathies: an American Heart Association scientific statement from the Council on Clinical Cardiology, Heart Failure and Transplantation Committee; Quality of Care and Outcomes Research and Functional Genomics and Translational Biology Interdisciplinary Working Groups; and Council on Epidemiology and Prevention, Circulation 113:1807–1816, 2006.

Yancy CW, Jessup M, Bozkurt B, et al: 2013 ACCF/AHA guideline for the management of heart failure: a report of the American College of Cardiology Foundation/American Heart Association Task Force on Practice Guidelines, Circulation 128:1810–1852, 2013.

10

Other Cardiac Topics

Jinnette Dawn Abbott, Sena Kilic

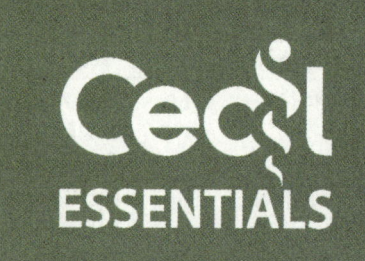

CARDIAC DISEASE IN PREGNANCY

Pregnancy is associated with dramatic changes in the cardiovascular system that may result in significant hemodynamic stress to the patient with underlying heart disease. During a normal pregnancy, plasma volume increases an average of 50%, beginning in the first trimester and peaking between the 20th and 24th weeks of gestation. This change is accompanied by increases in stroke volume, heart rate, and, accordingly, cardiac output. In addition, a concomitant fall in systemic vascular resistance and mean arterial pressure occurs because of the effects of gestational hormones on the vasculature and the creation of a low-resistance circulation in the pregnant uterus and placenta. During labor, uterine contractions result in a transient increase of up to 500 mL of blood in the central circulation, resulting in further increases in stroke volume and cardiac output. After delivery, intravascular volume and cardiac output increase further as compression of the inferior vena cava by the gravid uterus is relieved and extravascular fluid is mobilized. The American Heart Association guidelines for the prevention of cardiovascular disease in women identified pregnancy complications as risk factors for cardiovascular disease in women. Hypertensive disorders of pregnancy and gestational diabetes mellitus are independently associated with increased 10-year cardiovascular risk.

Most women with cardiovascular disease can complete a pregnancy and delivery with proper follow-up. While cardiac disease may sometimes be manifested for the first time in pregnancy, the symptoms and signs that may mimic cardiac disease often accompany the usual hemodynamic changes of pregnancy, including fatigue, reduced exercise tolerance, lower-extremity edema, distention of the neck veins, S_3 gallop, and new systolic murmurs. Differentiating symptoms produced by cardiac disease from those attributable to a normal pregnancy can be difficult. Under such circumstances, echocardiography can be a safe and helpful noninvasive test to assess cardiac structure and function in the pregnant patient.

Certain cardiac conditions, including pulmonary hypertension, cardiomyopathy, valvular heart disease and connective tissue disorders including Marfan syndrome with a dilated aortic root, are associated with a high risk for cardiovascular complications and maternal death and require special consideration and counseling. The risk for cardiac complications during pregnancy depends on the maternal conditions as summarized in Table 10.1.

Specific Cardiac Conditions
Valvular Heart Disease

Due to the declining incidence of rheumatic heart disease in Western countries, valvular heart disease is infrequent in North America but remains prevalent in developing countries. Bicuspid aortic stenosis and mitral stenosis are the most common valvular diseases encountered during pregnancy. When aortic stenosis complicates pregnancy, it is usually secondary to a congenital bicuspid aortic valve whereas mitral stenosis is the most common rheumatic valvular disease encountered during pregnancy. These valvular conditions tend to worsen during pregnancy due to the increased cardiac output and tachycardia. Congestive heart failure may develop as the pregnancy progresses and may be worsened by the onset of atrial fibrillation. Careful echocardiographic assessment is recommended, and the cornerstone of therapy for the symptomatic patient is β-blockade. In patients with symptoms refractory to medical therapy aortic balloon valvuloplasty for aortic stenosis or mitral balloon valvotomy for mitral stenosis can be considered. Mitral and aortic regurgitation are usually well tolerated in pregnancy provided the regurgitation is no more than moderate in severity, the woman is symptom-free before pregnancy, and the left ventricular function is normal.

Prosthetic valves. When selecting a prosthetic valve for women of childbearing age, careful consideration has to be made with regards to the type of valve. Mechanical valves have greater longevity but routinely involve the use of warfarin, which is associated with a higher chance of fetal loss, placental hemorrhage, and prosthetic valve thrombosis. Tissue valves are less thrombogenic but tend to degenerate after an average of 10 years, necessitating a re-operation, which carries certain operative risks including mortality.

There is no universal consensus on the management of a pregnancy when the mother has a mechanical valve prosthesis. Prepregnancy counseling should include a detailed discussion of the risks to the patient. During pregnancy, increased platelet adhesiveness, increased concentration of clotting factors, and decreased fibrinolysis increase the risk of maternal valve thrombosis and thromboembolism. Unfractionated heparin, used subcutaneously or intravenously, is begun in the first trimester, as soon as pregnancy is diagnosed, to minimize fetal exposure to the teratogenic effects of warfarin. It is usually continued until week 13 or 14 of pregnancy, when fetal embryogenesis is complete, after which warfarin is resumed. Continuing heparin throughout pregnancy has been shown to increase valve thrombosis risk to 33%. Low-molecular-weight heparin is an alternative to unfractionated heparin but its use remains controversial with no large prospective studies or evidence base to support its use and therapeutic monitoring.

Marfan Syndrome

Pregnant women with Marfan syndrome are at increased risk for aortic dissection and rupture, especially during the third trimester and the first postpartum month. Pregnancy is contraindicated in women with an aortic root diameter greater than 40 mm. Periodic echocardiographic surveillance every 6 to 8 weeks is recommended to monitor the mother's aortic root size and treatment with β-adrenergic blockers is recommended. Vaginal delivery is safe in patients with Marfan syndrome with an aortic diameter less than 40 mm. To

其他心脏疾病

周强 译 马业新 刘震宇 审校 郑金刚 通审

妊娠期心脏疾病

对于有基础心脏病的孕妇，妊娠相关心血管系统的骤然变化可能带来巨大的血流动力学挑战。正常妊娠时孕妇血容量平均增加50%，这一变化从妊娠早期开始、在妊娠20～24周时达峰，相应伴有每搏输出量、心率以及心输出量的增加。此外，妊娠激素作用于血管，在妊娠子宫和胎盘中形成低阻力循环，体循环血管阻力和平均动脉压也随之下降。在产程中，子宫收缩引起中心循环血容量一过性增加高达500 ml，导致每搏输出量和心输出量进一步增加。分娩后，子宫对下腔静脉的压迫得到缓解、血管外液转移到血管内，血容量和心输出量随之进一步增加。《美国心脏病学会女性心血管疾病防治指南》将妊娠并发症确定为女性心血管疾病的高危因素，妊娠高血压和妊娠糖尿病是10年心血管风险增加的独立危险因素。

通过适当的产前随访，大多数患有心血管疾病的孕妇能够安然度过妊娠和分娩。心脏疾病有时在妊娠期才首次暴露出来，出现疲劳、运动耐力降低、下肢水肿、颈静脉扩张、S_3奔马律和新发收缩期杂音等症状和体征，但这些表现也可能是妊娠期常见的血流动力学改变，而不是心脏病所致。因此，仅凭症状、体征难以准确鉴别究竟是心脏病还是正常妊娠状态所致，鉴于此，可采用超声心动图来安全、有效、无创地评估心脏结构和功能。

某些心脏疾病，包括肺动脉高压、心肌病、心脏瓣膜病等，以及结缔组织病，如马方综合征所致主动脉根部扩张，与心血管并发症和孕产妇死亡高风险相关，需要特别考虑和咨询。表10.1总结了孕产妇的妊娠期心脏并发症风险。

特定心脏疾病

心脏瓣膜病

西方国家的风湿性心脏病发病率不断下降，因此心脏瓣膜病在北美地区并不常见，但在发展中国家仍然很普遍。二叶主动脉瓣狭窄和二尖瓣狭窄是妊娠期最常面对的心脏瓣膜病。主动脉瓣狭窄使得妊娠情况复杂化，通常继发于先天性二叶主动脉瓣，而二尖瓣狭窄是妊娠期最常见的风湿性心脏瓣膜病。由于心输出量增加和心动过速，这些瓣膜疾病在妊娠期间往往会恶化。充血性心力衰竭可能随着妊娠的进程而出现，并可能因心房颤动的发作而恶化。推荐进行详细超声心动图评估。症状性患者治疗的基石是β受体阻滞剂。对药物治疗无效的症状性患者，可考虑对主动脉瓣狭窄患者行主动脉瓣球囊成形术、对二尖瓣狭窄患者行二尖瓣球囊成形术。如果二尖瓣或主动脉瓣反流不超过中度、妊娠前无症状且左心室功能正常，则患者通常在妊娠期能耐受。

人工瓣膜 为育龄妇女选择人工瓣膜时，必须仔细考虑瓣膜的类型。机械瓣寿命更长，但通常需要服用华法林，而华法林会增加流产、胎盘出血和人工瓣膜血栓形成的风险。组织（生物）瓣膜较少形成血栓，但平均使用寿命只有10年，需要再次手术，这就意味着一定的风险，甚至死亡。

对植入人工机械心脏瓣膜的妊娠母体，目前尚无管理共识，孕前咨询应包括对患者风险的详细讨论。妊娠期间，血小板黏附性增加、凝血因子浓度增加和纤溶减低会增加母体人工瓣膜血栓形成和栓塞的风险。从确定妊娠伊始、妊娠前3个月即应开始皮下或静脉应用普通肝素来替代华法林，以最大限度地减少胎儿暴露于华法林的致畸作用，通常应持续使用到妊娠13或14周、直至胚胎发育完成，之后恢复替换为华法林。有研究表明，整个妊娠期持续使用肝素可使人工机械瓣膜血栓形成风险增加33%。低分子量肝素是普通肝素的替代品，但其使用仍存在争议，因为没有大型前瞻性研究或证据支持其使用和治疗监测。

马方综合征

妊娠会增加马方综合征孕妇发生主动脉夹层和破裂的风险，尤其是在妊娠晚期和产后第1个月。主动脉根部内径大于40 mm的女性不应妊娠。建议对患有马方综合征的孕妇每6～8周进行一次超声心动图检查，以监测主动脉根部内径，并推荐使用β受体阻滞剂进行治疗。对于主动脉内径小于40 mm者，阴道分

TABLE 10.1 Specific Maternal Cardiac Conditions and Risk for Cardiac Complications During Pregnancy

Low Risk	Intermediate Risk	High Risk
Small left-to-right shunts	Large left-to-right shunt	New York Heart Association class III or IV symptoms
Repaired lesions without residual dysfunction	Unrepaired or palliated cyanotic congenital heart disease	Severe pulmonary hypertension
Mitral valve prolapse without regurgitation	Mechanical prosthetic valves	Marfan syndrome with aortic root dilation or major valvular disease
Bicuspid aortic valve without stenosis	Mitral or aortic valve stenosis	Severe aortic stenosis
Mild to moderate pulmonic stenosis	Severe pulmonic stenosis	History of peripartum cardiomyopathy with residual ventricular dysfunction
Valvular regurgitation with normal ventricular systolic function	Moderate to severe ventricular dysfunction	
	Unrepaired coarctation of the aorta	
	History of peripartum cardiomyopathy without residual ventricular dysfunction	

minimize pain and hemodynamic changes, epidural anesthesia and β-blockers or vasodilators should be used and forceps or vacuum use is recommended to shorten the second stage of labor. In patients with aortic diameter 40 mm or greater, delivery via elective C-section should be performed in a tertiary care center with cardiothoracic surgical expertise.

Congenital Heart Disease

Congenital heart disease is the predominant maternal cardiac disease in Western societies, and all patients with a history of congenital heart disease, whether or not they have had repair, should receive a detailed evaluation and appropriate counseling before conception. Patients with uncomplicated atrial or ventricular septal defects usually tolerate pregnancy without complications unless they have concomitant pulmonary hypertension or atrial fibrillation. In patients with pulmonary hypertension, pregnancy is contraindicated. The added volume load of pregnancy may potentially precipitate left ventricular failure in patients with large intracardiac shunts.

In women with coarctation of the aorta, symptoms may first present during pregnancy, typically as systemic hypertension. Therapeutic options such as antihypertensive therapy, percutaneous stenting of the coarctation, and surgical intervention are available and most women will have a successful pregnancy with proper care.

Women with uncorrected tetralogy of Fallot should undergo palliative or definitive repair before conception to improve maternal and fetal outcomes. Women with residual obstruction of the right ventricular outflow tract are at risk of worsening cyanosis and risk to both mother and fetus during pregnancy.

Heart Disease Arising During Pregnancy
Hypertension

Hypertension is the most common medical problem in pregnancy. It is defined as absolute blood pressure values greater than 140 mm Hg systolic or 90 mm Hg diastolic. The major forms of hypertension that may develop during pregnancy are essential or primary hypertension, gestational hypertension, preeclampsia superimposed on essential hypertension, and preeclampsia. Essential hypertension is defined as hypertension, without a secondary cause, present before pregnancy or that is diagnosed before week 20 of gestation. Gestational hypertension is new hypertension without proteinuria that occurs after the 20th week of gestation and resolves within 2 weeks after delivery.

The mainstay of treatment of hypertension in pregnancy is antihypertensive medications, which are usually effective in treating essential hypertension but not effective in preventing preeclampsia. Agents that have been safely used in pregnancy include hydralazine, α-methyldopa, clonidine, β-blockers, and labetalol. Diuretics should be used with caution because of the increased risk for placental hypoperfusion. When preeclampsia develops, typically characterized by hypertension and proteinuria, bedrest, salt restriction, and close monitoring are initiated and magnesium sulfate can be administered to prevent eclamptic seizures and prolong pregnancy to facilitate fetal maturity. Blood pressure usually normalizes rapidly with delivery.

Peripartum Cardiomyopathy

Peripartum cardiomyopathy (PCM) is a form of dilated cardiomyopathy that may begin during the last trimester of pregnancy or within 5 months of delivery in a previously healthy woman. The true incidence of the disease is unknown, but estimates conclude that 1 in every 2500 to 4000 pregnancies is affected in the United States. Although the cause of PCM is unknown, myocardial injury is thought to be immunologically mediated with inflammation playing a key role as evidenced by elevated serum markers of inflammation in many patients. Known risk factors include multiparity, black race, older maternal age and preeclampsia. Women usually exhibit symptoms and signs of congestive heart failure and cardiac imaging, usually with a transthoracic echocardiogram, establishes the diagnosis.

Management is similar to that for congestive heart failure (see Chapter 4) and usually includes the use of hydralazine, β-blockers, digoxin, and diuretics for symptom management and preload reduction. Diuretics may potentially reduce placental blood flow and must be used with caution. Angiotensin-converting enzyme inhibitors have been associated with increased fetal wastage in pregnant animals and aldosterone antagonists may have antiandrogenic effects on the fetus; therefore both classes of drugs should be avoided. Nitrates and inotropes may be necessary in severe cases and early fetal delivery may be necessary. Mechanical circulatory support may be necessary and cardiac transplantation may be considered in those cases refractory to mechanical circulatory support.

The outcome with PCM is variable. Left ventricular function normalizes in approximately 23% to 54% of women and death or progressive heart failure occurs in one third of affected women. The recurrence rate with subsequent pregnancies is 30%. In patients with full recovery of left ventricular function, mortality is negligible in subsequent pregnancies; however, women with a left ventricular ejection fraction less than 25% at diagnosis or persistent left ventricular dysfunction should be counseled against a subsequent pregnancy.

表 10.1 妊娠期特定心脏疾病和心脏并发症风险		
低危	中危	高危
小量左向右分流	大量左向右分流	Ⅲ或Ⅳ级纽约心功能症状
病变已矫正且未遗留功能障碍	未矫正或姑息治疗的发绀型先天性心脏病	严重的肺动脉高压
不伴反流的二尖瓣脱垂	机械人工瓣膜	马方综合征伴主动脉根部扩张或严重的心脏瓣膜病
无瓣膜狭窄的二叶主动脉瓣	二尖瓣或主动脉瓣狭窄	严重的主动脉瓣狭窄
轻至中度肺动脉狭窄	严重的肺动脉狭窄	围产期心肌病病史遗留心室功能不全
心室收缩功能正常的瓣膜反流	中至重度心室功能不全	
	未修复的主动脉缩窄	
	围产期心肌病病史未遗留心室功能不全	

娩是安全的。为了最大限度地减少疼痛和血流动力学变化，应使用硬膜外麻醉和 β 受体阻滞剂或血管扩张剂，并建议使用产钳或负压吸引以缩短第二产程。对于主动脉内径 ≥ 40 mm 的患者，应在有心胸外科专业支持的三级医疗中心选择剖宫产的方式分娩。

先天性心脏病

先天性心脏病是西方国家最常见的孕产妇心脏病。所有有先天性心脏病病史的患者，无论是否已完成矫正手术，都应在受孕前接受详细评估和适当咨询。非复杂性房间隔或室间隔缺损患者通常能耐受妊娠而无并发症，除非合并肺动脉高压或心房颤动。肺动脉高压患者不应妊娠。妊娠所致容量负荷增加可能会加速心内大量分流患者的左心室衰竭。

患有主动脉缩窄的女性，可能在妊娠期才第一次出现症状，通常为体循环高血压。降压治疗、经皮主动脉缩窄支架置入和手术干预都是可行的治疗措施，通过医护护航，大多数孕产妇都能安全度过妊娠期。

未经矫正的法洛四联症女性应在受孕前接受姑息性或根治性修复术，以改善孕产妇和胎儿的预后。右心室流出道残余梗阻的女性患者有发绀恶化的危险，在妊娠期间对孕产妇和胎儿都有风险。

妊娠引起的心脏病

高血压

高血压是妊娠期最常见的医疗问题，定义为绝对血压值收缩压大于 140 mmHg 和（或）舒张压大于 90 mmHg。妊娠期高血压的类型包括原发性高血压、妊娠高血压、原发性高血压合并先兆子痫，以及先兆子痫。原发性高血压是指妊娠前就有高血压，或妊娠 20 周前诊断的无继发性病因的高血压。妊娠高血压是指妊娠 20 周后出现的新发高血压、无蛋白尿，并在分娩后 2 周内血压回落。

妊娠高血压的主要治疗措施是使用降压药物，这些药物通常对治疗原发性高血压有效，但对预防先兆子痫无效。在妊娠期可安全使用的降压药包括肼屈嗪、α-甲基多巴、可乐定、β 受体阻滞剂和拉贝洛尔。利尿剂可能增加胎盘低灌注的风险，应谨慎使用。当先兆子痫发生时，典型表现有高血压和蛋白尿，应卧床休息、限盐和密切监测，使用硫酸镁预防子痫发作并延长妊娠期以促进胎儿成熟。分娩后血压通常会快速恢复正常。

围产期心肌病

围产期心肌病（PCM）为既往无心脏疾病的孕妇在妊娠晚期至分娩后 5 个月内发生的一种扩张型心肌病，其真实发病率尚不清楚，估计美国每 2500 ～ 4000 次妊娠发生 1 例。尽管 PCM 的病因尚不清楚，但心肌损伤被认为是免疫介导的，炎症在其中起着关键作用，因为临床上有许多患者可检测到血清炎症标志物升高。已知的患病危险因素包括多胎、黑人、高龄孕妇和先兆子痫。患者往往表现为充血性心力衰竭的症状和体征，通常由经胸超声心动图确定诊断。

PCM 的治疗可参见对充血性心力衰竭的治疗（第 4 章），通常用肼屈嗪、β 受体阻滞剂、地高辛和利尿剂来缓解症状和降低前负荷。利尿剂可能会减少胎盘血流量，须谨慎使用。血管紧张素转换酶抑制剂（ACEI）可能增加妊娠动物胎儿流产的发生率，醛固酮受体拮抗剂可能对胎儿有抗雄激素作用，应避免使用这两类药物。硝酸酯类和正性肌力药可用于严重患者，必要时应提前结束妊娠。重症患者可考虑机械循环支持，仍无效的患者可考虑心脏移植。

PCM 的预后在不同个体间差别很大。约 23% ～ 54% 的患者左心室功能恢复正常，但也有 1/3 出现心力衰竭恶化或死亡。再次妊娠时复发率为 30%。在左心室功能完全恢复的患者中，再次妊娠的死亡率低到可以忽略不计；但发病时左心室射血分数低于 25% 或左心功能不全持续存在的 PCM 患者不建议再次妊娠。

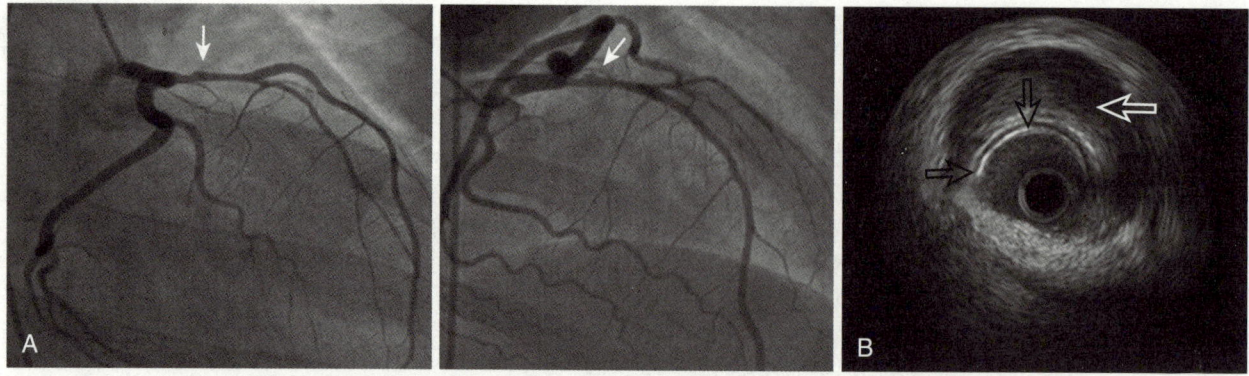

Fig. 10.1 Postpartum anterior wall myocardial infarction from spontaneous coronary dissection of the left anterior descending and diagonal arteries demonstrated by (A) left coronary angiography showing diffusely narrowed coronary lumen (proximal left anterior descending artery indicated by the *arrow*), and (B) intravascular ultrasound confirming hematoma in the medial-adventitial layer of the vessel. The imaging catheter is central in the lumen. *Black arrows* indicate the vessel media and the *white arrow* the hematoma. The intima of the vessel is thin and normal.

Spontaneous Coronary Artery Dissection

Spontaneous coronary artery dissection (SCAD) is defined as a separation of the arterial wall and subsequent coronary artery obstruction caused by the formation of an intramural hematoma that is not associated with atherosclerosis, trauma or iatrogenic injury (Fig. 10.1). While SCAD is the most common cause of pregnancy-associated myocardial infarction, pregnancy-associated SCAD represents a relatively small proportion of SCAD cases. The prevalence is 1.81 SCAD events per 100,000 pregnancies during pregnancy or in the postpartum period. SCAD has been reported as early as 5 weeks' gestation and up to a year or more postpartum, particularly in lactating women.

The cause of pregnancy-associated SCAD is not fully understood; however, hormonal changes of pregnancy are thought to alter the architecture of the arterial wall, weakening the wall and making it prone to rupture, intramural hematoma, and the subsequent development of clinical symptoms. Risk factors for pregnancy-associated SCAD include black race, chronic hypertension, lipid abnormalities, chronic depression, migraines, advanced maternal age, multiparty, and treatment for infertility.

Women with pregnancy-associated SCAD have poorer prognosis than women with SCAD not related to pregnancy. They have larger infarcts, more proximal artery dissections, and lower mean left ventricular ejection fraction immediately and at follow-up. Maternal complications of pregnancy-associated SCAD include cardiogenic shock, ventricular fibrillation, and mechanical circulatory support. In-hospital mortality has been reported to be as high as 4%.

CARDIAC TUMORS

Cardiac tumors are broadly divided into primary and secondary tumors. Primary cardiac tumors, defined as benign or malignant neoplasms that arise from any tissue of the heart, are extremely rare, with an autopsy incidence of 0.001% to 0.03%. Secondary, or metastatic, cardiac tumors are 30 times more common than primary tumors, with an autopsy incidence of 1.7% to 14%.

It is not uncommon for patients with cardiac tumors to initially have no symptoms or physical findings, but rather present with abnormalities on imaging. Alternatively, patients may present with a constellation of nonspecific symptoms or findings on physical examination.

The initial evaluation is typically imaging such as a two-dimensional transthoracic echocardiogram or magnetic resonance imaging (MRI). Once a mass is identified and described, additional imaging may be undertaken

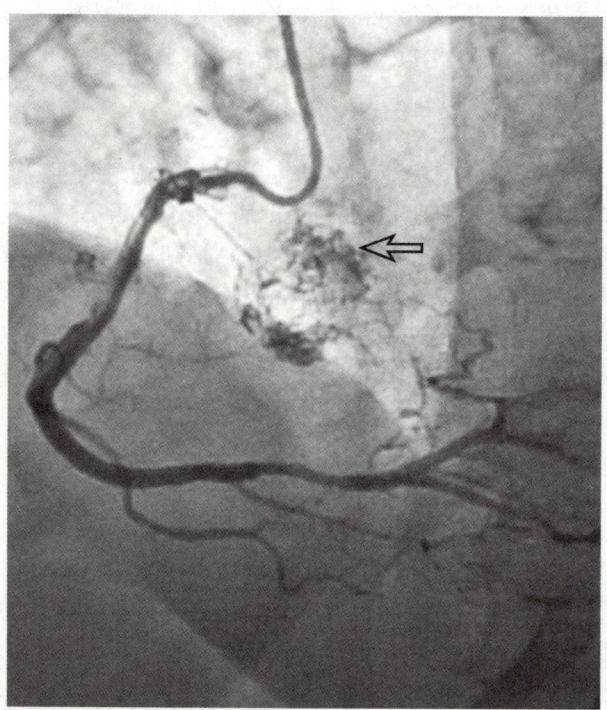

Fig. 10.2 Atrial myxoma vascularization identified on cardiac catheterization. Selective right coronary angiography demonstrates that the vascular supply to the tumor originates from atrial branches. The vascularized tumor is indicated by the *arrow*.

such as three-dimensional echocardiography with contrast, transesophageal echocardiography for anatomic information, MRI with gadolinium, coronary angiography to define coronary anatomy, position emission tomography (PET) for staging, and/or computed tomography (CT) to delineate other intrathoracic structures. When assessing a cardiac mass, the clinical context is critical to the diagnosis. The differential diagnosis of a cardiac mass is broad and includes tumors, thrombi, infection, and artifact.

Benign Primary Cardiac Tumors

Most primary cardiac tumors are benign, and myxoma is the most common primary tumor of the heart (Fig. 10.2). Most myxomas are

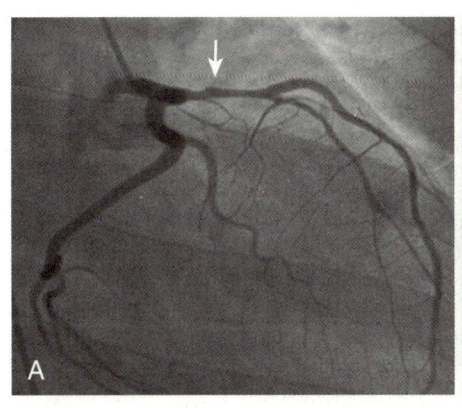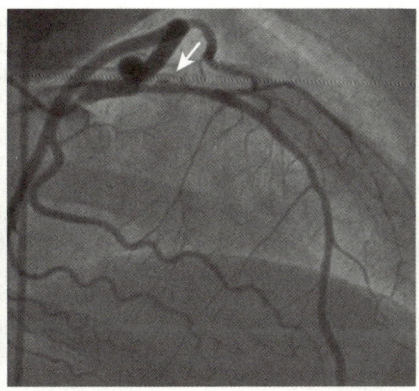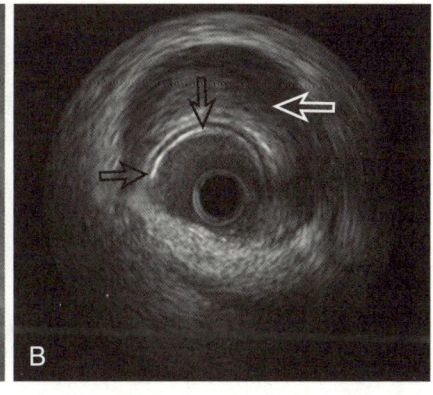

图 10.1　由左前降支和对角支自发夹层引起的产后前壁心肌梗死，左冠状动脉造影（A）显示冠脉管腔弥漫性狭窄（箭头所示为左前降支动脉近端），以及血管内超声检查（B）证实血管中-外膜层有血肿。成像导管位于管腔的中心。黑色箭头指示血管中膜，白色箭头指示血肿。血管内膜薄且正常

自发性冠状动脉夹层

自发性冠状动脉夹层（SCAD）是指动脉管壁层间分离从而形成壁内血肿，导致冠状动脉阻塞，与动脉粥样硬化、创伤或医源性损伤无关（图 10.1）。虽然 SCAD 是妊娠相关心肌梗死最常见的原因，但妊娠相关 SCAD 在 SCAD 病例中所占比例相对较小，孕妇在妊娠/产后期发生 SCAD 事件的比率为 1.81/10 万。据报道，SCAD 可早在妊娠第 5 周就发病，也可晚至产后 1 年或更长时间，后者尤见于哺乳期女性。

妊娠相关 SCAD 的病因尚不完全清楚。一般认为，妊娠期激素水平的变化可改变和削弱动脉壁结构，使其易于破裂、出现壁内血肿，最终导致临床症状。妊娠相关 SCAD 的危险因素包括黑人、慢性高血压、脂质异常、慢性抑郁症、偏头痛、高龄产妇、多胎（原文有误，multiparty 应为 multiparity）和对不孕症的治疗。

妊娠相关 SCAD 患者的预后比与妊娠无关 SCAD 的女性患者差，夹层位于冠脉更近端、心肌梗死面积更大、发病和随访期间平均左心室射血分数更低。妊娠相关 SCAD 母体的并发症包括心源性休克、心室颤动和需要机械循环支持。院内死亡率高达 4%。

心脏肿瘤

心脏肿瘤分为原发肿瘤和继发肿瘤。原发心脏肿瘤定义为起源于任何心脏组织的良性或恶性肿瘤，极为罕见，尸检检出率为 0.001%～0.03%。继发或转移性心脏肿瘤的发病率是原发性肿瘤的 30 倍，尸检检出率为 1.7%～14%。

由影像学检查而不是症状体征的线索发现心脏肿瘤，这种情况并非少见。有时患者只是表现出一些并不指向心脏疾病的非特异性症状而去做影像学检查，或甚至是常规体检，才偶然发现了心脏肿瘤。

一般先采用经胸二维超声心动图或磁共振成像（MRI）进行初步评估，识别肿块并进行初步描述后，

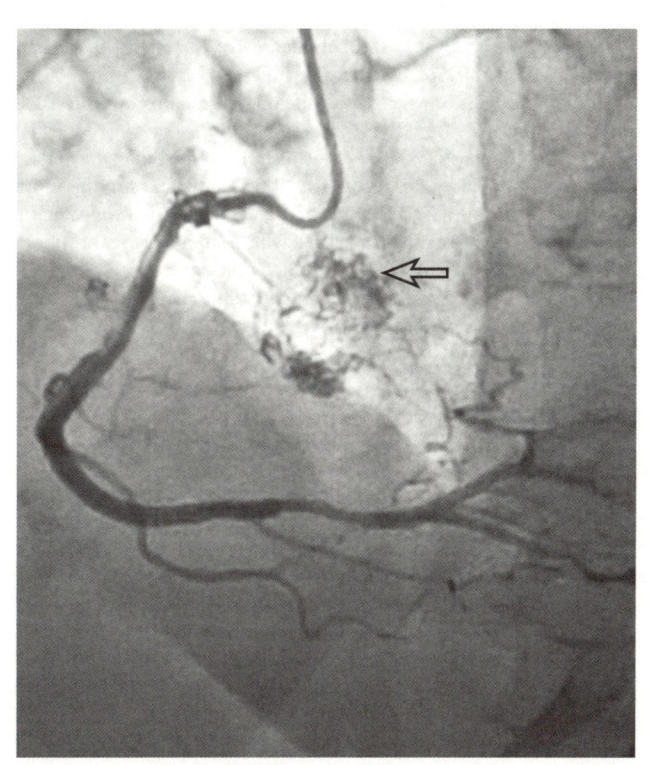

图 10.2　心导管检查发现心房黏液瘤的血管化。选择性右冠状动脉造影显示肿瘤的血管来源于心房支。箭头指示血管化的肿瘤

根据需要行进一步影像学检查，三维超声造影、经食管超声心动图（明确心脏解剖）、钆增强 MRI、冠状动脉造影（明确冠脉解剖）、正电子发射断层成像（PET）（用于肿瘤分期）和（或）计算机断层成像（CT）（显示其他胸腔内结构）。在评估心脏肿块时，临床背景对诊断至关重要。心脏肿块的鉴别诊断范围很广，包括肿瘤、血栓、感染和伪影。

原发心脏良性肿瘤

大多数原发心脏肿瘤都是良性的，其中最常见的是心脏黏液瘤（图 10.2）。大多数黏液瘤发生在左心

found in the left atrium. Less commonly, they may be found in the right atrium, right ventricle, and left ventricle in decreasing frequencies. While most myxomas occur sporadically, a familial pattern of myxomas can occur in an autosomal dominant manner. In a particular syndrome called the Carney complex, patients may present with cardiac myxomas, cutaneous myxomas, breast fibroadenomas, hyperpigmented nevi, hyperactive adrenal or testicular glands, and pituitary tumors. The Carney complex occurs in young individuals and should be considered in myxomas in atypical locations in the heart. Surgical removal is the only definitive treatment of cardiac myxomas. Myxomas tend to recur with rates varying from 5% to 14%; therefore, it is imperative that lifelong follow-up continue after surgical removal.

Less common benign tumors include rhabdomyomas, fibromas, lipomas, and papillary fibroelastomas. Rhabdomyomas are the most common cardiac tumors found in children and are usually located in the ventricle. They are often associated with a family history of tuberous sclerosis. Surgery can often be avoided unless the patient develops clinical evidence of arrhythmias and heart failure. Fibromas are composed of fibroblasts or collagen and typically occur in childhood. They are most often located on the interventricular septum and patients may present with chest pain, pericardial effusion, heart failure, arrhythmias, and sudden death. While both occur in the ventricle, the distinguishing feature of fibromas, in contrast to rhabdomyomas, is the presence of calcification. Lipomas are rare and occur most frequently in the left ventricle and the right atrium, although they can be found anywhere in the heart and the pericardium. They are frequently asymptomatic but can grow large enough to cause obstructive symptoms. Papillary fibroelastomas are pedunculate tumors with filiform attachments that typically arise from the aortic or mitral valve. They carry an elevated risk of embolic phenomena and, when situated on the aortic valve, can cause coronary ostial occlusion. Complete surgical resection is recommended because of the risk of systemic embolism. Recurrence rates are low and long-term anticoagulation is not recommended unless the patient has other indications.

Malignant Primary Cardiac Tumors

Malignant primary cardiac tumors commonly cause symptoms via three mechanisms: obstruction, embolization, and arrhythmia. Obstructive tumors can present with syncope, chest pain, dyspnea or heart failure. Pericardial invasion and tamponade are rarely the first manifestation of the disease. Primary cardiac sarcoma is the most common malignant primary cardiac tumor. Once diagnosed, treatment for cardiac sarcomas is primarily surgical with complete resection as the goal followed by adjacent chemotherapy. Cardiac sarcomas carry a very poor overall prognosis.

Secondary Cardiac Tumors

Cardiac metastases are common and can be found in up to 14% of patients dying with a known malignancy. Cardiac metastases can occur either by direct extension, by way of the bloodstream or lymphatics, or by intracavitary diffusion through the inferior vena cava (IVC). Metastases to the pericardium are most common, followed by epicardium, myocardium, and endocardium. Primary thoracic cancers, including breast and lung cancer, tend to invade the pericardium directly whereas abdominal and pelvic tumors reach the right atrium usually through the IVC. Renal cell carcinoma is the most common tumor to exhibit this tendency. In men and women, lung cancer is the most frequent cause of cardiac metastasis. In men, this is followed by esophageal cancer and lymphoma whereas in women it is followed by lymphoma and breast cancer.

The prognosis of metastatic cardiac tumors is poor, with 1-year mortality being 50%. Treatment therefore is primarily palliative and may include radiation therapy, chemotherapy, and surgical resection, if possible. Malignant pericardial effusion is typically managed with pericardiocentesis and may need a pericardiotomy to reduce subsequent reaccumulation of pericardial fluid.

TRAUMATIC HEART DISEASE

Traumatic heart disease can be categorized based on the mechanism of injury (Table 10.2).

Nonpenetrating Cardiac Trauma

Nonpenetrating or blunt cardiac trauma accounts for about 10% of all traumatic heart disease. Nonpenetrating cardiac trauma can manifest as a spectrum of pathology including septal rupture, free wall rupture, coronary artery thrombosis or dissection, rupture of the cordae tendinae or papillary muscle, pericarditis or cardiac tamponade, and arrhythmias. Commotio cordis is a type of nonpenetrating cardiac trauma that occurs more often in child athletes as a result of a projectile such as a ball striking the chest, resulting in ventricular fibrillation and sudden cardiac death.

Nonpenetrating cardiac trauma can present with clinically significant or clinically insignificant injury. Conduction disturbances are common and a screening 12-lead electrocardiogram (ECG) can be useful for initial evaluation. Sinus tachycardia is the most common ECG abnormality. Other possible findings on ECG include T-wave and ST-segment changes, bradycardia, first- and second-degree atrioventricular block, right bundle branch block, third-degree heart block, atrial fibrillation, premature ventricular complexes, ventricular tachycardia, and ventricular fibrillation. Elevated cardiac enzymes are not specific for blunt cardiac trauma and may be related to severity of noncardiac injury or underlying coronary disease. In one study, only 485 of patients with elevated troponin were clinically found to have significant blunt cardiac trauma. A negative troponin, however, had a negative predictive value of 93%. The major use of transthoracic echocardiography in the evaluation of nonpenetrating cardiac trauma is for the assessment of pericardial effusion, the presence of which is concerning for chamber rupture. Transesophageal echocardiography is a more sensitive test for the evaluation of more subtle features of blunt cardiac injury.

Most patients who present with suspected blunt cardiac injury can be managed with observation and monitoring. Patients in cardiogenic shock in whom structural injury is confirmed should be promptly referred to cardiothoracic surgery for surgical repair.

Penetrating Cardiac Trauma

Penetrating cardiac injury is the most common cause of significant cardiac injury, most often by firearms and knives. Due to their anterior location on the chest wall, the right and left ventricles are at the greatest risk for injury. Most penetrating cardiac injuries involve the myocardium, sparing additional structures, and are managed effectively with surgical intervention and rarely requiring reoperation for a residual defect.

Penetrating injury to the epigastrium and precordium should raise suspicion for penetrating cardiac injury. The clinical presentation

TABLE 10.2 Cardiac Trauma Categorized by Mechanism of Injury

Penetrating	Nonpenetrating (Blunt)
Stab wounds (e.g., knives, swords, ice picks)	Motor vehicle accident
Gunshot wounds (e.g., handguns, nail guns)	Vehicular-pedestrian accident
Shotgun wounds	Falls from height
Blast fragments	Crush (e.g., industrial accidents)
	Blast (e.g., explosives)

表 10.2　按损伤机制分类的心脏创伤	
穿透性外伤	非穿透性（顿挫）外伤
刺伤（如刀、剑、碎冰锥）	机动车事故
枪伤（如手枪、射钉枪）	车辆碰撞行人事故
霰弹枪伤	高处坠落
爆破碎片伤	挤压伤（如工业事故）
	爆炸伤（如炸药）

房。其他部位不太常见，按照发生频率降序依次为右心房、右心室和左心室。黏液瘤多数散发，也可以常染色体显性遗传的家族模式出现。在一种称为 Carney 复合体的特殊综合征，患者可表现为心脏黏液瘤、皮肤黏液瘤、乳腺纤维腺瘤、色素沉着痣、肾上腺或睾丸功能过度活跃以及垂体瘤。年轻患者在心脏非典型部位出现黏液瘤应考虑 Carney 复合体。手术切除是唯一治疗方案。黏液瘤复发率为 5%～14%，因此手术切除后必须终身随访。

较少见的良性肿瘤包括横纹肌瘤、纤维瘤、脂肪瘤和乳头状弹力纤维瘤。横纹肌瘤是儿童最常见的心脏肿瘤，通常发生于心室，常与结节性硬化症家族史有关，除非出现心律失常和心力衰竭，通常可以免于手术。纤维瘤由成纤维细胞或胶原组成，通常儿童期起病，常见于室间隔，患者可能会出现胸痛、心包积液、心力衰竭、心律失常和猝死。横纹肌瘤和纤维瘤都见于心室，但相比之下纤维瘤的显著特征是钙化。脂肪瘤很罕见，可发生于心脏和心包中的任何一处，但最常见于左心室和右心房，通常无症状，但瘤体增大可导致阻塞性症状。乳头状弹力纤维瘤是一种具有丝状附着物的带蒂肿瘤，通常发生在主动脉瓣或二尖瓣，有较高的栓塞症风险，当位于主动脉瓣上时可导致冠状动脉口堵塞；由于存在体循环栓塞的风险，建议进行手术切除。其复发率低，除非有其他抗凝治疗适应证，否则不建议长期抗凝。

原发心脏恶性肿瘤

原发心脏恶性肿瘤产生症状的机制主要是梗阻、栓塞和心律失常。阻塞性肿瘤可表现为晕厥、胸痛、呼吸困难或心力衰竭，很少以心包侵犯和心脏压塞为首发表现。原发性心脏肉瘤是最常见的原发心脏恶性肿瘤，确诊后应手术治疗，以完全切除为目标，然后进行辅助化疗。心脏肉瘤的总体预后非常差。

继发心脏肿瘤

肿瘤的心脏转移较常见，死于已知恶性肿瘤的患者中，有心脏转移者比例高达 14%。肿瘤向心脏的转移可通过血流或淋巴管直接蔓延，或通过下腔静脉（IVC）向心腔内扩散。心包转移最常见，其次是心外膜、心肌和心内膜。乳腺癌、肺癌等原发性胸部癌症往往直接侵犯心包，而腹部和盆腔肿瘤通常经过下腔静脉到达右心房，这种转移路径在肾细胞癌最常见。无论男女，肺癌都是心脏转移最常见的源肿瘤，其次是食管癌和淋巴瘤（男性），以及淋巴瘤和乳腺癌（女性）。

转移性心脏肿瘤的预后较差，1 年死亡率为 50%。因此，治疗主要是姑息性的，包括放疗、化疗和手术切除。恶性心包积液通常采用心包穿刺术，也可能需要采用心包切开术，以减少随后心包液体的再次聚积。

创伤性心脏疾病

创伤性心脏疾病可根据损伤机制进行分类（表 10.2）。

非穿透性心脏创伤

非穿透性心脏创伤或心脏顿挫伤约占所有创伤性心脏病的 10%。非穿透性心脏创伤的病理学改变包括室间隔穿孔、游离壁破裂、冠状动脉血栓形成/夹层、腱索/乳头肌断裂、心包炎/心脏压塞（亦称心包填塞），以及心律失常。心脏震荡就属于非穿透性心脏创伤，比如少儿运动员被抛射物（球类等）撞击胸部，导致心室颤动和心源性猝死。

非穿透性心脏创伤可有明显临床表现，也可为无明显临床表现的损伤。传导障碍很常见，筛查 12 导联心电图（ECG）可用于初始评估。窦性心动过速是最常见的心电图异常，其他包括 T 波和 ST 段改变、心动过缓、一度和二度房室传导阻滞、右束支传导阻滞、三度房室传导阻滞、心房颤动、室性早搏、室性心动过速和心室颤动。心脏标志物升高并不特异性指向心脏顿挫伤，也可能与严重的心脏外损伤或潜在冠状动脉疾病有关。在一项研究中，检测到肌钙蛋白升高的胸外伤患者中，仅 48%（原文有误，485 应为 48%）被证实存在心脏顿挫伤。然而，肌钙蛋白阴性的阴性预测值达 93%。经胸超声心动图在非穿透性心脏创伤中的主要作用是评估心包积液，如发现心包积液需警惕心脏破裂。经食管超声心动图是一种更敏感的检查，用于评估更细微的心脏顿挫伤。

大多数疑似心脏顿挫伤的患者可以先观察和监测；心源性休克患者一旦确诊有结构性损伤，应立即转至心胸外科进行手术修复。

穿透性心脏创伤

穿透性心脏创伤是最常见的严重心脏外伤，主要是枪伤和刀伤。右心室和左心室位于胸壁的前部，故而受伤风险最大。大多数穿透性心脏创伤主要是心肌受损，未累及其他附加结构，手术干预即可有效治疗，很少需要对残余缺陷进行再次手术。

对位于上腹和心前区的穿透性创伤，应考虑到穿透性心脏创伤的可能，其临床表现从生命体征平稳到

TABLE 10.3 Key Features of Available Left Ventricular Percutaneous Assist Devices

	IABP	Impella 2.5	Impella CP	Impella 5.0	TandemHeart	V-A ECMO
Mechanism	Aorta	LV → Aorta	LV → Aorta	LV → Aorta	LA → Aorta	RA → Aorta
Flow (L/min)	0.3-0.5	1.0-2.5	3.7-4.0	Max 5.0	2.5-5.0	3.0-7.0
Max implant time	—	7-10 days	7-10 days	2-3 weeks	2-3 weeks	3-4 weeks
Ability to oxygenate	No	No	No	No	No	Yes
Cardiac Power	↑	↑↑	↑↑	↑↑	↑↑	↑↑↑
Afterload	↓	↓	↓	↓	↑	↑↑↑
MAP	↑	↑↑	↑↑	↑↑	↑↑	↑↑
LVEDP	↓	↓	↓↓	↓↓	↓↓	↔
PCWP	↓	↓↓	↓↓	↓↓	↓↓	↔
LV preload	—	↓↓	↓↓	↓↓	↓↓	↓
Coronary perfusion	↑	↑	↑	↑	—	—

IABP, Intraaortic balloon pump; *LA*, left atrium; *LV*, left ventricle; *LVEDP*, left ventricular end-diastolic pressure; *MAP*, mean arterial pressure; *PCWP*, pulmonary capillary wedge pressure; *RA*, right atrium; *V-A ECMO*, veno-arterial extracorporeal membrane oxygenation.

could be varied from normal vital signs to circulatory collapse. This is because after a weapon injuring the myocardium and pericardium is withdrawn, blood filling the pericardium may not be able to escape. As pericardial fluid accumulates, ventricular filling is impaired and stroke volume decreases. In response to a decrease in stroke volume, there is a catecholamine surge resulting in tachycardia and increased right-sided filling pressures. As little as 60 mL to 100 mL of blood in the pericardial sac can result in clinical pericardial tamponade where the limits of distensibility are reached and there is bowing of the interventricular septum, further compromising left ventricular function, reducing cardiac output, and resulting in irreversible shock. The classic findings of Beck triad (muffled heart sounds, hypotension and distended neck veins) is rarely seen. Pulsus paradoxus (a fall in systolic blood pressure of 20 mm Hg or more during inspiration) and Kussmaul sign (increase in jugular venous distention on inspiration) may be present but not reliably predictive of pericardial tamponade. Narrowing of the pulse pressure, however, is a reproducible sign of tamponade. In the case of penetrating cardiac injury, definitive treatment involves surgical intervention.

PERCUTANEOUS MECHANICAL CIRCULATORY SUPPORT

Mechanical circulatory support (MCS) is a term that refers to mechanical pumps designed to assist or replace the function of the left ventricle, right ventricle or both ventricles of the heart. There are several MCS systems available including the intra-aortic balloon pump (IABP), extracorporeal membrane oxygenation (ECMO) or extracorporeal life support (ECLS), ventricular assist devices (VADs), and total artificial hearts (TAHs). Further details on the disease process and management of chronic heart failure are covered in Chapter 4. The following discussion will focus on temporary or percutaneous MCS as indicated in patients with cardiogenic shock refractory to medical therapy when the objective is rapid augmentation of cardiac output, reduction of ventricular filling pressures, and life support. Longer-term support, with VADs, TAHs, and cardiac transplantation are covered elsewhere. A comparison of the key features of the available percutaneous assist devices is summarized in Table 10.3.

Percutaneous Left Ventricular Assist Devices
Intra-Aortic Balloon Pump
The IABP remains the most commonly used form of circulatory support. A polyethylene helium-filled balloon is placed percutaneously through the femoral artery into the thoracic aorta, just distal to the left subclavian artery. Timing of balloon inflation and deflation is based on the ECG or the arterial waveform of the patient. The balloon inflates with the onset of diastole and deflates at the onset of left ventricular systole. Balloon inflation during diastole increases diastolic blood pressure, referred to as diastolic augmentation, allowing for maximal delivery of oxygenated blood to the coronary arteries. Deflation during systole decreases the afterload and myocardial oxygen consumption while modestly enhancing cardiac output. The IABP reduces myocardial oxygen demand but provides only modest ventricular unloading. Patients must have some left ventricular function and electrical stability for an IABP to be most effective because the device only results in an increase in cardiac output of 0.5 to 1.0 liter per minute.

The major contraindication for IABP is greater than mild aortic valve regurgitation because the diastolic inflation of the balloon may worsen the degree of regurgitation. Severe peripheral arterial disease or aortic disease increases the risk of vascular complication such as thromboembolism and lower extremity and visceral ischemia. Potential major complications include balloon leak, severe bleeding (e.g., retroperitoneal), thromboembolic events, major limb or visceral ischemia, vascular trauma, thrombocytopenia from platelet deposition in the IABP membrane, and infection.

Impella
The Impella (Abiomed, Danvers, Mass.) is a nonpulsatile axial flow Archimedes-screw pump that propels blood from the left ventricle into the proximal ascending aorta. Depending on the version used, these devices can deliver up to 5.0 L/min of maximal flow. Designed to be placed via the femoral artery, delivery can either be percutaneous (Impella 2.5 and CP) or via a surgical cutdown (Impella 5.0). At the tip of the catheter there is a flexible pigtail loop that stabilizes the device in the left ventricle. The main body of the device contains the pump inlet and outlet areas, motor housing, and pump pressure monitor. Unlike the IABP, the Impella does not require ECG or arterial pressure timing and therefore provides stability despite transient arrhythmias.

The hemodynamic effects of the Impella are to unload the left ventricle and increase forward flow, reducing myocardial oxygen consumption, improving mean arterial pressure, and reducing pulmonary capillary wedge pressure. Compared to the IABP, the Impella delivers a significant increase in cardiac output. Adequate right ventricular function is necessary to maintain left ventricular preload and hemodynamic support. In cases where there is significant biventricular failure or unstable ventricular arrhythmias, a concomitant right ventricular assist device may be necessary.

表 10.3 各种经皮左心室辅助装置的主要特点

	IABP	Impella 2.5	Impella CP	Impella 5.0	TandemHeart	V-A ECMO
机制	主动脉	左心室→主动脉	左心室→主动脉	左心室→主动脉	左心房→主动脉	右心房→主动脉
流量（L/min）	0.3~0.5	1.0~2.5	3.7~4.0	最大5.0	2.5~5.0	3.0~7.0
最长植入时间	—	7~10天	7~10天	2~3周	2~3周	3~4周
氧合能力	无	无	无	无	无	有
心脏功率	↑	↑↑	↑↑	↑↑	↑↑	↑↑↑
后负荷	↓	↓	↓	↓	↑	↑↑↑
MAP	↑	↑↑	↑↑	↑↑	↑↑	↑↑
LVEDP	↓	↓	↓↓	↓↓	↓↓	↔
PCWP	↓	↓↓	↓↓	↓↓	↓↓	↔
左室前负荷	—	↓↓	↓↓	↓↓	↓↓	↓
冠状动脉灌注	↑	↑	↑	↑	—	—

IABP：主动脉内球囊反搏；LVEDP：左心室舒张末期压力；MAP：平均动脉压；PCWP：肺毛细血管楔压；V-A ECMO：静脉-动脉模式体外膜肺氧合。

循环崩溃不等。当损伤心肌和心包的锐器被拔出后，血液充盈心包、无法排出。随着心包内液体的积聚，心室充盈受损，每搏输出量下降；为应对每搏输出量的减少，儿茶酚胺骤增，导致心动过速和右心充盈压增加。即使只有60~100 ml血液快速积聚在心包内都会导致心包填塞，此时心包达到伸展极限，室间隔推移使左心室功能受限，心输出量下降，导致不可逆休克。Beck三联征的典型表现（心音低沉、低血压和颈静脉怒张）很少见。奇脉（吸气相收缩压下降≥20 mmHg）和Kussmaul征（吸气相颈静脉明显扩张）可能会出现，但不能据此可靠预测心包填塞；脉压变小是可靠的心包填塞症状。穿透性心脏创伤需要手术干预。

经皮机械循环支持

机械循环支持（MCS）是指辅助或替代左心室、右心室或双心室功能的机械泵，包括主动脉内球囊反搏（IABP）、体外膜肺氧合（ECMO）或体外生命支持（ECLS）、心室辅助装置（VAD）和全人工心脏（TAH）。有关慢性心力衰竭疾病进程和治疗的更多内容见第4章。下文主要介绍临时或经皮MCS的临床应用，其适应证是药物治疗无效的心源性休克患者，目标是快速增加心输出量、降低心室充盈压、维持生命。长期循环支持，包括VAD、TAH和心脏移植将在其他章节介绍。表10.3总结并比较了各种经皮辅助装置的主要特性。

经皮左心室辅助装置
主动脉内球囊反搏

IABP仍然是最常用的循环支持手段。充氦气的聚乙烯球囊通过股动脉入路置入胸主动脉、置于左锁骨下动脉远端的胸主动脉腔内，根据患者的心电图或动脉压力波形触发充气和放气，在左心室舒张期开始时充气、左心室收缩期开始时放气。左心室舒张期球囊充气膨胀、舒张压升高，称为舒张期增压，得以最大限度地将含氧血液输送到冠状动脉。收缩期放气、降低左心室后负荷、减少心肌氧耗量，同时适度提高了心输出量。IABP降低了心肌耗氧，但仅能提供有限的心室减压。在有自主收缩舒张功能的左心室，IABP可使心输出量增加0.5~1.0 L/min，只有当患者具备一定左心室功能和心电稳定性时，IABP才能发挥作用。

IABP的主要禁忌证是轻度以上主动脉瓣反流，因为球囊在舒张期膨胀可加重反流。严重周围动脉疾病和主动脉疾病会增加血管并发症的风险，如血栓栓塞、下肢/内脏缺血。IABP的主要并发症包括球囊破裂、严重出血（如腹膜后）、血栓栓塞事件、肢体或内脏缺血、血管损伤、血小板沉积于IABP球囊膜引起的血小板减少症和感染。

Impella

Impella（Abiomed, Danvers, Mass.）是一种非脉动轴流阿基米德螺旋泵，能驱动血液从左心室进入近端升主动脉，可提供最高达5.0 L/min的血流量，不同型号仪器最大流量有所不同。Impella经股动脉置入，包括经皮（Impella 2.5和CP）和外科切开（Impella 5.0）两种方式，通过导管尖端一可活动的猪尾环稳定置于左心室中。Impella的主体包括泵入口和出口区、电机外壳和泵压力监测器。与IABP不同，Impella不需要心电图或动脉压力触发，因而可实现稳定输出，短暂心律失常不影响其工作。

Impella的血流动力学作用是左心室减压并增加前向血流，降低心肌氧耗量，提高平均动脉压，以及降低肺毛细血管楔压。与IABP相比，Impella可显著提高心输出量。使用Impella时必须有足够的右心室功能来维持左心室前负荷，这样才足以支持血流动力学。如果出现严重的双心室衰竭或不稳定的室性心律失常，可能需要合并使用右心室辅助装置。

Contraindications to the use of the Impella are the presence of a mechanical aortic valve, left ventricular thrombus, severe aortic stenosis, moderate to severe aortic insufficiency, severe peripheral arterial disease, and the inability to tolerate systemic anticoagulation. Possible complications of Impella use include limb ischemia, vascular complications, hemolysis due to mechanical erythrocyte shearing, and bleeding requiring blood transfusion.

TandemHeart

The TandemHeart (TandemLife, Pittsburgh, Penn.) is a percutaneous centrifugal pump that provides up to 4 L/min of mechanical circulator support via a continuous-flow centrifugal pump. The TandemHeart is inserted through the femoral vein and advanced across the interatrial septum into the left atrium. Oxygenated blood is then withdrawn from the left atrium via a 21-Fr inflow cannula and reinjected into the lower abdominal aorta or iliac arteries via a 15-Fr to 17-Fr outflow cannula. The need for transseptal puncture is a limitation to the widespread use of this device. The potential complications of the TandemHeart include the need for blood transfusion, sepsis/systemic inflammatory response syndrome, bleeding around the cannula, gastrointestinal bleeding, coagulopathy, stroke, left atrial perforation, and device-related limb ischemia.

Right Ventricular Support

Acute right ventricular (RV) failure may occur in a number of clinical settings such as acute myocardial infarction, fulminant myocarditis, acute pulmonary embolism, pulmonary hypertension, postcardiotomy shock, postcardiac transplantation, and following LVAD implantation. The mainstay of therapy for RV failure is inotropic and pulmonary vasodilator support and volume status optimization. Vasopressors are often used to maintain coronary perfusion pressure and inhaled nitric oxide can be used to reduce RV afterload. When these measures are insufficient to augment RV systolic function, mechanical circulatory support may be required to unload the RV, ensure adequate LV preload, and optimize tissue perfusion.

There are both surgical and percutaneous options for RV mechanical circulatory support. The surgical right ventricular assist device (RVAD) was associated with worse outcomes when compared to patients with RV failure who did not need an RVAD. Unfavorable outcome data and the need for repeat sternotomy for both insertion and removal of the device has limited clinical utilization. There are two percutaneous devices currently available for RV support: (1) Impella RP (Abiomed, Danvers, Mass.), an axial catheter-based pump and (2) the Protek Duo (Cardiac Assist Inc., Pittsburgh, Penn.), a catheter with an extracorporeal centrifugal pump. The Impella RP provides RV unloading with up to 4 L/min of continuous flow from the inlet in the inferior vena cava through a cannula to the outlet in the pulmonary artery. The pump is inserted via a 23-Fr sheath in the femoral vein into the atrium and across the tricuspid and pulmonic valves into the main pulmonary artery. The Protek Duo is a dual-lumen cannula that is inserted percutaneously via the internal jugular vein. The inflow lumen is positioned in the right atrium and the outflow lumen is positioned in the main pulmonary artery. The extracorporeal pump allows flows up to 5 L/min and an oxygenator can also be introduced into the circuit to allow for oxygenation support.

Extracorporeal Membrane Oxygenation

ECMO provides cardiopulmonary support in patients whose heart and/or lungs no longer provide adequate physiologic support. ECMO can be either veno-venous (V-V ECMO) for isolated pulmonary failure only or veno-arterial (V-A ECMO) for pulmonary and cardiac failure. Cannulas are placed in the right side of the heart, from the vena cava, to drain blood into the ECMO circuit for oxygenation. Blood can then either be returned to the right side of the heart in V-V ECMO or to the arterial system (proximal or distal aorta) in V-A ECMO. The bypass circuit in ECMO is composed of a centrifugal, nonpulsatile pump for blood propulsion, and a membrane oxygenator for gas exchange. V-A ECMO requires anticoagulation while V-V ECMO does not. Complications relate to bleeding, thromboembolism, and mechanical complications such as hemolysis and arterial insufficiency.

V-V ECMO offers gas exchange and is useful for conditions resulting in severe impairment of gas exchange such as ARDS or pulmonary embolism. V-V ECMO does not provide hemodynamic support. Alternatively, V-A ECMO provides additional hemodynamic support with flows sometimes exceeding 6 L/min depending on the cannula French size and length and properties of the pump. V-A ECMO alone, however, does not reduce ventricular wall stress and the use of a concomitant MCS such as IABP or percutaneous VAD is usually needed to vent or unload the left ventricle.

NONCARDAIC SURGERY IN THE PATIENT WITH CARDIOVASCULAR DISEASE

Noncardiac surgery in patients with known cardiovascular disease may be associated with an increased risk for death or cardiac complications such as MI, congestive heart failure, and arrhythmias. To determine an individual patient's risk for a procedure, the consulting physician must have knowledge of the type and severity of the patient's cardiac disease, the comorbid risk factors, and the type and urgency of surgery. In general, the preoperative evaluation and management are the same as in the nonoperative setting; for patients who are at risk, additional noninvasive and invasive testing may be performed if the results would affect treatment or outcome.

Estimation of a patient's perioperative risk can be determined by a careful clinical evaluation, including a history, physical examination, ECG, and type of surgery. Risk models can then be applied to guide the clinician with regards to additional testing and treatment. The most widely used risk model was developed in a study of 4315 patients 50 years or older undergoing major noncardiac procedures in a tertiary care teaching hospital and has been validated over the past 15 years. The index includes six independent predictors of complications in a revised cardiac risk index (RCRI): high-risk type of surgery, history of cerebrovascular disease, preoperative treatment with insulin, history of ischemic heart disease, history of congestive heart failure, and preoperative serum creatinine concentration greater than 2.0 mg/dL. The evaluating clinician can risk stratify the patients into low, intermediate, or high cardiovascular risk on the basis of having zero, one to two, or three or more risk factors, respectively. Another risk model was developed from the American College of Surgeons 2007 National Surgical Quality Improvement Program database (NSQIP), which identified five predictors of perioperative myocardial infarction or cardiac arrest: type of surgery, dependent functional status, abnormal creatinine level, American Society of Anesthesiologists class, and increasing age.

Once the clinical evaluation is complete and the type of surgery is known, the need for additional testing and treatment can be determined. Very high-risk patients are defined as those with recent myocardial infarction (within 60 days), unstable angina, decompensated heart failure, and hemodynamically important valvular disease. These patients are at very high risk of preoperative myocardial infarction, heart failure, fatal arrhythmia, and cardiac death. All such patients should be optimally treated and referred to a cardiologist for evaluation.

If emergency surgery is contemplated, little in the way of cardiac assessment can be performed, and recommendations may be directed at perioperative medical management and surveillance. If surgery is not urgent, additional evaluation is based on the clinical assessments of the risk and type of surgery.

Impella 的禁忌证包括：已置入机械主动脉瓣、左心室血栓、严重主动脉狭窄、中重度主动脉瓣关闭不全、严重周围动脉疾病、不能耐受全身抗凝治疗。并发症包括：肢体缺血、血管并发症、机械剪切作用所致红细胞损伤引起溶血，以及需要输血的出血。

TandemHeart

TandemHeart（TandemLife, Pittsburgh, Penn.）是一种经皮离心泵，通过离心泵驱动高达 4 L/min 持续流动的血液，提供机械循环支持。TandemHeart 从股静脉入路置入、穿过房间隔进入左心房，通过 21Fr 流入管从左心房抽取含氧血，经 15Fr~17Fr 流出管注入下腹主动脉或髂动脉。由于需要房间隔穿刺限制了其广泛使用。潜在并发症包括输血需求、感染中毒症/全身炎症反应综合征、鞘管周围出血、胃肠道出血、凝血功能障碍、卒中、左心房穿孔和装置相关的肢体缺血。

右心室支持

急性右心室（RV）衰竭可能发生在以下临床情况中：急性心肌梗死、急性暴发性心肌炎、急性肺栓塞、肺动脉高压、心脏切开术后休克、心脏移植术后和 LVAD 植入后。右心室衰竭的治疗主要包括正性肌力药和肺血管扩张剂，用以提供血流动力学支持和优化容量状态。血管升压药可维持冠状动脉灌注压，吸入一氧化氮可降低右心室后负荷。当药物治疗不足以增加右心室收缩功能时，可能需要机械循环支持进行右心室减压、保证左心室前负荷，并优化组织灌注。

右心室机械循环支持有外科和经皮介入两种方式。与不需要右心室辅助装置（RVAD）的右心室衰竭患者相比，应用外科 RVAD 的患者预后较差。鉴于数据显示置入 RVAD 的患者预后不良，且需要反复行胸骨切开术以置入和撤出机械装置，因此临床应用十分有限。目前有两种经皮介入装置可用于 RV 支持：① Impella RP（Abiomed, Danvers, Mass.），是一种基于导管的轴流泵；② Protek Duo（Cardiac Assist Inc., Pittsburgh, Penn.），是一种带有体外离心泵的导管。Impella RP 经股静脉置入 23Fr 鞘管，将泵送入心房，继而穿过三尖瓣和肺动脉瓣到达主肺动脉，通过一条入口起自下腔静脉、出口到肺动脉的套管提供高达 4 L/min 的连续血流，为右心室减轻负荷。Protek Duo 是一种双腔套管，从颈内静脉经皮置入，流入腔定位在右心房，流出腔定位在主肺动脉，体外泵提供高达 5 L/min 的血流量，并可将氧合器引入回路中，以提供氧合支持。

体外膜肺氧合

对心脏和（或）肺功能不能满足生理需求的患者，ECMO 可提供心肺支持。ECMO 有两种运行模式：静脉-静脉模式（V-V ECMO）用于仅有肺衰竭的患者，静脉-动脉模式（V-A ECMO）用于心肺功能衰竭的患者。ECMO 导管经腔静脉置入右心，从右心房抽吸血液到 ECMO 管路中进行氧合，然后含氧血液在 V-V ECMO 模式下送回右心、在 V-A ECMO 模式下送入动脉系统（近端或远端主动脉）。ECMO 的旁路管道由非脉冲离心泵（用于推动血液流动）和膜氧合器（用于气体交换）组成。V-A ECMO 需要抗凝，而 V-V ECMO 则不需要。并发症包括出血、血栓栓塞和机械并发症，例如溶血和肢端动脉供血不足。

V-V ECMO 提供气体交换，无血流动力学支持作用，适用于有严重气体交换障碍的情况，如急性呼吸窘迫综合征（ARDS）和肺栓塞。而 V-A ECMO 可提供血流动力学支持，根据管路内径、长度和离心泵的性能，血液流量可超过 6 L/min。然而，单独使用 V-A ECMO 并不能降低心室壁张力，通常需要合并使用其他 MCS，如 IABP 或经皮 VAD，以减轻左心室负荷或排空左心室。

心血管疾病患者的非心脏手术

有心血管疾病的患者接受非心脏手术可能会增加死亡或心脏并发症的风险，如心肌梗死、充血性心力衰竭和心律失常。当评估具体患者的手术风险时，会诊医生应了解该患者心脏疾病的类型和严重程度、共患疾病的风险因素，以及手术的类型和紧迫程度。术前评估和处理遵循一般常规即可；但对于围术期心血管风险较大的患者，可以根据治疗和预后需要增加额外的无创和有创性检查。

预测围术期风险主要包括对病史、体格检查、心电图和手术类型等临床情况的详细评估，并根据风险评估模型进行额外的检查和治疗。目前应用最广泛的非心脏手术围术期风险评估模型是一所三级教学医院通过对 4315 名 ≥ 50 岁接受重大非心脏手术的患者进行研究后开发出来的，并在过去 15 年中得到了验证。这项改良心脏风险评估指数（RCRI）包括 6 个独立危险因素：高风险手术、脑血管疾病史、术前胰岛素治疗、缺血性心脏病史、充血性心力衰竭病史和术前血清肌酐水平高于 2.0 mg/dl。临床医生可以根据有 0、1~2 或 ≥ 3 个危险因素，将患者评估为低、中、高心血管风险。另一个风险评估模型是从美国外科医师协会 2007 年国家外科质量改进项目数据库（NSQIP）中开发的，该数据库确定了围术期心肌梗死或心搏骤停的 5 个预测因素：年龄、手术类型、依赖性功能状态、血清肌酐水平异常，以及麻醉医师的级别。

当确定手术类型、完成临床评估后，可进一步完善相关检查和治疗。高危患者定义为近期心肌梗死（60 天内）、不稳定型心绞痛、失代偿性心力衰竭，以及造成了血流动力学影响的心脏瓣膜病患者。这些患者术前发生心肌梗死、心力衰竭、致命性心律失常和心源性死亡的风险非常高，都应该给予最佳治疗，并转诊给心血管专家进行评估。

紧急手术前很少有时间完善心脏评估，主要能做的是围术期严密监护和药物治疗。不太紧迫的手术则应根据临床评估的手术风险和手术类型安排进行额外的检查。

Disease-Specific Approaches
Ischemic Heart Disease

About 70% of MIs occur within the first 6 days after an operation, with the peak incidence between 24 and 72 hours. Multiple stresses associated with surgery such as volume shifts, anemia, and infection can increase the heart rate and blood pressure perioperatively and can provoke myocardial ischemia. Identification of known or symptomatic stable coronary artery disease or risk factors for coronary artery disease can guide further evaluation or changes in perioperative management.

Patients with stable angina represent a continuum from mild to severe. In mild cases, patients manifest angina only after strenuous exercise and do not have signs of left ventricular dysfunction. These patients can be stabilized with optimal medical therapy with aspirin, β-adrenergic blocking agents and statins. On the severe end of the continuum, patients with angina on mild exertion are at high risk for development of perioperative major cardiovascular events and warrant consideration of additional cardiovascular testing.

Coronary angiography and revascularization should be reserved for individuals in whom this treatment would otherwise result in significant improvement in symptoms or long-term survival. Current data do not support a clear benefit of preoperative coronary revascularization.

The preoperative management of patients with a history of recent coronary artery revascularization on antiplatelet therapy is challenging as clinicians balance the cardiac risks of discontinuing therapy with the bleeding risks of continuing antiplatelet agents. Several large observational studies have shown an increased risk of adverse cardiovascular events in patients undergoing noncardiac surgery, particularly within 6 weeks of receiving a coronary stent. While the risk extends to 12 months, it stabilizes without significant decrease in risk from 6 to 12 months. The American College of Cardiology (ACC) and American Heart Association (AHA) guidelines recommend the following algorithm for patients with a coronary stent. If surgery is elective and can be safely delayed, the optimal timing is 12 months after PCI. For those in whom surgery cannot be delayed and are within 30 days of bare metal or 6 months of a drug-eluting stent, dual-antiplatelet therapy with aspirin and $P2Y_{12}$ inhibitor should be continued. If the risk of bleeding is prohibitive, the $P2Y_{12}$ inhibitor is temporarily interrupted (for 5 to 7 days) and aspirin is continued throughout the perioperative period because typically aspirin provides benefits that outweigh the bleeding risk. Possible exceptions to this include intracranial procedures, transurethral prostatectomy, intraocular procedures, and operations with extremely high bleeding risk. In clinical practice, the decision is made with a multidisciplinary team approach considering a number of factors such as the risk of stent thrombosis if DAPT needs to be interrupted, the consequences of delaying the surgical procedure, the increased intra- and periprocedural bleeding risks, and possible consequences of such bleeding if DAPT is continued.

Heart Failure

Studies have shown that heart failure is associated with increased perioperative cardiac morbidity after noncardiac surgery. During the postoperative period, congestive heart failure most commonly occurs in the first 24 to 48 hours, when fluid administered during surgery is mobilized from the extravascular space. However, heart failure may also result from myocardial ischemia and new arrhythmias. Initial management includes identification and treatment of the underlying cause. In addition, intravenous diuretics usually provide rapid relief of pulmonary congestion. If heart failure is complicated by hypotension or poor urine output, insertion of a pulmonary artery catheter may be helpful to guide additional therapy.

Valvular Heart Disease

In regard to valvular heart disease the greatest risk for complications after noncardiac surgery is in those with aortic or mitral stenosis. Patients with symptomatic, severe aortic or mitral stenosis should be evaluated for valve replacement before high-risk noncardiac surgery. In patients with mild to moderate aortic or mitral stenosis, careful attention to volume status and heart rate control are necessary to optimize left ventricular filling and avoid pulmonary congestion. In patients with valve disease or prosthetic heart valves, prophylactic antibiotics are recommended if appropriate. Lifelong anticoagulation with an oral vitamin K antagonist (VKA) is recommended for all patients with mechanical prosthetic heart valves. In addition to the thrombogenic nature of the intravascular prosthetic material, mechanical valves create abnormal flow conditions and areas of high-shear stress, both of which can result in platelet activation leading to valve thrombosis and embolic events. The preoperative management of patients with mechanical heart valves in whom interruption of anticoagulation therapy is needed for diagnostic or surgical procedures should account for the type of procedure, risk factors, and type, location, and number of heart valve prostheses. The ACC/AHA guidelines recommend continuation of VKA anticoagulation with a therapeutic INR in patients undergoing minor procedures (such as dental extractions or cataract removal) where uncontrolled bleeding risk is low. The guidelines recommend bridging anticoagulation with either intravenous unfractionated heparin or subcutaneous low-molecular-weight heparin during the time interval when INR is subtherapeutic in patients who are undergoing invasive or surgical procedures with (1) mechanical aortic valves and any thromboembolic risk factor, (2) older-generation mechanical aortic valves, or (3) mechanical mitral valves.

Arrhythmias and Conduction Defects

Patients with symptomatic, high-grade conduction disturbances, such as third-degree atrioventricular (AV) block, have an increased perioperative risk for cardiac complications and should have a temporary pacemaker inserted before surgery. Patients with first-degree AV block, Mobitz type I AV block, or bifascicular block (right bundle branch block and left anterior fascicular block) do not require prophylactic pacemaker insertion.

Atrial arrhythmias such as atrial fibrillation are common after surgery and usually are not associated with significant complications if the ventricular rate is well controlled. Mounting evidence suggests that new-onset postoperative atrial fibrillation following noncardiac surgery carries a similar risk of thromboembolism as in patients with nonvalvular atrial fibrillation. Therefore, the long-term management of these patients should be similar with regards to anticoagulation.

Ventricular premature beats and nonsustained ventricular tachycardia are also common after noncardiac surgery and do not require specific therapy unless they are associated with myocardial ischemia or heart failure. In most instances, treatment of the underlying cause (e.g., hypoxia, metabolic abnormalities, ischemia, volume overload) results in significant improvement or resolution of the rhythm disturbance without specific antiarrhythmic therapy.

SUGGESTED READINGS

Brickner ME: Cardiovascular management in pregnancy: congenital heart disease, *Circulation* 130:273–282, 2014.

Butt JH, Olesen JB, Havers-Borgersen E, et al.: Risk of thromboembolism associated with atrial fibrillation following noncardiac surgery, *J Am Coll Cardiol* 72:2027–2036, 2018.

Douketis JD, Spyropoulos AC, Kaatz S, et al.: Perioperative bridging anticoagulation in patients with atrial fibrillation, *N Engl J Med* 373:823–833, 2015.

疾病-特异性治疗方案

缺血性心脏病

心肌梗死约70%发生于术后前6天、高峰期在术后24~72h。手术相关的多种应激因素如容量变化、贫血和感染使围术期心率增快、血压升高，并可能诱发心肌缺血。如患者已确诊稳定型冠心病，或当下有冠心病症状，或有多重心血管危险因素，则可根据这些信息进一步明确围术期风险，并指导围术期治疗。

稳定型心绞痛患者的症状从轻度到重度均有，轻症患者只在剧烈运动后才发作心绞痛、且没有左心室功能障碍的表现，可通过最佳药物治疗，如阿司匹林、β受体阻滞剂以及他汀类药物等来稳定病情。而严重心绞痛患者轻微活动即出现症状，其围术期心血管事件风险很高，应考虑进行额外的心血管检查。

冠状动脉造影和冠脉再血管化治疗适用于那些预计能明显缓解症状、改善长期生存的患者，对冠心病患者术前常规进行冠状动脉血运重建治疗无明显获益证据，目前不推荐。

对于近期进行冠状动脉血运重建、正在接受抗血小板治疗的患者，术前处理具有挑战性，临床医生必须权衡停用抗栓药物带来的心血管风险与继续使用抗栓药物的出血风险。数项大型观察性研究表明，近期做过冠状动脉支架治疗的患者非心脏手术围术期心血管不良事件风险增加，尤以6周内置入支架者为著；该风险延长至支架置入术后12个月，在第6~12个月期间，风险相对稳定且无显著下降。美国心脏病学会（ACC）和美国心脏协会（AHA）指南推荐按照以下流程处理冠状动脉支架置入患者：如为择期手术且可安全延迟，则最好推迟到PCI术后12个月再手术。30天内置入金属裸支架或60天内置入药物洗脱支架、且外科手术不能推迟的患者，术前继续使用阿司匹林和P2Y12抑制剂进行双联抗血小板治疗，如出血风险过高，则暂停P2Y12抑制剂5~7天，并在整个围术期继续服用阿司匹林，因为通常阿司匹林的应用获益大于出血风险。颅内手术、经尿道前列腺切除术、眼内手术和出血风险极高的手术不在此列。在临床实践中，应由多学科团队共同做出医疗决策，考量多种因素，包括：中断DAPT治疗带来的支架内血栓形成风险，推迟外科手术的后果，术中和围术期出血风险，以及继续DAPT治疗带来的出血风险等。

心力衰竭

研究表明，心力衰竭（心衰）与非心脏手术围术期心脏事件发生率增加有关。充血性心力衰竭最常发生于术后第24~48h，在此期间，术中输注的液体从血管外间隙被动员转移；心衰也可能是由心肌缺血和新发心律失常所致。应早期识别和治疗潜在病因；利尿剂通常能快速缓解肺充血。如有心衰合并低血压或尿量不足，插入肺动脉导管进行有创血流动力学监测有助于指导治疗。

心脏瓣膜病

在心脏瓣膜病患者中，非心脏手术并发症风险最大的是主动脉瓣狭窄或二尖瓣狭窄患者。症状性严重主动脉瓣或二尖瓣狭窄的患者应在高危非心脏手术前进行评估，看是否先完成瓣膜置换。对轻中度主动脉瓣或二尖瓣狭窄的患者应关注容量状态和心率控制的情况，以达到既保证左心室充盈又避免肺充血。对心脏瓣膜病或人工心脏瓣膜置换的患者推荐根据需要预防性应用抗生素。建议所有人工机械心脏瓣膜置换的患者口服维生素K拮抗剂（VKA）进行终身抗凝治疗，除血管内人工材料的致血栓形成特性外，机械瓣膜还导致异常血流状态和高剪切应力区域，两者共同导致血小板活化，引起瓣膜血栓形成和栓塞事件。人工机械心脏瓣膜患者在进行诊断性操作或外科手术前一般需要考虑中断抗凝治疗，术前权衡时应考虑有创操作或手术的类型、危险因素以及人工心脏瓣膜的类型、位置和数量。ACC/AHA指南建议，当操作或手术不太可能导致不可控出血时，比如拔牙、摘除白内障或小手术操作，应继续VKA抗凝治疗，维持INR在治疗范围。指南建议，对于接受侵入性操作或外科手术，具有①机械主动脉瓣合并任何血栓栓塞高危因素、②老一代机械主动脉瓣或③机械二尖瓣的患者，当INR值低于治疗水平时应使用静脉注射普通肝素或皮下注射低分子量肝素进行桥接抗凝治疗。

心律失常和传导障碍

症状性高度传导阻滞（如三度房室传导阻滞）患者围术期心脏并发症的风险增加，应在手术前植入临时起搏器。一度房室传导阻滞、莫氏Ⅰ型房室传导阻滞或双束支传导阻滞（包括右束支传导阻滞合并左前分支阻滞）的患者不需要预防性植入起搏器。

心房颤动等房性心律失常术后常见，如心室率得到控制，通常不会出现严重并发症。越来越多的证据表明，非心脏手术后新发心房颤动患者与非瓣膜性心房颤动患者血栓栓塞风险相近，因此应接受相似的长期抗凝治疗。

室性早搏和非持续性室性心动过速在非心脏手术后也很常见，除非与心肌缺血或心力衰竭有关，否则不需要特殊治疗。在大多数情况下，对基础病因（如缺氧、代谢异常、缺血、容量过载）的治疗可使心律失常得到显著改善或解决，并不需要特殊的抗心律失常治疗。

推荐阅读

Brickner ME: Cardiovascular management in pregnancy: congenital heart disease, *Circulation* 130:273–282, 2014.
Butt JH, Olesen JB, Havers-Borgersen E, et al.: Risk of thromboembolism associated with atrial fibrillation following noncardiac surgery, *J Am Coll Cardiol* 72:2027–2036, 2018.
Douketis JD, Spyropoulos AC, Kaatz S, et al.: Perioperative bridging anticoagulation in patients with atrial fibrillation, *N Engl J Med* 373:823–833, 2015.

Hayes SN, Kim ESH, Saw J, et al.: Spontaneous coronary artery dissection: current state of the science: a scientific statement from the American Heart Association, *Circulation* 137:e523–e557, 2018.

Huis In't Veld MA, Craft CA, Hood RE: Blunt cardiac trauma review, *Cardiol Clin* 36:183–191, 2018.

Maleszewski J, Anavekar N, Moynihan T, et al.: Pathology, imaging, and treatment of cardiac tumours, *Nat Rev Cardiol* 14:536–549, 2017.

Nanna M, Stergiopoulos K: Pregnancy complicated by valvular heart disease: an update, *J Am Heart Assoc* 3:e000712, 2014.

Nishimura RA, Otto CM, Bonow RO, et al.: 2014 AHA/ACC guideline for the management of patients with valvular heart disease: executive summary: a report of the American College of Cardiology/American Heart Association Task Force on Practice Guidelines, *Circulation* 129:2440–2492, 2014.

Hayes SN, Kim ESH, Saw J, et al.: Spontaneous coronary artery dissection: current state of the science: a scientific statement from the American Heart Association, *Circulation* 137:e523–e557, 2018.

Huis In't Veld MA, Craft CA, Hood RE: Blunt cardiac trauma review, *Cardiol Clin* 36:183–191, 2018.

Maleszewski J, Anavekar N, Moynihan T, et al.: Pathology, imaging, and treatment of cardiac tumours, *Nat Rev Cardiol* 14:536–549, 2017.

Nanna M, Stergiopoulos K: Pregnancy complicated by valvular heart disease: an update, *J Am Heart Assoc* 3:e000712, 2014.

Nishimura RA, Otto CM, Bonow RO, et al.: 2014 AHA/ACC guideline for the management of patients with valvular heart disease: executive summary: a report of the American College of Cardiology/American Heart Association Task Force on Practice Guidelines, *Circulation* 129:2440–2492, 2014.

11

Vascular Diseases and Hypertension

Thomas Sperry, Wanpen Vongpatanasin

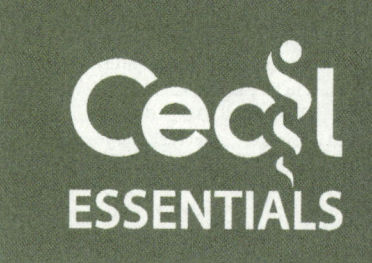

INTRODUCTION

Diseases of the systemic and pulmonary vasculature are among the most common clinical problems encountered in internal medicine. Yet these important diseases are not often given the emphasis they deserve; they fall between the cracks of traditional medical subspecialties. Early clinical recognition is important because effective therapy often can prevent or at least delay needless suffering and death. This chapter reviews the causes, clinical manifestations, diagnostic evaluations, and therapeutic approaches to the major forms of systemic and pulmonary vascular diseases, as well as arterial hypertension.

SYSTEMIC VASCULAR DISEASE

Peripheral Arterial Disease

Peripheral arterial disease (PAD) refers to atherosclerotic vascular disease of mainly the lower extremities. The prevalence increases with age, ranging from 2% to 6% for adults under the age of 60 years to 20% to 30% for those over age 70. As with coronary atherosclerosis, the major reversible risk factors are cigarette smoking, diabetes mellitus, hyperlipidemia, and hypertension. The diagnosis of PAD may at times be elusive, as only 30% to 50% of patients with PAD become symptomatic. PAD may present with symptoms of intermittent claudication, critical limb ischemia, or acute limb ischemia. Roughly 10% to 15% of patients present with the classic syndrome of intermittent claudication, which refers to ischemic muscle pain or weakness brought on by exertion and promptly relieved by rest. A larger proportion of PAD patients (50%) have more atypical leg symptoms different from classic claudication, which either may not limit an individual from walking or may not resolve within 10 minutes of rest. Claudication is also associated with a significant 10-year risk of morbidity and mortality. Approximately 10% to 20% of patients will develop worsening claudication or critical limb ischemia, 5% will require amputation, 10% to 20% will require revascularization, and up to 30% will die of a cardiovascular event (e.g., heart attack, stroke) as a result of concomitant coronary and/or cerebrovascular atherosclerosis. To minimize progression of PAD and avoid complications, risk factor modification is absolutely essential. This includes tight control of blood pressure (BP), plasma lipids, and blood glucose. Complete cessation of tobacco use is a must.

The diagnosis of PAD begins with a careful history and physical examination and is confirmed with noninvasive laboratory testing. Ischemic pain occurs in the leg muscles supplied by arterial segments that are distal to the site of stenosis. Calf claudication is the hallmark of femoral-popliteal disease, whereas discomfort in the thigh, hip, or buttock associated with impotence indicates aortoiliac disease (Leriche syndrome). Depending on the severity of the stenosis, the pain is experienced at a predictable walking distance and is promptly relieved by rest. Claudication must be differentiated from the pseudoclaudication of lumbar degenerative spinal canal stenosis. In the latter condition, walking can also aggravate leg pain, but it is not relieved simply by the cessation of exercise. Rather, assuming positions that minimize lumbar extension such as stooping forward or sitting alleviates the pain. The characteristic physical findings of PAD are absent or diminished pulses distal to the stenosis, bruits over the diseased artery, hair loss, thin shiny skin, and muscle atrophy. Severe ischemia causes pallor, cyanosis, decreased skin temperature, ulceration, and gangrene.

Noninvasive techniques are quite good in the diagnosis of PAD. The *ankle-brachial index* (ABI) is the ratio of the highest systolic BP measured from either the dorsalis pedis or posterior tibialis artery to the highest systolic BP obtained from the brachial artery of either arm using a Doppler stethoscope. The normal ABI range is 1.0 to 1.4. An ABI of 0.9 or less indicates PAD. This simple noninvasive test has a sensitivity and specificity of 68% to 84% and 84% to 99%, respectively, when compared to vascular imaging. In the occasional patient with a high likelihood of PAD but with borderline (between 0.9-1.0) or normal ABI, ABI obtained during exercise treadmill testing may prove useful in the diagnosis. In some patients with diabetes mellitus or renal failure, the media of the affected leg vessels become so heavily calcified that they resist compression except during very high levels of cuff inflation. The result is a falsely elevated ankle BP and an artificially normal or supernormal ABI of greater than 1.4 (Table 11.1). Measurement of toe BP to obtain toe-brachial index in that situation is recommended to verify presence of PAD. Patients with a toe-brachial index of less than or equal to 0.70 are considered to have hemodynamically significant PAD.

Duplex ultrasonography is an important adjunct to the ABI, with a similar sensitivity and specificity. This test is particularly useful to diagnose PAD in patients with noncompressible vessels from medial wall calcification. The Doppler velocity waveform remains abnormal, despite a spuriously normal or elevated ABI. Magnetic resonance (MR) angiography and computed tomographic (CT) angiography also

TABLE 11.1 Interpretation of Ankle-Brachial Index	
Ankle-Brachial Index	**Interpretation**
1.00-1.40	Normal
0.90-0.99	Borderline
0.70-0.89	Mild PAD
0.40-0.69	Moderate PAD
<0.40	Severe PAD
>1.40	Noncompressible vessels

PAD, Peripheral arterial disease.

血管疾病与高血压

陈改玲 耿嘉璐 译 里程楠 刘嘉慧 刘靖 审校 郑金刚 通审

引言

体循环血管和肺血管疾病是内科常见的临床问题之一。然而，这些重要疾病往往没有得到应有的重视，它们在传统医学亚专科的夹缝中生存。早期临床识别很重要，因为有效的治疗通常可以避免或至少延缓不必要的痛苦和死亡。本章回顾了主要的体循环血管病、肺血管疾病以及动脉高血压的原因、临床表现、诊断评估和治疗方法。

体循环血管疾病

周围动脉疾病

周围动脉疾病（PAD）是指主要发生在下肢的动脉粥样硬化性血管疾病。PAD 的患病率随年龄增长而升高，60 岁以下的成年人患病率为 2%～6%，70 岁以上的成年人患病率为 20%～30%。与冠状动脉粥样硬化一样，主要的可逆危险因素是吸烟、糖尿病、高脂血症和高血压。由于仅 30%～50% 的患者出现症状，因此 PAD 有时容易漏诊。PAD 可能表现为间歇性跛行、严重肢体缺血或急性肢体缺血症状。10%～15% 的患者出现典型的间歇性跛行综合征，即在劳累后出现缺血性肌肉疼痛或无力，休息后迅速缓解。更多的 PAD 患者（50%）出现不同于典型跛行的非典型腿部症状，这些症状可能不限制患者行走，也可能休息 10 min 内仍无法缓解。跛行还与 10 年的发病率和死亡率相关。10%～20% 的患者会出现跛行恶化或严重肢体缺血，5% 的患者需要截肢，10%～20% 的患者需要血运重建手术，高达 30% 的患者将因并发冠状动脉和（或）脑血管动脉粥样硬化而死于心血管事件（如心肌梗死、卒中）。为最大限度减缓 PAD 进展，避免并发症发生，危险因素干预是非常重要的，包括严格控制血压、血脂和血糖水平，必须完全戒烟。

PAD 的诊断首先需要仔细询问病史和进行体格检查，然后通过无创的实验室检查确诊。缺血性疼痛发生在动脉狭窄部位以远的腿部肌肉。小腿跛行是股-腘动脉疾病的典型症状，而伴有阳痿的大腿、髋部或臀部不适则提示主髂动脉疾病（Leriche 综合征）。根据动脉狭窄的严重程度，疼痛在可预测的行走距离内发生，经休息可迅速缓解。必须将跛行与腰椎退行性椎管狭窄引起的假性跛行区别开来。在后一种情况下，行走也会加重腿部疼痛，但并不会因为停止运动而缓解。相反，采取尽量减少腰椎伸展的体位，如弯腰前倾或坐位可以缓解疼痛。PAD 的特征性体征包括狭窄部位以远的脉搏减弱或消失、病变部位的血管杂音、毛发脱落、皮肤变薄发亮和肌肉萎缩。严重的缺血会导致苍白、发绀、皮温降低、溃疡和坏疽。

非侵入性技术在 PAD 的诊断中非常有效。踝臂指数（ABI）是使用多普勒听诊器测得足背动脉或胫后动脉的最高收缩压与任一上肢的肱动脉的最高收缩压之比。ABI 正常范围是 1.0～1.4。ABI 低于或等于 0.9 提示存在 PAD。与血管造影相比，这种简单的无创检查的敏感性和特异性分别为 68%～84% 和 84%～99%。在少数高度怀疑 PAD，但 ABI 值在边缘（0.9～1.0）或正常范围的患者，进行平板运动试验获得的 ABI 可能有助于诊断。在一些糖尿病或肾功能衰竭患者中，受累腿部血管钙化严重，除非袖带充气压力非常高，否则所测量的血管无法被压缩。结果是踝部血压假性升高，ABI 正常或高于正常，大于 1.4（表 11.1）。在这种情况下，建议测量脚趾部血压以获得趾踝指数，以确认是否存在 PAD。趾踝指数小于或等于 0.70 的患者被认为存在血流动力学意义上的 PAD。

双相超声波检查是 ABI 的重要辅助手段，其敏感性和特异性相似。对于血管壁钙化导致血管不可压缩的患者，该检查尤其有助于诊断 PAD。尽管 ABI 假性正常或升高，但 Doppler 速度波形仍然异常。磁共振（MR）血管成像和 CT 血管成像也能很好地观察血管

表 11.1 踝臂指数的释义

踝臂指数	释义
1.00～1.40	正常
0.90～0.99	临界
0.70～0.89	轻度 PAD
0.40～0.69	中度 PAD
< 0.4	重度 PAD
> 1.4	不可压缩的血管

PAD，周围动脉疾病

permit excellent visualization of vascular stenosis and identification of runoff vessels. With these noninvasive imaging modalities, spatial resolution is comparable with that of traditional invasive angiography, which now is reserved for patients undergoing revascularization.

The medical management of PAD includes lifestyle and risk factor modification, as well as antiplatelet therapy. Smoking cessation reduces the risk of limb loss, myocardial infarction, and death. Lipid-lowering therapy with high-intensity statin therapy should be initiated and intensified to reduce the rate of vascular events regardless of cholesterol levels. In addition, PAD patients with LDL-C greater than 70 mg/dL despite maximally tolerated statin therapy should be considered for additional lipid-lowering therapy such as ezetimibe. Those with persistently elevated LDL-C despite statin and ezetimibe may then be considered for PCSK9 inhibition. Antihypertensive medication should be initiated and intensified until BP is less than 130/80 mm Hg. Choice of antihypertensive regimen should be based on corresponding comorbidities, but there is some evidence to support the use of ACE inhibitors or angiotensin-receptor blockers. β-Adrenergic blockers do not reduce walking capacity or worsen intermittent claudication in patients with PAD. Aspirin reduces the risk of myocardial infarction, death, and stroke. However, clopidogrel is an effective alternative treatment and is more effective than aspirin in reducing cardiovascular events. Newer antiplatelet agents, such as ticagrelor, have not been proven to be more effective than clopidogrel in reducing cardiovascular events or limb ischemia in patients with symptomatic PAD. More recently, the combination of low-dose factor Xa inhibitor rivaroxaban (2.5 mg twice daily) and low-dose aspirin of (≤100 mg) was shown to reduce the risk of cardiovascular events and limb amputation in PAD patients when compared to low-dose aspirin alone. While the overall bleeding risk is increased with the combination therapy, fatal bleeding is not. Therefore, this combination should be considered in PAD patients with high cardiovascular risk but low bleeding risk. Each patient also needs an exercise prescription as exercise training improves walking capacity and quality of life. This exercise training should be conducted in a medical facility or clinic at a minimal frequency of three times weekly for 12 weeks, preferably for 30 to 45 minutes per session. Cilostazol, a phosphodiesterase-3 inhibitor, is effective in improving claudication symptoms but is not effective in preventing cardiovascular events. Side effects of cilostazol include headache, diarrhea, dizziness, and palpitation. However, cilostazol must be avoided in patients with congestive heart failure because its use in such patients may increase mortality. Pentoxifylline should not be used in PAD as it is no more effective than placebo for intermittent claudication.

Revascularization (percutaneous or surgical) is indicated for patients with severe claudication that is resistant to medical therapy, limb-threatening ischemia, or ischemia-induced impotence (Fig. 11.1). A variety of devices are now available for aortoiliac, femoropopliteal, and infrapopliteal percutaneous interventions, including drug-coated balloons, cutting balloons, laser atherectomy, self-expanding stents, and drug-coated stents. However, efficacy of these newer devices has not been directly compared to each other or to surgical revascularization. In general, surgical revascularization is more suitable for longer areas of stenosis and remains the best option for some patients. The decision between surgery versus endovascular intervention also depends on a patient's life expectancy and other comorbid conditions. Overall, the selection of surgery versus percutaneous intervention as the initial mode of revascularization in patients with limb-threatening ischemia is complex and should be a decision made amongst an interdisciplinary team of physicians.

Acute limb ischemia (ALI) is a vascular emergency. Sudden occlusion of a peripheral artery is caused by either arterial embolism or thrombosis in situ. Arterial emboli usually originate in the cardiac chambers in the setting of preexisting cardiac disease such as myocardial infarction (e.g., left ventricular mural thrombus), congestive heart failure, or atrial arrhythmias (e.g., left atrial thrombus in a patient with atrial fibrillation). Thrombosis in situ usually occurs in arteries with a preexisting severe stenosis in the setting of long-standing PAD with or without previous vascular surgery. Patients with arterial embolism usually experience sudden onset of symptoms without a history of claudication, whereas those with thrombosis in situ typically have a history of claudication that has previously been stable and then suddenly assumes a crescendo pattern over a period of days. In either case, the physical examination reveals a cold, cyanotic (bluish) extremity with absent pulses distal to the site of arterial occlusion and diminished

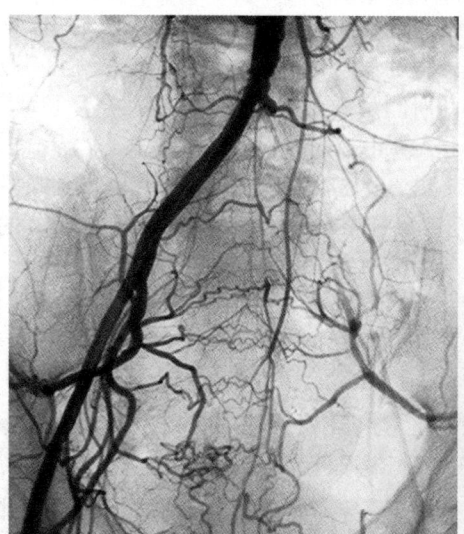 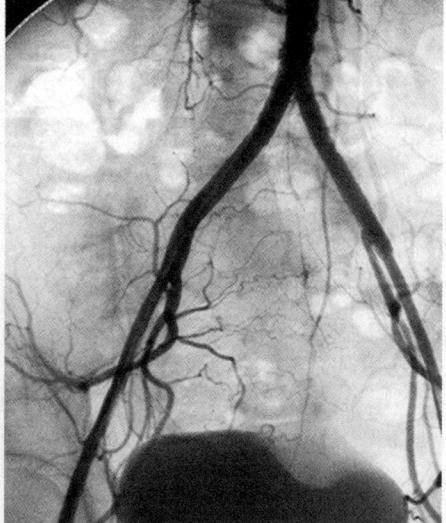

Fig. 11.1 Angiogram of the distal abdominal aorta and iliac arteries demonstrates an occluded left common iliac artery with extensive collateral circulation from the contralateral internal iliac artery *(left)*, which resolved after successful stent implantation *(right)*. (Courtesy of Bart Domatch, MD, Radiology Department, University of Texas Southwestern Medical Center, Dallas, Texas.)

狭窄情况并识别径流血管。这些无创成像技术的空间分辨率与传统的经皮血管造影术相当，而经皮血管造影术目前仅用于血运重建治疗的患者。

PAD 的内科治疗包括生活方式改善、控制危险因素及抗血小板治疗。戒烟可以降低截肢、心肌梗死和死亡的风险。不论血胆固醇水平如何，都应该启动并使用高强度他汀类降脂治疗，以降低血管事件的发生率。此外，在他汀类药物治疗达到最大耐受量的情况下，LDL-C 仍高于 70 mg/dl 的 PAD 患者，应考虑使用额外的降脂治疗，如依折麦布。尽管使用他汀类和依折麦布治疗，但 LDL-C 水平仍然持续升高的患者，可考虑使用 PCSK9 抑制剂。应启动强化降压药物治疗，直至血压低于 130/80 mmHg。降压方案的选择应基于相应的合并症，但有证据支持使用血管紧张素转换酶抑制剂或血管紧张素受体阻滞剂。β 受体阻滞剂不会降低 PAD 患者的行走能力或加重间歇性跛行。阿司匹林可以降低心肌梗死、死亡和卒中的风险。然而，氯吡格雷是一种有效的替代治疗，在降低心血管事件方面比阿司匹林更有效。在降低有症状的 PAD 患者心血管事件或肢体缺血方面，新型抗血小板药物如替格瑞洛尚未被证明比氯吡格雷更有效。最近，低剂量的 Xa 因子抑制剂利伐沙班（2.5 mg，每日两次）与低剂量的阿司匹林（≤ 100 mg）联合治疗与单独使用低剂量的阿司匹林相比，可降低 PAD 患者发生心血管事件和截肢的风险。尽管联合疗法会增加总体出血风险，但不会增加致命性出血风险。因此，对于心血管风险较高但出血风险低的 PAD 患者，应考虑联合治疗。还需为每个患者制定运动处方，因为运动训练可以提高行走能力和改善生活质量。这种运动训练应在医疗机构或诊所进行，每周最少 3 次，每次最好持续 30～45 min，持续 12 周。西洛他唑是一种磷酸二酯酶-3 抑制剂，可有效改善跛行症状，但对预防心血管事件无效。西洛他唑的副作用包括头痛、腹泻、头晕和心悸。然而，在充血性心力衰竭患者必须避免使用西洛他唑，因为此类患者使用可能会增加死亡率。己酮可可碱对间歇性跛行的疗效不优于安慰剂，因此不应用于 PAD 患者。

血运重建（经皮或手术）适用于药物治疗无效的严重跛行、可能导致截肢的缺血或缺血引起阳痿（图 11.1）。目前有多种器械可用于主髂动脉、股-腘动脉和腘下动脉经皮介入治疗，包括药物涂层球囊、切割球囊、激光斑块消蚀设备、自膨胀支架和药物涂层支架。然而，这些较新器械的疗效尚未与其他器械或血运重建手术进行比较。一般来说，外科血运重建手术更适用于较长的狭窄病变，对于某些患者仍然是最佳选择。选择外科手术还是血管内介入治疗，还取决于患者的预期寿命和其他合并症。总之，不论选择外科手术还是经皮介入治疗，作为肢体严重缺血患者的初始血管再通方式都是非常复杂的，应由跨学科医生团队共同决定。

急性肢体缺血（ALI）是一种血管急症。外周动脉突然闭塞通常由动脉栓塞或原位血栓形成引起。动脉栓子通常起源于心腔，发生在心肌梗死（如左心室壁血栓）、充血性心力衰竭或房性心律失常（如心房颤动患者的左心房血栓）等原有心脏病的情况下。原位血栓形成通常发生在已有严重动脉狭窄的长期慢性 PAD 患者，无论既往是否接受过血管手术治疗。动脉栓塞患者通常突然出现症状，且无间歇性跛行症状史，而原位血栓形成患者通常有稳定的间歇性跛行症状病史，在数天内突然加重。无论哪种情况，体格检查均可显示动脉闭塞部位远端肢体冰冷、发绀（发青），脉搏消失，运动和（或）

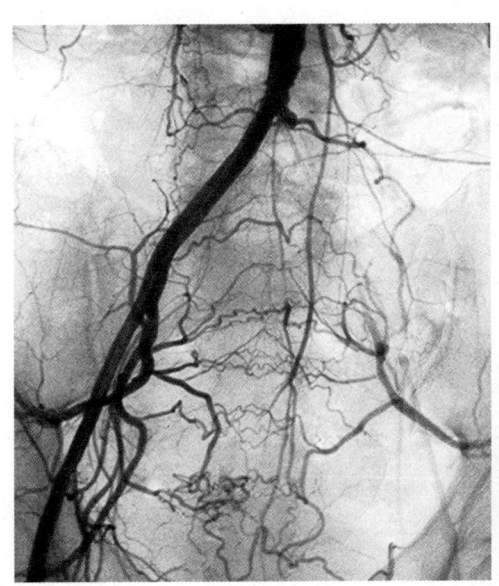 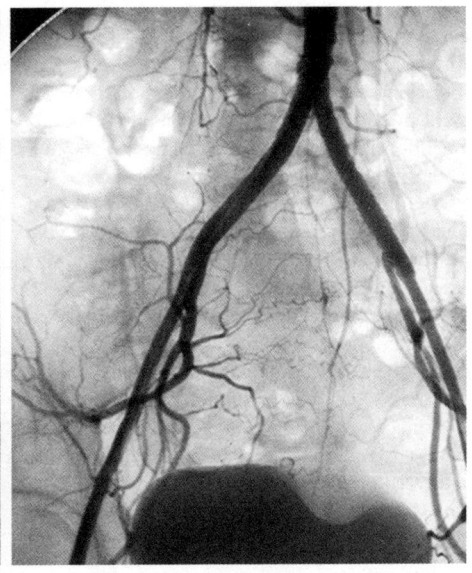

图 11.1 腹主动脉远端和髂动脉的血管造影显示，左侧髂总动脉闭塞，对侧髂内动脉（左图）有广泛的侧支循环，成功置入支架后侧支循环消失（右图）（授权自 Bart Domatch，MD，Radiology Department，University of Texas Southwestern Medical Center，Dallas，Texas.）

motor and/or sensory function. A handheld Doppler device is used to assess signals at different arterial segments and confirms the diagnosis of acute vascular occlusion. Anticoagulation should be initiated immediately with intravenous heparin titrated to maintain the activated partial thromboplastin time equal to 2.0 to 2.5 times control. Catheter-directed infusion of thrombolytic therapy offers a similar success rate in salvaging the limbs as surgical revascularization (thromboembolectomy or bypass surgery). However, survival rate is higher with catheter-based therapy, likely related to the multiple comorbidities of patients with ALI. Patients with irreversible tissue necrosis, regardless of the cause, should be treated with emergent amputation rather than revascularization to reduce the risk of kidney failure (myoglobinuria), sepsis, and multiorgan failure.

Aortic Aneurysm

An aortic aneurysm is commonly defined as a dilation of all three layers of the vessel to more than 50% of the expected normal diameter. The two main types are thoracic aortic aneurysms (TAA), which occur above the diaphragm, and abdominal aortic aneurysms (AAA), which occur below the diaphragm. Abdominal aortic aneurysm is a common vascular disease in older adults, affecting 4% to 8% of men and 0.5% to 1.5% of women over the age of 65 years. Thoracic aortic aneurysm is much less prevalent (0.4% to 0.5%). Besides age, the major risk factors for abdominal aortic aneurysms are cigarette smoking, hypertension, and a family history of aortic aneurysms. Atherosclerosis is responsible for most cases of abdominal aortic aneurysm, while other causes such as genetic (Marfan syndrome, Ehlers-Danlos syndrome, Loeys-Dietz, Turner syndrome, or bicuspid aortic valve), vasculitis with connective tissue disease (Takayasu's arteritis, giant-cell arteritis), chronic infection (syphilitic aortitis), and trauma may cause thoracic or abdominal aortic aneurysms. Abdominal aortic aneurysms gradually grow in size over time at an average rate of 1 to 4 mm per year. The risk of rupture is low until the diameter reaches 5 cm, and then it increases exponentially. The risk of aortic rupture is 1% per year for aneurysms between 3.5 and 4.9 cm in diameter and 5% per year for aneurysms larger than 5 cm.

Most cases of aortic aneurysms are asymptomatic and detected incidentally during routine screening or imaging for other indications. However, some patients with AAA may develop vascular complications such as aneurysm expansion with compression of adjacent structures. Occasionally, mural thrombi form within the aneurysm and embolize, causing acute occlusion of distal arterial segments. Patients with iliac aneurysm may develop hydronephrosis or recurrent urinary tract infection from ureteral compression. Others develop neurologic symptoms from compression of sciatic or femoral nerves. The classic physical finding is a pulsatile nontender mass below the umbilicus (distal to the origin of the renal arteries). In thin patients, normal aortic pulsations are often palpable but above the umbilicus. Hypotension and acute abdominal pain should prompt consideration of aneurysm rupture, which requires emergent operative repair. Duplex ultrasonography is an accurate and reliable diagnostic tool for abdominal aortic and iliac aneurysms. Routine screening for AAA with ultrasonography is recommended for all men between the ages of 65 and 75 years who have ever smoked or men above the age of 60 with family history of AAA among first-degree relatives. Such screening has a proven mortality benefit. CT and MR angiography allow visualization of the thoracic and abdominal aorta, as well as the iliac arteries and its branches (Fig. 11.2).

Medical treatment for aortic aneurysm includes smoking cessation, tight BP control to less than 130/80 mm Hg, and intensive statin therapy. Although transforming growth factor-β has been implicated in the pathogenesis of aortic aneurysm in Marfan syndrome, which is mediated by angiotensin-II receptor activation, losartan was not shown to more effective than beta adrenergic receptor blockade in reducing the rate of aortic root enlargement. β-Adrenergic blockade has not proven beneficial in patients with abdominal aortic aneurysm from other causes. Similarly, a randomized clinical trial failed to demonstrate superiority of angiotensin-converting enzyme inhibitors (ACEI) over calcium-channel blockers in preventing AAA expansion. However, small sample size and inclusion of patients with well-controlled hypertension may have limited the investigators' ability to detect a difference. Patients who develop symptoms from thoracic aneurysms of any size should undergo repair. For asymptomatic patients, presence of large aneurysms (diameter 5.5 cm or above) or rapid aneurysm expansion regardless of the size are also indications for aneurysm repair (Table 11.2). Open surgical repair remains the treatment of choice for thoracic aneurysms involving the aortic root, ascending aorta, or aortic arch. However, thoracic endovascular aortic repair (TEVAR) has now emerged as the procedure of choice for descending thoracic aneurysm given lower early morbidity and mortality compared to open surgical repair in several observational studies. Elective abdominal aortic aneurysm repair carries a perioperative mortality rate of 2% to 6%.

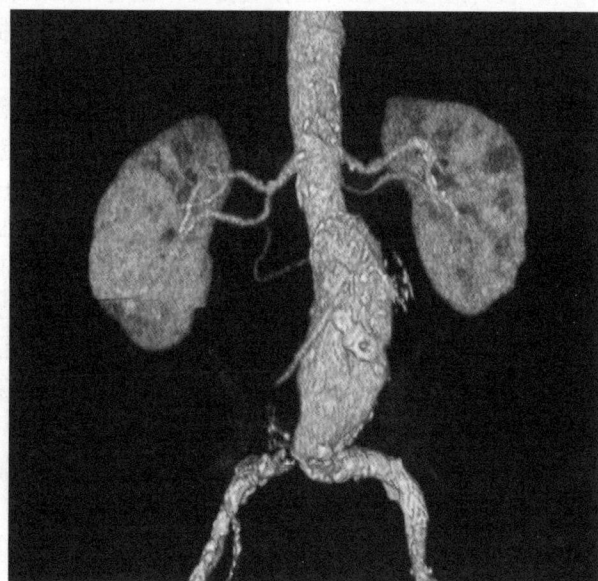

Fig. 11.2 CT angiogram of the distal abdominal aorta shows abdominal aortic aneurysm with the largest diameter of 6.2 cm and severe stenosis at the origin of the right common iliac artery. (Courtesy of Bart Domatch, MD, Radiology Department, University of Texas Southwestern Medical Center, Dallas, Texas.)

TABLE 11.2 Indications for Surgical Treatment of Arterial Aneurysms

Symptoms from expansion of aneurysm or compression of adjacent structure
Rupture of aneurysm
Rapid aortic aneurysm expansion of ≥1 cm per year
Asymptomatic with large size
  Thoracic aneurysm (ascending or descending aneurysm) with diameter >5.5 cm in adults
  For genetic cause of thoracic aneurysm (such as Marfan, Loeys-Dietz, Ehlers-Danlos, Turner syndrome, or bicuspid aortic valve), a lower diameter or aortic size may be considered (generally of at least 5 cm or >4.5 cm in the presence of family history of aortic dissection)
  Abdominal aorta >5.5 cm
  Iliac aneurysm >3 cm

感觉功能减弱。可使用手持式多普勒设备评估不同动脉节段的信号，以确认急性血管闭塞的诊断。一旦确诊，应立即开始抗凝治疗，静脉注射肝素，剂量滴定至维持活化部分凝血活酶时间于参考值的 2.0～2.5 倍。经导管输注溶栓治疗与外科血运重建（血栓切除术或搭桥手术）在挽救肢体方面的成功率相似。然而，基于导管的治疗具有更高的生存率，可能与急性肢体缺血患者的多种合并症降低有关。对于出现不可逆组织坏死的患者，无论病因如何，都应立即进行截肢治疗，而不是进行血运重建手术，以降低肾功能衰竭（肌红蛋白尿）、感染中毒症和多器官功能衰竭的风险。

主动脉瘤

主动脉瘤通常被定义为血管的所有三层都扩张到超过正常直径的 50% 以上。主要有两种类型：胸主动脉瘤（TAA），发生在膈肌上方；腹主动脉瘤（AAA），发生在膈肌下方。腹主动脉瘤是老年人常见的血管疾病，65 岁以上的老年人中，4%～8% 的男性和 0.5%～1.5% 的女性患这种疾病。胸主动脉瘤的发病率要低得多（0.4%～0.5%）。除年龄外，腹主动脉瘤的主要危险因素还包括吸烟、高血压和主动脉瘤家族史。动脉粥样硬化是大多数腹主动脉瘤的病因，其他病因如遗传因素（马方综合征、埃勒斯-当洛综合征、洛伊斯-迪茨综合征、特纳综合征或二叶主动脉瓣）、结缔组织病相关血管炎（大动脉炎、巨细胞动脉炎）、慢性感染（梅毒性主动脉炎）和外伤等都可能导致胸主动脉瘤或腹主动脉瘤。腹主动脉瘤的直径随时间的推移逐渐增大，平均每年增长 1～4 mm。在直径达到 5 cm 之前，破裂风险较低，然后破裂风险呈指数增加。直径在 3.5～4.9 cm 之间的动脉瘤每年主动脉破裂风险为 1%，直径大于 5 cm 的动脉瘤每年主动脉破裂风险为 5%。

大多数主动脉瘤患者无症状，是在常规筛查或因其他适应证的成像检查中被偶然发现。然而，一些 AAA 患者可能会出现血管并发症，如瘤体扩张并压迫邻近结构。偶尔，在动脉瘤内部形成附壁血栓并发生栓塞，导致远端动脉段急性闭塞。髂动脉瘤患者可能会因输尿管受压而出现肾积水或反复尿路感染。其他患者可能会因坐骨神经或股神经受压而出现神经症状。典型的体格检查结果是脐下（肾动脉起始处远端）有搏动性无压痛肿块。瘦弱患者脐上方通常可触及正常的主动脉搏动。低血压和急性腹痛应考虑动脉瘤破裂，需紧急手术修复。双相超声波检查是腹主动脉瘤和髂动脉瘤准确可靠的诊断工具。建议对所有 65～75 岁曾吸烟的男性、或 60 岁以上一级亲属中有 AAA 家族史的男性常规进行超声波筛查 AAA。已证实这样的筛查可降低死亡率。CT 和 MR 血管成像可以显示胸主动脉、腹主动脉以及髂动脉及其分支的情况（图 11.2）。

主动脉瘤的保守治疗包括戒烟、严格控制血压至低于 130/80 mmHg，以及强化他汀类药物治疗。虽然转化生长因子-β 被认为与马方综合征主动脉瘤发病机制有关，其被血管紧张素-Ⅱ 受体激活介导，但在降低主动脉根部扩张速度方面，并未证明氯沙坦比 β 受体阻滞剂更为有效。β 受体阻滞剂还未被证明对其他原因引起的腹主动脉瘤治疗有益。同样，一项随机临床试验也未能证明血管紧张素转换酶抑制剂（ACEI）在预防腹主动脉瘤扩大方面优于钙通道阻滞剂。然而，由于样本量较小，且纳入血压控制良好的高血压患者，这可能限制了研究人员检测差异的能力。无论瘤体大小，只要是因胸主动脉瘤而出现了症状，都应进行修复治疗。对于无症状患者，大的动脉瘤（直径≥ 5.5 cm），或无论大小但动脉瘤快速扩大也是行动脉瘤修复的指征（表 11.2）。对于累及主动脉根部、升主动脉或主动脉弓的胸主动脉瘤，开放手术修复仍是首选治疗方法。然而，多项观察性研究显示，胸主动脉血管内修复术（TEVAR）的早期发病率和死亡率低于开放手术修复治疗，因此已成为降主动脉瘤的首选治疗方法。选择性腹主动脉瘤修复术的围术期死亡率为 2%～6%。此

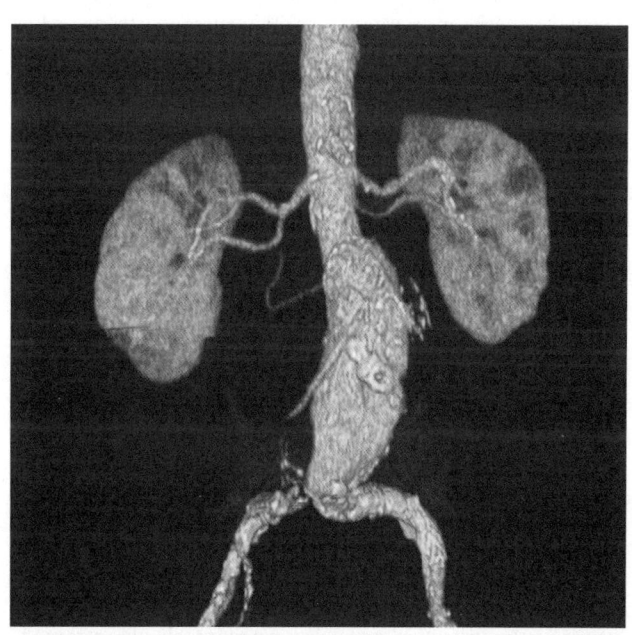

图 11.2　腹主动脉 CT 血管成像显示腹主动脉瘤，最大直径 6.2 cm，右髂总动脉起始部位严重狭窄（授权自 Bart Domatch，MD，Radiology Department，University of Texas Southwestern Medical Center，Dallas，Texas.）

表 11.2　动脉瘤的外科治疗适应证
动脉瘤扩张或压迫邻近结构引起了症状
动脉瘤破裂
主动脉瘤每年快速扩张≥ 1 cm
无症状但体积较大
胸主动脉瘤（升主动脉瘤或降主动脉瘤）直径＞ 5.5 cm（成人）
对于有胸主动脉瘤遗传病因（如马方、洛伊斯-迪茨、埃勒斯-当洛、特纳综合征或二叶主动脉瓣）的患者，即使主动脉直径较小（至少 5 cm 或有主动脉夹层家族史者＞ 4.5 cm）也应考虑手术
腹主动脉瘤＞ 5.5 cm
髂动脉瘤＞ 3 cm

Furthermore, a large randomized study failed to demonstrate any benefit of surgery in patients with aneurysms 4.0 to 5.4 cm in diameter. For these reasons, patients with small aortic aneurysms (4.0 to 5.4 cm in diameter) should be treated medically with close monitoring of aneurysm size with periodic imaging studies every 6 to 12 months (see Table 11.2).

Percutaneous endovascular aneurysm repair (EVAR) is an alternative method to open surgical repair for treatment of abdominal aortic aneurysm. EVAR offers lower perioperative death than surgical repair with equivalent long-term survival. However, EVAR should be reserved for patients with favorable anatomy who are able to return for follow-up visits and repeated imaging studies of the aneurysm sites to ensure that the stent graft is free from endovascular leaks or displacement.

Aortic Dissection

In aortic dissection, the intimal layer is torn from the aortic wall leading to the formation of a false lumen in parallel with the true lumen. Risk factors include hypertension, cocaine use, trauma, hereditary connective tissue disease (e.g., Marfan syndrome, Ehlers-Danlos syndrome), vasculitis (e.g., Takayasu's arteritis, giant-cell arteritis), Behçet's disease, bicuspid aortic valve, and aortic coarctation. Aortic dissection can be classified as types A and B (Stanford system). Type A dissection involves the ascending aorta, whereas type B dissection involves the distal aorta. The DeBakey system subdivides aortic dissection into three subtypes—types I, II, and III. Type 1 dissection involves the entire aorta, whereas type II involves only the ascending aorta and type III involves only the descending aorta. Aortic dissection involving the ascending aorta carries a high mortality rate of 1% to 2% per hour during the first 24 to 48 hours. Patients usually develop acute onset of severe chest or back pain. Abdominal pain, syncope, and stroke are common. Retrograde propagation of the dissection can cause pericardial tamponade or coronary artery dissection with acute myocardial infarction. Dissection involving the aortic valve causes acute severe aortic insufficiency with acute pulmonary edema. The dissection plane may propagate in an antegrade direction to compromise flow in the carotid and subclavian arteries, producing a stroke or acute upper limb ischemia. Patients with distal (type B) aortic dissection exhibit acute onset of back pain or chest pain often accompanied by lower extremity ischemia and ischemic neuropathy.

The physical findings include pulse deficits, neurologic deficits, or a diastolic murmur of aortic regurgitation. However, acute aortic regurgitation into an unprepared ventricle produces only a short, soft diastolic murmur that is often missed. The widened pulse pressure and associated physical findings of chronic aortic regurgitation are absent, and the clinical picture is that of an acutely ill patient with tachypnea, tachycardia, and a narrow pulse pressure. Hypotension, jugular venous distention, and pulsus paradoxus should prompt the diagnosis of pericardial tamponade. Transesophageal echocardiography, MR angiography, or CT angiography confirm the diagnosis by demonstrating an intimal flap that separates the true lumen from the false lumen (Fig. 11.3). Type A aortic dissection is uniformly fatal without emergent surgical repair. With surgery, mortality is reduced to 10% at 24 hours and 20% at 30 days. Patients with type B aortic dissection should be treated medically because 1-year survival is higher with medical therapy than it is with surgery (75% versus 50%). However, surgery is indicated if type B dissection compromises blood flow to the legs, kidneys, or other viscera. Tight control of BP is essential because aortic aneurysm was found to develop in 30% to 50% of patients with type B aortic dissection when studied over 4 years.

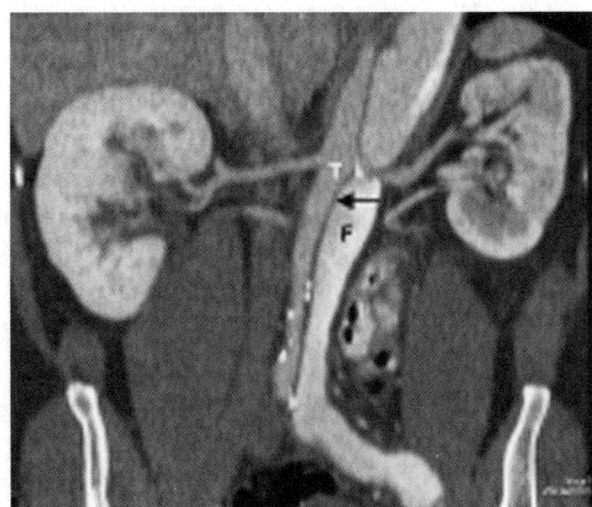

Fig. 11.3 CT angiogram of the aorta shows type B aortic dissection. The intimal flap *(arrow)* separates the true lumen *(T)* from the false lumen *(F)* and compromises blood flow to the right kidney causing renal atrophy and cortical thinning. (Courtesy of Bart Domatch, MD, Radiology Department, University of Texas Southwestern Medical Center, Dallas, Texas.)

Penetrating Aortic Ulcers and Intramural Hematoma

Penetrating aortic ulcers and intramural hematomas exhibit chest pain that is indistinguishable from that of aortic dissection. In contrast to aortic dissection, however, the pathologic condition is localized. No identifiable intimal flap and thus no branch vessel occlusion are produced. Disruption of the internal elastic lamina produces aortic ulcers that erode into the medial wall and protrude into the surrounding structures. Rupture of the vasa vasorum causes formation of localized hematoma underneath the adventitia with resultant asymmetric thickening of the aortic wall. Patients with either condition typically are older than those with aortic dissection, have a larger aortic size, and have a higher prevalence of abdominal aortic aneurysm. Aortic rupture is the major complication of both penetrating ulcers and intramural hematomas, particularly with those aneurysms located in the ascending aorta. The diagnosis is made with invasive angiography, CT angiography, or MR angiography (Fig. 11.4). Surgical intervention should be considered for ulcers and hematomas of the ascending aorta, deeply penetrating ulcers, or severely bulging hematomas, irrespective of their location. Ulcers and hematomas of the descending aortic may be managed successfully with β-adrenergic blockade and tight control of BP.

Other Arterial Diseases

Buerger's disease, or thromboangiitis obliterans is a nonatherosclerotic disease of the arteries, veins, and nerves of the arms and legs affecting mostly young men before the age of 45 years. The mechanism is unknown, but all patients have a history of heavy tobacco addiction. The presenting symptom is claudication of the feet, legs, hands, or arms. Multiple-limb involvement and superficial thrombophlebitis are common. The C-reactive protein and Westergren sedimentation rate typically are normal, and a search for serologic markers for connective tissue disease (e.g., antinuclear antibody or rheumatoid factor, antiphospholipid antibody) is negative. The diagnosis is based on the typical clinical presentation. If the presentation is atypical, then biopsy is needed to make the diagnosis. The histologic hallmark is inflammatory intramural thrombi within the arteries and veins with sparing of internal elastic lamina and other arterial wall structures. The most effective

外，一项大型随机研究未能证明手术治疗对瘤体直径为4.0～5.4 cm的患者有任何益处。因此，小主动脉瘤（直径4.0～5.4 cm）患者应接受药物治疗，同时每6～12个月定期进行影像检查，密切监测动脉瘤的大小（见表11.2）。

经皮血管内动脉瘤修复术（EVAR）是腹主动脉瘤开放手术修复的替代治疗方法。与手术修复相比，EVAR的围术期死亡率较低，长期存活率相当。然而，EVAR应限于解剖结构良好的患者，这些患者应能复诊并反复进行动脉瘤部位的成像检查，以确保支架没有发生内漏或移位。

主动脉夹层

主动脉夹层是主动脉壁内膜层撕裂，形成一个与真腔平行的假腔。危险因素包括高血压、使用可卡因、外伤、遗传性结缔组织病（如马方综合征、埃勒斯-当洛综合征）、血管炎（如大动脉炎、巨细胞动脉炎）、白塞病、二叶主动脉瓣和主动脉缩窄。主动脉夹层可分为A型和B型（Stanford分型）。A型夹层累及升主动脉，而B型夹层累及远端主动脉。DeBakey系统将主动脉夹层分为三个亚型：Ⅰ型、Ⅱ型和Ⅲ型。Ⅰ型夹层累及整个主动脉，而Ⅱ型只累及升主动脉，Ⅲ型只累及降主动脉。累及升主动脉的主动脉夹层在最初24～48 h内每小时的死亡率高达1%～2%。患者通常会急性发作剧烈胸痛或背痛。腹痛、晕厥和卒中为常见症状。夹层的逆撕可导致心包积液，或冠状动脉夹层而引起急性心肌梗死。累及主动脉瓣的夹层会导致急性严重主动脉瓣关闭不全，并出现急性肺水肿。夹层可能前行撕裂，影响颈动脉和锁骨下动脉的血流，导致卒中或急性上肢缺血。远端主动脉夹层（B型）患者通常会出现急性背痛或胸痛，常伴有下肢缺血和缺血性神经病变。

体格检查结果包括无脉、神经功能缺损或主动脉瓣反流的舒张期杂音。然而，急性主动脉瓣反流进入心室仅会产生短暂而轻柔的舒张期杂音，常常被漏诊。脉压增大和慢性主动脉瓣反流相关的体征均不存在，临床常表现为急性发病患者伴呼吸急促、心动过速和窄脉压。低血压、颈静脉充盈和奇脉提示心脏压塞。经食管超声心动图、磁共振血管成像或CT血管成像可通过显示将真腔与假腔分离的内膜片而确诊（图11.3）。A型主动脉夹层如不进行紧急手术修复，患者无法幸存。通过手术治疗，24 h死亡率降至10%，30天死亡率降至20%。B型主动脉夹层患者应接受药物治疗，因为药物治疗的1年生存率高于手术治疗（75% vs. 50%）。然而，如果B型主动脉夹层累及肢体、肾脏或其他内脏器官的血供，则应进行手术治疗。严格控制血压至关重要，因为在对B型主动脉夹层患者进行为期4年的研究后发现，30%～50%的患者会发展成主动脉瘤。

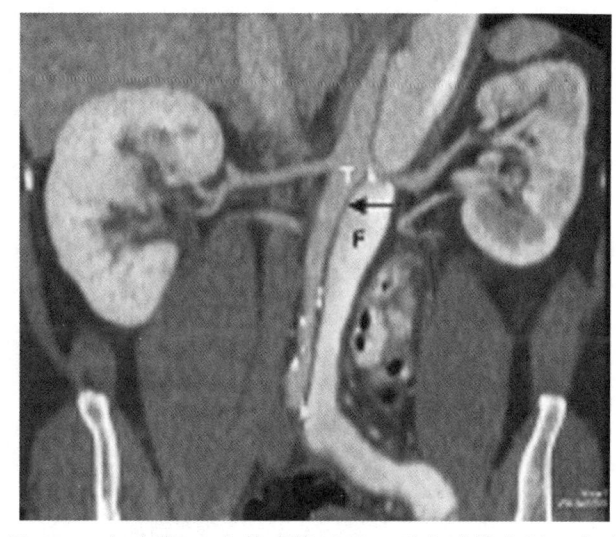

图11.3 主动脉CT血管成像显示B型主动脉夹层。内膜片（箭头）将真腔（T）与假腔（F）分开，影响右肾的血供，导致肾萎缩和皮质变薄（授权自Bart Domatch, MD, Radiology Department, University of Texas Southwestern Medical Center, Dallas, Texas.）

穿透性主动脉溃疡和壁内血肿

穿透性主动脉溃疡和壁内血肿表现出的胸痛与主动脉夹层无法区分。然而，与主动脉夹层不同的是，穿透性主动脉溃疡病变部位是局部的。没有可识别的内膜片，因此不会发生分支血管闭塞。内弹力膜的破裂产生主动脉溃疡，侵蚀到中膜壁并突出到周围结构中。血管滋养动脉的破裂会在血管外膜下形成局部血肿，导致主动脉壁的不对称增厚。有这两种情况的患者通常比主动脉夹层患者年龄更大，主动脉内径更大，腹主动脉瘤患病率更高。主动脉破裂是穿透性溃疡和壁内血肿的主要并发症，尤其是位于升主动脉的动脉瘤。通过侵入性血管造影、CT血管成像或MR血管成像（图11.4）进行诊断。对于升主动脉溃疡和血肿、深度穿透性溃疡或严重突起的血肿，无论其位置如何，都应考虑手术治疗。降主动脉的溃疡和血肿可通过β受体阻滞剂和严格控制血压来成功管理。

其他动脉疾病

Buerger病，或称血栓闭塞性脉管炎，是一种非动脉粥样硬化性疾病，好发于四肢动脉、静脉和神经，主要发生于年龄在45岁以下的年轻男性。发病机制不明，但所有患者都有严重的烟瘾史。主要症状是脚、腿、手或臂的活动障碍（claudication）。多肢体受累和浅表血栓性静脉炎很常见。C反应蛋白和魏氏法红细胞沉降率通常正常，结缔组织病的血清标志物（如抗核抗体或类风湿因子、抗磷脂抗体）的检测结果为阴性。诊断基于典型的临床表现。如果表现不典型，则需要进行活检才能确诊。组织学特征是动脉和静脉内有炎性壁内血栓，内

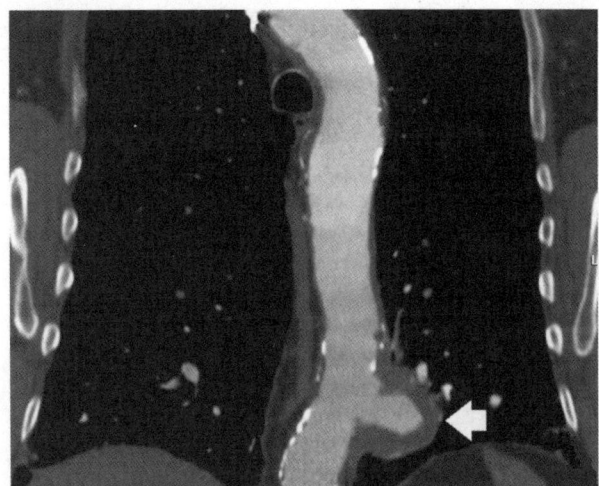

Fig. 11.4 CT angiogram of the descending thoracic aorta shows a large penetrating aortic ulcer above the diaphragm *(arrow)*. (Courtesy of Bart Domatch, MD, Radiology Department, University of Texas Southwestern Medical Center, Dallas, Texas.)

treatment for Buerger's disease is complete tobacco abstinence. The prostacyclin analog iloprost constitutes adjunctive therapy to reduce limb ischemia and improve wound healing.

Raynaud's phenomenon is a vasospastic disease of the small arteries of mainly the fingers and toes. Primary (idiopathic) Raynaud's phenomenon occurs in the absence of underlying disorders. Secondary Raynaud's phenomenon occurs in association with connective tissue diseases (e.g., scleroderma, polymyositis, rheumatoid arthritis, systemic lupus erythematosus), as well as with repeated mild physical trauma (e.g., use of jackhammers), certain drugs (e.g., antineoplastic chemotherapeutic agents, interferon, monamine-reuptake inhibitors such as tricyclic antidepressants, serotonin agonists), and Buerger's disease. Patients usually complain of recurrent episodes of digital ischemia, with a characteristic white-blue-red color sequence. Pallor is followed by cyanosis if ischemia is prolonged and then by erythema (reactive hyperemia) when the episode resolves. Episodes are precipitated by cold temperature or emotional stress. Physical examination can be entirely normal between attacks with normal radial, ulnar, and pedal pulses. Some patients may have digital ulcers or thickening of fat pad (sclerodactyly). Patients should be instructed to avoid cold temperatures and dress warmly. Calcium-channel blockers (CCBs) reduce the frequency and severity of vasospastic episodes.

Giant-cell arteritis is an immune-mediated vasculitis predominantly involving medium-sized and large arteries such as the subclavian artery, axillary artery, and aorta of the older adult with a strong male predominance. Approximately 40% of patients with giant-cell arteritis also have polymyalgia rheumatica, a syndrome characterized by severe stiffness and pain originating in the muscles of the shoulders and pelvic girdle. Patients may exhibit headache from temporal arteritis, jaw claudication from ischemia of the masseter muscles, or visual loss from involvement of the ophthalmic artery. Chest pain suggests the coexistence of aortic aneurysm or dissection. Physical findings include low-grade fever, scalp tenderness in the temporal area, pale and edematous fundi, or a diastolic murmur of aortic regurgitation. BP difference of more than 15 mm Hg between arms suggests subclavian artery stenosis. Laboratory findings include significantly elevated C-reactive protein and Westergren sedimentation rate plus anemia. The diagnosis is confirmed by histologic examination of the arterial tissue (frequently from temporal artery biopsy), showing infiltration of lymphocytes and macrophages (i.e., giant cells) in all layers of the vascular wall. High-dose corticosteroids are highly effective and should be initiated immediately when the diagnosis is suspected to prevent potentially permanent blindness. To minimize complications from long-term corticosteroid administration, the steroid dose should be tapered to find the lowest dose needed to suppress symptoms, which often wane. Every attempt should be made to discontinue corticosteroids over time, and treatment with methotrexate or the interleukin-6 receptor antagonist tocilizumab may be used as steroid sparing agents.

Takayasu's arteritis is an idiopathic granulomatous vasculitis of the aorta, its main branches, and the pulmonary artery. This condition is particularly common in young women of Asian descent, but it also occurs in non-Asian women and men. The inflammatory process in the vascular wall can lead to stenosis and/or aneurysm formation. Hypertension, as a result of renal artery stenosis or aortic coarctation, is the most common manifestation and is present in as many as 80% of affected individuals. Because the vascular involvement is so widespread, patients may have symptoms and signs of coronary ischemia, congestive heart failure, stroke, vertebrobasilar insufficiency, or intermittent claudication. Physical findings include bruits over the subclavian arteries or aorta, as well as diminished brachial pulses and thus a low brachial artery BP. The diagnosis is based primarily on this clinical presentation. First-line treatment is with corticosteroids. Other immunosuppressive agents such as methotrexate or cyclophosphamide are often added to prevent disease progression and relapse, and newer biologics such as anti-TNF inhibitors (infliximab, etanercept) provide a viable alternative. Immunosuppressive therapy does not cause regression of preexisting vascular stenoses or aneurysms. For this reason, percutaneous or surgical revascularization is usually required.

Arteriovenous (AV) fistulas are abnormal vascular communications that shunt blood flow from the arterial system directly into the venous system, bypassing the capillary beds that normally ensure optimal tissue perfusion and nutrient exchange. AV fistulas may be congenital, as in AV malformation (AVM), or acquired. The main causes of acquired AV fistula are penetrating trauma (e.g., gunshot, knife wound) and surgically created shunts for hemodialysis access. Patients may exhibit a pulsatile mass, symptoms related to compression of an adjacent organ, or bleeding from spontaneous rupture of an AVM. Systolic and diastolic bruits or thrills may be detectable over the fistula or AVM. An AVM in skeletal muscle may lead to bone malformation or a pathologic fracture, whereas AVM in the brain may result in neurologic deficits or seizures. High-output heart failure is another complication from a large AVM or fistula. MR angiography, CT angiography, or conventional angiography confirms the diagnosis. Depending on the size and location of the AVM, treatment options include surgical resection, transcatheter embolization, or pulse laser irradiation. Patients with acquired AV fistulas from trauma usually need surgical closure.

PULMONARY VASCULAR DISEASE

Pulmonary hypertension is characterized by elevated mean pulmonary artery pressure (PAP) of greater than 20 mm Hg at rest. The many causes of pulmonary hypertension are summarized in Table 11.3.

Patients with pulmonary hypertension not only have an elevated pulmonary arterial pressure but also a low cardiac output, causing symptoms of exertional dyspnea, fatigue, and syncope. Pulmonary capillary wedge pressure is usually normal (≤15 mm Hg) except in patients with pulmonary hypertension due to impaired left ventricular systolic or diastolic function or left-sided valvular heart disease.

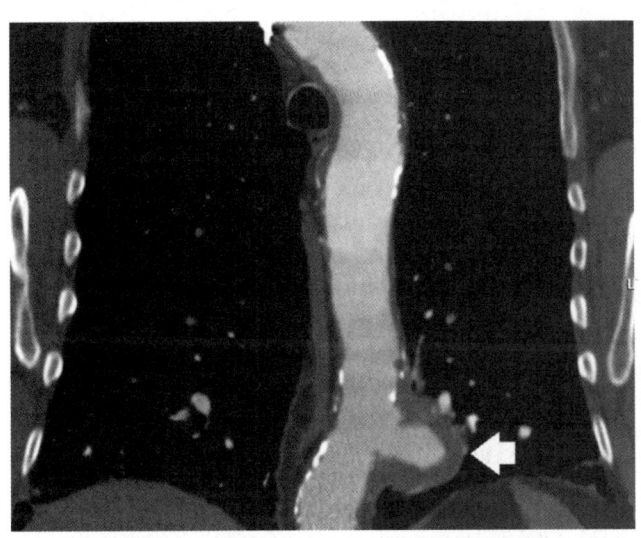

图 11.4 胸降主动脉 CT 血管成像显示在横膈肌上方有一个大的穿透性主动脉溃疡（箭头）（授权自 Bart Domatch, MD, Radiology Department, University of Texas Southwestern Medical Center, Dallas, Texas.）

弹力膜层和其他动脉壁结构不受影响。对于 Buerger 病最有效的治疗方法是严格戒烟。前列环素类似物伊洛前列素是辅助疗法，可减轻肢体缺血并改善伤口愈合。

雷诺现象是一种主要发生在手指和脚趾小动脉的血管痉挛性疾病。原发性（特发性）雷诺现象在没有潜在疾病情况下发生。继发性雷诺现象与结缔组织疾病（如硬化症、多发性肌炎、类风湿关节炎、系统性红斑狼疮）以及反复轻度物理创伤（如使用手提钻）、某些药物（如抗肿瘤化疗药物、干扰素、单胺再摄取抑制剂如三环类抗抑郁药、5-羟色胺激动剂）和 Buerger 病有关。患者通常主诉反复发作的手指缺血，呈现典型的白-蓝-红的颜色顺序。如果缺血时间较长，会出现苍白，然后是发绀，发作缓解后出现红斑（反应性充血）。低温或情绪紧张会诱发发病。在发作间歇期，体格检查可能完全正常，尺动脉、桡动脉和足动脉脉搏正常。一些患者可能有手指溃疡或脂肪垫增厚（硬结）的症状。应指导患者避免低温，并注意保暖。钙通道阻滞剂（CCB）可以减少血管痉挛发作的频率和严重程度。

巨细胞动脉炎是一种免疫介导的血管炎，主要累及中型和大型动脉，如锁骨下动脉、腋动脉和主动脉，老年人、男性多见。大约 40% 的巨细胞动脉炎患者伴有多发性风湿痛，这是一种以严重的肩部和骨盆肌肉僵硬和疼痛为特征的综合征。患者可能会因颞动脉炎而出现头痛，因咀嚼肌缺血而出现下颌跛行，或者眼动脉受累引起视力丧失。胸痛提示同时存在主动脉瘤或夹层。体格检查结果包括低热、颞部头皮触痛、眼底苍白水肿或主动脉瓣反流的舒张期杂音。两臂血压相差超过 15 mmHg 提示锁骨下动脉狭窄。实验室检查结果包括明显升高的 C 反应蛋白和魏氏法红细胞沉降率以及贫血。通过对动脉组织进行组织学检查（通常是颞动脉活检），显示血管壁各层均有淋巴细胞和巨噬细胞（即巨细胞）浸润，即可确诊。高剂量皮质类固醇激素疗效显著，一旦疑诊此病，应立即开始使用，以防止潜在的永久性失明。为尽量减少长期使用皮质类固醇引起的并发症，应逐渐减少类固醇剂量，以找到抑制症状（症状通常会减轻）所需的最低剂量。应尽量停用皮质类固醇，并可使用甲氨蝶呤或白细胞介素-6 受体拮抗剂托西单抗作为激素的替代药物。

大动脉炎是主动脉及其主要分支和肺动脉的特发性肉芽肿性血管炎。这种疾病尤其常见于亚裔年轻女性，但也发生在非亚裔女性和男性中。血管壁的炎症过程可导致狭窄和（或）动脉瘤形成。肾动脉狭窄或主动脉缩窄导致的高血压是最常见的临床表现，多达 80% 的患者会出现这种情况。由于血管受累范围广泛，患者可能出现冠状动脉缺血、充血性心力衰竭、卒中、椎-基底动脉供血不足或间歇性跛行的症状和体征。体征包括锁骨下动脉或主动脉杂音，以及肱动脉脉搏减弱，因此肱动脉血压偏低。诊断主要基于这一临床表现。一线治疗是使用皮质类固醇。通常还会添加其他免疫抑制剂，如甲氨蝶呤或环磷酰胺，以防止疾病进展和复发，较新的生物制剂如抗 TNF 抑制剂（英夫利昔单抗、依那西普）也是一种可行的替代疗法。免疫抑制治疗不能使已有的血管狭窄或动脉瘤消退。因此，通常需行经皮或外科血运重建术。

动静脉瘘是异常的血管通路，将血液从动脉系统直接引流到静脉系统，绕过了通常确保最佳组织灌注和营养交换的毛细血管床。动静脉瘘可以是先天性的，如动静脉畸形（AVM），也可以是后天获得的。后天获得的动静脉瘘的主要原因包括穿透性外伤（如枪击、刀伤）和为血液透析而手术建立的分流通路。患者可能出现搏动性肿块、与邻近器官受压有关的症状或因 AVM 自发破裂而出血。在动静脉瘘或动静脉畸形处可检测到收缩期和舒张期杂音或震颤。骨骼肌内的动静脉畸形可能导致骨骼畸形或病理性骨折，而脑部的动静脉畸形可能导致神经功能缺损或癫痫发作。高输出量性心力衰竭是大型动静脉畸形或动静脉瘘的另一种并发症。磁共振血管成像、CT 血管成像或常规血管造影可以确定诊断。根据动静脉畸形的大小和位置，治疗选择包括外科切除、经导管栓塞或脉冲激光照射。外伤引起的后天动静脉瘘通常需要外科闭合术。

肺血管疾病

肺动脉高压的特征是静息状态下平均肺动脉压（PAP）大于 20 mmHg。肺动脉高压的众多原因总结于表 11.3。

肺动脉高压患者不仅肺动脉压升高，而且心输出量降低，导致运动时呼吸困难、疲劳和晕厥等症状。肺毛细血管楔压通常正常（≤ 15 mmHg），但因左心室收缩或舒张功能障碍或左心室心脏瓣膜病引起的肺动脉高压患者除外。

TABLE 11.3 Classification of Pulmonary Hypertension

Category 1: Pulmonary Arterial Hypertension (PAH)
Primary pulmonary hypertension (PPH) or idiopathic pulmonary hypertension (IPAH):
  Sporadic
  Familial
PPH associated with:
  Connective tissue disease
  Congenital heart disease
  Portal hypertension
  Human immunodeficiency viral infection
  Drugs and toxins: Anorexigens, cocaine, methamphetamine

Category 2: Pulmonary Venous Hypertension
Left ventricular heart failure
Left ventricular valvular heart disease

Category 3: Pulmonary Hypertension Associated With Chronic Respiratory Disease or Hypoxemia
Chronic obstructive pulmonary disease
Obstructive sleep apnea

Category 4: Pulmonary Hypertension Associated With Chronic Venous Thromboembolism
Left ventricular valvular heart disease

Category 5: Pulmonary Hypertension Due to Miscellaneous Disorders Directly Affecting the Pulmonary Vasculature
Sarcoidosis, histiocytosis X, compression of pulmonary vessels (adenopathy, tumor, fibrosing mediastinitis)

Pulmonary Arterial Hypertension

Pulmonary arterial hypertension (PAH) is caused by a combination of pulmonary vasoconstriction, endothelial cell and/or smooth muscle proliferation, intimal fibrosis, and thrombosis in the pulmonary capillaries and arterioles. PAH is either idiopathic (primary pulmonary hypertension [PPH]) or secondary to connective tissue disease, congenital heart disease, portal hypertension, or human immunodeficiency viral (HIV) infection, as well as anorexigenic drugs or toxins. Connective tissue diseases, particularly scleroderma, are the most common secondary causes of PAH.

Patients with mild PAH can be asymptomatic, but patients with more advanced disease complain of exertional dyspnea, chest pain, syncope, or presyncope. Orthopnea is an uncommon symptom associated with PAH and more commonly identified in patients with pulmonary hypertension from left-sided heart disease. Physical findings include a left parasternal lift, loud pulmonary component of the second heart sound, murmur of tricuspid or pulmonic regurgitation, hepatomegaly, peripheral edema, or ascites. Associated ECG abnormalities indicate right ventricular hypertrophy, right atrial enlargement, or right axis deviation. Echocardiography provides important information about the severity of the pulmonary hypertension (i.e., estimated pulmonary artery pressure, right ventricular dimensions and function) and its potential causes (e.g., left ventricular failure, valvular lesions, congenital heart disease with left-to-right shunts). Pulmonary function tests, ventilation-perfusion (V̇/Q̇) lung scans, polysomnography or overnight oximetry, autoantibody tests, HIV serology, and liver-function tests also should be performed to determine other potential causes. Right ventricular catheterization should be performed in all patients with suspected PAH. Under basal conditions in the catheterization laboratory, an elevated mean pulmonary artery pressure exceeding 20 mm Hg, a pulmonary capillary wedge pressure below 15 mm Hg, and a pulmonary vascular resistance exceeding 3 units confirm the diagnosis. Acute vasodilator drug challenge should be performed during right ventricular catheterization to guide appropriate treatment.

Without treatment, the prognosis of PAH is poor with a median survival of less than 3 years. Patients with high-risk features for clinical deterioration or death, including poor functional capacity, history of syncope, or right ventricular failure, should be treated with intravenous epoprostenol (a prostacyclin analog) because of its proven efficacy to improve exercise capacity and overall survival. Other prostacyclin analogs such as beraprost, treprostinil, and iloprost or prostacyclin-receptor agonists such as selexipag are also effective in reducing pulmonary artery pressure and improving exercise capacity. Other classes of medications approved for treatment of PAH include drugs that target the endothelin pathway and nitric oxide (NO) pathway. Currently available endothelin-receptor antagonists (ERAs) include bosentan, ambrisentan, macitentan. Drugs in the NO pathway include soluble guanyl cyclase stimulators (riociguat), and phosphodiesterase (PDE)5 inhibitors (sildenafil, tadalafil). Combination therapy of two to three drugs from different classes improves exercise capacity when compared to monotherapy and should be considered in patients with severe disease or those who fail to improve with monotherapy. Oral calcium-channel blockers (CCBs) are indicated only for the small subset of patients with mild-to-moderate symptoms who demonstrate significant reduction in pulmonary pressure with acute CCB challenge (decrease in mean PAP of at least 10 mm Hg to an absolute level of less than 40 mm Hg without a decrease in cardiac output). Supplemental home oxygen is indicated for all patients with hypoxemia. Travel to high elevations exacerbates hypoxia, and relocation to sea level improves symptoms. Oral anticoagulation should be considered for patients with PAH, particularly in those with a chronic indwelling central venous catheter for intravenous epoprostenol. Iron status should be monitored regularly to avoid iron deficiency anemia to prevent further deterioration in functional capacity. Diuretics should be prescribed for patients with peripheral edema or hepatic congestion. Lung transplantation is recommended only for patients in whom severe symptoms occur despite intensive medical therapy.

VENOUS THROMBOEMBOLIC DISEASE

Venous thromboembolism (VTE) encompasses both deep vein thrombosis (DVT) and pulmonary embolism (PE). Among the adult United States population, the overall combined annual incidence is as high as 2 new cases per 1000 persons. The incidence of VTE is higher in men than it is in women and higher in African Americans and white individuals than it is in Asians and Hispanics. Over 150 years ago, Dr. Rudolf Virchow recognized three predisposing factors: (1) endothelial damage, (2) venous stasis, and (3) hypercoagulation (Virchow's triad). Endothelial damage is common with surgery or trauma, venous stasis is common with prolonged bedrest or immobilization (leg cast), and hypercoagulation is more prevalent with cancer, oral estrogen use, and pregnancy. Trousseau syndrome consists of migratory thrombophlebitis with noninfectious vegetations on the heart valves (marantic endocarditis) typically in the setting of mucin-secreting adenocarcinoma. Dr. Trousseau, a pathologist, diagnosed his own pancreatic carcinoma on the basis of the association that now bears his name. Hypercoagulable states include hereditary diseases such as deficiencies in antithrombin III, protein C, or protein S; mutation in factor V gene (factor V Leiden) or factor II gene (prothrombin G20210A); as well as

表 11.3 肺动脉高压的分类

1. 动脉型肺动脉高压（PAH）

   原发性肺动脉高压（PPH）或特发性肺动脉高压（IPAH）：
   - 散发性
   - 家族性

   疾病相关的 PPH：
   - 结缔组织病
   - 先天性心脏病
   - 门静脉高压
   - 人类免疫缺陷病毒感染
   - 药物和毒素：厌氧菌、可卡因、甲基苯丙胺

2. 肺静脉高压
   - 左心室心力衰竭
   - 左心室心脏瓣膜病

3. 慢性呼吸疾病或低氧血症相关的肺动脉高压
   - 慢性阻塞性肺疾病
   - 阻塞性睡眠呼吸暂停

4. 慢性静脉血栓栓塞相关的肺动脉高压
   - 左心室心脏瓣膜病

5. 其他直接影响肺血管的疾病所致的肺动脉高压
   - 结节病、组织细胞增生症X、肺血管受压（腺病、肿瘤、纤维性纵隔炎）

动脉型肺动脉高压

动脉型肺动脉高压（PAH）是由肺血管收缩、内皮细胞和（或）平滑肌增生、内膜纤维化以及肺毛细血管和小动脉中的血栓形成所引起的。PAH 可以是特发性[原发性肺动脉高压（PPH）]，也可以是由结缔组织病、先天性心脏病、门静脉高压或人类免疫缺陷病毒（HIV）感染以及食欲抑制药物或毒素引起的继发性肺动脉高压。结缔组织病，尤其是硬皮病，是肺动脉高压最常见的继发性原因。

轻度 PAH 患者可能没有症状，但病情较为严重的患者会出现劳力性呼吸困难、胸痛、晕厥或晕厥前症状。端坐呼吸是 PAH 相关的不常见症状，更常见于左心病变引起的肺动脉高压患者。体格检查结果包括左侧胸骨旁抬高、第二心音肺动脉瓣音增强、三尖瓣或肺动脉瓣反流杂音、肝大、外周水肿或腹水。相关的心电图异常表现为右心室肥厚、右心房增大或电轴右偏。超声心动图提供了有关肺动脉高压严重程度（如估计的肺动脉压力、右心室直径和功能）及其潜在原因（如左心衰竭、瓣膜病变、左右分流的先天性心脏病）的重要信息。还应进行肺功能检查、通气-灌注（$\dot{V}/\dot{Q}$）肺扫描、多导睡眠监测或夜间血氧饱和度监测、自身抗体检测、HIV 血清学检查和肝功能检测，以确定其他潜在病因。对于疑似 PAH 的所有患者应进行右心室导管检查。在导管室的基础条件下，如果平均肺动脉压超过 20 mmHg、肺毛细血管楔压低于 15 mmHg，并且肺血管阻力超过 3 单位，即可确诊。在右心室导管检查期间应进行急性血管扩张药物试验，以指导适当的治疗。

如不进行治疗，PAH 的预后很差，中位生存期不到 3 年。具有临床恶化或死亡高风险特征（包括活动耐量减低、晕厥史或右心室衰竭）的患者，应接受静脉注射依前列醇（一种前列环素类似物）治疗，因其已被证实可改善运动能力和总体生存率，在降低肺动脉压力和改善运动能力方面也有效。其他前列环素类似物，如贝前列素、曲前列尼尔和伊洛前列素，或前列环素受体激动剂，如司来帕格，也能有效降低肺动脉压力并提高运动能力。其他被批准用于治疗 PAH 的药物包括靶向内皮素通路和一氧化氮（NO）通路的药物。目前可用的内皮素受体拮抗剂（ERA）包括波生坦、安贝生坦和马昔腾坦。NO 通路中的药物包括可溶性鸟苷酸环化酶激动剂（利奥西呱）、磷酸二酯酶 V 型抑制剂（西地那非、他达拉非）。与单药治疗相比，2～3 种不同类别药物联合治疗可提高运动能力，病情严重或单药治疗无效的患者应考虑联合治疗。口服钙通道阻滞剂（CCB）仅适用于表现出急性 CCB 试验后肺动脉压显著降低（平均 PAP 降低至少 10 mmHg，且绝对水平降低至 40 mmHg 以下，同时无心输出量下降）的轻至中度症状患者。所有低氧血症患者均应接受补充家庭氧疗。前往高海拔地区会加重低氧血症，而迁回海平面地区则会改善症状。PAH 患者应考虑口服抗凝药，尤其是长期留置中心静脉导管注射依前列醇的患者。应定期监测铁状态，以避免铁缺乏性贫血，以防运动能力及心功能进一步恶化。有外周水肿或肝淤血患者应服用利尿剂。肺移植仅推荐于接受强化药物治疗后仍出现严重症状的患者。

静脉血栓栓塞症

静脉血栓栓塞症（VTE）包括深静脉血栓形成（DVT）和肺栓塞（PE）。在美国成年人中，每年的总发病率高达每 1000 人中新增 2 例。VTE 的发病率男性高于女性，非裔美国人和白人的发病率高于亚洲人和西班牙裔人。150 多年前，Rudolf Virchow 博士发现三个易发因素：①内皮损伤，②静脉淤滞，③高凝状态（Virchow 三联征）。内皮损伤在手术或创伤中很常见，静脉淤滞常见于长期卧床或固定（腿部打石膏），而高凝状态多见于癌症、口服雌激素和妊娠。Trousseau 综合征包括游走性血栓性静脉炎伴非感染性心脏瓣膜赘生物（非细菌性血栓性心内膜炎），通常发生在黏液腺癌患者。Trousseau 医生是一名病理学家，他根据这些关系给自己确诊了胰腺癌，这一综合征也因此以他命名。高凝状态包括遗传性疾病，如抗凝血酶Ⅲ、蛋白 C 或蛋白 S 缺乏；凝血因子 V 基因（因子 V Leiden）或凝血因子Ⅱ基因（凝血酶原 G20210A）的突变；以及

hyperhomocysteinemia. However, a thorough search for identifiable risk factors will come up negative in 25% to 50% of patients with VTE.

Deep Vein Thrombosis

Most DVT starts in the calf veins. Without treatment, 15% to 30% of these clots propagate to the proximal calf veins. The risk of a subsequent PE is much higher with proximal DVT than with clots confined to the distal calf vessels (40% to 50% versus 5% to 10%, respectively). Involvement of the upper extremities is much less common, but subclavian and/or axillary vein thrombosis also can lead to PE in as many as 30% of affected individuals. The same risk factors that cause lower extremity DVT also cause upper extremity DVT. In addition, other specific causes of upper extremity DVT include traumatic damage of the vessel intima from heavy exertion such as rowing, wrestling, or weight lifting (Paget-Schroetter syndrome), from extrinsic compression at the level of thoracic inlet (thoracic outlet obstruction), or from insertion of central venous catheters or pacemakers. Pain and/or swelling are the major complaints from patients with DVT; however, a large number of patients with DVT are asymptomatic, particularly if the DVT is restricted to the calf. Patients with upper-extremity DVT can develop the superior vena caval syndrome of facial swelling, blurred vision, and dyspnea. Thoracic outlet obstruction can compress the brachial plexus leading to unilateral arm pain associated with hand weakness. Physical examination frequently reveals tenderness, erythema, warmth, and swelling below the site of thrombosis. Pain with dorsiflexion of the foot (Homan's sign) may be present, but the low sensitivity and the low specificity limit its usefulness in the diagnosis of lower extremity DVT. A palpable tender cord, dilated superficial veins, and low-grade fever occur in some patients. Upper extremity DVT can cause brachial plexus tenderness in the supraclavicular fossa and atrophic hand muscles. For patients with probable thoracic outlet obstruction, several provocative tests should be performed. Adson test is positive if the radial pulses weaken during inspiration and during extension of the arm of the affected side while rotating the head to the same side. Wright test is positive if the radial pulses become weaker and painful symptoms are reproduced while abducting the shoulder of the affected side with the humerus externally rotated.

The laboratory diagnosis of DVT includes measurement of D-dimers, which are fibrin degradation products. D-dimer elevation is a highly sensitive indicator of DVT that can be performed rapidly in the emergency department. In a patient with low to intermediate probability, a negative D-dimer test effectively excludes the diagnosis of DVT. However, the test is not specific and can be elevated in many other conditions frequently encountered in hospitalized patients (e.g., inflammation, recent surgery, malignancy). Duplex ultrasonography can be used to demonstrate the presence of a blood clot and/or noncompressibility of the affected veins proximal to the site of occlusion. Duplex ultrasonography has greater sensitivity in detecting proximal DVT (90% to 100%) than distal DVT (40% to 90%) of the lower extremities. With upper extremity DVT, acoustic shadowing of the clavicle may obscure detection of thrombosis in subclavian vein segments. MR angiography is particularly helpful in making the diagnosis of upper extremity DVT and pelvic vein thrombosis. Contrast venography is the conventional gold standard test, but it is invasive and technically difficult in patients with edematous extremities. Therefore, invasive venography should be reserved for patients in whom the clinical suggestion is high, despite negative or inconclusive results from noninvasive imaging.

Patients with DVT should be treated initially with subcutaneous low-molecular-weight heparin (LMWH), or subcutaneous selective factor Xa inhibitor fondaparinux to prevent thrombus propagation and to maintain the patency of venous collaterals. Oral administration of factor Xa inhibitors, rivaroxaban or apixaban, may also be used in the initial monotherapy without pretreatment with heparin. In contrast, other direct anticoagulants such as dabigatran and edoxaban should be started only after an initial parenteral heparin or fondaparinux therapy for 3 to 5 days. Intravenous unfractionated heparin (UFH) should be given to only selected patients with DVT, such as those with severe renal failure (creatinine clearance of <30 mL/minute) in whom LMWH and fondaparinux are contraindicated or those with hemodynamic instability who may require thrombolytic therapy or invasive intervention. Intravenous UFH should be given as a bolus, followed by continuous infusion to maintain an activated partial thromboplastin time of at least 1.5 times the control value. LMWH and fondaparinux has a longer half-life than UFH and can be given once or twice daily with similar efficacy. Oral anticoagulation should be initiated after the acute phase. In general, direct anticoagulants (DOACs) including dabigatran, rivaroxaban, apixaban, and edoxaban are preferred over warfarin because of lower risk of intracranial hemorrhage without compromising antithrombotic efficacy. If warfarin is chosen, it should be initiated without delay with an overlap period with LMWH, UFH, or fondaparinux therapy and titrated until the international normalized ratio (INR) reaches a value between 2 and 3. DOACs, however, have rapid onset of action and should be started at the discontinuation of UFH, LMWH, or fondaparinux without overlap period to avoid bleeding complication. After the acute phase, oral anticoagulants should be continued for 3 months in most patients. Lifelong anticoagulation should be considered in patients with unprovoked proximal DVT (either first episode or recurrent event) as well as patients with cancer-associated DVT with low to moderate bleeding risk. Furthermore, avoidance of frequent clinic visits to monitor INR during the initial period of warfarin titration is another major advantage of DOACs. When DVT is confined to the calf, the risk of PE is lower than proximal DVT. Therefore, anticoagulants should be started only in patients with severe symptoms or those with high-risk features for clot expansion, such as elevated D-dimer, large thrombus with greater than 5 cm in length, multiple vein involvement, history of thromboembolic events or active cancer, unprovoked DVT, or inpatient status. Oral anticoagulants should be continued for 3 months in most patients. In the absence of severe symptoms or risk factors for clot extension, patients with isolated distal DVT should be treated conservatively without anticoagulation with close monitoring via serial imaging of the deep veins for 2 weeks.

When upper extremity DVT occurs in the subclavian veins or axillary veins in patients who are severely symptomatic but otherwise healthy with low risk of bleeding, catheter-directed thrombolysis should be considered as it carries lower risk of bleeding than systemic thrombolytic therapy. The purpose of thrombolysis is to prevent or minimize the post-thrombotic syndrome, which includes chronic arm pain, swelling, hyperpigmentation, and ulceration from residual venous obstruction. In asymptomatic patients with occlusion in the more distal location, anticoagulation is preferred. If anticoagulation is stopped prematurely for any reason, aspirin should be considered in the absence of contraindication as it has been shown to reduce recurrent venous thromboembolism by 20% to 40% without increased risk of bleeding.

Catheter-based direct thrombolysis is effective in restoring venous patency and reducing post-thrombotic syndrome of venous congestion but increases risk of bleeding. Therefore, it should be considered for patients with iliofemoral DVT of recent onset who have low risk of bleeding. Vena cava filters are effective in reducing the incidence of PE, but they increase the risk of recurrent DVT. Consequently, IVC filters should be removed after 3 months. In patients treated with anticoagulation, addition of an IVC filter to anticoagulation offers no additional benefit in reducing recurrent venous thromboembolism compared

高同型半胱氨酸血症。然而，对可识别的危险因素进行全面筛查，25%～50%的VTE患者呈阴性结果。

深静脉血栓形成

大多数DVT始于小腿静脉。如不治疗，15%～30%的患者血栓会扩展到近端小腿静脉。与局限于远端小腿静脉的血栓相比，近端深静脉血栓形成引发肺栓塞的风险要高得多（分别为40%～50%和5%～10%）。上肢受累的情况要少得多，但锁骨下和（或）腋静脉血栓形成也可导致多达30%的患者发生肺栓塞。导致下肢深静脉血栓形成的危险因素同样也会导致上肢深静脉血栓形成。此外，导致上肢深静脉血栓形成的其他特殊原因还包括划船、摔跤或举重等剧烈运动（Paget-Schroetter综合征）、胸廓入口处的外力压迫（胸廓出口梗阻）或置入中心静脉导管或心脏起搏器导致血管内膜受损。疼痛和（或）肿胀是DVT患者的主要症状；然而，许多DVT患者并无症状，尤其是当深静脉血栓仅限于小腿时。上肢深静脉血栓形成患者会出现上腔静脉综合征，表现为面部肿胀、视物模糊和呼吸困难。胸廓出口阻塞可压迫臂丛神经，导致单侧上臂疼痛并伴有手无力。体格检查经常会发现血栓形成部位下方有触痛、红斑、发热和肿胀。足部外翻时可能会出现疼痛（霍曼征），但其敏感性和特异性较低，限制了其对下肢深静脉血栓的诊断作用。一些患者可出现可触及的压痛条索、扩张的浅静脉和低热。上肢深静脉血栓形成可导致锁骨上窝臂丛压痛和手部肌肉萎缩。对于可能存在胸廓出口梗阻的患者，应进行几种激发试验。在进行斜角肌压迫试验（Adson试验）时，如果吸气期患侧手臂向同侧头部旋转时患侧桡动脉脉搏减弱，则为阳性。如果肱骨外旋时患侧肩部外展，桡动脉搏动减弱且再现疼痛症状，则过度外展试验（Wright试验）阳性。

DVT的实验室诊断包括检测纤维蛋白降解产物D-二聚体。D-二聚体升高是DVT的高度敏感指标，可以在急诊科迅速完成检测。对于中低概率的患者，D-二聚体检测阴性可有效排除DVT的诊断。然而，该检测并不具有特异性，住院患者经常出现的许多其他情况下（如炎症、近期手术、恶性肿瘤等）D-二聚体也会升高。双相超声波检查可用于确诊血栓和（或）病变静脉阻塞部位近端的不可压缩性。双相超声波检查对下肢近端DVT的检查灵敏度（90%～100%）高于远端DVT（40%～90%）。对于上肢DVT，锁骨的声影可能会影响锁骨下静脉的血栓检查。磁共振血管成像尤其有助于上肢深静脉血栓和盆腔静脉血栓的诊断。应用造影剂的静脉造影是传统的金标准检查方法，但对于肢体水肿的患者来说，这种方法具有侵入性且技术上困难。因此，有创静脉造影应推荐给那些尽管无创影像检查结果为阴性或不确定，但临床高度提示该病的患者。

DVT患者首先应接受皮下注射低分子量肝素（LMWH）或皮下注射选择性Xa因子抑制剂磺达肝癸钠，以防止血栓扩展并保持静脉通畅。口服Xa因子抑制剂利伐沙班或阿哌沙班也可以在初始单药治疗时使用，无需预先使用肝素。相比之下，其他直接抗凝药物，如达比加群和艾多沙班，应在初始胃肠外用肝素或磺达肝癸钠治疗3～5天后才开始使用。静脉注射普通肝素（UFH）应仅用于特定的DVT患者，如严重肾功能衰竭（肌酐清除率＜30 ml/min）且禁用LMWH和磺达肝癸钠的患者，或血流动力学不稳定且可能需要溶栓治疗或侵入性干预的患者。静脉注射UFH时应先一次性静脉推注给药，然后持续输注以维持活化部分凝血活酶时间至少为参考值的1.5倍。LMWH和磺达肝癸钠的半衰期比UFH长，每天给药一次或两次，疗效相似。口服抗凝药物治疗应在急性期后开始。一般来说，因较低颅内出血风险且不影响抗血栓疗效，直接抗凝剂（DOAC）包括达比加群、利伐沙班、阿哌沙班和艾多沙班优先于华法林。如果选择华法林，则应立即开始使用，并与LMWH、UFH或磺达肝癸钠治疗重叠一段时间，直到国际标准化比值（INR）达到2～3之间。然而，DOAC起效迅速，应在停用UFH、LMWH或磺达肝癸钠后立即开始使用，无需重叠期，以避免出血并发症。急性期后，大多数患者应继续口服抗凝药3个月。对于无诱因的近端DVT（首次发作或复发）以及癌症相关DVT但中低出血风险的患者，应考虑终生抗凝。此外，DOAC的另一个主要优势是无需监测INR，避免了使用华法林的初始阶段频繁门诊监测INR。当DVT局限于小腿时，发生PE的风险低于近端DVT。因此，只有症状严重或具有血栓扩展高风险特征（如D-二聚体升高、长达5 cm以上的大血栓、多静脉受累、静脉血栓栓塞病史、活动性癌症、无诱因DVT或住院）的患者才应开启使用抗凝药物。对于大多数患者，口服抗凝剂应持续应用3个月。在没有严重症状或血栓扩展风险因素的情况下，孤立的远端DVT患者应在连续2周的深静脉影像监测下保守治疗，不使用抗凝剂。

当上肢DVT发生在锁骨下静脉或腋静脉，患者症状严重但身体其他方面健康，出血风险低，应考虑导管引导溶栓治疗，因为这种治疗出血风险低于全身溶栓治疗。溶栓治疗的目的是预防或最大限度减少血栓后综合征，包括慢性手臂疼痛、肿胀、色素沉着和由残余静脉阻塞引起的溃疡。对于无症状的远端闭塞患者，首选抗凝治疗。如果因任何原因提前停止抗凝治疗，在无禁忌证的情况下应考虑使用阿司匹林，因为研究表明阿司匹林可减少20%～40%的复发性静脉血栓栓塞风险而不增加出血风险。

导管直接溶栓能有效恢复静脉通畅和减少静脉充血的血栓后综合征，但会增加出血风险。因此，对于新近发病的出血风险较低的髂股DVT患者，应考虑使用这种方法。腔静脉滤器能够有效降低肺栓塞的发生率，但会增加复发性DVT的风险。因此，应在3个月后移除腔静脉滤器。对于接受抗凝治疗的患者，在抗凝治疗的基础上置入腔静脉滤器与单独抗凝治疗相比，

to anticoagulation alone. Therefore, it should be considered only in patients in whom anticoagulation is contraindicated.

Pulmonary Embolism

PE occurs when a thrombus dislodges from the deep veins of the upper or lower extremities. Pulmonary vascular resistance and pulmonary arterial pressure increase from two mechanisms: (1) anatomic reduction in cross-sectional area of the pulmonary vascular bed and (2) functional hypoxia-induced pulmonary vasoconstriction. The pressure overload on the right ventricle can lead to dilation, hypokinesis, and tricuspid regurgitation. When severe, elevated right ventricular end-diastolic pressure can compress the right coronary artery, causing subendocardial ischemia. In acute PE, areas of lung tissue are ventilated but underperfused. This $\dot{V}/\dot{Q}$ mismatch and the resultant redistribution of pulmonary blood flow from the obstructed pulmonary artery to other lung regions with lower $\dot{V}/\dot{Q}$ ratios cause arterial hypoxemia. In patients with a patent foramen ovale, hypoxemia worsens when the sudden elevation in right atrial pressure causes right-to-left shunting across the foramen.

The classic symptoms of acute PE are the sudden onset of dyspnea and pleuritic chest pain. Additional symptoms include anginal chest pain from right ventricular ischemia, hemoptysis from pulmonary infarction, and syncope or presyncope from massive PE with acute right ventricular failure (cor pulmonale). The most common physical findings are tachypnea and tachycardia. Additional physical findings include a right ventricular lift, inspiratory crackles, a loud pulmonary component of the second sound, expiratory wheezing, and a pleural rub. Symptoms and signs of proximal DVT are present in 10% to 20% of patients. Arterial blood gas analysis often reveals hypoxemia, respiratory alkalosis, and a high alveolar-to-arterial oxygen tension gradient. However, normal arterial blood gases values do not exclude the diagnosis. The most common finding with ECG analysis is sinus tachycardia. Atrial fibrillation, premature atrial contraction, and supraventricular tachycardia are less common. Other ECG changes suggest acute right ventricular strain. These include the S1-Q3-T3 pattern, a new right bundle branch block or right-axis deviation, and P-wave pulmonale. However, these findings are present in only 30% of patients with even massive PE. Common but nonspecific abnormalities with chest radiographic studies include atelectasis, pleural effusion, and pulmonary infiltrates. Less common but more specific radiographic findings include Hampton's hump (i.e., wedge-shaped infiltrate in the peripheral lung field), which is indicative of pulmonary infarction and Westermark's sign (decreased vascularity). The plasma D-dimer test is elevated in most patients with PE as a result of activation of the endogenous fibrinolytic system, which is not sufficient to dissolve the clot. Commercially available D-dimer assays have a high sensitivity and negative predictive value but low specificity, particularly with increasing age. Therefore, it is important to use age-adjusted cut-off values (age × 10 μg/L) in patients older than 50 years old to improve specificity without compromising sensitivity of detection to above 97%. A normal age-adjusted D-dimer test effectively excludes the diagnosis of PE in patients in whom the clinical suggestion is low or intermediate. However, it should not be used to screen patients with high index of suspicion because of low negative predictive value. Elevated levels of cardiac troponin I and troponin T and other markers of myocardial injury can be found in patients with PE and are indicative of right ventricular dysfunction and a poor prognosis. Similarly, elevated natriuretic peptides, including B-type natriuretic peptide (BNP) and N-terminal pro-BNP have been shown to be predictive of adverse outcomes.

CT angiography is the imaging modality of choice in patients with suspected PE and high clinical probability because of its excellent visualization of the pulmonary artery (Fig. 11.5). The resolution of 1 mm

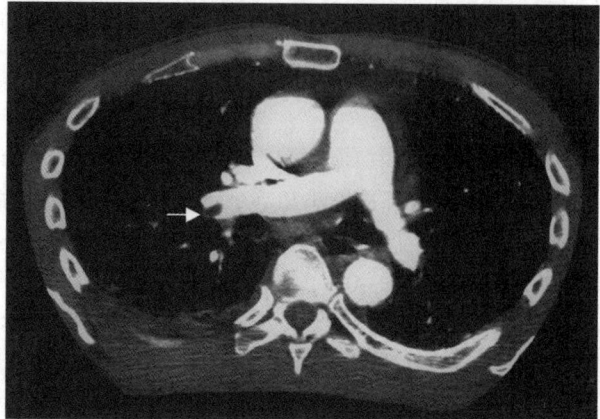

Fig. 11.5 Spiral chest CT angiogram shows a large thrombus in the right main pulmonary artery *(arrow)*. (Courtesy of Michael Landay, MD, Department of Radiology, University of Texas Southwestern Medical Center, Dallas, Texas.)

or less rivals that of conventional invasive angiography. The speed of the newer generation of scanners allows acquisition of all images within a single breath-hold, avoiding respiratory motion artifacts. The overall negative predictive value of multidetector CT angiography exceeds 99%. A negative CT excludes the diagnosis of PE and eliminates the need for further diagnostic testing. The CT scan also permits detection of other pathologic conditions involving the lung parenchyma, pleura, and mediastinal structures. Such pathologic findings may mimic PE and constitute alternative causes of chest pain and dyspnea. The requirement for intravenous injection of iodinated contrast material restricts applicability to those without a history of kidney disease or an allergic reaction to contrast dye. In such patients, $\dot{V}/\dot{Q}$ scan is a more suitable imaging modality. A completely normal $\dot{V}/\dot{Q}$ scan effectively excludes the diagnosis without further testing. However, less than 10% of $\dot{V}/\dot{Q}$ scans are interpreted as definitively normal. In patients in whom a moderate or high level of clinical probability of PE exists, a high-probability $\dot{V}/\dot{Q}$ scan has a diagnostic accuracy of 90% to 100%; however, a low or intermediate probability scan is no more helpful than a coin flip. Fig. 11.6 presents an algorithm for the work-up of PE based on current evidence. Echocardiography may directly detect thrombi in the right atrium, right ventricle, or pulmonary artery or indirectly demonstrate right ventricular dysfunction, signifying presence of hemodynamically significant emboli. Therefore, it is helpful in diagnosis of PE in patients with hypotension or shock. Invasive pulmonary angiography should be reserved for patients in whom noninvasive testing is inconclusive.

Once diagnosis of PE is made, clinical risk assessment should be made to guide treatment approach. Patients with low risk based on stable hemodynamic parameters without history of cardiovascular disease or excessive bleeding risk for anticoagulation treatment may be suitable for outpatient treatment or a brief inpatient observation. Similar to the treatment of DVT described previously, oral direct anticoagulants with or without initial parenteral therapy are preferred over warfarin because of lower risk of intracranial bleeding and increased ease of use associated with DOACs. PE patients with moderate to high risk features for cardiovascular decompensation (Table 11.4) should be admitted and monitored closely (PESI class III-V, or simplified PESI of at least 1). Aggressive parenteral therapy is preferred when patients have one or more features of high clinical risk. Thrombolytic therapy with recombinant tissue plasminogen activator (rt-PA) is indicated for patients with hypotension or shock. In patients with right

在减少复发性静脉血栓栓塞方面并没有额外益处。因此，只有在抗凝治疗禁忌的患者中才考虑使用。

肺栓塞（PE）

当血栓从上肢或下肢深静脉脱落时，就会发生肺栓塞。肺血管阻力和肺动脉压力增加有两种机制：①解剖学上肺血管床横截面积缩小；②功能性缺氧引起的肺血管收缩。右心室压力超负荷会导致扩张、运动减低和三尖瓣反流。在严重情况下，右心室舒张末压升高会压迫右冠状动脉，造成心内膜下缺血。在急性肺栓塞时，肺组织区域通气但血流灌注不足。这种$\dot{V}/\dot{Q}$不匹配以及由此导致的肺血流从阻塞的肺动脉重新分配到其他$\dot{V}/\dot{Q}$比较低的肺部区域，导致动脉低氧血症。在卵圆孔未闭患者中，当右心房压力突然升高引起经卵圆孔的右向左分流时，低氧血症会加重。

急性 PE 的典型症状是突然出现的呼吸困难和胸膜炎性胸痛。其他症状包括右心室缺血引起的心绞痛、肺梗死引起的咯血，以及大块 PE 并发急性右心室衰竭（肺源性心脏病）引起的晕厥或晕厥先兆症状。最常见的体征是呼吸急促和心动过速。其他体征还包括右心室抬举、吸气性爆裂音、肺动脉瓣区第二心音亢进、呼气性哮鸣音和胸膜摩擦音。10%～20% 患者出现近端 DVT 的症状和体征。动脉血气分析通常会显示低氧血症、呼吸性碱中毒和肺泡-动脉氧张力梯度过高。然而，动脉血气值正常并不能排除诊断。心电图分析最常见的发现是窦性心动过速；心房颤动、房性期前收缩和室上性心动过速较少见。其他提示急性右心室负荷增加的 ECG 表现包括 S1-Q3-T3 模式、新发右束支传导阻滞或电轴右轴以及肺型 P 波。然而，即使大面积 PE 患者，这些发现也仅存在于 30% 的患者中。常见但非特异性的胸部 X 线异常包括肺不张、胸腔积液和肺浸润。较少见但更具特异性的胸部 X 线检查结果包括驼峰征（即外周肺野的楔形浸润），提示肺梗死和韦斯特马征（血管减少）。大多数 PE 患者的血浆 D-二聚体检测值都会升高，这是内源性纤维蛋白溶解系统激活的结果，但这种激活不足以溶解血栓。市售的 D-二聚体检测具有较高的敏感性和阴性预测值，但特异性较低，尤其是随着年龄的增长。因此，对于 50 岁以上的患者，使用年龄调整后的截断值（年龄×10 μg/L）非常重要，可以在提高诊断特异性的同时又不影响检测敏感性达到 97% 以上。对于临床提示为低度或中度的患者，年龄调整后的正常 D-二聚体检测值可有效排除 PE 诊断。然而不应将其用于高度怀疑的患者的筛查，由于这时阴性预测值较低。PE 患者中可以发现心肌肌钙蛋白 I 和肌钙蛋白 T 及其他心肌损伤标志物水平升高，表明右心室功能障碍和预后不良。同样，B 型利钠肽（BNP）和 N 末端 BNP 前体升高也预示着不良预后。

CT 血管成像是疑似 PE 和临床高度可能性患者的首选成像方式，因为它能很好地显示肺动脉（图 11.5）。

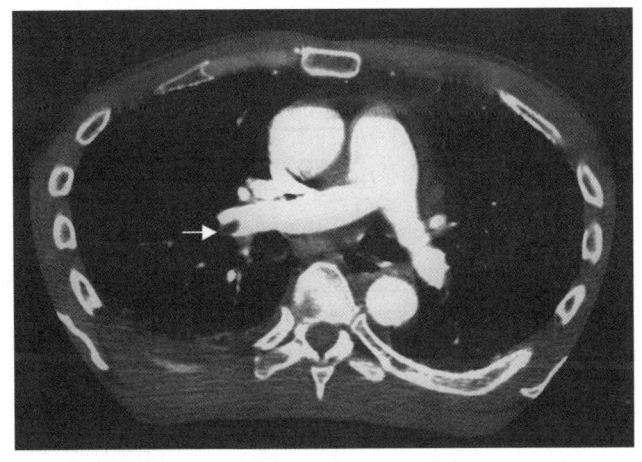

图 11.5　胸部螺旋 CT 血管成像显示右主肺动脉大块血栓（箭头）（授权自 Michael Landay, MD, Department of Radiology, University of Texas Southwestern Medical Center, Dallas, Texas.）

1 mm 或更小的分辨率可与传统有创血管造影相媲美。新一代扫描仪的速度允许在单次屏气中获取所有图像，避免了呼吸运动伪影。多层 CT 血管成像的总体阴性预测值超过 99%。阴性 CT 可排除 PE 诊断，并确认无需进一步诊断检查。CT 扫描还可以检查涉及肺实质、胸膜和纵隔结构的其他病理情况，某些病理结果可能与 PE 相似，是胸痛和呼吸困难的其他病因。静脉注射碘造影剂的使用要求，限制了其适用范围，适用于无肾脏疾病史或无造影剂过敏史患者。对于有肾脏疾病或造影剂过敏患者，$\dot{V}/\dot{Q}$ 扫描是更合适的影像检查。如果 $\dot{V}/\dot{Q}$ 扫描完全正常，则无需进一步检查即可有效排除诊断。然而，只有不到 10% 的 $\dot{V}/\dot{Q}$ 扫描报告为明确正常。对于临床上中度或高度 PE 可能性的患者，高概率 $\dot{V}/\dot{Q}$ 扫描结果的诊断准确率可达 90%～100%；然而，低中概率扫描结果对诊断并不比抛硬币更有帮助。图 11.6 是基于现有证据提出的 PE 的诊断流程。超声心动图可以直接检测右心房、右心室或肺动脉中的血栓，或间接显示右心室功能障碍，表明存在对血流动力学有重大影响的栓子。因此，它有助于诊断伴有低血压或休克患者的 PE。侵入性肺动脉造影应仅用于无创检查结果不明确的患者。

一旦确诊 PE，应进行临床风险评估以指导治疗方案。血流动力学参数稳定、无心血管疾病史或过高的抗凝治疗出血风险的低风险患者适合门诊治疗或短暂的住院观察。与前文所述的 DVT 治疗类似，口服直接抗凝药物联合或不联合初始胃肠外抗凝治疗优于华法林，因为 DOAC 相关的颅内出血风险较低，而且更易于使用。具有中高风险的心血管失代偿特征（表 11.4）PE 患者，应住院密切监测（PESI 分级Ⅲ～Ⅴ或简化 PESI 分级至少为 1）。当患者具有一项或多项高风险临床特征时，应首选积极的胃肠外治疗。对伴有低血压或休克的患者，推荐使用重组组织型纤溶酶原激活物（rt-PA）进行溶栓治疗。对仅有右心室扩大或功能障碍而无低血压的患者（称次大面积 PE），溶栓疗法可降

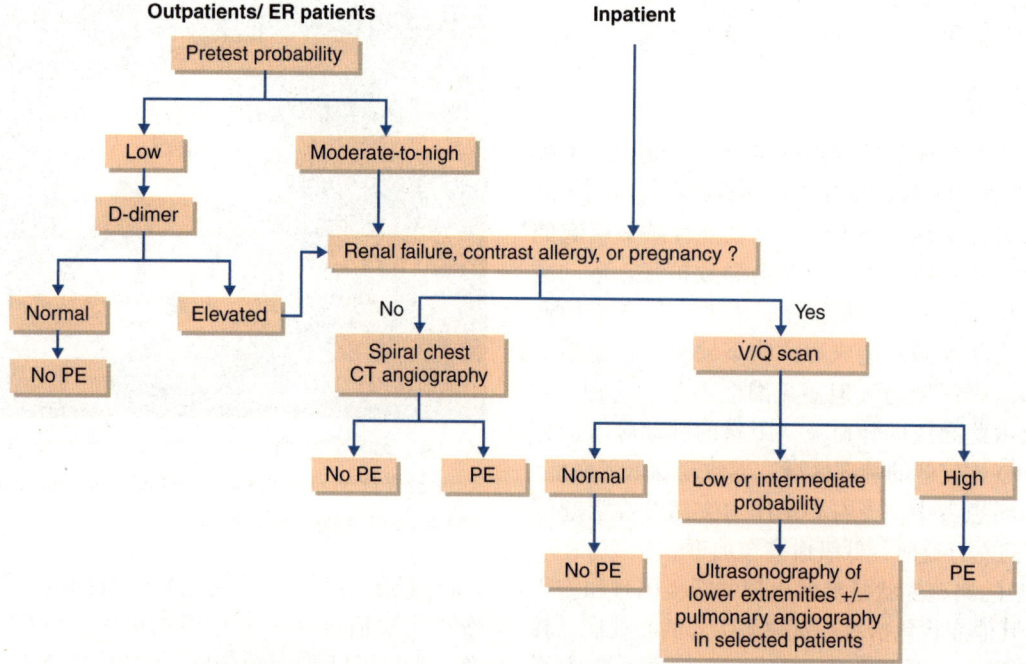

Fig. 11.6 Diagnostic algorithm for patients with suggested pulmonary embolism (PE).

TABLE 11.4 Pulmonary Embolism Severity Index (PESI)		
Parameter	Original[a]	Simplified[a]
Age	Years	1 (for age >80 yrs)
Male sex	+10	—
Cancer	+30	1
Chronic heart failure	+10	1
Chronic pulmonary disease	+10	
HR at least 110 bpm	+20	1
SBP <100 mm Hg	+30	1
Respiratory rate >30 breaths per min	+20	—
Temperature <36° C	+20	—
Altered mental status	+60	—
Arterial oxyhemoglobin saturation <90%	+20	1

[a]Original: Total Score Class
≤65: I
66-85: II
86-105: III
106-125: IV
>125: V
Simplified:
0= low risk
≥1 = high risk

ventricular enlargement or dysfunction alone without hypotension (known as submassive PE), thrombolytic therapy reduces the risk of hemodynamic decompensation at the cost of increased risk of major hemorrhage and stroke. Thus, anticoagulation alone is preferred in most cases of submassive PE. After initial treatment with heparins or fondaparinux in high-risk patients, DOACs should be administered in a similar manner to treatment of DVT. If warfarin therapy is chosen instead of DOACs, parenteral anticoagulation should be administered until a therapeutic INR of 2 to 3 is reached. Surgical or percutaneous removal of emboli should be considered in patients with massive PE who have contraindications for thrombolytic therapy.

The time necessary to continue anticoagulation after an acute PE or DVT episode depends on the presence or absence of reversible risk factors for recurrent VTE. Patients with a history of trauma or surgery generally have a low rate of recurrent VTE; therefore, warfarin can be discontinued after 3 months of administration. Patients with cancer and VTE should be treated initially with subcutaneous fixed-dose LMWH for 3 to 6 months because of its greater efficacy than warfarin in preventing recurrent thromboembolism in this setting. Preliminary studies indicated that DOACs are as effective as LMWH in preventing thromboembolic events though the bleeding risk is higher with DOACs. After this initial period, treatment with LMWH or DOACs should be continued indefinitely unless the cancer is cured. Patients with unprovoked PE with low risk of bleeding should be treated with oral anticoagulation for more than 3 months while those with high bleeding risk should be on treatment for at least 3 months. Beyond 3 months, aspirin is an alternative to long-term warfarin and should be considered for patients who have contraindication for anticoagulation or high bleeding risk.

Venous Thromboembolism Prophylaxis

Patients who are at high risk for VTE should receive pharmacologic prophylaxis. Subcutaneous LMWH is generally preferred over subcutaneous UFH because of a modest reduction in venous thromboembolism in high-risk patients. UFH is usually reserved for patients with creatinine clearance less than 30 mL/min). Patients at high risk include those who are hospitalized with acute medical illness—particularly congestive heart failure, acute respiratory illness, acute inflammatory diseases—those who are expected to be immobilized for 3 days or longer, or patients with previous VTE. Major surgery, either elective or emergent, is an important indication for VTE prophylaxis. Subcutaneous LMWH has a marginal advantage over UFH in preventing symptomatic DVT in patients undergoing general surgery, gynecologic surgery, or neurosurgery in some but not all studies. However, LMWH is more effective

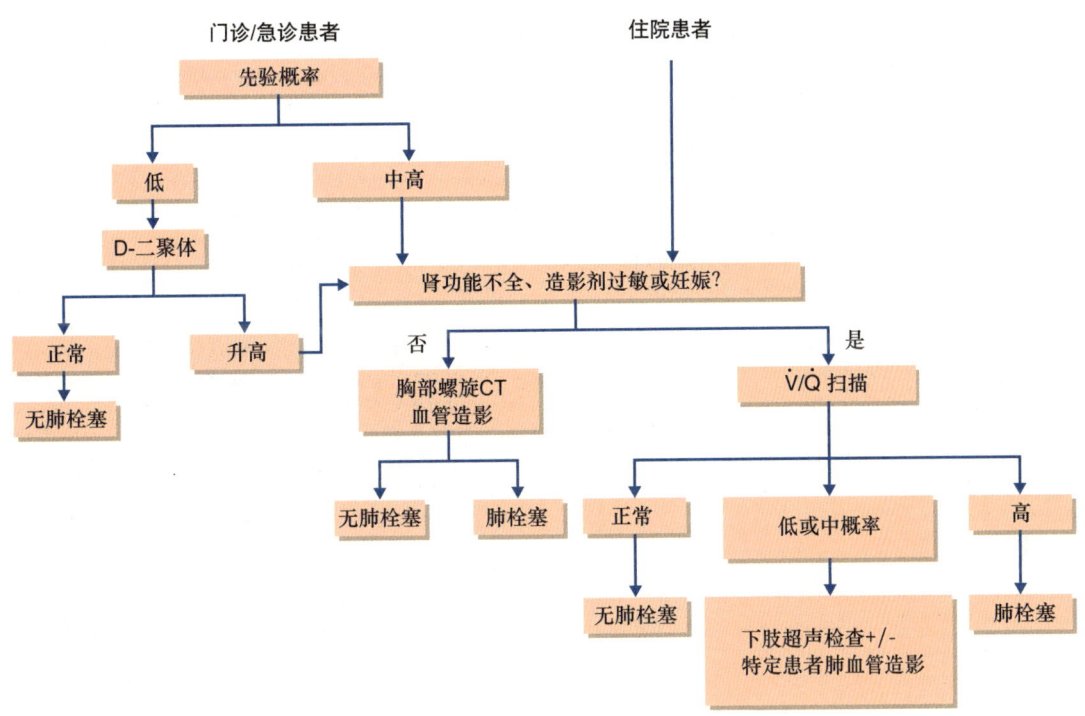

图 11.6 疑诊肺栓塞（PE）患者的诊断流程

急性 PE 或 DVT 发作后继续抗凝的治疗时间取决于是否存在可逆性复发 VTE 的危险因素。有外伤或手术史的患者复发 VTE 的风险通常较低，因此，华法林可在用药 3 个月后停用。癌症和 VTE 患者最初应皮下注射固定剂量 LMWH 治疗 3～6 个月，因为 LMWH 在预防复发性血栓栓塞方面比华法林更有效。初步研究表明，DOAC 在预防血栓栓塞事件方面与 LMWH 同样有效，尽管 DOAC 的出血风险更高。初期治疗后，除非癌症已治愈，否则应长期使用 LMWH 或 DOAC 治疗。对无诱因 PE 且出血风险低的患者应口服抗凝治疗 3 个月以上，而出血风险高的患者应至少接受 3 个月的口服抗凝治疗。超过 3 个月后，阿司匹林是长期华法林治疗的替代药物，对于有抗凝禁忌证或出血风险高的患者也应考虑使用阿司匹林。

表 11.4 肺栓塞严重程度指数（PESI）		
因素	原始版本[a]	简化版本
年龄	岁数	1（年龄＞80 岁）
男性	+10	—
癌症	+30	1
慢性心力衰竭	+10	1
慢性肺疾病	+10	—
心率至少 110 次 / 分	+20	1
收缩压＜ 100 mmHg	+30	1
呼吸频率＞ 30 次 / 分	+20	—
体温＜ 36℃	+20	—
精神状态改变	+60	—
动脉血氧合血红蛋白饱和度＜ 90%	+20	1

[a] 原始版本：总评分分级
≤ 65：Ⅰ
66～85：Ⅱ
86～105：Ⅲ
106～125：Ⅳ
＞ 125：Ⅴ
简化版本：0 ＝低危；≥ 1 ＝高危

低血流动力学失代偿的风险，但代价是增加严重出血和卒中风险。因此，大多数次大面积 PE 患者仅推荐抗凝治疗。高危患者在使用肝素或磺达肝癸钠进行初始治疗后，应按照 DVT 的类似方法使用 DOAC 治疗。如果选择华法林治疗而不是 DOAC，则应同时进行胃肠外抗凝治疗，直到 INR 达到 2～3。对于有溶栓治疗禁忌证的大面积 PE 患者，应考虑手术或经皮介入取栓治疗。

静脉血栓栓塞症预防

VTE 高危患者应接受药物治疗预防。皮下注射 LMWH 通常优于皮下 UFH，因为其在高危患者中能适度降低静脉血栓栓塞的发生率。普通肝素通常推荐用于肌酐清除率小于 30 ml/min 的患者。高危患者包括因急性内科疾病（尤其是充血性心力衰竭、急性呼吸道疾病、急性炎症性疾病）住院的患者，预计需要 3 天或更长时间不能活动的患者或既往有 VTE 史的患者。大手术无论是择期还是急诊手术，都是 VTE 预防的重要指征。在某些但并非所有研究中，在接受普外科手术、妇科手术或神经外科手术的患者中，皮下注射 LMWH 在预防症状性 DVT 方面比 UFH 显示出微弱优势。然而，LMWH 比 UFH 和调整剂量的华法林（INR 在 2～3 之间）更有效，

than UFH and adjusted dose warfarin (INR between 2-3) and is preferred for prevention of DVT in orthopedic surgery such as hip surgery or total knee replacement because of superior efficacy (level of evidence A). DOACs, such as dabigatran, rivaroxaban, and apixaban, have similar efficacy and safety when compared with LMWH in preventing VTE after knee surgery without increasing perioperative bleeding. Efficacy of DOACs in preventing VTE after hip surgery relative to LMWH has not been directly tested in the randomized trials. DVT prophylaxis should be continued for 10 to 14 days after knee surgery and 35 days after hip surgery. Patients undergoing major cancer surgery should receive continued prophylaxis after discharge up to 28 days. Mechanical prophylaxis with intermittent pneumatic compression has not been shown to confer additional benefit in preventing VTE in medical, surgical, and trauma ICU patients when used in combination with pharmacologic thromboprophylaxis versus pharmacologic thromboprophylaxis alone. However, it should be considered in patients with high risk of bleeding in whom anticoagulation is contraindicated.

ARTERIAL HYPERTENSION

Arterial hypertension is the leading cause of death in the world, affecting 103 million adults in the United States and 1.4 billion people worldwide. It is the most common cause for an outpatient visit to a physician and the most easily recognized treatable risk factor for stroke, myocardial infarction, heart failure, peripheral vascular disease, aortic dissection, atrial fibrillation, and end-stage kidney disease. Despite this knowledge and unequivocal scientific proof that treating hypertension with medication dramatically reduces its attendant morbidity and mortality, hypertension remains untreated or undertreated in the majority of affected individuals in all countries, including those with the most advanced systems of medical care. The 2017 American Heart Association/American College of Cardiology guideline has introduced the new threshold for diagnosis and treatment of hypertension to less than 130/80 mm Hg while most other countries in the world have continued the old thresholds of less than 140/90 mm Hg in their guidelines. Fewer than one in two Americans with hypertension have their blood pressure treated and controlled to below the new 130/80 mm Hg guideline. Globally, hypertension control rates among treated individuals have plateaued at the range below 70% since the mid-2000s (Fig 11.7). Thus, hypertension remains one of the world's great public health problems. The asymptomatic nature of the condition impedes early detection, which requires regular BP measurement. Because most cases of hypertension cannot be cured, BP control requires lifelong treatment with prescription medications, which can be costly. Effective hypertension management requires continuity of care by a regular and knowledgeable medical provider, as well as sustained active participation by an educated patient. This section reviews the most important principles in the early detection and effective treatment of hypertension.

Initial Evaluation for Hypertension

The initial evaluation for hypertension needs to accomplish three goals: (1) staging of BP, (2) assessing the patient's overall cardiovascular risk, and (3) detecting clues of secondary hypertension. The initial clinical data needed to accomplish these goals are obtained through a thorough history and physical examination, routine blood tests, a spot (preferably first morning) urine specimen, and a resting 12-lead ECG. Home BP monitoring is indicated in most patients to confirm the diagnosis of hypertension and to exclude white coat syndrome. In most cases, home BP or 24-hour ambulatory BP monitoring provides helpful additional data about the time-integral burden of BP on the cardiovascular system.

Goal 1: Accurate Assessment of Blood Pressure

Across populations, the risks of heart disease and stroke increase continuously and logarithmically with increasing levels of systolic and diastolic BPs at or above 115/75 mm Hg (Fig. 11.8). Thus, the dichotomous separation of *normal* from *high* BP is artificial. BP is currently staged as normal, elevated, or hypertension based on the average of two or more readings taken on at least two separate occasions. When a patient's average systolic and diastolic pressures fall into different stages, the higher stage applies (Table 11.5). *Elevated BP* is designated as BP in the 120 to 129 mm Hg systolic in the presence of diastolic BP below 80 mm Hg. Individuals with elevated BP are at higher risk for progression into hypertension and cardiovascular events.

BP normally varies dramatically throughout a 24-hour period. To minimize variability in readings, BP should be measured at least twice after 5 minutes of rest with the patient seated, the back supported, and the arm bare and at heart level. The most common mistake in measuring BP is using a standard-issue cuff that is too small for a large arm, producing spuriously elevated readings. Most overweight adults will require a large adult cuff. Tobacco and caffeine should be avoided for at least 30 minutes. To avoid underestimation of systolic pressure in older adults who may have an *auscultatory gap* as a result of arteriosclerosis, radial artery palpation should be performed to estimate systolic pressure; then the cuff should be inflated to a value 20 mm Hg higher than the level that obliterates the radial pulse and deflated at a rate of 3 to 5 mm Hg per second. BP should be measured in both arms and after 5 minutes of standing, the latter to exclude a significant postural fall in BP, particularly in older persons and in those with diabetes or other conditions (e.g., Parkinson's disease) that predispose the patient to autonomic insufficiency.

However, out-of-office readings either with home or ambulatory BP monitoring are required to accurately assess a person's typical BP. Because of the anxiety of going to the physician, BPs often are higher in the physician's office than when measured at home or during normal daily life outside the home. Self-monitoring of BP outside of the physician's office actively engages a patient in his or her own health care and provides a better estimate of a person's usual BP for medical decision making. BP should be measured in early morning and evening times. Three BP readings should be obtained during each measurement, separated by at least 1 minute. Because the first BP tends to be the highest, average BP should be used to assess home BP. Many electronic home monitors are available, but only a handful of models have been rigorously validated against mercury sphygmomanometry and can be recommended.

Ambulatory monitoring provides automated measurements of BP over a 24- or 48-hour period while patients are engaged in their usual activities, including sleep (Fig. 11.9). The *normal limits of 24-hour ambulatory BP*, which are corresponding to office BP of 130/80 mm Hg, are a mean daytime BP of less than 130/80 mm Hg, mean nighttime BP of 110/65 mm Hg, and a mean 24-hour BP of less than 125/75 mm Hg. To avoid undertreating hypertension, these lower treatment thresholds must be used when incorporating ambulatory monitoring in medical decision making. With self-monitoring of BP at home, an average value of less than 130/80 mm Hg should be considered the upper limit of normal.

Up to one third of patients with elevated office BPs have normal home or ambulatory BPs. If the 24-hour BP profile is completely normal and no target organ damage has occurred despite consistently elevated office readings, then the patient has *office only*, or *white coat*, hypertension, presumably the result of a transient adrenergic response to the measurement of BP in the physician's office (see Fig. 11.9). In other patients, office readings underestimate ambulatory BP,

并且由于其卓越的疗效（证据级别为 A），LMWH 是骨科手术（如髋关节手术或全膝关节置换术）中预防 DVT 的首选药物。DOAC 如达比加群、利伐沙班和阿哌沙班与 LMWH 相比，在预防膝关节手术后的 VTE 方面具有相似的疗效和安全性，且不会增加围术期出血。尚无随机试验直接比较 DOAC 与 LMWH 在预防髋关节手术后 VTE 方面的有效性。膝关节手术后 DVT 预防应继续 10～14 天，髋关节手术后应继续 35 天。接受大型癌症手术的患者在出院后应继续预防治疗长达 28 天。在内科、外科和创伤重症监护病房患者中，间歇性充气加压机械预防与药物预防血栓联合使用与单独药物预防血栓相比，并没有显示出在预防 VTE 方面有额外的获益。然而，对于高出血风险且抗凝禁忌的患者，应考虑使用机械预防。

动脉高血压

动脉高血压是世界上最主要的死因，影响着美国 1.03 亿成年人和全世界 14 亿人。动脉高血压是门诊患者就医的最常见原因，也是卒中、心肌梗死、心力衰竭、周围血管疾病、主动脉夹层、心房颤动和终末期肾脏病最容易识别且可治疗的危险因素。尽管有这些知识，且明确的科学证据也表明，通过药物治疗高血压能显著降低与其相关的疾病发病率和死亡率，但在所有国家，包括拥有最先进医疗体系的国家，大多数高血压患者仍未得到治疗或治疗不足。2017 年美国心脏协会 / 美国心脏病学会指南已将高血压诊断和治疗的新阈值调整为＜ 130/80 mmHg，而世界上大多数其他国家的指南仍沿用＜ 140/90 mmHg 的旧阈值。在美国每两名高血压患者中，只有不到一人接受降压治疗并控制在新标准 130/80 mmHg 以下。在全球范围内，自 2000 年代中期以来，接受治疗的高血压患者的血压控制率稳定在 70% 以下（图 11.7）。高血压仍然是全球重大公共卫生问题之一。高血压的无症状的特征阻碍了早期发现，这就需要定期测量血压。由于大多数高血压无法治愈，因此需要终身服药来控制血压，这可能带来高昂的成本。有效的高血压管理需要由医疗服务提供者提供连续和专业的护理，并需要受过教育的患者的持续积极参与。本部分回顾早期发现和有效治疗高血压的最重要原则。

高血压的初始评估

高血压的初始评估需要实现三个目标：①血压分级，②评估患者整体心血管风险，以及③检测继发性高血压的线索。实现这些目标所需的初步临床资料可通过全面的病史和体格检查、常规血液化验、单次尿液标本（最好是晨起第一次尿液标本）和静息 12 导联心电图获得。大多数患者都需要进行家庭血压监测，以确认高血压的诊断并排除白大衣高血压。在大多数情况下，家庭血压或 24 h 动态血压监测可提供血压对心血管系统影响的有用额外数据。

目标 1：准确评估血压

在不同人群中，随着收缩压和舒张压达到或超过 115/75 mmHg，心脏病和卒中风险以对数形式持续增加（图 11.8）。因此，将正常血压与高血压二分法是人为的。目前，根据至少两次不同场合测量血压的两次或两次以上读数的平均值，将血压分为正常、升高或高血压。当患者的平均收缩压和舒张压属于不同分级时，采用较高分级（表 11.5）。血压升高定义为收缩压在 120～129 mmHg 之间并且舒张压低于 80 mmHg。血压升高的个体发展为高血压及发生心血管事件风险更高。

正常情况下，血压在 24 h 内会有很大变化。为了最大限度地减小血压测量值的变化，患者应休息 5 min 后至少测量血压两次，测量时应保持坐位、背部支撑、手臂裸露且与心脏处于同一水平线上，测量血压最常见的错误是使用标准袖带去测量手臂较粗的患者，这会导致读数虚假升高。大多数超重成年人需要大号袖带。测量前至少 30 min 内应避免吸烟和摄入咖啡因。老年人可能因动脉硬化而出现听诊间断（auscultatory gap），为避免低估老年人收缩压，应进行桡动脉触诊以估计收缩压；然后将袖带充气至比桡动脉脉搏消失的压力高 20 mmHg，并以每秒 3～5 mmHg 柱的速度放气。应测量双臂血压和站立 5 min 后的血压，后者是为了排除显著的直立性低血压（亦称体位性低血压），尤其是老年人和患有糖尿病或其他疾病（如帕金森病）的患者，容易出现自主神经功能不全所致的直立性低血压。

然而，需要在诊室外通过家庭或动态血压监测才能准确评估患者的血压。由于存在就诊时的焦虑，在诊室测量的血压往往高于家中或户外日常生活中测量的血压值。在诊室外自我监测血压可使患者积极参与自身的健康管理，为治疗决策提供更好的日常血压数据。血压应在早晨和晚上测量。每次测量应该获得三次血压读数，每次测量血压至少相隔 1 min。因为第一次血压往往是最高的，所以应该使用平均血压来评估家庭血压。有许多家用电子血压计可供选择，但只有少数几种经过与水银血压计严格校验的型号推荐使用。

动态监测可提供 24 h 或 48 h 内患者日常活动（包括睡眠）时的血压自动测量值（图 11.9）。与诊室血压 130/80 mmHg 相对应，24 h 动态血压的正常范围是日间平均血压低于 130/80 mmHg，夜间平均血压低于 110/65 mmHg，24 h 平均血压低于 125/75 mmHg。为避免高血压治疗不足，治疗决策应结合动态血压监测，必须使用这些较低的治疗阈值。在家中自我监测血压时，应将平均值 130/80 mmHg 视为正常值上限。

在诊室血压升高的患者中，高达 1/3 的患者家庭或动态血压监测血压是正常的。如果 24 h 血压完全正常，尽管诊室血压读数持续升高，但没有靶器官损害，则患者为诊室高血压或白大衣高血压，推测可能是患者在诊室测量血压时短暂肾上腺素能反应的结果（见图 11.9）。而其他患者，诊室血压读数低于动态血压，这

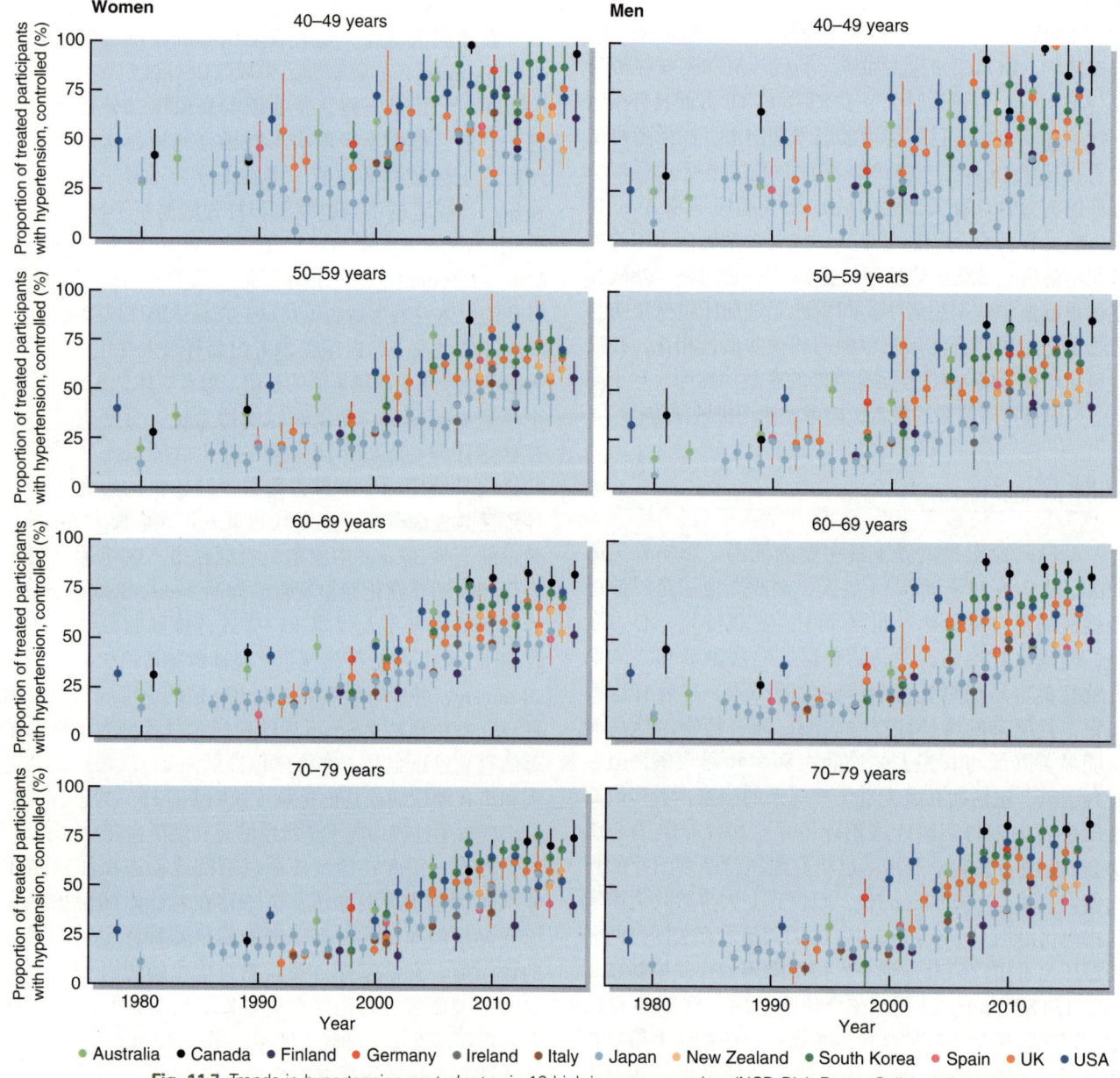

Fig. 11.7 Trends in hypertension control rates in 12 high-income countries. (NCD Risk Factor Collaboration [NCD-RisC], Lancet July 2019;10199:639-651.)

presumably because of sympathetic overactivity in daily life owing to job or home stress, tobacco use, or other adrenergic stimulation that dissipates when coming to the office (Fig. 11.10). Such documentation prevents underdiagnosing and undertreating this *masked hypertension*, which is also associated with high cardiovascular risks and identified in 10% of hypertensive patients in general, up to 40% of those with diabetes, and 70% of African American patients with hypertensive kidney disease.

Goal 2: Cardiovascular Risk Stratification

The great majority of patients with BPs in the prehypertensive or hypertensive range will have one or more additional modifiable risk factors for atherosclerosis (e.g., hypercholesterolemia, cigarette smoking, diabetes). The Pooled Cohort Equations (PCEs) is now recommended to estimate the 10-year risk of ASCVD (atherosclerotic cardiovascular disease) among patients without history of cardiovascular disease in hypertensive patients. Patients with 10-year ASCVD risk of 10% or higher with BP of at least 130/80 mm Hg should be started on antihypertensive drug treatment without delay. In addition to ASCVD risk, presence of target organ involvement, such as left ventricular hypertrophy or proteinuria, which are not captured by PCEs but should be considered as a high-risk feature.

Goal 3: Identification of Secondary (Identifiable) Causes of Hypertension

A thorough search for secondary causes is not cost-effective in most patients with hypertension, but it becomes critically important in two circumstances: (1) when a compelling cause is found on the initial evaluation, or (2) when the hypertensive process is so severe that

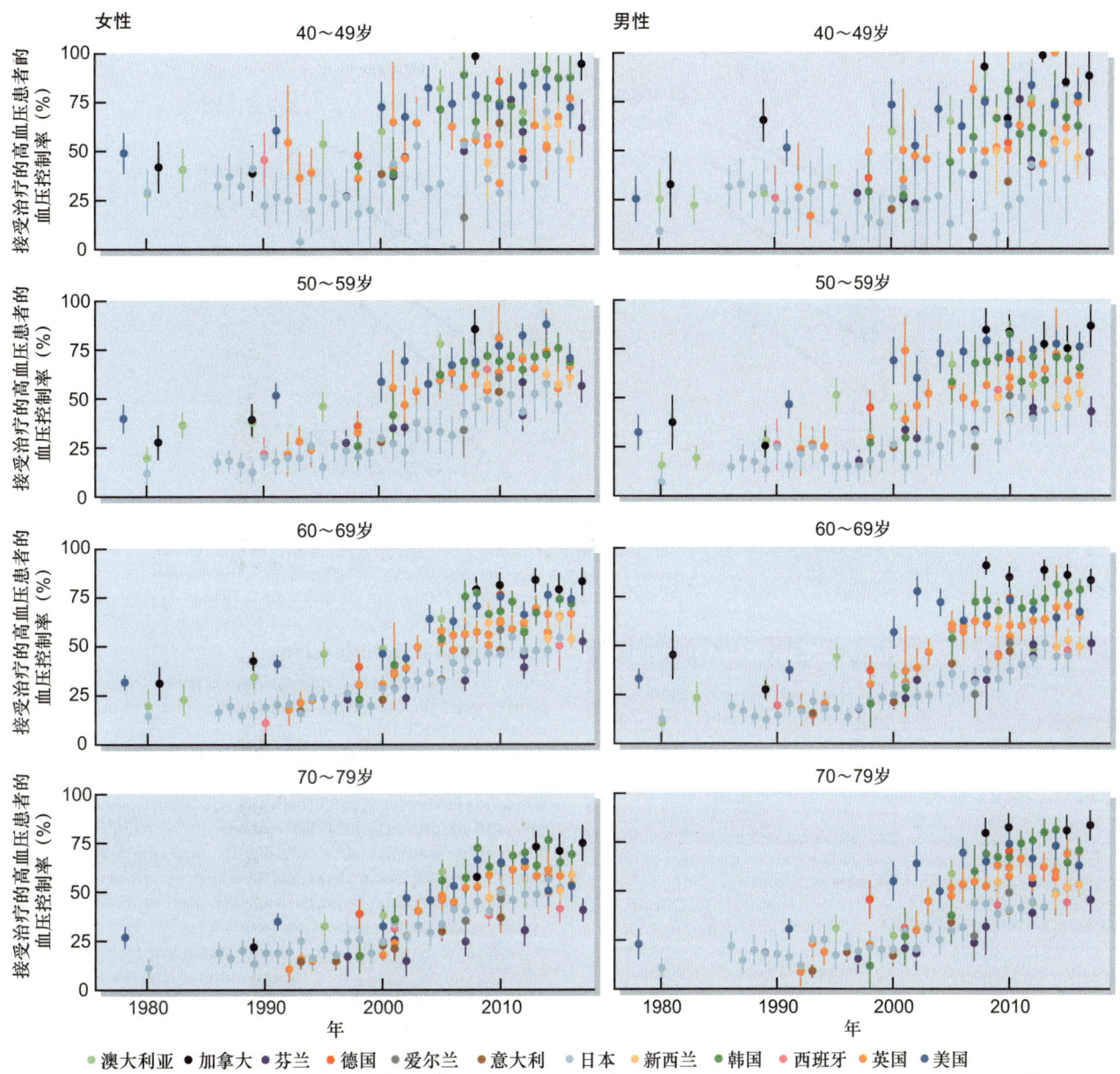

图 11.7 12 个高收入国家的高血压控制率变化趋势 [NCD Risk Factor Collaboration (NCD-RisC), Lancet July 2019; 10199: 639-651.]

可能是由于日常生活中交感神经过度激活造成的,原因包括工作或家庭压力、吸烟或其他肾上腺素能刺激,而这些刺激在就诊时会消失(图 11.10)。前述血压监测记录可以防止对此种隐匿性高血压诊断与治疗不足。隐匿性高血压也与高心血管风险有关,在 10% 的普通高血压患者、高达 40% 的糖尿病患者和 70% 的非裔美国高血压肾病患者中存在隐匿性高血压。

目标 2:心血管风险分层

绝大多数血压处于高血压前期或高血压的患者有一个或多个可改变的动脉粥样硬化危险因素(如高胆固醇血症、吸烟、糖尿病)。目前推荐使用集合队列方程(PCE)来评估无心血管疾病史的高血压患者的 10 年 ASCVD(动脉粥样硬化性心血管疾病)风险。10 年 ASCVD 风险为 10% 或更高的患者且血压至少为 130/80 mmHg 时应立即开始抗高血压药物治疗。除了 ASCVD 风险外,还应考虑是否存在靶器官损害,如左心室肥厚或蛋白尿,PCE 无法获得这些因素,但应将其视为高风险特征。

目标 3:继发性(可识别)高血压病因的识别

对大多数高血压患者来说,彻底查找继发性病因并不符合成本效益,但在两种情况下却至关重要:①在初始评估中发现有较强的临床线索,或者②当高血压非

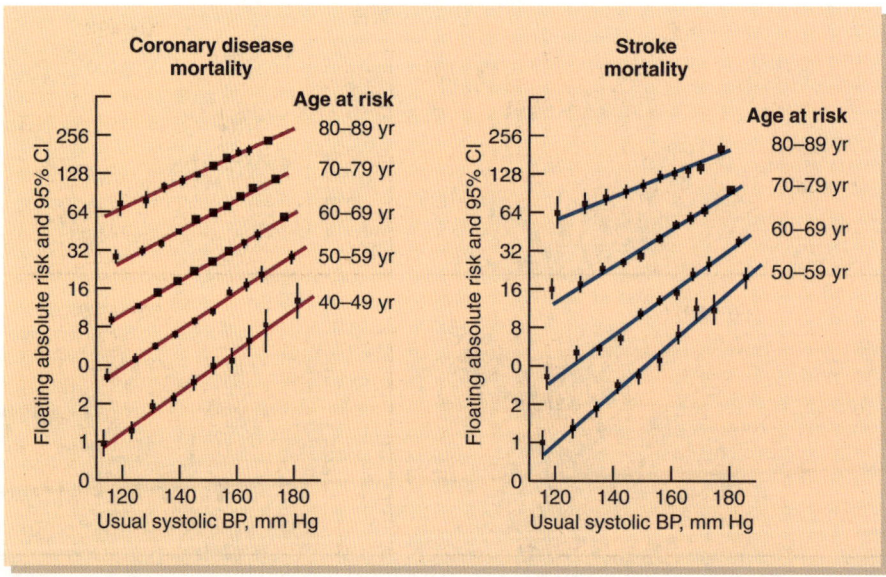

Fig. 11.8 Age-specific relevance of usual blood pressure to vascular mortality. Increased risk of myocardial infarction and stroke was observed with increasing levels of systolic BP beginning at the level of 115 mm Hg. (From Lewington S, et al. Age-specific relevance of usual blood pressure to vascular mortality: A meta-analysis of individual data for one million adults in 61 prospective studies. The Lancet 2002:360:1903-1913.)

TABLE 11.5 Staging of Office Blood Pressure[a]

Blood Pressure Category	Systolic Blood Pressure (mm Hg)	Diastolic Blood Pressure (mm Hg)
Normal	<120	and <80
Elevated	120-129	and <80
Stage 1 hypertension	130-139	or 80-89
Stage 2 hypertension	≥140	or ≥90

[a]Calculation of seated blood pressure is based on the mean of two or more readings on at least two separate occasions.
From Whelton PK, Carey RM, Aronow WS, et al. 2017 ACC/AHA/AAPA/ABC/ACPM/AGS/APhA/ASH/ASPC/NMA/PCNA guideline for the prevention, detection, evaluation, and management of high blood pressure in adults: a report of the American College of Cardiology/American Heart Association Task Force on Clinical Practice Guidelines. Circulation 2018. 138(17):e426-e483.

it either is refractory to intensive multiple-drug therapy or requires hospitalization. Table 11.6 summarizes the major causes of secondary hypertension that should be suggested on the basis of a good history, physical, and routine laboratory tests.

Renal Parenchymal Hypertension

Chronic kidney disease is the most common cause of secondary hypertension. Hypertension is present in more than 85% of patients with chronic kidney disease and is a major factor causing their increased cardiovascular morbidity and mortality. The mechanisms causing the hypertension include an expanded plasma volume and peripheral vasoconstriction, with the latter caused by both activation of vasoconstrictor pathways (renin-angiotensin and sympathetic nervous systems) and inhibition of vasodilator pathways (nitric oxide). Renal insufficiency should be considered when microalbuminuria of more than 30 mg/gram of creatinine is present or when the estimated glomerular filtration rate (eGFR) is below 60 mL/min/1.73 m².

Renovascular Hypertension

Unilateral or bilateral renal artery stenosis is present in less than 2% of patients with hypertension in a general medical practice but up to 30% in patients with medically refractory hypertension. The main causes of renal artery stenosis are atherosclerosis (85% of patients), typically in older adults with other clinical manifestations of systemic atherosclerosis and fibromuscular dysplasia (15% of patients), typically in women between the ages of 15 and 50 years. Unilateral renal artery stenosis leads to underperfusion of the juxtaglomerular cells, thereby producing renin-dependent hypertension even though the contralateral kidney is able to maintain normal blood volume. In contrast, bilateral renal artery stenosis (or unilateral stenosis with a solitary kidney) constitutes a potentially reversible cause of progressive renal failure and volume-dependent hypertension. The following clinical clues increase the suggestion of renovascular hypertension: any hospitalization for urgent or emergent hypertension; recurrent *flash* pulmonary edema; recent worsening of long-standing, previously well-controlled hypertension; severe hypertension in a young adult or in an adult after 50 years of age; precipitously and progressively worsening of renal function in response to angiotensin-converting enzyme (ACE) inhibition or angiotensin II-receptor blockade (ARB); unilateral small kidney by any radiographic study; extensive peripheral arteriosclerosis; or a flank bruit. The diagnosis is confirmed by noninvasive testing with MR or spiral computed tomographic (CT) angiography (Fig. 11.11). Renal artery angioplasty often cures fibromuscular dysplasia. Atherosclerotic renal artery stenosis should be treated with intensive medical management of atherosclerotic risk factors (hypertension, lipids, smoking cessation). Revascularization should be considered for the following indications: (1) medically refractory hypertension, (2) progressive renal failure on medical therapy, and (3) bilateral renal artery stenosis or stenosis of a solitary functioning kidney.

Primary Aldosteronism

The most common causes of primary aldosteronism are (1) a unilateral aldosterone-producing adenoma and (2) bilateral adrenal hyperplasia. Because aldosterone is the principal ligand for the mineralocorticoid

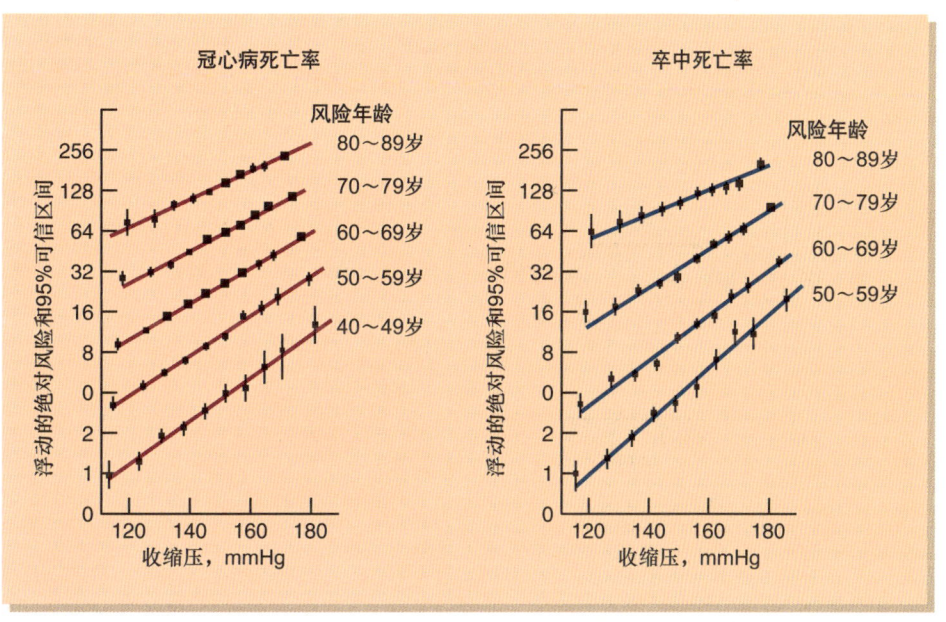

图11.8 平日血压与血管死亡率的年龄特异相关性。随着收缩压从 115 mmHg 开始升高，心肌梗死和卒中的风险增加（引自 Lewington S，et al. Age-specific relevance of usual blood pressure to vascular mortality：A meta-analysis of individual data for one million adults in 61 prospective studies. The Lancet 2002：360：1903-1913.）

表11.5	诊室血压分级[a]	
血压类型	收缩压（mmHg）	舒张压（mmHg）
正常	<120	和<80
升高	120～129	和<80
1级高血压	130～139	或80～89
2级高血压	≥140	或≥90

[a] 血压为不同时间所测血压两次或两次以上读数的平均值
引自 Whelton PK，Carey RM，Aronow WS，et al. 2017 ACC/AHA/AAPA/ABC/ACPM/AGS/APhA/ASH/ASPC/NMA/PCNA guideline for the prevention, detection, evaluation, and management of high blood pressure in adults：a report of the American College of Cardiology/American Heart Association Task Force on Clinical Practice Guidelines. Circulation 2018. 138（17）：e426-e483.

常严重，多种药物强化治疗无效或需要住院治疗。表11.6 总结了基于详细病史、体格检查和常规实验室检查获得提示的继发性高血压的主要病因。

肾实质性高血压

慢性肾脏病是继发性高血压最常见的原因。超过 85% 的慢性肾脏病患者存在高血压，高血压是导致心血管疾病发病率和死亡率增加的主要因素。引起高血压的机制包括血容量增加和周围血管收缩，后者由血管收缩通路（肾素-血管紧张素和交感神经系统）的激活和血管扩张通路（一氧化氮）的抑制引起。当尿微量白蛋白/肌酐超过 30 mg/g 或估算肾小球滤过率低于 60 ml/（min·1.73 m^2）时，应考虑肾功能不全。

肾血管性高血压

在一般临床诊疗中只有不到 2% 的高血压患者存在单侧或双侧肾动脉狭窄，但在药物难治性高血压患者中，这一比例高达 30%。肾动脉狭窄的主要原因是动脉粥样硬化（85% 的患者），多发生在伴有其他全身性动脉粥样硬化临床表现的老年人中，另一原因是纤维肌性发育不良（15% 的患者），通常为 15～50 岁的女性。单侧肾动脉狭窄导致肾小球旁细胞灌注不足，从而产生肾素依赖性高血压，即使对侧肾脏能够维持正常的血容量。相反，双侧肾动脉狭窄（或单侧肾动脉狭窄伴孤立肾）是进行性肾衰竭和容量依赖性高血压的潜在可逆原因。以下临床线索提示肾血管性高血压的可能性：任何因高血压亚急症或急症住院的病例；反复发作的一过性肺水肿；既往长期控制良好的高血压近期恶化；年轻人或 50 岁以后的成年人患重度高血压；血管紧张素转换酶抑制剂（ACEI）或血管紧张素 II 受体阻滞剂（ARB）导致肾功能急剧和进行性恶化；通过任何放射学检查发现单侧肾脏较小；广泛周围动脉硬化；或者是侧腹部杂音。可通过无创磁共振（MR）或螺旋计算机断层成像（CT）血管成像等非侵入性检查证实诊断（图11.11）。肾动脉成形术常用于治疗纤维肌性发育不良。动脉粥样硬化性肾动脉狭窄应对动脉粥样硬化危险因素（高血压、高脂血症、吸烟等）进行强化干预治疗。具有以下适应证的患者应考虑血运重建术：①药物难治性高血压，②药物治疗后出现进行性肾衰竭，③双侧肾动脉狭窄或有功能的孤立肾动脉狭窄。

原发性醛固酮增多症

原发性醛固酮增多症最常见的原因是：①单侧肾上腺醛固酮瘤，②双侧肾上腺皮质增生症。由于醛固酮是远端肾单位中盐皮质激素受体的主要配体，过量

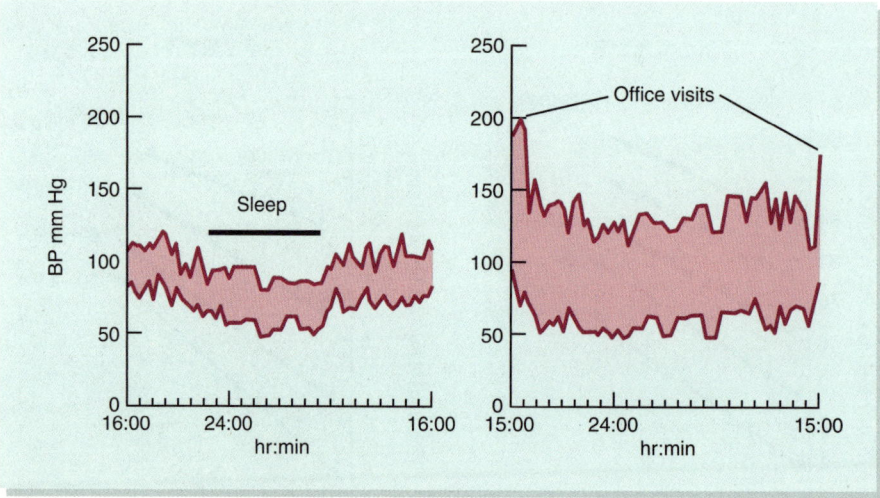

Fig. 11.9 Twenty-four hour ambulatory blood pressure (BP) monitor tracings in two different patients. (A) Optimal blood pressure (BP) in a healthy 37-year-old woman. The normal variability in BP, the nocturnal dip in BP during sleep, and the sharp increase in BP on awakening are noted. (B) Pronounced white coat effect in an 80-year-old woman referred for evaluation of medically refractory hypertension. Documentation of the white coat effect prevented overtreatment of the patient's isolated systolic hypertension.

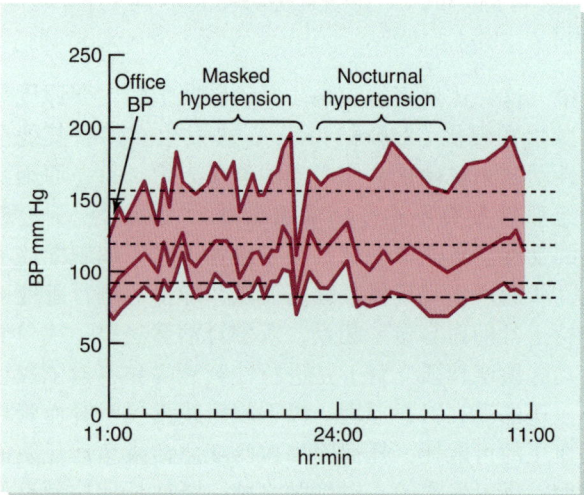

Fig. 11.10 Twenty-four hour ambulatory blood pressure (BP) monitor tracing shows both masked hypertension and nocturnal hypertension in a 55-year-old man with stage 3 chronic kidney disease. Treatment with three different antihypertensive medications in this patient produced an office BP of 125/75 mm Hg, which seems to be at goal. However, progressive hypertensive heart disease and deterioration of renal function suggested masked hypertension. Ambulatory monitoring revealed that the patient's treated BP was much higher out of the office, documenting both masked hypertension (ambulatory BP of 175/95 mm Hg) and sustained nocturnal hypertension (BP of 175/90 mm Hg). Additional medication was added. (Courtesy of Ronald G. Victor, MD, Hypertension Division, Department of Internal Medicine, University of Texas Southwestern Medical Center, Dallas, Texas.)

receptor in the distal nephron, excessive aldosterone production causes excessive renal Na^+-K^+ exchange, often resulting in hypokalemia. The diagnosis should always be suggested when hypertension is accompanied by either unprovoked hypokalemia (serum K^+ less than 3.5 mmol/L in the absence of diuretic therapy) or a tendency to develop excessive hypokalemia during diuretic therapy (serum K^+ less than 3.0 mmol/L). However, more than one third of patients do not have hypokalemia on initial presentation, and the diagnosis should be considered in any patient with refractory hypertension. The diagnosis is confirmed by the demonstration of nonsuppressible hyperaldosteronism during salt loading, followed by adrenal vein sampling to distinguish between a unilateral adenoma and bilateral hyperplasia. Laparoscopic adrenalectomy is the treatment of choice for unilateral aldosterone-producing adenoma, whereas pharmacologic mineralocorticoid-receptor blockade with eplerenone is the treatment for bilateral adrenal hyperplasia.

Mendelian Forms of Hypertension

Nine very rare forms of severe early-onset hypertension are inherited as Mendelian traits. In each case, the hypertension is mineralocorticoid-induced and involves excessive activation of the epithelial sodium channel (*ENaC*), the final common pathway for reabsorption of sodium from the distal nephron. The resultant salt-dependent hypertension can be caused by both gain-of-function mutations of *ENaC* (Liddle's syndrome) or the mineralocorticoid receptor (i.e., a rare form of pregnancy-induced hypertension) and by increased production or decreased clearance of mineralocorticoids. These include aldosterone (glucocorticoid-remediable aldosteronism), deoxycorticosterone (17-hydroxylase deficiency), and cortisol (syndrome of apparent mineralocorticoid excess). Mutations in the potassium channel subunit KCNJ5 and chloride channel CLCN2 have been linked to familial aldosteronism by increasing aldosterone release and or increasing proliferation of zona glomerulosa cells.

Pheochromocytoma and Paraganglioma

Pheochromocytomas are rare catecholamine-producing tumors of the adrenal chromaffin cells. Paragangliomas are even rarer extra-adrenal catecholamine-producing or nonfunctional tumors of sympathetic and parasympathetic ganglia. The diagnosis should be suggested when hypertension is accompanied by paroxysms of headaches, palpitations, pallor, or diaphoresis. However, the most common presentation of pheochromocytoma is an adrenal incidentaloma, an incidental adrenal mass discovered unexpectedly on abdominal imaging for another indication. In some patients,

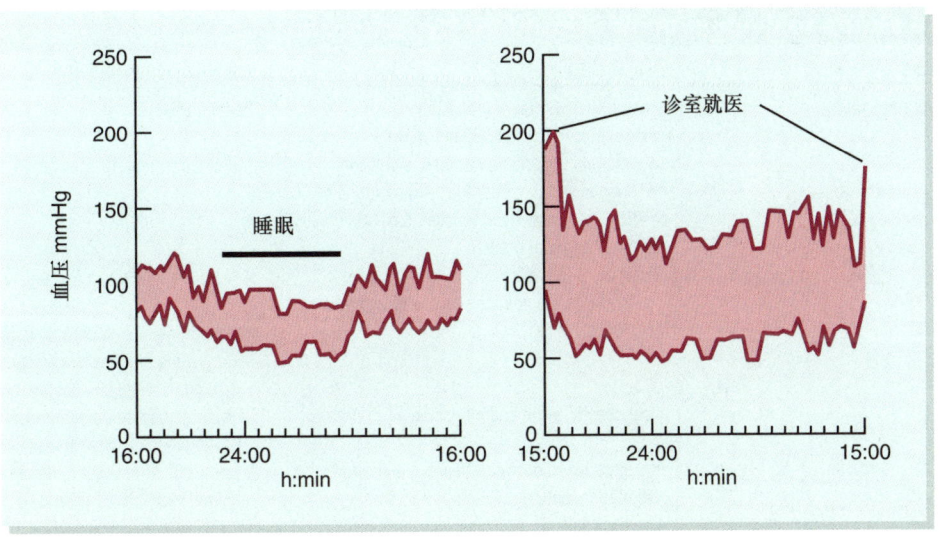

图 11.9 两名不同患者的 24 h 动态血压监测记录。左图为 37 岁健康女性的最佳血压。值得注意的是血压的正常变化，夜间睡眠时血压下降，醒来时血压急剧上升。右图为一名 80 岁女性在接受药物难治性高血压评估时出现明显的白大衣效应。对白大衣效应的捕捉和记录避免了对患者的单纯收缩期高血压的过度治疗

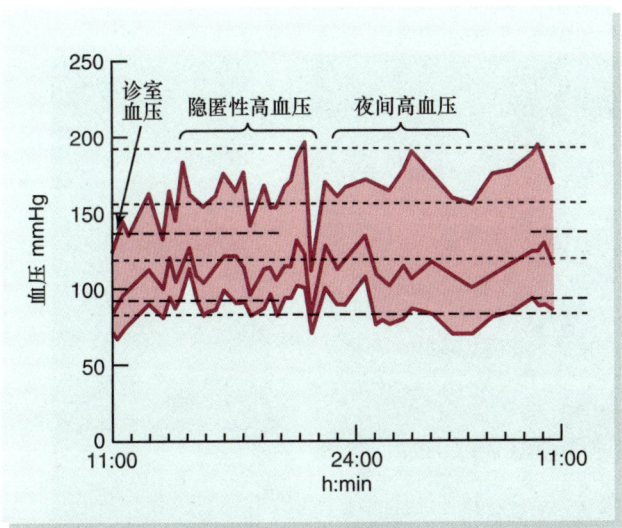

图 11.10 24 h 动态血压监测记录显示，一名 55 岁慢性肾脏病 3 期的男性患者同时存在隐匿性高血压和夜间高血压。通过 3 种不同的降压药物治疗，该患者的诊室血压降至 125/75 mmHg，似乎达到了目标。然而，进行性高血压心脏病和肾功能的恶化提示隐匿性高血压的存在。动态血压监测显示，患者接受治疗后的血压在诊室外要高得多，监测记录了隐匿性高血压（动态血压为 175/95 mmHg）和持续的夜间高血压（血压为 175/90 mmHg）。由此加用了额外的药物（授权自 Ronald G. Victor，MD，Hypertension Division，Department of Internal Medicine，University of Texas Southwestern Medical Center，Dallas，Texas.）

产生的醛固酮会导致肾脏 Na^+-K^+ 交换过多，常引起低钾血症。当高血压伴有不明原因的低钾血症（在没有利尿治疗的情况下血清 K^+ 低于 3.5 mmol/L）或在利尿治疗期间存在严重低钾血症（血清 K^+ 低于 3.0 mmol/L）的倾向时，应考虑此诊断。然而，超过 1/3 的患者在初次就诊时没有低钾血症，因而任何难治性高血压患者都应考虑该诊断。诊断的确认是在盐负荷期间出现不可抑制的高醛固酮症，然后进行肾上腺静脉取血，以区分单侧腺瘤和双侧增生。腹腔镜肾上腺切除术是针对单侧肾上腺醛固酮瘤的治疗方法，而依普利酮这类盐皮质激素受体阻滞剂药物则是针对双侧肾上腺增生的治疗方法。

高血压的孟德尔遗传性状

9 种非常罕见的严重早发性高血压是以孟德尔特征遗传的。在每种情况下，高血压都是由盐皮质激素诱导的，涉及上皮钠通道（ENaC）的过度激活，这是从远端肾单位重吸收钠的最终共同途径。由此产生的盐依赖性高血压可能是由 ENaC（利德尔综合征）或盐皮质激素受体（一种罕见的妊娠期高血压）的功能获得性突变以及盐皮质激素的产生增加或清除减少引起的。这些激素包括醛固酮（糖皮质激素可抑制性醛固酮增多症）、脱氧皮质酮（17-羟化酶缺乏症）和皮质醇（表象性盐皮质激素过多综合征）。钾通道亚基 KCNJ5 和氯通道 CLCN2 的突变与家族性醛固酮增多症有关，因为它会增加醛固酮的释放和（或）增加球状带细胞的增殖。

嗜铬细胞瘤和副神经节瘤

嗜铬细胞瘤是罕见的肾上腺嗜铬细胞产生儿茶酚胺的肿瘤。副神经节瘤则是更为罕见的肾上腺外产生儿茶酚胺或无功能的交感神经节和副交感神经节肿瘤。当高血压伴有阵发性头痛、心悸、面色苍白或出汗等症状时，应考虑该诊断。然而，嗜铬细胞瘤最常见的表现是肾上腺偶发瘤，即因其他病症在腹部影像学检查时，意外发现的肾上腺肿块。在一些患者中，嗜铬

TABLE 11.6	Guide to Evaluation of Secondary Hypertension	
Probable Diagnosis	**Clinical Clues**	**Diagnostic Testing**
Renal parenchymal hypertension	Estimated GFR <60 mL/min/1.73 m² Urine albumin:creatinine >30 mg/g	Renal ultrasound
Renovascular disease	New elevation in serum creatinine, significant elevation in serum creatinine with initiation of ACEI or ARBs, refractory hypertension, flash pulmonary edema, abdominal bruit	MR or CT angiography, invasive angiogram
	Coarctation of the aorta pulses, arm BP >leg BP, chest bruits, rib notching on chest radiograph	Arm pulses >leg chest MR or CT, aortogram
Primary aldosteronism	Hypokalemia, refractory hypertension	Plasma renin and aldosterone, 24-hr urine potassium, 24-hr urine aldosterone and potassium after salt loading, adrenal CT scan, adrenal vein sampling
Cushing's syndrome	Truncal obesity, wide and blanching	24-hr urine cortisol, purple striae, muscle weakness, dexamethasone suppression test, adrenal CT scan
Pheochromocytoma	Spells of paroxysmal hypertension, palpitations, perspiration, pallor Pain in the head Diabetes	Plasma and 24-hr urine metanephrines and catecholamines, adrenal CT scan
Obstructive sleep apnea	Loud snoring, daytime somnolence, obesity, large neck	Sleep study

ACEI, Angiotensin-converting enzyme inhibitor; *ARBs*, angiotensin-receptor blockers; *BP*, blood pressure; *CT*, computed tomography; *GFR*, glomerular filtration rate; *MR*, magnetic resonance.

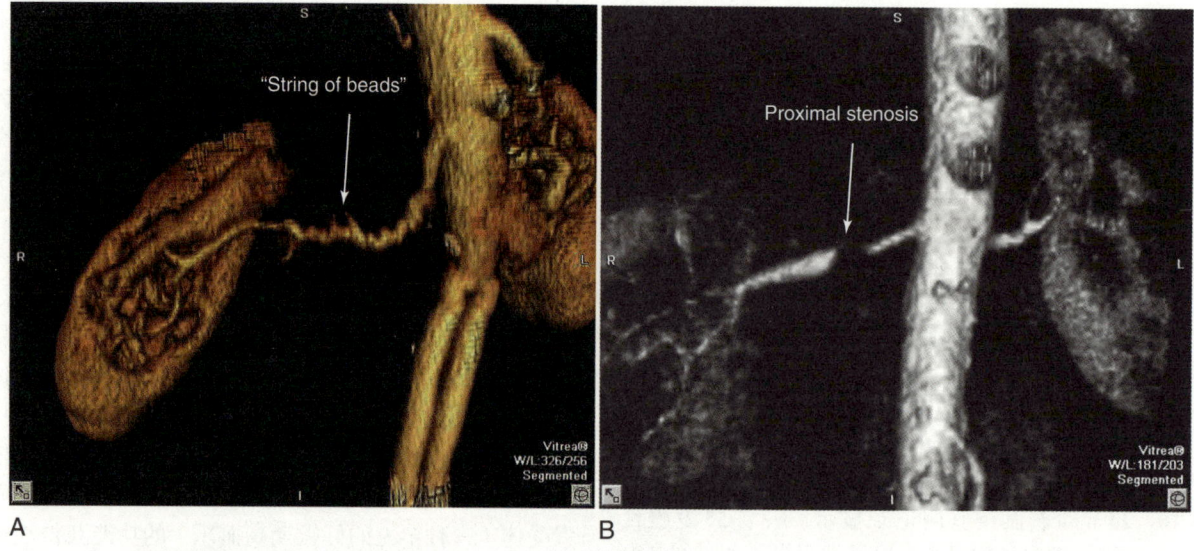

Fig. 11.11 Computed tomography (CT) angiogram with three-dimensional reconstruction. (A) Classic *string-of-beads* lesion of fibromuscular dysplasia. (B) Severe proximal atherosclerotic stenosis of the right renal artery. (Courtesy of Bart Domatch, MD, Radiology Department, University of Texas Southwestern Medical Center, Dallas, Texas.)

pheochromocytoma is misdiagnosed as panic disorder. A family history of early-onset hypertension may suggest pheochromocytoma as part of the multiple endocrine neoplasia syndromes or familial paraganglioma. If the diagnosis is missed, then outpouring of catecholamines from the tumor can cause an unsuspected hypertensive crisis during unrelated radiologic or surgical procedures; the perioperative mortality exceeds 80% in such patients.

Laboratory confirmation of pheochromocytoma is made by demonstrating elevated levels of plasma or urinary metanephrines; these are methylated derivatives of norepinephrine and epinephrine that are made in the adrenal medulla and continually leak out into the plasma even between blood pressure spikes. Pheochromocytomas are typically large adrenal tumors that can usually be localized by CT or MR imaging, although nuclear scanning with specific isotopes that localize to chromaffin tissue is occasionally needed to identify smaller tumors and paragangliomas.

Treatment of these tumors is surgical resection. Patients must receive adequate preoperative management with α-blockade followed by β-blockade and volume expansion to prevent the hemodynamic swings that can occur during surgical manipulation of the tumor. For unresectable tumors, chronic therapy with the α-adrenergic blocker phenoxybenzamine is usually effective.

表 11.6 继发性高血压评估指南		
可能的诊断	临床线索	诊断检查
肾实质性高血压	估测 GFR < 60 ml/(min · 1.73 m^2) 尿白蛋白/肌酐 > 30 mg/g	肾脏超声
肾血管疾病	血清肌酐新近升高，开始使用 ACEI 或 ARB 后血清肌酐显著升高，难治性高血压，一过性肺水肿，腹部杂音	MR 或 CT 血管成像，侵入性血管造影
	主动脉缩窄脉搏，上肢血压>下肢血压，胸部杂音，胸片上肋骨切迹	上肢脉搏>下肢脉搏，胸部 MR 或 CT、主动脉造影
原发性醛固酮增多症	低钾血症，难治性高血压	血浆肾素和醛固酮，24 h 尿钾，盐负荷后 24 h 尿醛固酮和尿钾，肾上腺 CT 扫描，肾上腺静脉取血
库欣综合征	向心性肥胖，体型宽大，苍白，紫纹，肌肉无力（译者注：原表位置有误）	24 h 尿皮质醇，地塞米松抑制试验、肾上腺 CT 扫描
嗜铬细胞瘤	阵发性高血压，心悸，出汗，面色苍白 头痛 糖尿病	血浆和 24 h 尿甲氧基肾上腺素和儿茶酚胺，肾上腺 CT 扫描
阻塞性睡眠呼吸暂停	打鼾，白天嗜睡，肥胖，脖子粗大	睡眠监测

ACEI，血管紧张素转换酶抑制剂；ARB，血管紧张素受体阻滞剂；CT，计算机断层成像；GFR，肾小球滤过率；MR，磁共振。

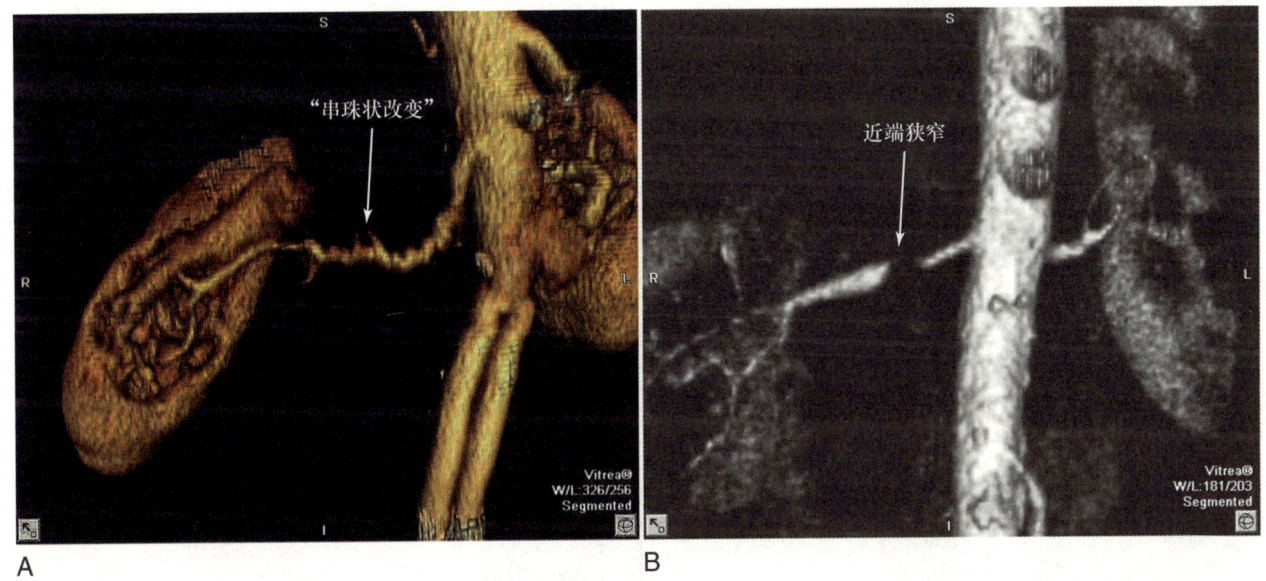

图 11.11 三维重建的 CT 血管成像。（A）典型的纤维肌性发育不良的串珠状改变。（B）右肾动脉近端严重的动脉粥样硬化性狭窄（授权自 Bart Domatch, MD, Radiology Department, University of Texas Southwestern Medical Center, Dallas, Texas.）

细胞瘤被误诊为惊恐障碍。早发性高血压的家族史可能表明嗜铬细胞瘤是多发性内分泌腺瘤综合征或家族性副神经节瘤的一部分。如果误诊，那么肿瘤中儿茶酚胺的大量分泌可能会在不相关的放射学或外科操作过程中引起无法预料的高血压危象；此类患者的围术期死亡率超过 80%。

实验室确诊嗜铬细胞瘤的方法是检测血浆或尿液中甲氧基肾上腺素的升高水平；这些是去甲肾上腺素和肾上腺素的甲基化衍生物，在肾上腺髓质中产生，即使在血压骤升的间歇期也会不断分泌到血浆中。嗜铬细胞瘤是典型的大的肾上腺肿瘤，通常可以通过 CT 或 MR 成像定位，但有时需要使用特定同位素定位于嗜铬组织进行核扫描，以识别较小的肿瘤和副神经节瘤。

这些肿瘤的治疗方法是手术切除。患者必须接受充分的术前治疗：先接受 α 受体阻滞剂治疗，再使用 β 受体阻滞剂并进行扩容治疗，以防止在肿瘤手术操作过程中可能发生的血流动力学波动。对于无法切除的肿瘤，使用 α 受体阻滞剂酚苄明进行长期治疗通常是有效的。

TABLE 11.7 Oral Antihypertensive Agents

Drug	Dose Range, Total mg/day (Doses Per Day)	Drug	Dose Range, Total mg/day (Doses Per Day)
Diuretics		Ramipril	2.5-20 (1)
Thiazide Diuretics		Trandolapril	1-8 (1)
Hydrochlorothiazide (HCTZ)	6.25-50 (1)		
Chlorthalidone	12.5-25 (1)	**Angiotensin-Receptor Blockers**	
Indapamide	1.25-5 (1)	Azilsartan	40-80 mg (1)
Metolazone	2.5-5 (1)	Candesartan	8-32 (1)
		Eprosartan	400-800 (1-2)
Loop Diuretics		Irbesartan	150-300 (1)
Furosemide	20-160 (2)	Losartan	25-100 (2)
Torsemide	2.5-20 (1-2)	Olmesartan	5-40 (1)
Bumetanide	0.5-2 (2)	Telmisartan	20-80 (1)
Ethacrynic acid	25-100 (2)	Valsartan	80-320 (1-2)
Potassium-Sparing		**Direct Renin Inhibitor**	
Amiloride	5-20 (1)	Aliskiren	75-300 (1)
Triamterene	25-100 (1)		
Spironolactone	12.5-400 (1-2)	**α-Blockers**	
Eplerenone	25-100 (1-2)	Doxazosin	1-16 (1)
		Prazosin	1-40 (2-3)
β-Blockers		Terazosin	1-20 (1)
Acebutolol	200-800 (2)	Phenoxybenzamine	20-120 (2) for pheochromocytoma
Atenolol	25-100 (1)		
Betaxolol	5-20 (1)	**Central Sympatholytics**	
Bisoprolol	2.5-20 (1)	Clonidine	0.2-1.2 (2-3)
Carteolol	2.5-10 (1)	Clonidine patch	0.1-0.6 (weekly)
Metoprolol	50-450 (2)	Guanabenz	2-32 (2)
Metoprolol XL	50-200 (1-2)	Guanfacine	1-3 (1) (q hs)
Nadolol	20-320 (1)	Methyldopa	250-1000 (2)
Nebivolol	5-40 (1)	Reserpine	0.05-0.25 (1)
Penbutolol	10-80 (1)		
Pindolol	10-60 (2)	**Direct Vasodilators**	
Propranolol	40-180 (2)	Hydralazine	10-200 (2)
Propranolol LA	60-180 (1-2)	Minoxidil	2.5-100 (1)
Timolol	20-60 (2)		
		Fixed-Dose Combinations	
β/α-Blockers		Aliskiren/HCTZ	75-300/12.5-25 (1)
Labetalol	200-2400 (2)	Amiloride/HCTZ	5/50 (1)
Carvedilol	6.25-50 (2)	Amlodipine/benazepril	2.5-5/10-20 (1)
		Amlodipine/valsartan	5-10/160-320 (1)
Calcium-Channel Blockers		Amlodipine/olmesartan	5-10/20-40 (1)
Dihydropyridines		Atenolol/chlorthalidone	50-100/25 (1)
Amlodipine	2.5-10 (1)	Azilsartan/chlorthalidone	40-80/12.5-25 (1)
Felodipine	2.5-20 (1-2)	Benazepril/HCTZ	5-20/6.25-25 (1)
Isradipine CR	2.5-20 (2)	Bisoprolol/HCTZ	2.5-10/6.25 (1)
Nicardipine SR	30-120 (2)	Candesartan/HCTZ	16-32/12.5-25 (1)
Nifedipine XL	30-120 (1)	Enalapril/HCTZ	5-10/25 (1-2)
Nisoldipine	10-40 (12)	Eprosartan/HCTZ	600/12.5-25 (1)
		Fosinopril/HCTZ	10-20/12.5 (1)
Nondihydropyridines		Irbesartan/HCTZ	15-30/12.5-25 (1)
Diltiazem CD	120-540 (1)	Losartan/HCTZ	50-100/12.5-25 (1)
Verapamil HS	120-480 (1)	Olmesartan/amlodipine	20-40/5-10 (1)
		Olmesartan/HCTZ	20-40/12.5-25 (1)
Angiotensin-Converting Enzyme Inhibitors		Olmesartan/amlodipine/HCTZ	20-40/5-10/12.5-25 (1)
Benazepril	10-80 (12)	Spironolactone/HCTZ	25/25 (1/2-1)
Captopril	25-150 (2)	Telmisartan/HCTZ	40-80/12.5-25 (1)
Enalapril	2.5-40 (2)	Trandolapril/verapamil	2-4/180-240 (1)
Fosinopril	10-80 (1-2)	Triamterene/HCTZ	37.5/25 (1/2-1)
Lisinopril	5-80 (1-2)	Valsartan/HCTZ	80-160/12.5-25 (1)
Moexipril	7.5-30 (1)	Valsartan/amlodipine/HCTZ	80-160/5-10/12.5-25 (1)
Perindopril	4-16 (1)		
Quinapril	5-80 (1-2)		

表 11.7 口服抗高血压药物

药品	剂量范围：总毫克/天（每日用药次数）	药品	剂量范围：总毫克/天（每日用药次数）
利尿剂		雷米普利	2.5～20（1）
噻嗪类利尿剂		群多普利	1～8（1）
氢氯噻嗪	6.25～50（1）	**血管紧张素受体阻滞剂**	
氯噻酮	12.5～25（1）	阿齐沙坦	40～80 mg（1）
吲达帕胺	1.25～5（1）	坎地沙坦	8～32（1）
美托拉宗	2.5～5（1）	依普沙坦	400～800（1～2）
袢利尿剂		厄贝沙坦	150～300（1）
呋塞米	20～160（2）	氯沙坦	25～100（2）
托拉塞米	2.5～20（1～2）	奥美沙坦	5～40（1）
布美他尼	0.5～2（2）	替米沙坦	20～80（1）
依他尼酸	25～100（2）	缬沙坦	80～320（1～2）
保钾药		**直接肾素抑制剂**	
阿米洛利	5～20（1）	阿利吉仑	75～300（1）
氨苯蝶啶	25～100（1）	**α受体阻滞剂**	
螺内酯	12.5～400（1～2）	多沙唑嗪	1～16（1）
依普利酮	25～100（1～2）	哌唑嗪	1～40（2～3）
β受体阻滞剂		特拉唑嗪	1～20（1）
醋丁洛尔	200～800（2）	酚苄明	20～120（2）用于治疗嗜铬细胞瘤
阿替洛尔	25～100（1）	**中枢交感神经阻滞剂**	
倍他洛尔	5～20（1）	可乐定	0.2～1.2（2～3）
比索洛尔	2.5～20（1）	可乐定贴剂	0.1～0.6（每周）
卡替洛尔	2.5～10（1）	胍那苄	2～32（2）
美托洛尔	50～450（2）	胍法辛	1～3（1）（每晚睡前）
美托洛尔 XL	50～200（1～2）	甲基多巴	250～1000（2）
纳多洛尔	20～320（1）	利血平	0.05～0.25（1）
奈必洛尔	5～40（1）	**直接血管扩张剂**	
喷布洛尔	10～80（1）	肼屈嗪	10～200（2）
吲哚洛尔	10～60（2）	米诺地尔	2.5～100（1）
普萘洛尔	40～180（2）	**固定剂量组合**	
普萘洛尔 LA	60～180（1～2）	阿利吉仑/氢氯噻嗪	75～300/12.5～25（1）
噻吗洛尔	20～60（2）	阿米洛利/氢氯噻嗪	5/50（1）
β/α受体阻滞剂		氨氯地平/贝那普利	2.5～5/10～20（1）
拉贝洛尔	200～2400（2）	氨氯地平/缬沙坦	5～10/160～320（1）
卡维地洛	6.25～50（2）	氨氯地平/奥美沙坦	5～10/20～40（1）
钙通道阻滞剂		阿替洛尔/氯噻酮	50～100/25（1）
二氢吡啶类		阿齐沙坦/氯噻酮	40～80/12.5～25（1）
氨氯地平	2.5～10（1）	贝那普利/氢氯噻嗪	5～20/6.25～25（1）
非洛地平	2.5～20（1～2）	比索洛尔/氢氯噻嗪	2.5～10/6.25～25（1）
伊拉地平 CR	2.5～20（1）	坎地沙坦/氢氯噻嗪	16～32/12.5～25（1）
尼卡地平 SR	30～120（2）	依那普利/氢氯噻嗪	5～10/25（1～2）
硝苯地平 XL	30～120（1）	依普沙坦/氢氯噻嗪	600/12.5～25（1）
尼索地平	10～40（12）	福辛普利/氢氯噻嗪	10～20/12.5（1）
非二氢吡啶类		厄贝沙坦/氢氯噻嗪	15～30/12.5～25（1）
地尔硫䓬 CD	120～540（1）	氯沙坦/氢氯噻嗪	50～100/12.5～25（1）
维拉帕米 HS	120～480（1）	奥美沙坦/氨氯地平	20～40/5～10（1）
血管紧张素转换酶抑制剂		奥美沙坦/氢氯噻嗪	20～40/12.5～25（1）
贝那普利	10～80（12）	奥美沙坦/氨氯地平/氢氯噻嗪	20～40/5～10/12.5～25（1）
卡托普利	25～150（2）	螺内酯/氢氯噻嗪	25/25（1/2～1）
依那普利	2.5～40（2）	替米沙坦/氢氯噻嗪	40～80/12.5～25（1）
福辛普利	10～80（1～2）	群多普利/维拉帕米	2～4/180～240（1）
赖诺普利	5～80（1～2）	氨苯蝶啶/氢氯噻嗪	37.5/25（1/2～1）
莫昔普利	7.5～30（1）	缬沙坦/氢氯噻嗪	80～160/12.5～25（1）
培哚普利	4～16（1）	缬沙坦/氨氯地平/氢氯噻嗪	80～160/5～10/12.5～25（1）
喹那普利	5～80（1～2）		

XL，缓释；LA，长效；CR，控释；SR，持续释放；CD，缓释长效；HS，延迟释放。

Pheochromocytoma is a great masquerader and the large differential diagnosis includes causes of neurogenic hypertension such as sympathomimetic agents (cocaine, methamphetamine), baroreflex failure, and obstructive sleep apnea. A history of surgery and radiation therapy for head-and-neck tumors suggests the possibility of baroreceptor damage. Loud snoring, obesity, and somnolence suggest obstructive sleep apnea. Weight loss, continuous positive airway pressure, and corrective surgery improve BP control in some patients with sleep apnea.

Other causes of secondary hypertension include nonsteroidal anti-inflammatory drugs (NSAIDs), hypothyroidism, hyperthyroidism coarctation of the aorta, and immunosuppressive drugs, especially cyclosporine and tacrolimus.

TREATMENT OF HYPERTENSION

Prescription medication is the cornerstone of treating hypertension. Lifestyle modification should be used as an adjunct but not as an alternative to life-saving BP medication. Most dietary sodium (Na^+) comes from processed foods, and daily salt consumption should be reduced to less than 4 grams, which is equivalent to 1500 mg or 65 mmol of Na^+. The **Dietary Approach to Stop Hypertension** (DASH diet), which is rich in fresh fruits and vegetables (for high potassium content) and low-fat dairy products, has been shown to lower BP in feeding trials. Other lifestyle modifications that can lower BP include weight loss in overweight patients with hypertension, regular aerobic exercise, smoking cessation, and moderation in alcohol intake.

The list of antihypertensive drugs marketed for the treatment of hypertension in the United States is shown in Table 11.7. Major contraindications and side effects of these drugs are summarized in Table 11.8.

Patients With Uncomplicated Hypertension

The three first-line drug classes for uncomplicated hypertension are: (1) CCB, (2) ACEI or ARB, and (3) thiazide diuretic. The 2017 ACC/AHA high blood pressure guideline, recommended any one of these three drug classes as initial therapy for most patients with hypertension. It also recommended initiating therapy with two first-line drugs of different classes, either as separate agents or in a fixed-dose combination for individuals with BP more than 20/10 mm Hg above their target goal. β-Blockers are not recommended as first-line therapy unless patients have other compelling indications (such as heart failure or ischemic heart disease) because it is inferior to three first-line drug classes in preventing target organ damage and cardiovascular events. In contrast, the European Society of Hypertension endorses β-blocker as the first-line agent, arguing that the most effective drugs are those that the patient will tolerate and take. Long-term patient adherence is best with an ARB, intermediate with an ACEI or CCB, and worst with a thiazide. Initiation of single pill combination therapy is encouraged as it allows BP control to reach target goal faster and improves long-term adherence. The European Society of Hypertension advocates a treatment strategy that is based on the patient's age and ethnicity. It recommends upfront combination therapy of RAS blocker (either an ACE inhibitor or an ARB) with a CCB or diuretic except in frail older adults with mild hypertension, in whom a monotherapy is recommended.

A growing body of evidence from clinical trials emphasizes the overriding importance of lowering BP with combinations of drugs rather than belaboring the choice of a single, best agent to begin therapy. Primary hypertension is multifactorial, and typically several medications (at least two or more) with different mechanisms of action (see Table 11.7) are required simultaneously to reach BP goal. In most patients with hypertension, low-dose combination drug therapy is the only way to control BP adequately and to minimize side effects. With many classes of antihypertensive medication, the dose-response relationship for BP is rather flat. Most of the BP lowering occurs at the lower end of the dose range. However, many of the side effects are steeply dose-dependent, becoming problematic mainly at the high end of the clinical dose range. Thus, low-dose combinations achieve therapeutic synergy and minimize side effects. Fixed-dose combinations reduce pill burden and cost.

One highly effective well-tolerated combination is a CCB plus an ACEI or ARB. A large benefit of combination therapy with an ACEI plus a dihydropyridine CCB over the combination of an ACEI plus a thiazide diuretic is reducing cardiovascular events in high-risk patients. In contrast, the combination of ARB plus an ACEI or direct renin inhibitor ("dual renin-angiotensin system blockade") should be avoided because it results in deterioration of renal function and increases risk of hypotension without added cardiovascular benefit.

Kaiser-Permanente of Northern California, a large managed care organization, has increased the control of hypertension among its membership over the past decade from 44% to an astounding 80% by: increasing access with walk-in BP checks by medical assistants, registry rounds to identify and contact patients with elevated office BP, and institution of a system-wide simple medication treatment protocol that features once-daily combination therapy.

Along with antihypertensive medication, statin therapy should be strongly considered as an integral part of most antihypertensive regimens in patients with 10-year ASCVD risk of at least 7.5%.

Hypertension in African Americans

Hypertension disproportionately affects African Americans. The explanation is unknown, but the dominant importance of environmental factors is indicated by geographic variation in hypertension prevalence among African-origin and European-origin populations. Hypertension is rare among Africans living in Africa and is more prevalent in several European countries than it is in the United States. As monotherapy for hypertension, an ACEI (or ARB) generally yields a smaller decrease in BP in black African patients than it does in non-black patients and thus affords less protection against stroke. However, when an ACEI or ARB is used in combination with a CCB or a diuretic, antihypertensive efficacy is amplified and ethnic differences disappear. In addition, combination of CCB with an ACEI (or ARB) or a diuretic is superior to combination of ACEI and diuretics in lowering BP in this population. Nevertheless, an ACEI-based treatment should be considered in African American patients with hypertensive nephrosclerosis as it slows the deterioration in renal function.

Hypertensive Nephrosclerosis

Hypertension is the second most common cause of chronic kidney disease, accounting for over 25% of cases. Hypertensive nephrosclerosis is the result of persistently uncontrolled hypertension, causing chronic glomerular ischemia. Typically, proteinuria is mild (<0.5 g/24 hr). Nondiabetic chronic kidney disease is a compelling indication for ACEI-based or ARB-based antihypertensive therapy. ACEIs cause greater dilation of the efferent renal arterioles, thereby minimizing intraglomerular hypertension. In contrast, arterial vasodilators such as dihydropyridine CCBs, when used without an ACEI or ARB, preferentially dilate the afferent arteriole and impair renal autoregulation. Glomerular hypertension can result if systemic BP is not sufficiently lowered. The ACEI should be withdrawn only if the rise in serum creatinine exceeds 30% of the baseline value or the serum K increases to greater than 5.6 mmol/L.

嗜铬细胞瘤是一种伪装性很强的疾病，需要进行大量的鉴别诊断，包括神经源性高血压，如拟交感神经药物（可卡因、甲基苯丙胺）、压力反射衰竭和阻塞性睡眠呼吸暂停；头颈部肿瘤手术和放射治疗史提示可能存在压力感受器损伤；大声打鼾、肥胖和嗜睡提示存在阻塞性睡眠呼吸暂停。减重、持续气道正压通气和矫正手术可改善部分睡眠呼吸暂停患者的血压控制。

继发性高血压的其他病因包括非甾体抗炎药（NSAID）、甲状腺功能减退、甲状腺功能亢进、主动脉缩窄和免疫抑制药物，尤其是环孢素和他克莫司。

高血压的治疗

处方药是治疗高血压的基石。生活方式调整应作为辅助手段，而不是挽救生命的降压药的替代方案。膳食中的钠（Na^+）大多数来自加工食品，每日盐摄入量应减少到 4 g 以下，相当于 1500 mg 或 65 mmol Na^+。终止高血压的膳食疗法（DASH饮食）富含新鲜水果、蔬菜（钾含量高）和低脂乳制品，已在饮食试验中证明可以降低血压。其他可以降低血压的生活方式调整包括减重（超重高血压患者）、定期进行有氧运动、戒烟和适量饮酒。

美国市场上销售的用于治疗高血压的降压药物清单如表 11.7 所示。这些药物的主要禁忌证和副作用总结于表 11.8 中。

无合并症高血压患者

治疗无合并症高血压的三种一线药物是：①钙通道阻滞剂（CCB），② ACEI 或 ARB，和③噻嗪类利尿剂。2017 年美国心脏病学会/美国心脏协会（ACC/AHA）高血压指南推荐将这三类药物中的任何一种作为大多数高血压患者的起始治疗。指南还建议，对于血压超过目标值 20/10 mmHg 以上的患者，应使用两种不同类别的一线药物进行起始治疗，可以分开使用，也可以以固定剂量组合使用。除非患者有其他强适应证（如心力衰竭或缺血性心脏病），否则不建议将 β 受体阻滞剂作为一线治疗，因为其在预防靶器官损伤和心血管事件方面的作用不如三种一线药物。与此相反，欧洲高血压协会认可 β 受体阻滞剂作为一线药物，并认为最有效的药物是患者能够耐受和服用的药物。长期治疗患者依从性最好的药物是 ARB，其次是 ACEI 或 CCB，最差的是噻嗪类药物。鼓励以单片复方开始治疗，因为它可以让血压更快地达到目标，并改善长期依从性。欧洲高血压协会提倡根据患者的年龄和种族制订治疗策略。它建议以肾素-血管紧张素系统（RAS）阻滞剂（ACEI 或 ARB）与 CCB 或利尿剂联合治疗作为起始治疗，但患轻度高血压的虚弱老年人除外，这类患者推荐使用单药治疗。

越来越多的临床试验证据强调了通过联合用药降低血压的重要性，而不是纠结于选择一种最佳的药物开始治疗。原发性高血压是多因素的，通常需要同时使用几种作用机制不同的药物（至少两种或以上）（见表 11.7）才能达到血压目标。对于大多数高血压患者，低剂量药物联合治疗是充分控制血压和尽量减少副作用的唯一方法。对于许多种类的降压药物而言，降压作用的剂量-反应关系相当平缓。大多数在剂量范围的低限时就可以产生降压作用。然而，许多副作用则是随着剂量增加显著增加的，主要在临床剂量范围的高限时出现问题。因此，低剂量的联合用药实现了治疗协同作用，并将副作用降至最低。固定剂量组合可以减少药物负担和成本。

一种高效且耐受性良好的用药组合是 CCB 联合 ACEI 或 ARB。与 ACEI 和噻嗪类利尿剂联合使用相比，ACEI 和二氢吡啶类 CCB 联合治疗的一大优势是可以减少高危患者的心血管事件。相反，应避免使用 ARB 联合 ACEI 或直接肾素抑制剂（"双重 RAS 阻断"）治疗，因为这会导致肾功能恶化并增加低血压风险，且不会带来额外的心血管获益。

北加州凯撒医疗集团（Kaiser-Permanemte）是一家大型医疗照护组织，在过去 10 年中，该组织通过以下方式将其成员的高血压控制率从 44% 提高到惊人的 80%：增加医疗助理免预约血压检查的机会；登记巡查以识别和联系诊室血压升高的患者；以及制订以每日一次复方治疗为特色的全系统简单药物治疗方案。

对于动脉粥样硬化性心血管疾病（ASCVD）10 年风险为 7.5% 以上的患者，除了降压药物外，应积极考虑将他汀类药物治疗作为大多数降压方案的组成部分。

非裔美国人的高血压

高血压对非裔美国人的影响尤为严重。其原因尚不清楚，但非裔和欧裔人群中高血压患病率的地理差异表明了环境因素的主导作用。居住在非洲的非洲人中高血压很少见，而在欧洲几个国家中高血压的患病率比美国更高。作为高血压的单药治疗，ACEI（或 ARB）在非洲黑人患者中产生的血压下降幅度通常小于非黑人患者，因此对卒中的保护作用较小。但是，当 ACEI 或 ARB 与 CCB 或利尿剂联合使用时，降压效果会增强，种族差异会消失。此外，在该人群中，CCB 与 ACEI（或 ARB）或利尿剂联合使用在降低血压方面优于 ACEI 和利尿剂联合使用。尽管如此，患有高血压肾硬化症的非裔美国患者仍应考虑使用基于 ACEI 的治疗，因为它可以减缓肾功能的恶化。

高血压肾硬化症

高血压是慢性肾脏病的第二大常见病因，占总数的 25% 以上。高血压肾硬化症是高血压长期未得到控制的结果，会导致慢性肾小球缺血。通常会出现轻度的蛋白尿（< 0.5 g/24 h）。非糖尿病性慢性肾脏病是 ACEI 或 ARB 降压治疗的强适应证。ACEI 扩张肾出球小动脉的作用更强，从而最大限度地减少肾小球内高血压。相反，动脉血管扩张剂如二氢吡啶类 CCB，在未与 ACEI 或 ARB 联合使用时，会优先扩张入球小动脉并对肾脏的自身调节造成损害。如果全身血压没有充分降低，则会导致肾小球高血压。只有当血清肌酐升高值超过基线值的 30% 或血钾升高至 5.6 mmol/L 以上时，才应停用 ACEI。

TABLE 11.8 Major Contraindications and Side Effects of Antihypertensive Drugs

Drug Class	Major Contraindications	Side Effects
Diuretics		
Thiazides	Gout	Insulin resistance, new onset type 2 diabetes (especially in combination with β-blockers)
		Hypokalemia, hyponatremia
		Hypertriglyceridemia
		Hyperuricemia, precipitation of gout
		Erectile dysfunction (more than other drug classes)
		Potentiate nondepolarizing muscle relaxants
		Photosensitive dermatitis
Loop diuretics	Hepatic coma	Interstitial nephritis
		Hypokalemia
		Potentiate succinylcholine
		Potentiate aminoglycoside ototoxicity
Potassium-sparing diuretics	Serum K >5.5 mEq/L	Fatal hyperkalemia if used with salt substitutes, ACE inhibitors, ARBs, high-potassium foods, NSAIDs
	GFR <30 mg/mL/1.73 m^2	
β-Blockers	Heart block	Insulin resistance, new onset type 2 diabetes (especially in combination with thiazides)
	Asthma	Heart block, acute decompensated CHF
	Depression	Bronchospasm
	Cocaine and/or methamphetamine abuse	Depression, nightmares, fatigue
		Cold extremities, claudication (β2 effect)
		Stevens-Johnson syndrome
		Agranulocytosis
ACEIs	Pregnancy	Cough
	Bilateral renal artery stenosis	Hyperkalemia
	Hyperkalemia	Angioedema
		Leukopenia
		Fetal toxicity
		Cholestatic jaundice (rare fulminant hepatic necrosis if the drug is not discontinued)
ARBs	Pregnancy	Hyperkalemia
	Bilateral renal artery stenosis	Angioedema (very rare)
	Hyperkalemia	Fetal toxicity
Direct Renin Inhibitors	Pregnancy	Hyperkalemia
	Bilateral renal artery stenosis	Diarrhea
	Hyperkalemia	Fetal toxicity
Dihydropyridine CCBs	As monotherapy in chronic kidney disease with proteinuria	Headaches
		Flushing
		Ankle edema
		CHF
		Gingival hyperplasia
		Esophageal reflux
Nondihydropyridine CCBs	Heart block	Bradycardia, AV block (especially with verapamil)
	Systolic heart failure	Constipation (often severe with verapamil)
		Worsening of systolic function, CHF
		Gingival edema and/or hypertrophy
		Increase cyclosporine blood levels
		Esophageal reflux
α-Blockers	Monotherapy for hypertension	Orthostatic hypotension
	Orthostatic hypotension	Drug tolerance (in the absence of diuretic therapy)
	Systolic heart failure	Ankle edema
	Left ventricular dysfunction	CHF
		First-dose effect (acute hypotension)
		Potentiate hypotension with PDE5 inhibitors (e.g., sildenafil)
Central sympatholytics	Orthostatic hypotension	Depression, dry mouth, lethargy
		Erectile dysfunction (dose dependent)

Continued

表 11.8　降压药物的主要禁忌证和副作用

药物类别	主要禁忌证	副作用
利尿剂		
噻嗪类药物	痛风	胰岛素抵抗，新发 2 型糖尿病（特别是与 β 受体阻滞剂联合） 低钾血症，低钠血症 高甘油三酯血症 高尿酸血症，痛风发作 勃起功能障碍（多于其他药物类别） 增强非去极化肌肉松弛剂的作用 光敏性皮炎
袢利尿剂	肝昏迷	间质性肾炎 低钾血症 增强琥珀胆碱的作用 增强氨基糖苷的耳毒性
保钾利尿剂	血清钾 > 5.5 mmol/L GFR < 30 mg/(ml·1.73 m^2)	如果与盐替代品、ACEI、ARB、高钾食物、NSAID 合用会导致致死性高钾血症
β 受体阻滞剂	心脏传导阻滞 哮喘 抑郁 可卡因和（或）甲基苯丙胺滥用	胰岛素抵抗，新发 2 型糖尿病（特别是与噻嗪类药物合用） 心脏传导阻滞，急性失代偿性 CHF 支气管痉挛 抑郁，噩梦，疲劳 四肢冰冷，跛行（β2 受体阻滞的效应） 史蒂文斯-约翰逊（Stevens-Johnson）综合征 粒细胞缺乏症
ACEI	妊娠 双侧肾动脉狭窄 高钾血症	咳嗽 高钾血症 血管性水肿 白细胞减少 胎儿毒性 淤积性黄疸（若不停药可能引发罕见的暴发性肝坏死）
ARB	妊娠 双侧肾动脉狭窄 高钾血症	高钾血症 血管性水肿（非常罕见） 胎儿毒性
直接肾素抑制剂	妊娠 双侧肾动脉狭窄 高钾血症	高钾血症 腹泻 胎儿毒性
二氢吡啶类 CCB	慢性肾病伴蛋白尿的单药治疗	头痛 潮红 踝关节水肿 CHF 牙龈增生 食管反流
非二氢吡啶类 CCB	心脏传导阻滞 收缩期心力衰竭	心动过缓，房室传导阻滞（尤其维拉帕米） 便秘（维拉帕米常加重症状） 收缩功能恶化，CHF 牙龈水肿和（或）肥大 环孢素血药浓度升高 食管反流
α 受体阻滞剂	高血压单药治疗 直立性低血压 收缩性心力衰竭 左心室功能不全	直立性低血压 药物耐受（无利尿剂治疗时） 踝关节水肿 CHF 首剂效应（急性低血压） 合用 PDE5 抑制剂（如西地那非）加重低血压
中枢交感神经阻滞剂	直立性低血压	抑郁，口干，嗜睡 勃起功能障碍（剂量依赖性）

TABLE 11.8 Major Contraindications and Side Effects of Antihypertensive Drugs—cont'd		
Drug Class	Major Contraindications	Side Effects
Direct vasodilators	Orthostatic hypotension	Rebound hypertension with clonidine withdrawal Coombs positive hemolytic anemia and elevated LFTs with α-methyldopa Reflex tachycardia Fluid retention Hirsutism, pericardial effusion with minoxidil Lupus with hydralazine

ACE, Angiotensin-converting enzyme; *ARBs,* angiotensin-receptor blockers; *AV,* arteriovenous; *CCBs,* calcium channel blockers; *CHF,* congestive heart failure; *GFR,* glomerular filtration rate; *LFTs,* liver function tests; *MI,* myocardial infarction; *NSAIDs,* nonsteroidal anti-inflammatory drugs; *PDE5,* phosphodiesterase type 5.

Hypertensive Patients With Diabetes

Compared with its 25% prevalence in the general adult population, hypertension is present in 75% of patients with diabetes and is a major factor contributing to excessive risk of myocardial infarction, stroke, heart failure, microvascular complications, and diabetic nephropathy progressing to end-stage renal disease. The Action to Control Cardiovascular Risk in Diabetes blood pressure trial (ACCORD BP) failed to show benefit of lowering systolic BP below 120 mm Hg in patients with type 2 diabetes mellitus in terms of reducing overall mortality or cardiovascular mortality. However, the risk of stroke was reduced by 60% in these patients. ACCORD trial also tested intensive versus standard glycemic targets (glycated hemoglobin <6% versus 7.0% to 7.9%). A more recent analysis has demonstrated benefit of intensive BP lowering in lowering cardiovascular events in diabetic patients in the standard glycemia arm but not in the intensive glycemic arm. Increased hypoglycemic events associated with intensive glycemic control may negate potential cardiovascular benefit of intensive BP lowering in this population. The Systolic Blood Pressure Intervention Trial (SPRINT), which was conducted in nondiabetic patients and has similar study design to the ACCORD trial, showed benefit of intensive BP lowering in patients with prediabetes. Consequently, the 2017 ACC/AHA guideline endorses a BP target of less than 130/80 mm Hg for diabetic patients. The 2019 American Diabetes Association endorses lower targets only in diabetic patients with 10-year ASCVD risk of greater than 15%. In general, an ACEI or ARB plus a CCB is an excellent combination to treat hypertension in patients with diabetes. Thiazide diuretics and standard β-blockers exacerbate glucose intolerance, whereas the vasodilating β-blockers such as carvedilol and nebivolol have neutral or possibly beneficial effects.

Hypertensive Patients With Coronary Artery Disease

To lower myocardial oxygen demands in patients with coronary disease, the antihypertensive regimen should reduce BP without causing reflex tachycardia. For this reason, a β-blocker is often prescribed in conjunction with a dihydropyridine CCB such as amlodipine. β-Blockers are indicated for patients with hypertension who have sustained a myocardial infarction and for most heart failure patients with reduced ejection fraction (HFrEF). In contrast, diuretics are recommended as the first therapy in heart failure patients with preserved ejection fraction (HFpEF) with evidence of volume overload. After euvolemia is achieved, ACEIs, ARBs, or spironolactone may be considered in patients with persistently elevated BP. In patients with stable coronary artery disease, a cardioprotective effect of ACE inhibition has also been demonstrated in patients with moderate cardiovascular risk profiles but not in those with lower risk profiles.

Isolated Systolic Hypertension in Older Adults

In developed countries, systolic pressure rises progressively with age; if individuals live long enough, then almost all (>90%) develop hypertension. Diastolic pressure rises until the age of 50 years and decreases thereafter, producing a progressive rise in pulse pressure (i.e., systolic pressure minus diastolic pressure) (Fig. 11.12).

Different hemodynamic faults underlie hypertension in younger and older persons. Patients who develop hypertension before 50 years of age typically have *combined systolic and diastolic hypertension*: systolic pressure greater than 140 mm Hg *and* diastolic pressure greater than 90 mm Hg. The main hemodynamic fault is vasoconstriction at the level of the resistance arterioles. In contrast, the majority of patients who develop hypertension after 50 years of age have *isolated systolic hypertension*: systolic pressure greater than 140 mm Hg but diastolic pressure less than 90 mm Hg (often less than 80 mm Hg). In isolated systolic hypertension, the primary hemodynamic fault is decreased distensibility of the aorta and other large conduit arteries (see Fig. 11.12). Collagen replaces elastin in the elastic lamina of the aorta, an age-dependent process that is accelerated by atherosclerosis and hypertension. The cardiovascular risk associated with isolated systolic hypertension is related to pulsatility, the repetitive pounding of the blood vessels with each cardiac cycle and a more rapid return of the arterial pulse wave from the periphery, both begetting more systolic hypertension. In the United States and Europe, the majority of uncontrolled hypertension occurs in older patients with isolated systolic hypertension. A BP of 160/60 mm Hg (pulse pressure of 100 mm Hg) carries twice the risk of fatal coronary heart disease as 140/110 mm Hg (pulse pressure of 30 mm Hg) (Fig. 11.13).

In older persons with isolated systolic hypertension, lowering systolic pressure from higher than 160 to lower than 150 mm Hg reduces the risks of stroke, myocardial infarction, and overall cardiovascular mortality; it also reduces heart failure admissions and slows the progression of dementia. Trial data do not yet exist in older persons to determine whether the treatment of isolated elevations in systolic pressure below 140 mm Hg is beneficial; however, in the absence of such data, treatment may be warranted to prevent progression of systolic hypertension if patients can tolerate treatment without side effects such as orthostatic hypotension.

The combination of a low-dose thiazide diuretic with a dihydropyridine CCB or with an ACEI reduces the risk of CV events in older patients with isolated systolic hypertension. According to the 2017 ACC/AHA high BP guideline, chlorthalidone is the preferred thiazide diuretic given its long half-life and more consistent reduction in cardiovascular events in clinical trials than other thiazide diuretics. To prevent orthostatic hypotension, medication should be titrated to standing BP and one low-dose medication should be started at a time.

表 11.8 降压药物的主要禁忌证和副作用（续表）		
药物类别	主要禁忌证	副作用
直接血管扩张剂	直立性低血压	停用可乐定后出现反弹性高血压 α-甲基多巴引起的 Coombs 阳性溶血性贫血和 LFT 结果升高 反射性心动过速 液体潴留 米诺地尔引起的多毛、心包积液 肼屈嗪引起的狼疮

ACEI，血管紧张素转换酶抑制剂；ARB，血管紧张素受体阻滞剂；CCB，钙通道阻滞剂；CHF，充血性心力衰竭；GFR，肾小球滤过率；LFT，肝功能检测；MI，心肌梗死；NSAID，非甾体抗炎药；PDE5，5 型磷酸二酯酶。

高血压合并糖尿病患者

普通成人的高血压患病率为 25%，与之相比，75% 的糖尿病患者患有高血压，是导致心肌梗死、卒中、心力衰竭、微血管并发症和糖尿病肾病进展为终末期肾病风险增高的一个主要因素。控制糖尿病患者心血管风险行动-血压试验（ACCORD BP）未显示将 2 型糖尿病患者的收缩压降至 120 mmHg 以下对降低总死亡率或心血管死亡率有益。然而，这些患者的卒中风险降低了 60%。ACCORD 试验还对比了强化与标准血糖目标（分别为糖化血红蛋白 < 6% 和 7.0% ~ 7.9%）治疗方案。最近的一项分析表明，在标准血糖治疗组中，强化降压有利于减少糖尿病患者心血管事件，而在强化血糖治疗组中则不然。与强化血糖控制相关的低血糖事件增加可能会抵消强化降压对该人群心血管的潜在益处。在非糖尿病患者中进行的收缩压干预试验（SPRINT），具有与 ACCORD 试验相似的研究设计，表明强化降压对糖尿病前期患者有益。因此，2017 年 ACC/AHA 指南支持糖尿病患者的血压目标低于 130/80 mmHg。但 2019 年美国糖尿病协会仅支持 10 年 ASCVD 风险大于 15% 的糖尿病患者的血压降低至这一目标。一般来说，ACEI 或 ARB 联合 CCB 是治疗糖尿病患者高血压的优秀组合。噻嗪类利尿剂和标准 β 受体阻滞剂会加重葡萄糖耐受不良，而具有血管舒张作用的 β 受体阻滞剂如卡维地洛和奈比洛尔则具有中性或可能有益的作用。

合并冠状动脉疾病的高血压患者

为了降低冠状动脉疾病患者的心肌氧耗量，降压方案应在降压的同时而又不引起反射性心动过速。因此，β 受体阻滞剂通常与二氢吡啶类 CCB（如氨氯地平）联合使用。β 受体阻滞剂适用于有心肌梗死病史的高血压患者和大多数射血分数降低的心力衰竭患者。相比之下，对于有容量超负荷证据的射血分数保留型心力衰竭患者，推荐使用利尿剂作为首选治疗。当实现容量负荷平衡后，在血压持续升高的患者中可考虑使用 ACEI、ARB 或螺内酯。在稳定的冠状动脉疾病患者中，ACEI 在中等心血管风险的患者中也有心脏保护作用，但在低风险的患者中则没有。

老年人单纯收缩期高血压

在发达国家，收缩压随年龄的增长而逐渐升高；如果寿命足够长，那么几乎所有人（> 90%）都会患上高血压。舒张压在 50 岁以前会随年龄一直升高，此后逐渐降低，导致脉压（即收缩压与舒张压差值）逐渐升高（图 11.12）。

不同的血流动力学异常是年轻人和老年人高血压的基础。50 岁以前发生高血压的患者通常合并收缩期和舒张期高血压：即收缩压大于 140 mmHg，舒张压大于 90 mmHg。主要的血流动力学紊乱是阻力小动脉的血管收缩。相反，大多数 50 岁以后发生高血压的患者为单纯收缩期高血压：即收缩压大于 140 mmHg，舒张压小于 90 mmHg（通常小于 80 mmHg）。在单纯收缩期高血压中，主要的血流动力学紊乱是主动脉和其他大动脉的扩张性降低（见图 11.12）。胶原蛋白取代了主动脉弹性层中的弹性蛋白，这是一个与年龄相关的过程，而动脉粥样硬化和高血压会加速这一过程。与单纯收缩期高血压相关的心血管风险与搏动有关，每个心动周期血管的重复搏动和从外周更快速度返回的动脉脉搏波，两者都会导致更显著的收缩期高血压。在美国和欧洲，大多数未控制的高血压发生在老年单纯收缩期高血压患者中。血压为 160/60 mmHg（脉压为 100 mmHg）患者发生致命性冠心病的风险是血压为 140/110 mmHg（脉压为 30 mmHg）患者的 2 倍（图 11.13）。

在老年单纯收缩期高血压患者中，将收缩压从 160 mmHg 以上降低到 150 mmHg 以下可以降低卒中、心肌梗死和心血管总体死亡风险；还可以减少心力衰竭的入院率，并减缓痴呆症的进展。目前暂无研究证据表明在老年单纯收缩压升高的患者中，将收缩压降至 140 mmHg 以下能否获益。然而，在缺乏此类数据的情况下，如果患者能够耐受治疗而无诸如直立性低血压等副作用，则可能需要治疗以防止收缩期高血压的进展。

小剂量噻嗪类利尿剂与二氢吡啶类 CCB 或 ACEI 联合使用可以降低老年单纯收缩期高血压患者发生心血管事件的风险。根据 2017 年 ACC/AHA 高血压指南，氯噻酮是首选的噻嗪类利尿剂。由于其半衰期长，在临床试验中比其他噻嗪类利尿剂更能持续地减少心血管事件。为防止出现直立性低血压，应根据站立血压进行药物滴定，每次应只启用一种小剂量药物。

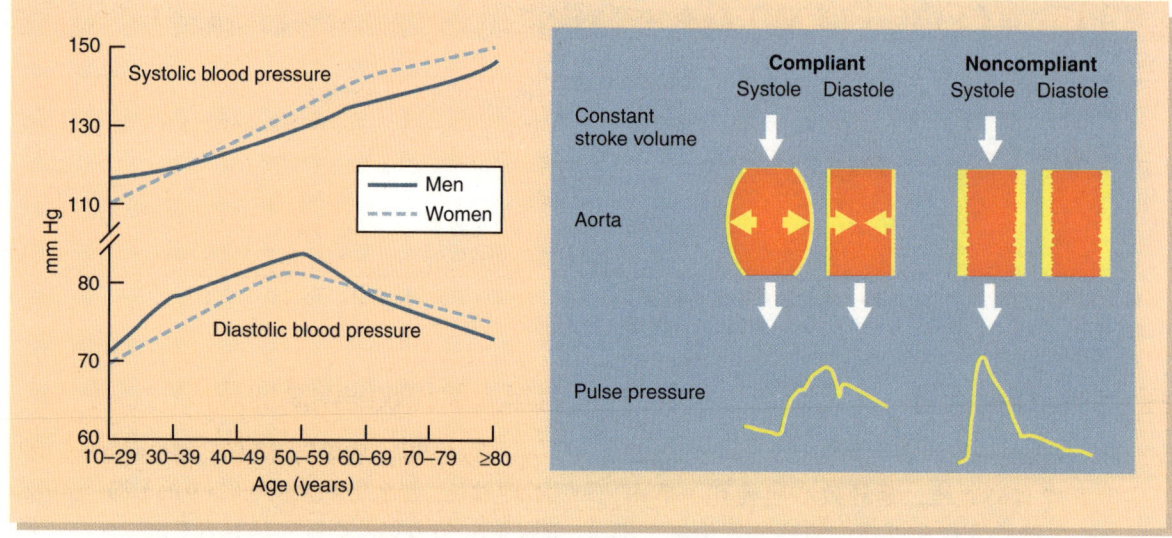

Fig. 11.12 Age-dependent changes in systolic and diastolic blood pressure (BP) in the United States *(left panel)*. Schematic diagram explains the relation between aortic compliance and pulse pressure *(right panel)*. (*Left panel,* From Burt V, Whelton P, Rocella EJ, et al: Prevalence of hypertension in the U.S. adult population: Results from the Third National Health and Nutrition Examination Survey, 1988–1991. Hypertension 25:305-313, 1995. *Right panel,* Courtesy of Dr. Stanley Franklin University of California at Irvine. Used with permission.)

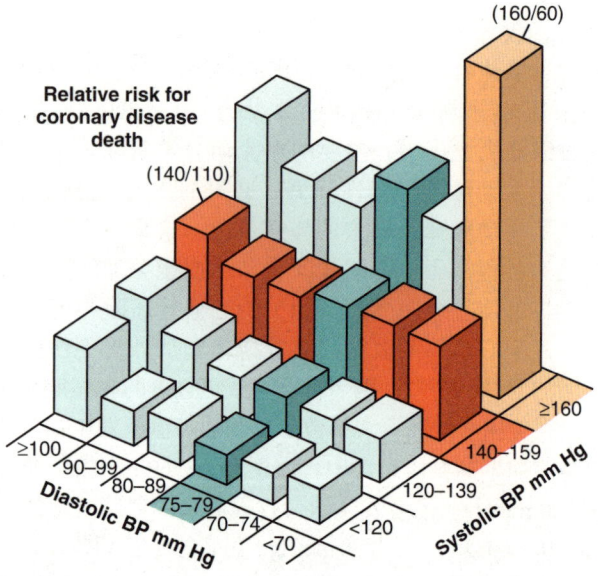

Fig. 11.13 Joint influences of systolic blood pressure (SBP) and diastolic BP on coronary heart disease (CHD) risk in the Multiple Risk Factor Intervention Trial. (Neaton JD, Wentworth D: Serum cholesterol, blood pressure, cigarette smoking, and death from coronary heart disease: Overall findings and differences by age for 316,099 white men. Arch Intern Med 152:56-64, 1992.)

Blood Pressure Lowering for Secondary Prevention of Stroke

Most neurologists do not recommend BP reduction during an acute stroke unless BP is extremely elevated (see section Acute Severe Hypertension). After the acute phase, BP should be lowered with a thiazide diuretic, adding an ACEI or additional drugs as needed to achieve BP lower than 140/90 mm Hg; whether BP should be lowered further remains unsettled. Lower BP target of less than 130/80 mm Hg for patients may be reasonable for patients with transient ischemic attack or lacuna infarct to prevent intracranial hemorrhage.

Blood Pressure Lowering for Prevention of Cognitive Impairment

Increasing number of studies have shown that high BP and other cardiovascular risk factors such as hyperlipidemia predisposes not only to increased cardiovascular damage but also brain injury and cognitive impairment in older adults, which is independent of stroke (i.e., what is good for the heart is good for the brain). The recent SPRINT MIND clinical trial showed that intensive lowering of systolic BP to below 120 mm Hg in adults with high cardiovascular risk but without history of stroke prevents development of cognitive impairment. There was no significant reduction in new cases of dementia but the trial was limited by short duration of follow-up. Additional studies are needed to clarify optimal BP target to prevent cognitive dysfunction in hypertensive adults.

Hypertensive Disorders of Women

Oral contraceptives cause a small increase in BP in most women but rarely cause a large increase into the hypertensive range. If hypertension develops, oral contraceptive therapy should be discontinued in favor of other methods of contraception. Oral estrogen replacement therapy seems to cause a small increase in BP. In contrast, transdermal estrogen (which bypasses first-pass hepatic metabolism) seems to avoid this side effect.

Hypertension, the most common nonobstetric complication of pregnancy, is present in 10% of all pregnancies. Of these women, one third are caused by chronic hypertension and two thirds are due to preeclampsia, which is defined as an increase in BP to 140/90 mm Hg or greater after the twentieth week of gestation accompanied by proteinuria (>300 mg/24 hr) and pathologic edema. This is sometimes accompanied by seizures (eclampsia) and the multisystem HELLP syndrome of hemolysis (H), elevated liver enzymes (EL), and low

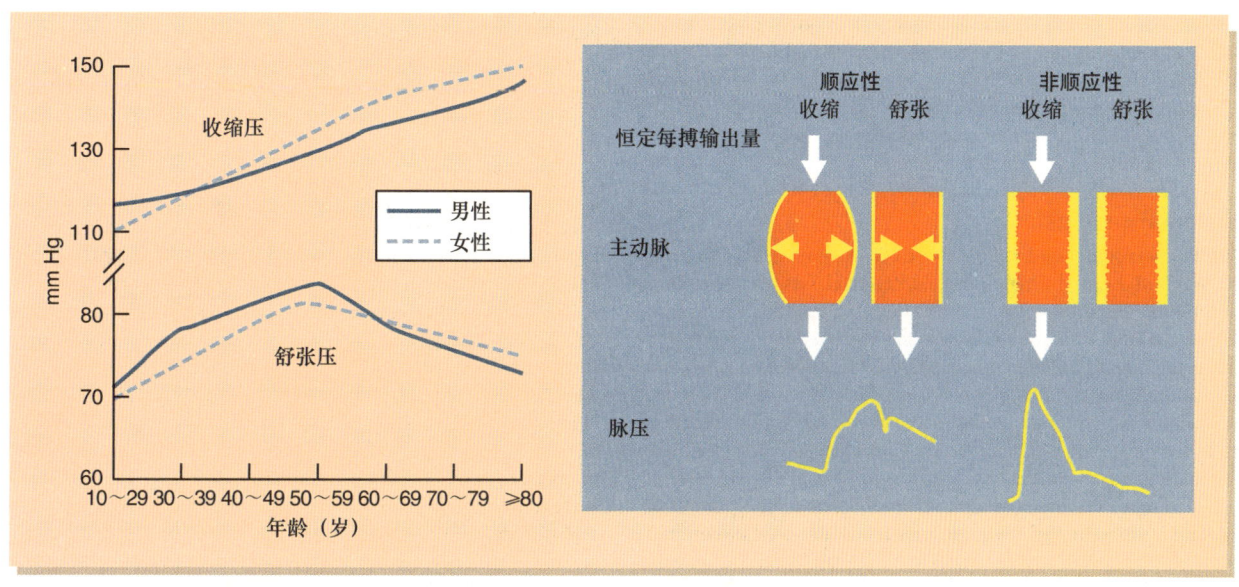

图 11.12 美国人收缩压和舒张压的年龄依赖性变化（左图）。主动脉顺应性与脉压的关系原理示意图（右图）。（左图，引自 Burt V，Whelton P，Rocella EJ，et al：Prevalence of hypertension in the U.S. adult population：Results from the Third National Health and Nutrition Examination Survey, 1988-1991. Hypertension 25：305-313，1995. 右图，授权自 Dr. Stanley Franklin University of California at Irvine. 经允许使用）

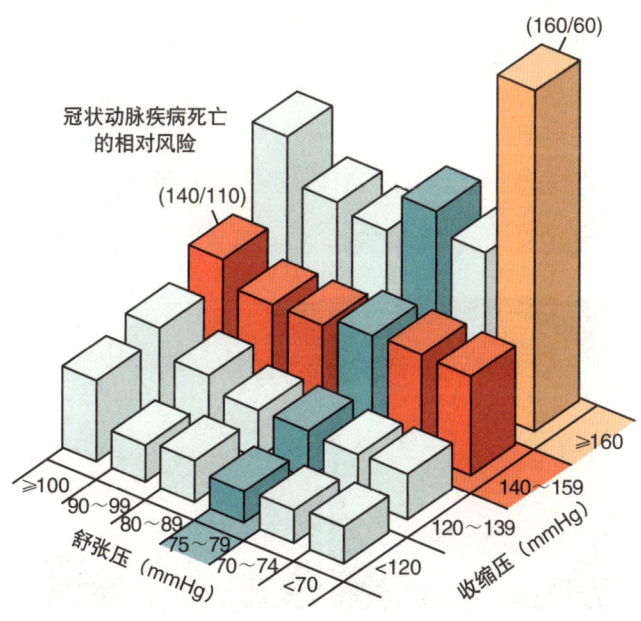

图 11.13 多危险因素干预试验中收缩压和舒张压对冠心病风险的共同影响（Neaton JD, Wentworth D：Serum cholesterol, blood pressure, cigarette smoking, and death from coronary heart disease：Overall findings and differences by age for 316,099 white men. Arch Intern Med 152：56-64，1992.）

降低血压对卒中的二级预防

大多数神经科医生不建议在急性卒中期间降低血压，除非血压急剧升高（见"急性重症高血压"部分）。急性期后，应使用噻嗪类利尿剂降低血压，并根据需要添加 ACEI 或其他药物以使血压低于 140/90 mmHg；是否应该进一步降低血压仍未确定。为防止颅内出血，对于短暂性脑缺血发作或腔隙性梗死的患者，低于 130/80 mmHg 的更低血压目标可能是合理的。

降低血压可以预防认知障碍

越来越多的研究表明，高血压和其他心血管危险因素如高脂血症，不仅会加重老年人的心血管损伤，还容易导致脑损伤和认知障碍，这与卒中无关（即对心脏有影响的，对大脑也有影响）。最近的 SPRINT MIND 临床试验表明，在没有卒中史的心血管高危成人中，强化降压将收缩压降至 120 mmHg 以下可以预防认知障碍的发生。但因随访时间短，试验中新发痴呆病例没有显著减少。尚需要进一步的研究来阐明预防成人高血压患者认知障碍的最佳血压目标。

女性高血压疾病

口服避孕药会使大多数女性血压小幅升高，但很少会使血压大幅升高到高血压范围。如果出现高血压，应停止口服避孕药治疗，转而采用其他避孕方法。口服雌激素替代疗法似乎也会导致血压小幅升高。相比之下，经皮雌激素（绕过肝首过代谢）似乎可以避免这种副作用。

高血压是最常见的妊娠非产科并发症，占所有妊娠的 10%。在这些妇女中，1/3 是由慢性高血压引起的，2/3 则是由于子痫前期。子痫前期的定义是妊娠 20 周后血压升高至 140/90 mmHg 或以上，并伴有蛋白尿（＞300 mg/24 h）和病理性水肿。高血压有时还伴有癫痫发作（子痫）和多系统 HELLP 综合征，包括溶血（H）、肝酶升高（EL）和血小板减少（LP）。尽管先兆子痫病

platelets (LP). Although the cause remains an enigma, preeclampsia is the most common cause of maternal mortality and perinatal mortality. Nifedipine and α-methyldopa are considered to be first-line drug therapy for preeclampsia and chronic hypertension in pregnancy. Labetalol is also effective in lowering BP but may result in intrauterine growth restriction.

Resistant Hypertension

Defined as persistence of usual BP above 140/90 mm Hg despite treatment with full doses of three or more different classes of medications in rational combination and including a diuretic, *resistant hypertension* is the most common reason for referral to a hypertension specialist. In practice, the majority of these patients have pseudoresistant hypertension due to: (1) *white coat aggravation*, a white coat reaction superimposed on chronic hypertension that is well-controlled with medication outside the physician's office; (2) an inadequate medical regimen; (3) nonadherence to medication, which is present in 30% to 60% of patients using direct measurement of drugs levels in the plasma or urine; and (4) ingestion of pressor substances. Common shortcomings of the medical regimen include under-treatment of hypertension with monotherapy and clonidine, a potent central sympatholytic that causes rebound hypertension between doses particularly with PRN dosing. Several common causes of pseudoresistant hypertension are related to the patient's behavior: medication nonadherence, recidivism with lifestyle modification (e.g., obesity, a high-salt diet, excessive alcohol intake), or habitual use of pressor substances such as sympathomimetics (e.g., tobacco, cocaine, methamphetamine, phenylephrine-containing cold or herbal remedies) or NSAIDs, with the latter causing renal sodium retention. Once these behavioral factors have been excluded, the search should begin for secondary hypertension.

The most common forms of secondary hypertension include obstructive sleep apnea, chronic kidney disease, and primary aldosteronism. Either a loop diuretic such a furosemide or a potent thiazide-type diuretic such as chlorthalidone may be required to control hypertension in patients with resistant hypertension and chronic kidney disease. The treatment of primary aldosteronism was discussed earlier. After excluding pseudoresistant hypertension and secondary hypertension, some patients have severe drug-resistant primary hypertension. Fourth- and fifth-line therapy includes a vasodilating β-blocker and spironolactone (even in the absence of primary aldosteronism). Percutaneous catheter-based renal denervation is proposed as a novel interventional approach to treat drug-resistant hypertension. Although the initial results raised enormous enthusiasm, subsequent randomized controlled trials have been disappointing as the magnitude of reduction in BP is modest (less than 10 mm Hg) when compared to the sham control arm. A number of studies that use other neuromodulation techniques, such as baroreflex activation, to reduce overall sympathetic tone beyond renal sympathetic activity alone, are being conducted to determine BP outcome in this population.

Acute Severe Hypertension

Of all the patients in the emergency department, 25% have an elevated BP. *Hypertensive emergencies* are acute, often severe elevations in BP that are accompanied by acute or rapidly progressive target organ dysfunction such as myocardial or cerebral ischemia or infarction, pulmonary edema, or renal failure. *Hypertensive urgencies* are severe elevations in BP without severe symptoms and without evidence of acute or progressive target organ dysfunction. Thus, the key distinction and approach to the patient depends on the state of the patient and the assessment of target organ damage, not simply the absolute level of BP. The full-blown clinical picture of a hypertensive emergency is a critically ill patient with a BP greater than 220/140 mm Hg, headaches, confusion, blurred vision, nausea and vomiting, seizures, heart failure, oliguria, and grade III or IV hypertensive retinopathy (Fig. 11.14). Hypertensive emergencies require immediate admission in an intensive care unit (ICU) for intravenous therapy and continuous BP monitoring, whereas hypertensive urgencies can often be managed with oral medications and appropriate outpatient follow-up in 24 to 72 hours. The most common hypertensive cardiac emergencies include hypertension associated with acute aortic dissection, coronary artery bypass graft surgery, acute myocardial infarction, and unstable angina. Other hypertensive emergencies include those accompanying eclampsia, head trauma, severe body burns, postoperative bleeding from vascular suture lines, and epistaxis that cannot be controlled with anterior and posterior nasal packing. Neurologic hypertensive emergencies, which include acute ischemic stroke, hemorrhagic stroke, subarachnoid hemorrhage, and hypertensive encephalopathy, can be difficult to distinguish from one another. Hypertensive encephalopathy is characterized by severe hypertensive retinopathy (i.e., retinal hemorrhages and exudates, with or without papilledema) and a posterior leukoencephalopathy affecting mainly the white matter of the parieto-occipital regions as seen on cerebral MR imaging or CT scanning. A new focal neurologic deficit suggesting a stroke-in-evolution demands a much more conservative approach to correcting the elevated BP.

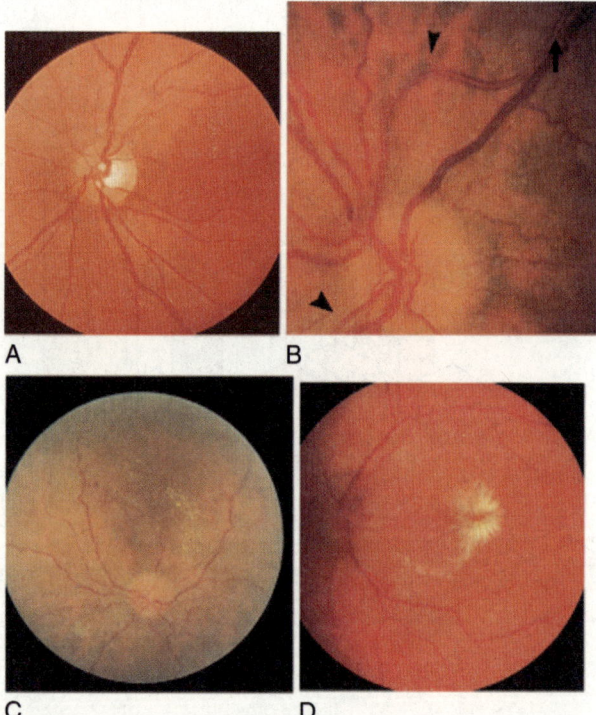

Fig. 11.14 Hypertensive retinopathy is traditionally divided into four grades. (A) Grade 1 shows very early and minor changes in a young patient; increased tortuosity of a retinal vessel and increased reflectiveness (silver wiring) of a retinal artery are seen at the 1-o'clock position in this view. Otherwise, the fundus is completely normal. (B) Grade 2 also shows increased tortuosity and silver wiring *(arrowheads)*. In addition, *nipping* of the venules at arteriovenous (AV) crossings is visualized *(arrow)*. (C) Grade 3 shows the same changes as grade 2 plus flame-shaped retinal hemorrhages and soft *cotton-wool* exudates. (D) In grade 4, swelling of the optic disc (papilledema) is observed, retinal edema is present, and hard exudates may collect around the fovea, producing a typical *macular star*. (From Forbes CD, Jackson WF: Color atlas and text of clinical medicine, 3rd ed. London, Mosby, 2003, with permission.)

因仍不明确，却是产妇死亡和围产期死亡的最常见原因。硝苯地平和 α- 甲基多巴被认为是治疗先兆子痫和妊娠合并慢性高血压的一线药物。拉贝洛尔也可有效降低血压，但可能导致宫内生长受限。

难治性高血压

难治性高血压定义为在合理联合足量使用三种或三种以上不同类别降压药物（其中包括一种利尿剂）治疗后，血压仍持续高于 140/90 mmHg，这是高血压患者转诊至高血压专科医生的最常见原因。实际上，这些患者中的大多数为假性难治性高血压，原因如下：①白大衣效应加重导致，即诊室外控制良好的高血压，由于白大衣效应的叠加，而表现为难治性高血压；②药物治疗方案不恰当；③药物依从性差，在直接检测血浆或尿液中的药物水平时，30%～60% 的患者存在这种情况；④摄入升压物质。药物治疗方案的常见缺点是高血压的治疗不充分，包括单药治疗和可乐定治疗。其中，可乐定是一种强效的中枢交感神经阻滞剂，在两次给药之间，尤其是在按必要时使用（pro re nata，PRN）给药的情况下，会导致高血压反弹。假性难治性高血压的几种常见原因与患者的行为有关：不坚持服药、生活方式改善后的反复（如肥胖、高盐饮食、过量饮酒）或习惯性使用升压物质，如拟交感神经药（如烟草、可卡因、甲基苯丙胺、含苯肾上腺素的感冒药或草药）或 NSAID，后者会导致肾脏的钠潴留。一旦排除了这些行为因素，就应该开始对继发性高血压进行筛查。

最常见的继发性高血压包括阻塞性睡眠呼吸暂停、慢性肾脏病和原发性醛固酮增多症。对于难治性高血压和慢性肾脏病患者，可能需要使用袢利尿剂（如呋塞米）或强效噻嗪类利尿剂（如氯噻酮）控制高血压。原发性醛固酮增多症的治疗已在前文讨论过。排除假性难治性高血压和继发性高血压后，一些患者为严重的药物难治性原发性高血压。四线和五线治疗包括血管扩张性 β 受体阻滞剂和螺内酯（即使在没有原发性醛固酮增多症的情况下）。基于经皮导管的去肾神经术被推荐作为一种治疗药物难治性高血压的新型介入方法。尽管最初的研究结果引起了极大的关注，但随后的随机对照试验结果令人失望，因为与假手术对照组相比，血压降低的幅度很小（小于 10 mmHg）。目前正在开展多项研究，利用其他神经调节技术，如压力反射激活来降低除肾交感神经活动之外的整体交感神经张力，以确定在这类人群中的降压疗效。

急性重症高血压

急诊科的所有患者中，25% 有血压升高。高血压急症是急性的，通常有严重的血压升高，伴有急性或快速进展的靶器官功能障碍，如心肌或脑的缺血或梗死、肺水肿或肾衰竭。高血压亚急症则是血压的严重升高，但没有严重症状，也没有急性或进展性靶器官功能障碍的证据。因此，对患者的甄别和处理关键取决于患者的状态和对靶器官损伤的评估，而不仅仅是血压的绝对水平。极端高血压急症的临床表现是血压高于 220/140 mmHg 的危重患者，伴有头痛、意识模糊、视物模糊、恶心呕吐、癫痫、心力衰竭、少尿以及 3 级或 4 级的高血压视网膜病变（图 11.14）。高血压急症需要立即入住重症监护病房（ICU）进行静脉注射治疗和持续的血压监测，而高血压亚急症通常可以口服药物和适当门诊随访 24～72 h。最常见的心脏性高血压急症包括高血压相关的急性主动脉夹层、冠状动脉旁路移植手术、急性心肌梗死和不稳定型心绞痛。其他高血压急症包括伴有子痫、头部创伤、严重身体灼烧感、术后血管缝合线出血以及无法通过前后鼻填塞控制的鼻出血。神经性高血压急症包括急性缺血性卒中、出血性卒中、蛛网膜下腔出血和高血压脑病，彼此之间很难区分。高血压脑病的特征是严重的高血压性视网膜病变（即视网膜出血和渗出，伴或不伴视乳头水肿）和 MR 成像或 CT 扫描可见的后脑白质病，主要影响脑顶枕区白质。如果出现新的局灶性神经功能缺损，表明卒中正在进展，需要采取更为保守的方法来纠正血压升高。

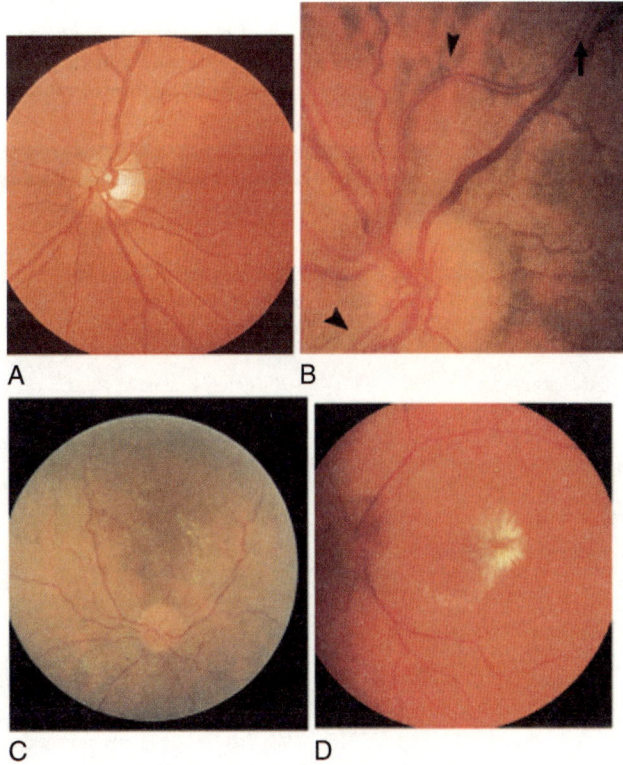

图 11.14 高血压视网膜病变传统上分为四级。（A）1 级显示年轻患者的非常早期和轻微的变化；在此视图中，在 1 点钟位置可见视网膜血管迂曲和视网膜动脉反光增强（银线）。除此之外，眼底完全正常。（B）2 级也显示视网膜血管迂曲和银线（箭头）。此外，可见动静脉交叉处的小静脉被压迫（箭头）。（C）3 级显示与 2 级相同的变化，加上火焰状视网膜出血和软性棉絮状渗出物。（D）在 4 级中，观察到视盘肿胀（视乳头水肿），存在视网膜水肿，并且硬性渗出物可能聚集在中央凹周围，形成典型的黄斑星芒状渗出（引自 Forbes CD, Jackson WF: Color atlas and text of clinical medicine, 3rd ed. London, Mosby, 2003, with permission.）

In most other hypertensive emergencies, the goal of parenteral therapy is to achieve a controlled and gradual lowering of BP. The rapidity of BP reduction is highly dependent on clinical presentation. Patients with acute aortic dissection require rapid reduction to the 120/80 mm Hg range almost immediately to reduce shear stress and prevent further intimal tear in the aortic wall, which could be life-threatening. On the other hand, patients with acute ischemic stroke who are not candidates for intravenous thrombolysis or endovascular treatment should not be treated with antihypertensive agents unless BP is 220/120 mm Hg or higher. Following initial therapy, a more conservative BP reduction goal to no more than 15% during the first 24 hours after onset of stroke is recommended. In those who are candidates for thrombolysis, however, BP should be less than 185/110 mm Hg before administration of intravenous tissue plasminogen activator and should be maintained below 180/105 mm Hg for at least the first 24 hours after initiating drug therapy. The widely cited goal of BP lowering by 10% in the first hour and by an additional 15% over the next 3 to 12 hours is limited to patients who present with hypertensive encephalopathy or other presentations. Unnecessarily rapid correction of the elevated BP to completely normal values places the patient at high risk for worsening cerebral, cardiac, and renal ischemia. In chronic hypertension, cerebral autoregulation is reset to higher-than-normal BPs. This compensatory adjustment prevents tissue overperfusion (i.e., increased intracranial pressure) at very high BPs, but it also predisposes the patient to tissue underperfusion (i.e., cerebral ischemia) when an elevated BP is lowered too quickly.

Parenteral agents for the treatment of hypertensive emergency are summarized in Table 11.9. Sodium nitroprusside, a nitric oxide donor, is the most popular agent because it can be titrated rapidly to control BP. Intravenous nitroglycerin, another nitric oxide donor, is indicated mainly for hypertension in the setting of acute coronary syndrome or decompensated heart failure. Nicardipine is a parenteral dihydropyridine CCB that is particularly useful in the postoperative cardiac patient and patients with renal failure to avoid the thiocyanate toxicity with nitroprusside. Clevidipine is another intravenous CCB with shorter half-life than nicardipine of only 1 minute. Fenoldopam is a selective dopamine-1-receptor agonist that causes both systemic and renal vasodilation, as well as increased glomerular filtration, natriuresis, and diuresis. Intravenous labetalol is an effective treatment of a hypertensive crisis particularly in the setting of myocardial ischemia with preserved ventricular function.

Most patients in the emergency department with hypertensive urgencies are either nonadherent with their medical regimen or are being treated with an inadequate regimen. To expedite the necessary changes in medications, outpatient follow-up should be arranged within 72 hours. To manage the patient during the short-interim period, effective oral medication includes labetalol, clonidine, or captopril, which is a short-acting ACEI.

BPs greater than 160/110 mm Hg are a common incidental finding among patients in emergency departments and other acute care settings for urgent medical or surgical care of symptoms that are unrelated to BP (e.g., musculoskeletal pain, orthopedic injury). In these settings, the elevated BP is more often the first indication of chronic hypertension than a simple physiologic stress reaction, providing an important opportunity to initiate primary care referral for formal evaluation and treatment of chronic hypertension. Home and ambulatory BP monitoring are indicated to determine whether the patient's BP normalizes completely once the acute illness has resolved.

TABLE 11.9 Parenteral Agents for Management of Hypertensive Emergencies

Agent	Dose	Onset of Action	Precautions
Parenteral Vasodilators			
Sodium nitroprusside	0.25-10 mcg/kg/min IV infusion	Immediate	Thiocyanate toxicity with prolonged use
Nitroglycerin	5-100 mcg/min IV infusion	2-5 min	Headache, tachycardia, tolerance
Nicardipine	5-15 mg/hr IV infusion	1-5 min	Protracted hypotension after prolonged use
Clevidipine	1-21 mg/hr IV infusion	2-4 min	Tachycardia
Fenoldopam mesylate	0.01-0.3 mcg/kg/min IV infusion	1-5 min	Headache, tachycardia, increased intraocular pressure
Hydralazine	5-10 mg as IV bolus or 10-40 mg IM; repeat every 4-6 hrs	10 min IV; 20 min IM	Unpredictable and excessive falls in tachycardia; angina exacerbation; blood pressure
Enalaprilat	0.625-1.25 mg every 6 hr IV bolus	15-60 min	Unpredictable and excessive falls in blood pressure; acute renal failure in patients with stenosis bilateral renal artery
Parenteral Adrenergic Inhibitors			
Labetalol	20-80 mg as slow IV injection every 10 min, or 0.5-2.0 mg/min IV as infusion	5-10 min	Bronchospasm, heart block, orthostatic hypotension
Metoprolol	5 mg IV every 10 min for three doses	5-10 min	Bronchospasm, heart block, heart failure, exacerbation of cocaine-induced myocardial ischemia
Esmolol	500 mcg/kg IV over 3 min; then 25-100 mg/kg/min as IV infusion	1-5 min	Bronchospasm, heart block, heart failure
Phentolamine	5-10 mg IV bolus every 5-15 min	1-2 min	Tachycardia, orthostatic hypotension

IM, Intramuscular; *IV*, intravenous.

在大多数其他高血压急症中，注射药物治疗的目标是实现血压的控制和逐渐降低。血压降低的速度在很大程度上取决于临床表现。急性主动脉夹层患者需要立即将血压快速降低至 120/80 mmHg 范围，以减少剪切应力，防止主动脉壁内膜进一步撕裂，否则可能危及生命。另一方面，不适合静脉溶栓或介入治疗的急性缺血性卒中患者不应使用降压药物治疗，除非血压达到 220/120 mmHg 或更高。初始治疗后，建议将血压降低目标定为更为保守的水平，即在卒中发作后的前 24 h，降压目标不超过 15%。然而，对于适合溶栓治疗的患者，在静脉注射组织型纤溶酶原激活剂之前，应控制血压低于 185/110 mmHg，并且在开始药物治疗后至少前 24 h 内应维持在 180/105 mmHg 以下。广泛引用的降压目标是在第一小时内血压降低 10%，在接下来的 3～12 h 内再降低 15%，但这一目标仅限于患有高血压脑病或伴有其他表现的患者。不必要地将升高的血压快速纠正至完全正常水平，会使患者面临较高的脑、心脏和肾脏缺血恶化风险。在慢性高血压中，脑的自动调节会将其重置为高于正常的血压值。这种代偿性调节可防止血压非常高时出现组织过度灌注（即颅内压升高），但当升高的血压降低得太快时，也容易使患者出现组织灌注不足（即脑缺血）。

治疗高血压急症的注射药物总结于表 11.9。硝普钠是一种一氧化氮供体，因其可以快速滴定以控制血压，是最常用的药物。硝酸甘油是另一种一氧化氮供体，静脉注射主要用于急性冠脉综合征或失代偿性心力衰竭情况下的高血压。尼卡地平是一种注射用二氢吡啶类 CCB，特别适用于心脏病术后患者和肾功能衰竭患者，以避免硝普钠引起的硝普盐毒性。氯维地平是另一种静脉注射的 CCB，其半衰期比尼卡地平短，仅为 1 min。非诺多泮是一种选择性多巴胺-1 受体激动剂，可引起体循环和肾脏血管扩张，以及增加肾小球滤过、促进排钠和利尿。静脉注射拉贝洛尔是治疗高血压危象的有效方法，特别是在心肌缺血伴心室功能保留的情况下。

急诊科大多数高血压亚急症患者或是不依从药物治疗方案，或是治疗不充分。为了加速必要的药物更换，应在 72 h 内安排门诊随访。为了在短期内管理患者，有效的口服药物包括拉贝洛尔、可乐定或短效 ACEI 类药物卡托普利。

在急诊科和其他急症救治机构中，患者因与血压无关的症状（如肌肉骨骼疼痛、骨科损伤）而接受紧急内科或外科治疗时，偶然发现血压超过 160/110 mmHg 的情况十分常见。在这些情况下，血压升高通常提示慢性高血压，而非简单的生理应激反应，这为启动初级保健转诊以进行慢性高血压的正式评估和治疗提供了重要机会。而家庭和动态血压监测可用于确定急性疾病缓解后患者的血压是否完全恢复正常。

表 11.9 治疗高血压急症的注射剂

药物	剂量	起效	注意事项
注射用血管扩张剂			
硝普钠	0.25～10 μg/（kg·min）静脉滴注	即刻	硝普盐长期使用毒性
硝酸甘油	5～100 μg/min 静脉滴注	2～5 min	头痛、心动过速、耐受性
尼卡地平	5～15 mg/h 静脉滴注	1～5 min	长期使用后持续低血压
氯维地平	1～21 mg/h 静脉滴注	2～4 min	心动过速
甲磺酸非诺多泮	0.01～0.3 μg/（kg·min）静脉滴注	1～5 min	头痛、心动过速、眼压升高
肼屈嗪	5～10 mg 静脉推注或 10～40 mg 肌内注射；每 4～6 h 重复一次	静脉注射 10 min 肌内注射 20 min	心动过速时出现不可预测和过度的心率下降；心绞痛恶化；注意血压变化
依那普利	每 6 h 0.625～1.25 mg 静脉推注	15～60 min	不可预测和过度的血压降低；双侧肾动脉狭窄患者的急性肾衰竭
注射用肾上腺素能抑制剂			
拉贝洛尔	20～80 mg，每 10 min 缓慢静脉注射，或 0.5～2.0 mg/min 静脉滴注	5～10 min	支气管痉挛、心脏传导阻滞、直立性低血压
美托洛尔	5 mg 静脉注射，每 10 min 1 次，共 3 次	5～10 min	支气管痉挛、心脏传导阻滞、心力衰竭、可卡因引起的心肌缺血加重
艾司洛尔	500 μg/kg 静脉注射，超过 3 min；之后 25～100 μg/（kg·min）静脉滴注（译者注：原文 25～100 mg/kg/min 有误）	1～5 min	支气管痉挛、心脏传导阻滞、心力衰竭
酚妥拉明	5～10 mg 静脉推注，每 5～15 min 1 次	1～2 min	心动过速，直立性低血压

PROGNOSIS

One of the most important prognostic factors in hypertension is ECG or echocardiographic LVH, with the latter already present in as many as 25% of patients with newly diagnosed hypertension. LVH predisposes the patient to heart failure, atrial fibrillation, and sudden cardiac death.

Because of their relatively short duration (typically <5 years), randomized controlled trials underestimate the lifetime protection against premature disability and death afforded by several decades of antihypertensive therapy in clinical practice. In the Framingham Heart Study, treating hypertension for 20 years in middle-aged adults reduced total cardiovascular mortality by 60%, which is considerably greater than the results of most randomized trials despite the less intense treatment guidelines when therapy was initiated in the 1950s through the 1970s.

PROSPECTS FOR THE FUTURE

- Further delineation of genetic causes of hypertension and application of this research to the treatment and prevention of hypertension, including development of pharmacologic and nonpharmacologic therapy that target the various signaling pathways in hypertension
- Determination of antihypertensive drug classes that are most effective in preventing dementia and cognitive decline
- Evaluation of the comparative efficacy and safety of DOACs against LMWH in preventing VTE in patients with active malignancy
- Further assessment of safety and efficacy of combination of direct anticoagulants and antiplatelet therapy in patients with atrial fibrillation, venous thromboembolism, and vascular disease

SUGGESTED READINGS

Arabi YM, Al-Hameed F, Burns KEA, et al: Adjunctive intermittent pneumatic compression for venous thromboprophylaxis, *N Engl J Med* 380:1305–1315, 2019.

Gerhard-Herman MD, Gornik HL, Barrett C, et al: 2016 AHA/ACC guideline on the management of patients with lower extremity peripheral artery disease: a report of the American College of Cardiology/American Heart Association Task Force on Clinical Practice Guidelines, Circulation 135:e726–e779, 2017.

Group SMIftSR, Williamson JD, Pajewski NM, et al: Effect of intensive vs standard blood pressure control on probable dementia: a randomized clinical trial, JAMA 321:553–561, 2019.

Kearon C, Akl EA, Ornelas J, et al: Antithrombotic therapy for VTE disease: chest guideline and expert panel report, Chest 149:315–352, 2016.

Konstantinides SV, Meyer G, Becattini C, et al: 2019 ESC Guidelines for the diagnosis and management of acute pulmonary embolism developed in collaboration with the European Respiratory Society (ERS): the Task Force for the diagnosis and management of acute pulmonary embolism of the European Society of Cardiology (ESC), Eur Respir J 54(3):1901647, 2019.

Ojji DB, Mayosi B, Francis V, et al.: Comparison of dual therapies for lowering blood pressure in black africans, N Engl J Med 380:2429–2439, 2019.

Simonneau G, Montani D, Celermajer DS, et al: Haemodynamic definitions and updated clinical classification of pulmonary hypertension, Eur Respir J 53, 2019.

Vongpatanasin W: Resistant hypertension: a review of diagnosis and management, JAMA 311(21):2216–2224, 2014.

Vongpatanasin W, Ayers C, Lodhi H, et al.: Diagnostic thresholds for blood pressure measured at home in the context of the 2017 hypertension guideline, Hypertension 72:1312–1319, 2018.

Whelton PK, Carey RM, Aronow WS, et al: 2017 ACC/AHA/AAPA/ABC/ACPM/AGS/APhA/ASH/ASPC/NMA/PCNA Guideline for the prevention, detection, evaluation, and management of high blood pressure in adults: Executive summary: A report of the American College of Cardiology/American Heart Association task force on clinical practice guidelines, Circulation 138:e426–e483, 2018.

Williams B, Mancia G, Spiering W, et al: 2018 ESC/ESH Guidelines for the management of arterial hypertension, Eur Heart J 39:3021–3104, 2018.

预后

影响高血压预后最重要的因素之一是心电图或超声心动图提示的左心室肥厚（LVH），后者已经出现在多达 25% 的新确诊的高血压患者中。LVH 易使患者发生心力衰竭、心房颤动和心源性猝死。

由于持续时间相对较短（通常 < 5 年），随机对照试验低估了临床实践中长达数十年的降压治疗对预防过早残疾和死亡的终身保护作用。在弗雷明汉心脏研究中，对中年高血压患者进行长达 20 年的降压治疗，使心血管疾病的总死亡率降低了 60%。这一结果比大多数随机试验的结果要高得多，尽管该研究起始于 20 世纪 50 年代到 70 年代，当时还没有那么严格的治疗指南。

未来展望

- 进一步阐明高血压的遗传机制，并将这项研究应用于高血压的治疗和预防。包括针对高血压各种信号通路的药物和非药物治疗的发展
- 确定在预防痴呆和认知能力下降方面最有效的降压药物类别
- 评估比较直接口服抗凝药与低分子量肝素在预防活动性恶性肿瘤患者静脉血栓栓塞方面的疗效和安全性
- 在心房颤动、静脉血栓栓塞和血管疾病患者中，进一步评估联合使用直接抗凝剂和抗血小板治疗的安全性和有效性

推荐阅读

Arabi YM, Al-Hameed F, Burns KEA, et al: Adjunctive intermittent pneumatic compression for venous thromboprophylaxis, N Engl J Med 380:1305–1315, 2019.

Gerhard-Herman MD, Gornik HL, Barrett C, et al: 2016 AHA/ACC guideline on the management of patients with lower extremity peripheral artery disease: a report of the American College of Cardiology/American Heart Association Task Force on Clinical Practice Guidelines, Circulation 135:e726–e779, 2017.

Group SMIftSR, Williamson JD, Pajewski NM, et al: Effect of intensive vs standard blood pressure control on probable dementia: a randomized clinical trial, JAMA 321:553–561, 2019.

Kearon C, Akl EA, Ornelas J, et al: Antithrombotic therapy for VTE disease: chest guideline and expert panel report, Chest 149:315–352, 2016.

Konstantinides SV, Meyer G, Becattini C, et al: 2019 ESC Guidelines for the diagnosis and management of acute pulmonary embolism developed in collaboration with the European Respiratory Society (ERS): the Task Force for the diagnosis and management of acute pulmonary embolism of the European Society of Cardiology (ESC), Eur Respir J 54(3):1901647, 2019.

Ojji DB, Mayosi B, Francis V, et al.: Comparison of dual therapies for lowering blood pressure in black africans, N Engl J Med 380:2429–2439, 2019.

Simonneau G, Montani D, Celermajer DS, et al: Haemodynamic definitions and updated clinical classification of pulmonary hypertension, Eur Respir J 53, 2019.

Vongpatanasin W: Resistant hypertension: a review of diagnosis and management, JAMA 311(21):2216–2224, 2014.

Vongpatanasin W, Ayers C, Lodhi H, et al.: Diagnostic thresholds for blood pressure measured at home in the context of the 2017 hypertension guideline, Hypertension 72:1312–1319, 2018.

Whelton PK, Carey RM, Aronow WS, et al: 2017 ACC/AHA/AAPA/ABC/ACPM/AGS/APhA/ASH/ASPC/NMA/PCNA Guideline for the prevention, detection, evaluation, and management of high blood pressure in adults: Executive summary: A report of the American College of Cardiology/American Heart Association task force on clinical practice guidelines, Circulation 138:e426–e483, 2018.

Williams B, Mancia G, Spiering W, et al: 2018 ESC/ESH Guidelines for the management of arterial hypertension, Eur Heart J 39:3021–3104, 2018.

索引 Index

A

Abdominal aortic aneurysm (AAA), 278
ABI. *See* Ankle-brachial index
Abnormal automaticity, 194-196
Accessory pathways, 214
Acquired long QT syndrome, 238
Actin, of myocytes, 8
Action potential, cardiac, 194, 196f
Acute coronary syndrome, 172-180
 clinical presentation of, 172
 definition of, 172
 diagnosis of, 172-176, 174f-176f
 differential diagnosis of, 176-178
 epidemiology of, 172
 pathology of, 172
 prognosis of, 180
 treatment of, 178-180
Acute fibrillation, after myocardial infarction, 186
Acute limb ischemia, 276-278
Acute pericarditis, 242, 244t
Acyanotic heart disease, 106-118
Adenosine
 as antiarrhythmic agent, 204
 coronary blood flow and, 12-14
 as vasodilator, 68
Adenosine triphosphate (ATP), 6-8
 coronary blood flow and, 12-14
Calcium
 myocardial contraction and, 8
Adrenal hyperplasia
 primary aldosteronism and, 296-298
Adrenal tumors
 adenoma
  aldosterone-producing, 296-298
African Americans
 hypertension in, 304
Afterload, 12, 12t
Aldosterone antagonist, for heart failure, 96
Aldosteronism
 glucocorticoid-remediable, 298
 primary, 296-298, 300t, 312
Ambulatory electrocardiographic recording, 56-58
Ambulatory monitoring, in arrhythmias, 198
Anasarca, 24
Aneurysm (s)
 aortic, 278-280, 278f, 278t
 aortic coarctation and, 114
Angina equivalent, dyspnea as, 22
Angina pectoris, 156-172
 clinical presentation of, 156-158, 158t
 definition of, 156
 diagnosis and differential diagnosis of, 158-162, 160f-162f, 164t
 microvascular, with normal coronary arteries, 170
 pathology of, 156
 prognosis of, 170-172
 treatment for, 162-168
  medical management in, 162-166, 164t
  medications for, 166t
  revascularization therapy for, 166-168
 unstable. *See* Unstable angina
 variant. *See* Variant angina

Page numbers followed by "f" indicate figures, "t" indicate tables, and "b" indicate boxes.

A

腹主动脉瘤（AAA），279
ABI 参见踝臂指数
异常自律性，195-197
旁路，215
获得性长QT间期综合征，239
肌动蛋白，心肌细胞，9
动作电位，心脏，195，197f
急性冠脉综合征，173-181
 临床表现，173
 定义，173
 诊断，173-177，175f-177f
 鉴别诊断，177-179
 流行病学，173
 病理学，173
 预后，181
 治疗，179-181
急性心房颤动，心肌梗死后，187
急性肢体缺血，277-279
急性心包炎，243，245t
非发绀型心脏病，107-119
腺苷
 抗心律失常药物，205
 冠状动脉血流，13-15
 血管扩张剂，69
三磷酸腺苷（ATP），7-9
 冠状动脉血流，13-15
钙
 心肌收缩，9
肾上腺皮质增生
 原发性醛固酮增多症，297-299
肾上腺肿瘤
 腺瘤
  醛固酮瘤，297-299
非裔美国人
 高血压，305
后负荷，13，13t
醛固酮受体拮抗剂，治疗心力衰竭，97
醛固酮增多症
 糖皮质激素可抑制性，299
 原发性，297-299，301t，313
动态心电图记录，57-59
动态监测，心律失常，199
全身性水肿，25
动脉瘤
 主动脉瘤，279-281，279f，279t
 主动脉缩窄，115
"心绞痛样"胸痛，呼吸困难，23
心绞痛，157-173
 临床表现，157-159，159t
 定义，157
 诊断和鉴别诊断，159-163，161f-163f，165t
 冠状动脉正常的微血管性心绞痛，171
 病理学，157
 预后，171-173
 治疗，163-169
  药物治疗，163-167，165t
  药物，167t
  血运重建治疗，167-169
 不稳定型 参见不稳定型心绞痛
 变异型 参见变异型心绞痛

页码数字中，"f"代表"图","t"代表"表格","b"代表"框"。

Angioplasty, renal artery 　　for fibromuscular dysplasia, 296 Angiotensin-converting enzyme (ACE) inhibitors 　　contraindications to, 306t-308t 　　for hypertension, 302t 　　side effects of, 306t-308t Angiotensin-receptor blockers (ARBs) 　　contraindications to, 306t-308t 　　for hypertension, 302t 　　side effects of, 306t-308t Ankle-brachial index (ABI), 274, 274t Antiarrhythmic drugs 　　for atrial fibrillation, 224-226, 226f 　　characteristics of, 200t 　　class I, 200-202 　　class II, 202 　　class III, 202-204 　　class IV, 202 　　classification of, 198-200, 198t 　　side effects of, 202t Antiarrhythmics Versus Implantable Defibrillators (AVID) trial, 234 Anticoagulation 　　in acute limb ischemia, 276-278 　　atrial fibrillation and, 222-224 　　for deep vein thrombosis, 286 　　for mitral stenosis, 132 　　in pulmonary arterial hypertension, 284 　　for pulmonary embolism, 290 Antidromic atrioventricular reentrant tachycardia, 214 Antihypertensive agents, 302t 　　for acute severe hypertension, 314, 314t 　　contraindications and side effects of, 306t-308t 　　in hypertensive emergencies, 314t 　　lifetime protection from, 316 Aorta 　　intramural hematoma of, 280 　　Takayasu's arteritis of, 282 Aortic aneurysm, 278-280, 278f, 278t Aortic coarctation, 112-114 Aortic dissection, 280, 280f 　　pain in, 20 Aortic regurgitation, 136-138, 138t 　　carotid pulse and, 32 　　clinical presentation of, 136-138 　　definition of, 136 　　diagnosis of, 138 　　etiology of, 136 　　murmur of, 20 　　natural history of, 136-138 　　pathophysiology of, 136 　　physical examination for, 138 　　tetralogy of Fallot and, 118 　　treatment for, 138 　　ventricular septal defects and, 110 Aortic root enlargement, in Marfan syndrome, β-adrenergic blockade 　　for, 278-280 Aortic stenosis, 124-128, 126f, 128t 　　carotid pulse and, 32 　　clinical presentation of, 124 　　definition and etiology of, 124 　　diagnosis of, 126 　　murmurs in, 36 　　natural history of, 124 　　noncardiac surgery inpatient with, 270 　　pathophysiology of, 124 　　physical examination of, 124-126 　　in pregnancy, 258 　　treatment of, 126-128 Aortic ulcers, penetrating, 280, 282f	肾动脉成形术 　　纤维肌发育不良，297 血管紧张素转换酶抑制剂 　　禁忌证，307t-309t 　　高血压，303t 　　副作用，307t-309t 血管紧张素受体阻滞剂（ARB） 　　禁忌证，307t-309t 　　高血压，303t 　　副作用，307t-309t 踝臂指数（ABI），275，275t 抗心律失常药物 　　心房颤动，225-227，227f 　　特点，201t 　　Ⅰ类，201-203 　　Ⅱ类，203 　　Ⅲ类，203-205 　　Ⅳ类，203 　　分类，199-201，199t 　　副作用，203t 抗心律失常药物对比植入式除颤器（AVID）试验，235 抗凝治疗 　　急性肢体缺血，277-279 　　心房颤动，223-225 　　深静脉血栓形成，287 　　二尖瓣狭窄，133 　　肺动脉高压，285 　　肺栓塞，291 逆向型房室折返性心动过速，215 降压药物，303t 　　急性重症高血压，315，315t 　　禁忌证和副作用，307t-309t 　　高血压急症，315t 　　终身保护作用，317 主动脉 　　壁内血肿，281 　　大动脉炎，283 主动脉瘤，279-281，279f，279t 主动脉缩窄，113-115 主动脉夹层，281，281f 　　疼痛，21 主动脉瓣反流，137-139，139t 　　颈动脉搏动，33 　　临床表现，137-139 　　定义，137 　　诊断，139 　　病因，137 　　杂音，21 　　自然病程，137-139 　　病理生理学，137 　　体格检查，139 　　法洛四联症，119 　　治疗，139 　　室间隔缺损，111 主动脉根部扩张，见于马方综合征，β受体阻滞剂，279-281 主动脉瓣狭窄，125-129，127f，129t 　　颈动脉搏动，33 　　临床表现，125 　　定义和病因，125 　　诊断，127 　　杂音，37 　　自然病程，125 　　非心脏手术患者，271 　　病理生理学，125 　　体格检查，125-127 　　妊娠期主动脉瓣狭窄，259 　　治疗，127-129 穿透性主动脉溃疡，281，283f

Aortic valve
    anatomy of, 4
    fibroelastoma of, 264
    opening of, 10f
Aortic valve replacement (AVR), for stenosis, 126
Arrhythmias
    after myocardial infarction, 186
    associated with fibromas, 264
    cardiac, 194-240
        basic cellular electrophysiology in, 194-198, 196f
        bradycardia, 204-212, 208f-210f
        cardioversion and defibrillation for, 204
        classification of, 194
        management of, 198-204
        mechanisms of, 194-198, 196f
        syncope, 228, 230t, 232f
        tachycardias, 212-228, 216f-218f, 226f
        ventricular, sudden cardiac death and, 228-238, 232f, 232t-234t, 236f
    noncardiac surgery inpatient with, 270
    palpitations associated with, 22
    from trauma, 264
Arrhythmogenic right ventricular cardiomyopathy (ARVC), 236, 236f
Arterial embolism, acute limb ischemia in, 276-278
Arterial hypertension, 292-304, 294f
    in African Americans, 304
    initial evaluation for, 292-296
        assessment of blood pressure, 292-294, 296f-298f, 296t
        risk stratification in, 294
        secondary causes of hypertension and, 294-296, 300t
    peripheral arterial disease with, 274
    stroke risk in, 292, 296f
Arterial pressures, in normal cardiac cycle, 8-10
Arterial pulse, 28-32, 30f
Arterial switch procedure, for transposition of great arteries, 120
Arteriovenous malformation, 282
Arteritis
    Takayasu's, 282
    temporal, 282
Aspirin
    in peripheral arterial disease, 276
    for reduction of atrial fibrillation-related stroke, 222
Atherosclerosis, 150
    renal artery stenosis in, 296, 300f
    risk factors for, 150-152
Atherosclerotic plaque, 150
Atrial arrhythmias, 218-222, 218f
    tetralogy of Fallot and, 118
Atrial fibrillation, 16, 218f, 222-228
    acute management of, 224
    anticoagulation and, 222-224
    with aortic valve stenosis, 116
    atrial septal defects and, 108
    electrical cardioversion of, 224
    heart failure and, management of, 96-98
    mechanisms of, 222
    mitral stenosis and, 132
    overview and classification, 222
    pharmacologic conversion of, 224
    surgical ablation of, 226-228
    Wolff-Parkinson-White syndrome and, 216-218, 216f
Atrial Fibrillation Follow-up Investigation of Rhythm Management (AFFIRM) trial, 226
Atrial flutter, 212-214
    atypical, 220-222
    typical, 218f, 220
Atrial pressure, 10
    left, 10, 10f, 12t
    right, 10f, 12t, 14

主动脉瓣
    解剖学，5
    弹力纤维瘤，265
    开放，11f
主动脉瓣置换（AVR），治疗主动脉瓣狭窄，127
心律失常
    心肌梗死后，187
    纤维瘤相关性，265
    心律失常，195-241
        基础细胞电生理学，195-199，197f
        心动过缓，205-213，209f-211f
        心脏复律和除颤，205
        分类，195
        处理，199-205
        机制，195-199，197f
        晕厥，229，231t，233f
        心动过速，213-229，217f-219f，227f
        室性心律失常和心源性猝死，229-239，233f，233t-235t，237
    非心脏手术患者，271
    心悸，23
    创伤，265
致心律失常型右心室心肌病（ARVC），237，237f
动脉栓塞，急性肢体缺血，277-279
动脉高血压，293-305，295f
    非裔美国人，305
    初始评估，293-297
        血压评估，293-295，297f-299f，297t
        风险分层，295
        继发性高血压病因，295-297，301t
    周围动脉疾病，275
    卒中风险，293，297
动脉压，正常心动周期，9-11
动脉脉搏，29-33，31f
动脉调转术，治疗大动脉转位，121
动静脉畸形，283
动脉炎
    大动脉炎，283
    颞动脉炎，283
阿司匹林
    周围动脉疾病，277
    降低心房颤动相关卒中发生率，223
动脉粥样硬化，151
    肾动脉狭窄，297，301f
    危险因素，151-153
动脉粥样硬化斑块，151
房性心律失常，219-223，219f
    法洛四联症，119
心房颤动，17，219f，223-229
    急性期治疗，225
    抗凝治疗，223-225
    主动脉瓣狭窄，117
    房间隔缺损，109
    心脏电复律，225
    心力衰竭患者心房颤动的处理，97-99
    机制，223
    二尖瓣狭窄，133
    概述和分类，223
    药物复律，225
    外科消融治疗，227-229
    WPW综合征，217-219，217f
心房颤动节律管理的随访研究（AFFIRM）试验，227
心房扑动，213-215
    非典型，221-223
    典型，219f，221
心房压，11
    左心房压，11，11f，13t
    右心房压，11f，13t，15

Atrial septal defects, 106-108, 108f
Atrioventricular blocks
　2∶1, 210f, 212
　first-degree, 210, 210f
　high-grade, 210f, 212
　noncardiac surgery inpatient with, 270
　second-degree, 210-212, 210f
　third-degree, 210f, 212
Atrioventricular conduction, disturbances in, 208-212, 210f
Atrioventricular nodal reentry tachycardia, 214, 216f
Atrioventricular (AV) node, 6, 204-206
　autonomic influences on, 6
Atrioventricular reentrant tachycardia
　antidromic, 214
　orthodromic, 214
Atrioventricular septal defects, complete, 110-112
Augmented leads, 44
Auscultation, 32-42
　abnormal heart sounds in, 34-38, 34t-36t, 36f-38f
　categories, 38, 38t-40t
　murmurs in, 38-42
　normal heart sounds in, 34
　other cardiac sounds, 42
　prosthetic heart sounds, 42
　shape of, 38, 40f
　techniques in, 32-34, 34t
Auscultatory gap, 292
Austin-Flint murmur, 42, 138
Autonomic nervous system, 6
　and systemic vascular tone, 14
AVR. See Aortic valve replacement
Axial reference system, 46

B

Balloon angioplasty, for aortic coarctation, 112-114
Baroreflex loop, 14
Becker sign, in chronic severe regurgitation, 140t
Bicuspid aortic valves
　aortic coarctation and, 112
　aortic stenosis and, 124
Bioprosthetic valves, for aortic stenosis, 126, 128f
Bisferiens pulse, 32
α-blockers
　contraindications to, 306t-308t
　for hypertension, 302t
　side effects of, 306t-308t
β-blockers
　for aortic regurgitation, 138
　for aortic root enlargement, in Marfan syndrome, 278-280
　contraindications to, 306t-308t
　for heart failure, 96
　for hypertension, 302t
　formitral stenosis, 132
　for penetrating aortic ulcers and intramural hematoma, 280
　side effects of, 306t-308t
Blood flow
　regulation of
　　coronary, 12
　　systemic, 14
Blood pressure
　age-dependent changes in systolic and diastolic, 308, 310f
　arterial, regulation of, 12
　assessment of, 292-294
　　ambulatory, 292, 298f
　estrogen replacement therapy and, 310
　oral contraceptives, 310
Bloodvessels
　normal structure and function of, 4-14
Bradycardia, 204-212

房间隔缺损，107-109, 109f
房室传导阻滞
　2∶1, 211f, 213
　一度, 211, 211f
　高度, 211f, 213
　非心脏手术患者, 271
　二度, 211-213, 211f
　三度, 211f, 213
房室传导，障碍, 209-213, 211f
房室结折返性心动过速, 215, 217f
房室（AV）结, 7, 205-207
　自主神经影响, 7
房室折返性心动过速
　逆向型, 215
　顺向型, 215
房室间隔缺损，完全性, 111-113
加压肢体导联, 45
听诊, 33-43
　异常心音, 35-39, 35t-37t, 37f-39f
　分类, 39, 39t-41t
　杂音, 39-43
　正常心音, 35
　其他心音, 43
　人工瓣膜音, 43
　形态, 39, 41f
　技巧, 33-35, 35t
听诊间断, 293
Austin-Flint 杂音, 43, 139
自主神经系统, 7
　体循环血管张力, 15
AVR 参见主动脉瓣置换术
心电轴参考系统, 47

B

球囊血管成形术，治疗主动脉缩窄, 113-115
压力反射环, 15
Becker 征，见于严重慢性主动脉瓣反流, 141t
二叶主动脉瓣
　主动脉缩窄, 113
　主动脉瓣狭窄, 125
生物瓣，治疗主动脉瓣狭窄, 127, 129f
双峰脉, 33
α 受体阻滞剂
　禁忌证, 307t-309t
　高血压, 303t
　副作用, 307t-309t
β 受体阻滞剂
　主动脉瓣反流, 139
　主动脉根部扩张，见于马方综合征, 279-281
　禁忌证, 307t-309t
　心力衰竭, 97
　高血压, 303t
　二尖瓣狭窄, 133
　穿透性主动脉溃疡和壁内血肿, 281
　副作用, 307t-309t
血流量
　调节
　　冠状动脉, 13
　　体循环, 15
血压
　收缩压和舒张压的年龄依赖性变化, 309, 311f
　动脉调节, 13
　评估, 293-295
　　动态血压, 293, 299f
　雌激素替代疗法, 311
　口服避孕药, 311
血管
　正常结构和功能, 5-15
心动过缓, 205-213

anatomy and physiology in, 204-206
atrioventricular conduction disturbances in, 208-212, 210f
autonomic regulation of heart rate in, 206
sinus node dysfunction in, 206-208, 208f
Bradycardia-tachycardia syndrome, 206-208, 208f
Broadbent sign, 32
Bruce protocol, 68
Brugada syndrome, 236f, 238
Bundle branch blocks, 50, 52f
Bundle branches, 6

C

Calcium
    myocardial contraction and, 8, 8f
Calcium channel blockers, 202, 202t
    contraindications to, 306t-308t
    for hypertension, 302t
    for hypertensive emergencies, 314t
    side effects of, 306t-308t
Cannon a wave, 26-28
Cardiac catheterization, 72-78
    in aortic coarctation, 112
    in aortic valve stenosis, 116
    in atrial septal defects, 108
    in constrictive pericarditis, 246
    left heart, 74-76, 76f
    right heart, 76-78, 78f, 80t
    in ventricular septal defects, 110
Cardiac cycle, 8-10, 10f
Cardiac index, 10
Cardiac output, 10
Cardiac performance, 10-12
    factors affecting, 12t
Cardiac tamponade, 242-244
Cardiac trauma
    nonpenetrating, 264, 264t
    penetrating, 264-266, 264t
Cardiac tumors, 262-264, 262f
Cardiogenic shock, myocardial infarction and, 188
Cardiomyopathies, 250-256, 250t. See also Heart failure
    arrhythmogenic right ventricular, 254-256
    dilated, 250-252
    hypertrophic, 252-254, 254f
    new-onset, 88
    restrictive, 254, 256t
    types of, 82
    unclassified, 256
Cardiovascular disease (CVD)
    clinical presentation of, 16-24
    definition and epidemiology of, 16
    diagnosis and physical examination, 24-42
        of arterial pressure and pulse, examination, 28-32, 30f
        auscultation, 32-42
        chamber abnormalities and ventricular hypertrophy, 48-50, 48f, 50t
        general, 24-26
        of jugular venous pulsations, 26-28, 28f
        precordium, examination of, 32
    diagnostic tests and procedures for, 44-80
        abnormal electrocardiographic patterns, 48-52, 50t
        abnormalities of the ST segment and T wave, 52, 56f
        ambulatory electrocardiographic recording, 56-58
        cardiac catheterization, 72-78
        chest radiography, 58, 60f
        computed tomography, 72, 74f
        echocardiography, 58-60, 60f-64f
        electrocardiography, 44-46
        interventricular conduction delays, 50, 50t, 52f
        magnetic resonance imaging, 62-64, 68f-70f
        myocardial ischemia and infarction, 50-52, 54f, 56t

解剖学和生理学，205-207
房室传导障碍，209-213，211f
自主神经系统的心率调节，207
窦房结功能障碍，207-209，209f
心动过缓-心动过速综合征，207-209，209f
Broadbent 征，33
布鲁斯方案，69
Brugada 综合征，237f，239
束支传导阻滞，51，53f
束支，7

C

钙
    心肌收缩，9，9f
钙通道阻滞剂，203，203t
    禁忌证，307t-309t
    高血压，303t
    高血压危象，315t
    副作用，307t-309t
大炮 A 波，27-29
心导管检查，73-79
    主动脉缩窄，113
    主动脉瓣狭窄，117
    房间隔缺损，109
    缩窄性心包炎，247
    左心，75-77，77f
    右心，77-79，79f，81t
    室间隔缺损，111
心动周期，9-11，11f
心脏指数，11
心输出量，11
心功能，11-13
    影响因素，13t
心脏压塞，243-245
心脏创伤
    非穿透性，265，265t
    穿透性，265-267，265t
心脏肿瘤，263-265，263f
心源性休克，心肌梗死，189
心肌病，251-257，251t；参见心力衰竭
    致心律失常型右心室（心肌病），255-257
    扩张型，251-253
    肥厚型，253-255，255f
    新发，89
    限制型，255，257t
    类型，83
    未分类的（心肌病），257
心血管疾病（CVD）
    临床表现，17-25
    定义和流行病学，17
    诊断和体格检查，25-43
        动脉血压和脉搏检查，29-33，31f
        听诊，33-43
        腔室异常和心室肥厚，49-51，49f，51t
        一般情况，25-27
        颈静脉搏动，27-29，29f
        心前区检查，33
    诊断性检查和方法，45-81
        异常心电图，49-53，51t
        ST 段和 T 波异常，53，57f
        动态心电图，57-59
        心导管检查，73-79
        胸部 X 线检查，59，61f
        计算机断层成像，73，75f
        超声心动图，59-61，61f-65f
        心电图，45-47
        室内传导延迟，51，51t，53f
        磁共振成像，63-65，69f-71f
        心肌缺血和梗死，51-53，55f，57t

nuclear cardiology, 62, 66f
    stress imaging, 68-72
    stress testing, 64-68, 70t
evaluation of, 16-42
pathology of, 16
Cardioversion
    of atrial fibrillation, 224
    direct current, 204
Carvedilol, for hypertensive patients with diabetes, 308
Catecholaminergic polymorphic ventricular tachycardia, 238
Catheter ablation
    for arrhythmias, 204
    for atrial fibrillation, 226f, 228
    for atrioventricular nodal reentry tachycardia, 214
    of atrioventricular node, 228
    in Wolff-Parkinson-White syndrome, 218
Central cyanosis, 24
Central sympatholytics, 302t
    contraindications and side effects of, 306t-308t
$CHADS_2$ score, 222
Channelopathies
    genetic testing for, 238
Chest pain, 18-20
    cardiovascular causes of, 18t
    ischemic, hypertrophic cardiomyopathy and, 252
    noncardiac causes of, 20t
    recurrent, myocardial infarction and, 186, 186t
Chest radiography
    for aortic valve stenosis, 116
    in cardiovascular disease, 58, 60f
    for patent ductus arteriosus, 114
    in pericardial effusions, 244
    in pulmonary embolism, 288
Chordaetendineae, anatomy of, 4
Chronotropic incompetence, 206
Chronotropy, 6
Cilostazol, in peripheral arterial disease, 276
Circulation, systemic, physiology of, 14
Circulatory pathway, 4, 6f
Circulatory physiology, 8-10, 10f
Claudication, 32, 274
    in Buerger's disease, 280-282
    jaw, 282
    in Takayasu's arteritis, 282
Clopidogrel
    in peripheral arterial disease, 276
Coarctation of aorta, 22
Co-dominant circulation, 4
Color Doppler imaging, 58-60, 62f
Complete heart block, 22, 210f, 212
Computed tomographic angiography (CTA)
    of aortic aneurysm, 278, 278f
    of aortic dissection, 280, 280f
    of aortic ulcer, penetrating, 280, 282f
    multidetector, in pulmonary embolism, 288, 290f
    in peripheral arterial disease, 274-276
    in pulmonary embolism, 288, 288f
    of renal artery stenosis, 296, 300f
    in pericardial effusions, 244
    in pulmonary embolism, 288, 288f
Conduction defects, noncardiac surgery inpatient with, 270
Conduction system, cardiac, 4-6
    blood supply of, 4
    cells of, 6
Congenital heart disease, 16, 106-122
    acyanotic, 106-118
    aortic coarctation, 112-114
    aortic valve stenosis, 116-118
    atrial septal defects, 106-108, 108f

心脏核素检查，63，67f
    负荷成像，69-73
    负荷试验，65-69，71t
评估，17-43
病理学，17
心脏复律
    心房颤动，225
    直流电复律，205
卡维地洛，治疗合并糖尿病的高血压患者，309
儿茶酚胺敏感性多形性室性心动过速，239
导管消融
    心律失常，205
    心房颤动，227f，229
    房室结折返性心动过速，215
    导管消融房室结，229
    WPW综合征，219
中心性发绀，25
中枢交感神经阻滞剂，303t
    禁忌证和副作用，307t-309t
$CHADS_2$ 评分，223
离子通道病
    基因检测，239
胸痛，19-21
    心血管病因，19t
    缺血性，肥厚型心肌病，253
    非心脏病因，21t
    复发性胸痛，心肌梗死，187，187t
胸部X线
    主动脉瓣狭窄，117
    心血管疾病，59，61f
    动脉导管未闭，115
    心包积液，245
    肺栓塞，289
腱索，解剖，5
变时功能不全，207
变时性，7
西洛他唑，治疗周围动脉疾病，277
体循环，生理机制，15
循环途径，5，7f
循环系统生理机制，9-11，11f
跛行（活动障碍），33，275
    血栓闭塞性脉管炎，281-283
    下颌，283
    大动脉炎，283
氯吡格雷
    周围动脉疾病，277
主动脉缩窄，23
均衡优势循环，5
彩色多普勒成像，59-61，63f
完全性心脏传导阻滞（完全性阻滞），23，211f，213
CT血管成像（CTA）
    主动脉瘤，279，279f
    主动脉夹层，281，281f
    主动脉溃疡，穿透性，281，283f
    多层CTA，肺栓塞，289，291f
    周围动脉疾病，275-277
    肺栓塞，289，289f
    肾动脉狭窄，297，301f
    心包积液，245
    肺栓塞，289，289f
传导障碍，非心脏手术患者，271
心脏传导系统，5-7
    血液供应，5
    细胞，7
先天性心脏病，17，107-123
    非发绀型，107-119
    主动脉缩窄，113-115
    主动脉瓣狭窄，117-119
    房间隔缺损，107-109，109f

atrioventricular septal defects, complete, 110-112
cyanotic, 118-122
patent ductus arteriosus, 108f, 114
in pregnancy, 260
pulmonary valve stenosis, 114-116
surviving to adulthood, 108t
tetralogy of Fallot, 118, 120f
transposition of great arteries, 118-122
ventricular septal defects, 108-110, 108f
Congenital long QT syndrome, 236-238, 236f
Congestive heart failure, 16
Constrictive pericarditis, 246, 246f
restrictive cardiomyopathy *versus*, 256t
Contractility, cardiac, 12, 12t
myocardial oxygen consumption and, 12
Coronary artery disease (CAD), 16
hypertension and, 296f, 308
stress testing, 64-68, 70t
Coronary circulation, physiology of, 12-14
Coronary heart disease, 150-192. *See also* Angina pectoris; Myocardial infarction
clinical presentations of, 154-190
definition and epidemiology of, 150
pathology of, 152-154, 156f
prognosis, 190-192
risk factors for, 150-152, 152t
Coronary sinus, unroofed, 106
Corrigan pulse, 32
in chronic severe regurgitation, 140t
Corticosteroids
for giant-cell arteritis, 282
for Takayasu's arteritis, 282
Cough, 24
Coumadin, for stroke prevention, 224
Cyanosis, 24
Cyanotic heart disease, 118-122

D

D-dimer test
in deep vein thrombosis, 286
in pulmonary embolism, 288
Deep vein thrombosis, 286-288
Defibrillation, 204
Delayed after depolarizations (DADs), 196
Delta waves, 214-216
Diabetes
hypertensive patients with, 308
Diastole, 4, 8-10
Diastolic dysfunction, 16
Diastolic murmur, 42
in ventricular septal defects, 110
Diastolic rumbles, 42
Dicrotic notch, 30
Digoxin
as antiarrhythmic agent, 204
for heart failure, 96
Dilated cardiomyopathy, 250-252, 250t
Direct renin inhibitors, 302t
contraindications and side effects of, 306t-308t
Disopyramide, 200-202, 200t-202t
Diuretics
for aortic regurgitation, 138
contraindications to, 306t-308t
for heart failure, 96
for hypertension, 302t
for mitral stenosis, 132
in pulmonary arterial hypertension, 284
side effects of, 306t-308t
for tricuspid stenosis, 136
Dofetilide, 202t, 204

房室间隔缺损，完全性，111-113
发绀型，119-123
动脉导管未闭，109f，115
妊娠期，261
肺动脉瓣狭窄，115-117
存活至成年，109t
法洛四联症，119，121f
大动脉转位，119-123
室间隔缺损，109-111，109f
先天性长QT间期综合征，237-239，237
充血性心力衰竭，17
缩窄性心包炎，247，247f
限制型心肌病 *vs.* 缩窄性心包炎，257t
收缩力，心肌，13，13t
心肌氧耗量，13
冠状动脉疾病（CAD），17
高血压，297f，309
负荷试验，65-69，71t
冠状动脉循环，生理机制，13-15
冠心病，151-193；参见心绞痛；心肌梗死
临床表现，155-191
定义和流行病学，151
病理学，153-155，157f
预后，191-193
危险因素，151-153，153t
无顶冠状窦，107
水冲脉，33
慢性主动脉瓣反流，141t
皮质类固醇
巨细胞动脉炎，283
大动脉炎，283
咳嗽，25
香豆素，预防卒中，225
发绀，25
发绀型心脏病，119-123

D

D-二聚体
深静脉血栓，287
肺栓塞，289
深静脉血栓形成，287-289
除颤，205
延迟后除极（DAD），197
delta波，215-217
糖尿病
高血压患者，309
舒张期，5，9-11
舒张功能障碍，17
舒张期杂音，43
室间隔缺损，111
舒张期隆隆样杂音，43
重搏切迹，31
地高辛
抗心律失常药，205
心力衰竭，97
扩张型心肌病，251-253，251t
直接肾素抑制剂，303t
禁忌证和副作用，307t-309t
丙吡胺，201-203，201t-203t
利尿剂
主动脉瓣反流，139
禁忌证，307t-309t
心力衰竭，97
高血压，303t
二尖瓣狭窄，133
肺动脉高压，285
副作用，307t-309t
三尖瓣狭窄，137
多非利特，203t，205

Doppler, 62f
    in peripheral arterial disease, 274-276
Down syndrome, atrioventricular septal defects and, 110
Dronedarone, 202t, 204, 226
Duroziez sign, in chronic severe regurgitation, 140t
Dysplasia, 236
Dyspnea
    in cardiac disease, 20-22
    paroxysmal nocturnal, 20-22

E

Early afterdepolarizations (EADs), 196
Early repolarization, 52
Echocardiography, 58-60, 60f-64f
    in aortic stenosis, 124-126
    enhanced with intravenous ultrasound contrast agent, 64f
    in mitral stenosis, 132
    in pulmonary arterial hypertension, 284
    in pulmonary embolism, 288
Eclampsia, 310-312
Ectopic atrial tachycardia, 220
Ectopy, ventricular, 228
Edema, 22-24
Effusive constrictive pericarditis, 248
Eisenmenger's syndrome
    atrioventricular septal defects with, 112
    patent ductus arteriosus and, 114
    ventricular septal defects with, 110
Ejection clicks, 38
Ejection sounds, 36-38
Electrocardiography, 44-46, 46f
    abnormalities of the ST segment and T wave, 52, 56f
    in acute pericarditis, 242
    in aortic coarctation, 112
    in aortic valve stenosis, 116
    in arrhythmias, 198
    in atrial septal defects, 108
    in atrioventricular septal defects, 112
    augmented leads, 44
    axis, 46, 48f
    in bundle branch blocks, 50, 52f
    in dilated cardiomyopathy, 252
    in fascicular block, 50, 50t
    intervals, 44-46
    lead positioning for, 44, 46f-48f
    in left bundle branch blocks, 50, 52f
    in myocarditis, 248
    in patent ductus arteriosus, 114
    patterns, abnormal, 48-52
        chamber abnormalities and ventricular hypertrophy, 48-50, 48f, 50t
        interventricular conduction delays, 50, 50t, 52f
        myocardial ischemia and infarction, 50-52, 54f, 56t
    in pericardial effusions, 244, 246f
    precordial leads in, 46, 48f
    in PSVT, 214
    in pulmonary valve stenosis, 116
    for ST elevation myocardial infarction, 182
    in tetralogy of Fallot, 118
    in transposition of great arteries, 120
    in trauma, 264
    in ventricular septal defects, 110
Electrophysiologic testing, for arrhythmias, 198
Encephalopathy
    hypertensive, 312
Endocarditis
    in Trousseau's syndrome, 284-286
    patent ductus arteriosus and, 114
    ventricular septal defects and, 110
Endomyocardial biopsy, 78

多普勒，63f
    周围动脉疾病，275-277
唐氏综合征，房室间隔缺损，111
决奈达隆，203t，205，227
Duroziez征，见于慢性主动脉瓣反流，141t
发育不良，237
呼吸困难
    心脏病，21-23
    夜间阵发性，21-23

E

早期后除极（EAD），197
早复极，53
超声心动图，59-61，61f-65f
    主动脉瓣狭窄，125-127
    经静脉注射超声造影剂，65f
    二尖瓣狭窄，133
    肺动脉高压，285
    肺栓塞，289
子痫，311-313
异位性房性心动过速，221
室性异位搏动，229
水肿，23-25
渗出性缩窄性心包炎，249
艾森门格综合征
    房室间隔缺损，113
    动脉导管未闭，115
    室间隔缺损，111
喀喇音，39
喷射音，37-39
心电图，45-47，47f
    ST段和T波异常，53，57f
    急性心包炎，243
    主动脉缩窄，113
    主动脉瓣狭窄，117
    心律失常，199
    房间隔缺损，109
    房室间隔缺损，113
    加压肢体导联，45
    电轴，47，49f
    束支传导阻滞，51，53f
    扩张型心肌病，253
    分支阻滞，51，51t
    间期，45-47
    导联定位，45，47f-49f
    左束支传导阻滞，51，53f
    心肌炎，249
    动脉导管未闭，115
    异常心电图，49-53
        腔室异常和心室肥厚，49-51，49f，51t
        室内传导延迟，51，51t，53f
        心肌缺血和梗死，51-53，55f，57t
    心包积液，245，247
    心前区导联，47，49f
    PSVT，215
    肺动脉瓣狭窄，117
    ST段抬高型心肌梗死，183
    法洛四联症，119
    大动脉转位，121
    创伤，265
    室间隔缺损，111
电生理检查，针对心律失常，199
脑病
    高血压脑病，313
心内膜炎
    Trousseau综合征，285-287
    动脉导管未闭，115
    室间隔缺损，111
心内膜心肌活检，79

Endothelin, 14
Endothelin-receptor antagonists (ERAs), for pulmonary arterial hypertension, 284
Endovascular aneurysm repair (EVAR), percutaneous, 280
Epicardium, 4
Eplerenone
　for adrenal hyperplasia, 296-298
Event recorder, 58
Exercise
　in peripheral arterial disease, 276
External event monitors, 198
Extracorporeal membrane oxygenation (ECMO), 266t, 268

F

Fascicular block, 50
　electrocardiographic manifestations of, 50t
Fatigue
　in cardiac disease, 24
Fenoldopam, 314, 314t
Fibroelastoma, cardiac, 264
Fibromas, cardiac, 264
Fibromuscular dysplasia (FMD), 296, 300f
Filling pressures
　atrial, 10
　　left, 10, 10f, 12t
　　right, 10f, 12t, 14
　ventricular, 10-12
First-degree atrioventricular block, 210, 210f
Flecainide, 200t-202t, 202
Flow-dependent vasodilation, 12-14
Focal atrial tachycardia, 212-214, 218f, 220
Fondaparinux
　for deep vein thrombosis, 286
　for pulmonary embolism, 288-290
Frank-Starling law, 84, 86f
Functional status
　assessment of, 18
　classification of, 26t

G

Gap junctions, 194
Genetic testing
　for channelopathies, 238
Gerhard sign, in chronic severe regurgitation, 140t
Giant cell arteritis (GCA), 282
Giant cell myocarditis, 248
Glucocorticoid-remediable aldosteronism, 298
Great arteries, transposition of, 118-122

H

Hampton's hump, 288
HAS-BLED (hypertension, abnormal renal/liver function, stroke, bleeding history or predisposition, labile international normalized ratio, elderly, drugs/alcohol) score, 222
Heart
　blood supply of, 4
　conduction system of, 4-6
　　blood supply of, 4
　　cells of, 6
　contraction of, 8-14, 8f
　hemodynamic changes in, 10
　innervation of, 6
　muscle physiology of, 8-14, 8f
　normal structure and function of, 2-14
　trauma to, 264-266, 264t
　tumors of, 262-264, 262f
Heart disease, traumatic, 264-266, 264t
Heart failure, 82-104
　ACCF/AHA stages of, 82-84

内皮素，15
内皮素受体拮抗剂（ERA），治疗肺动脉高压，285
经皮血管内动脉瘤修复术（EVAR），281
心外膜，5
依普利酮
　肾上腺增生，297-299
事件记录器，59
运动
　周围动脉疾病，277
外部事件监视器，199
体外膜肺氧合（ECMO），267t，269

F

分支阻滞，51
　心电图表现，51t
乏力
　心脏病，25
非诺多泮，315，315t
弹力纤维瘤，心脏，265
纤维瘤，心脏，265
纤维肌性发育不良（FMD），297，301f
充盈压
　心房压力，11
　　左心房压力，11，11f，13t
　　右心房压力，11f，13t，15
　心室压力，11-13
一度房室传导阻滞，211，211f
氟卡尼，201t-203t，203
血流依赖性血管舒张，13-15
局灶性房性心动过速，213-215，219f，221
磺达肝癸钠
　深静脉血栓形成，287
　肺栓塞，289-291
Frank-Starling 定律，85，87f
心功能
　活动能力测评，19
　分级，27t

G

缝隙连接，195
基因检测
　离子通道病，239
Gerhard 征，见于慢性主动脉瓣反流，141t
巨细胞动脉炎（GCA），283
巨细胞性心肌炎，249
糖皮质激素可抑制性醛固酮增多症，299
大动脉转位，119-123

H

驼峰征，289
HAS-BLED（高血压、肝肾功能异常、卒中、出血史或出血倾向、国际标准化比值不稳定、老年人、药物/酒精滥用）评分，223
心脏
　血液供应，5
　传导系统，5-7
　　血供，5
　　细胞，7
　收缩，9-15，9f
　血流动力学变化，11
　神经分布，7
　心肌生理特点，9-15，9f
　正常结构和功能，3-15
　创伤，265-267，265t
　肿瘤，263-265，263f
心脏疾病，创伤性，265-267，265t
心力衰竭，83-105
　ACCF/AHA 分期，83-85

acute, precipitating factors for, 88
acute decomposition, diagnosis and management of, 86-104
acute management for, 90-92
    diuresis, 90
advanced therapy for, 98-102
causes of, 82, 84t
definition and classification of, 82-84
device therapy for, 96-98, 98f
exam findings for, 88
functional impairment and, 82-84, 86t
future directions for, 104
guideline-directed medical therapy, 92-96, 94f
heart transplant for, 102, 102f
hemodynamic profiles and, 84, 86f
history of, 86-88
hypertrophic cardiomyopathy and, 252
inotropic support for, 100
laboratory data and imaging for, 88-90, 90f-92f
mechanical circulatory support, 100-102, 102t
myocardial infarction and, 186
noncardiac surgery inpatient with, 270
NYHA functional classification of, 84
palliative care for, 102-104
pathophysiology of, 84-86
    adaptive neurohormonal response, 84-86
    Frank-Starling law, 84, 86f
in pregnancy
    aortic stenosis, 258
    mitral stenosis, 258
symptoms of, 86-88
Heart rate (HR), 6
    autonomic regulation of, 206
    myocardial oxygen consumption and, 12, 12t
Heart sounds
    abnormal, 34-38, 34t-36t, 36f-38f
    normal, 34
    prosthetic, 42
HELLP syndrome, 310-312
Hematoma
    intramural, aortic, 280
Hemochromatosis, 82
Heparin
    for acute limb ischemia, 276-278
    for deep vein thrombosis, 286
    in pulmonary embolism, 288-290
High-grade atrioventricular blocks, 210f, 212
High-pressure baroreceptors, 14
Hills sign, in chronic severe regurgitation, 140t
His, bundle of, 6
Holosystolic murmurs, 42
    in atrial septal defects, 106-108
    in atrioventricular septal defects, 112
    in tetralogy of Fallot, 118
    in ventricular septal defects, 110
Holter monitoring, in arrhythmias, 198
Homan's sign, 286
Hydralazine
    for heart failure, 96
    reduction of afterload by, 12
17-Hydroxylase deficiency, 298
Hypertension
    acute severe, 312-314, 312f, 314t
    in African Americans, 304
    aortic coarctation and, 112
    in chronic kidney disease, 304, 312
    coronary artery disease with, 308
    with diabetes, 308
    isolated systolic, in older adults, 308, 310f
    masked, 294

急性心衰加重的诱发因素，89
急性失代偿心衰的诊断和治疗，87-105
急性期管理，91-93
    利尿，91
高阶治疗，99-103
病因，83，85t
定义和分类，83-85
器械治疗，97-99，99f
体格检查结果，89
功能障碍，83-85，87t
未来方向，105
指南指导的药物治疗，93-97，95f
心脏移植，103，103f
血流动力学特征，85，87f
病史，87-89
肥厚型心肌病，253
正性肌力药物支持，101
实验室和影像学检查，89-91，91f-93f
机械循环支持，101-103，103t
心肌梗死，187
非心脏手术患者，271
NYHA 心功能分级，85
缓和医疗，103-105
病理生理学，85-87
    适应性神经激素反应，85-87
    Frank-Starling 定律，85，87f
妊娠期
    主动脉瓣狭窄，259
    二尖瓣狭窄，259
症状，87-89
心率（HR），7
    自主神经系统调节，207
    心肌氧耗量，13，13t
心音
    异常，35-39，35t-37t，37f-39f
    正常，35
    人工，43
HELLP 综合征，311-313
血肿
    主动脉壁内，281
血色病，83
肝素
    急性肢体缺血，277-279
    深静脉血栓形成，287
    肺栓塞，289-291
高度房室传导阻滞，211f，213
高压压力感受器，15
Hills 征，见于慢性主动脉瓣反流，141t
希氏束，7
全收缩期杂音，43
    房间隔缺损，107-109
    房室间隔缺损，113
    法洛四联症，119
    室间隔缺损，111
Holter 监测，心律失常，199
霍曼征，287
肼屈嗪
    心力衰竭，97
    减小后负荷，13
17-羟化酶缺乏症，299
高血压
    急性重症，313-315，313f，315t
    非裔美国人，305
    主动脉缩窄，113
    慢性肾脏病，305，313
    合并冠状动脉疾病，309
    合并糖尿病，309
    单纯收缩期（高血压），老年人，309，311f
    隐匿性，295

Mendelian forms of, 298
oral contraceptives, 310
in pregnancy, 260, 310-312
prognosis of, 316
prospects for future of, 316
pseudoresistant, 312
renal parenchymal, 296
renovascular, 296
resistant, 312
secondary causes of, 294-296, 300t
treatment of, 304-314
    with lifestyle modification, 304
    lifetime protection from, 316
    for secondary prevention of stroke, 310
uncomplicated, 304
vascular disease and, 274-316
in women, 310-312
Hypertensive emergencies, 312, 314t
Hypertensive encephalopathy, 312
Hypertensive nephrosclerosis, 304
Hypertensive retinopathy, 312, 312f
Hypertensive urgencies, 312
Hypocalcemia
    electrocardiographyin, 52
Hypoglycemia
    syncope and, 22
Hypokalemia
    electrocardiographyin, 52

I

Ibutilide, 202t, 204
Idiopathic ventricular tachycardia, 234-236
Iloprost, in Buerger's disease, 280-282
Impella, 266-268
Innocent murmurs, 34, 38
Inotropy, 6, 12

J

Jpoint, 46
Jugular venous pulsations, examination of, 26-28

K

Korotkoff sounds, 30
Kussmaul sign, 26
Kyphoscoliosis, 32

L

Labetalol, for hypertensive crisis, 314
Laplace's law,wall stress and, 12
Left atrioventricular valve regurgitation, atrioventricular septal defects and, 112
Left bundle branch blocks, 50, 52f
Left ventricular dysfunction
    tetralogy ofFallot and, 118
Left ventricular failure, 20-22, 30f
Left ventricular hypertrophy, aortic stenosis and, 124-126
Left ventricular outflow tract, 22
Left-dominant circulation, 4
Leriche syndrome, 274
Liddle's syndrome, 298
Lidocaine, 200t-202t, 202
Lifestyle modifications
    for lowering blood pressure, 304
Lipoma, cardiac, 264
Long QT syndrome
    acquired, 238
    congenital, 236-238, 236f

孟德尔遗传性状，299
口服避孕药，311
妊娠（高血压），261，311-313
预后，317
未来展望，317
假性难治性，313
肾实质性，297
肾血管性，297
难治性，313
继发性病因，295-297，301t
治疗，305-315
    生活方式调整，305
    终身保护，317
    卒中的二级预防，311
无合并症，305
血管疾病，275-317
女性（高血压），311-313
高血压急症，313，315t
高血压脑病，313
高血压肾硬化症，305
高血压性视网膜病变，313，313f
高血压亚急症，313
低钙血症
    心电图，53
低血糖
    晕厥，23
低钾血症
    心电图，53

I

伊布利特，203t，205
特发性室性心动过速，235-237
伊洛前列素，治疗血栓闭塞性脉管炎，281-283
Impella，267-269
无害性杂音，35，39
收缩力，7，13

J

J点，47
颈静脉搏动检查，27-29

K

Korotkoff音，31
Kussmaul征，27
脊柱后侧凸，33

L

拉贝洛尔，治疗高血压危象，315
拉普拉斯定律，室壁应力，13
左房室瓣反流，房室间隔缺损，113
左束支传导阻滞，51，53f
左心室功能不全
    法洛四联症，119
左心衰竭，21-23，31f
左心室肥厚，主动脉瓣狭窄，125-127
左心室流出道，23
左优势循环，5
Leriche综合征，275
利德尔综合征，299
利多卡因，201t-203t，203
生活方式调整
    降低血压，305
脂肪瘤，心脏，265
长QT间期综合征
    获得性，239
    先天性，237-239，237

Long RP tachycardia, 214
Low-density lipoproteins (LDL) cholesterol
    in coronary heart disease, 150
    in peripheral arterial disease, 276
Lown-Ganong-Levine syndrome, 214
Low-pressure baroreceptors, 14
Lung transplantation
    for pulmonary hypertension, arterial, 284

M

Machinery murmurs, 42
Magnetic resonance imaging (MRI)
    in tetralogy of Fallot, 118, 120f
    in transposition of great arteries, 120
Marfan syndrome
    β-blockers in, for aortic root enlargement, 278-280
    in pregnancy, 258-260
Mayne sign, in chronic severe regurgitation, 140t
Mechanical circulatory support (MCS), 266
Metabolic syndrome, 150
α-Methyldopa, for hypertension, in pregnancy, 310-312
Mid-diastolic murmur, atrial septal defects and, 106-108
Mitral regurgitation, 138-144
    clinical presentation of, 140
    definition and etiology of, 138-140, 140f-142f
    diagnosis of, 142-144
    mechanisms of, 142t
    natural history of, 140
    pathophysiology of, 140, 142f
    physical examination for, 140-142
    treatment of, 144, 144f
Mitral stenosis, 128-132, 130f
    clinical presentation of, 132
    definition and etiology of, 128
    diagnosis of, 132
    natural history of, 132
    noncardiac surgery inpatient with, 270
    pathophysiology of, 128-132
    physical examination for, 132
    in pregnancy, 258
    recommendations for, 134t
    stages of, 134t
    treatment of, 132
Mitral valve, 4
    in auscultation, 32-34
    fibroelastoma of, 264
    opening of, 10f
Mitral valve prolapse, 142
Mobitz type I second-degree atrioventricular block, 210-212, 210f
Mobitz type II second-degree atrioventricular block, 210f, 212
Mueller sign, in chronic severe regurgitation, 140t
Multifocal atrial tachycardia, 218, 218f
Murmurs, 38-42
    in aortic coarctation, 112
    in aortic regurgitation, 138
    in aortic (valve) stenosis, 116, 126
    in atrial septal defects, 106-108
    in atrioventricular septal defects, 112
    in hypertrophic cardiomyopathy, 252
    innocent, 34, 38
    maneuvers affecting, 34t
    in mitral regurgitation, 140
    in patent ductus arteriosus, 114
    physiologic, 34
    in pulmonary arterial hypertension, 284
    in pulmonary valve stenosis, 114-116
    in tetralogy of Fallot, 118
    in transposition of great arteries, 120
    venous hums, 42

长RP间期心动过速，215
低密度脂蛋白（LDL）胆固醇
    冠心病，151
    周围动脉疾病，277
Lown-Ganong-Levine综合征，215
低压压力感受器，15
肺移植
    肺动脉高压，285

M

机械性杂音，43
磁共振成像（MRI）
    法洛四联症，119，121f
    大动脉转位，121
马方综合征
    β受体阻滞剂，主动脉根部扩张，279-281
    妊娠期，259-261
Mayne征，见于慢性主动脉瓣反流，141t
机械循环支持（MCS），267
代谢综合征，151
α-甲基多巴，治疗妊娠高血压，311-313
舒张中期杂音，房间隔缺损，107-109
二尖瓣反流，139-145
    临床表现，141
    定义和病因，139-141，141f-143f
    诊断，143-145
    机制，143t
    自然病程，141
    病理生理学，141，143f
    体格检查，141-143
    治疗，145，145f
二尖瓣狭窄，129-133，131f
    临床表现，133
    定义和病因，129
    诊断，133
    自然病程，133
    非心脏手术患者，271
    病理生理学，129-133
    体格检查，133
    妊娠期，259
    指南推荐，135t
    分期，135t
    治疗，133
二尖瓣，5
    听诊，33-35
    弹力纤维瘤，265
    开放，11f
二尖瓣脱垂，143
莫氏I型二度房室传导阻滞，211-213，211f
莫氏II型二度房室传导阻滞，211f，213
Mueller征，见于慢性主动脉瓣反流，141t
多源性房性心动过速，219，219f
杂音，39-43
    主动脉缩窄，113
    主动脉瓣反流，139
    主动脉瓣狭窄，117，127
    房间隔缺损，107-109
    房室间隔缺损，113
    肥厚型心肌病，253
    无害性杂音，35，39
    动作（对杂音的）影响，35t
    二尖瓣反流，141
    动脉导管未闭，115
    生理性，35
    肺动脉高压，285
    肺动脉瓣狭窄，115-117
    法洛四联症，119
    大动脉转位，121
    静脉营营音，43

in ventricular septal defects, 110
Muscle
    cardiac, 8-14, 8f
Myocardial disease, 248-256
    cardiomyopathies, 250-256, 250t, 254f, 256t
    myocarditis, 248
Myocardial infarction
    cardiac catheterization and noninvasive testing for, 190
    complications of, 186-190
    electrocardiographic monitoring of, 190
    and left bundle branch block, 50
    mechanical complications of, 188
    patient education and rehabilitation for, 192
    predictors of sudden cardiac death after, 234t
    risk stratification after, 190
    secondary prevention of, 190-192
    ST segment and T wave abnormalities in, 50-52, 54f, 56f
    thromboembolic complications of, 188-190
Myocardial ischemia
    due to obstructive CAD, 18
Myocardial oxygen consumption, 12
Myocardial perfusion, imaging for, 72
Myocarditis, 248
Myocardium, 6-8
    structure, 6-8
Myocytes
    anatomy of, 6-8
    contraction of, 8
Myofibrils, cardiac, 6-8
Myosin, of cardiac myocytes, 8, 8f

N

Nephrosclerosis, hypertensive, 304
Neurocardiogenic syncope, 22
New York Heart Association Functional Classification, 24
Nicardipine, for hypertensive crisis, 314, 314t
Nitrates
    for heart failure, 96
Nitric oxide
    as coronary vasodilator, 14
Nitroglycerin
    for hypertensive crisis, 314, 314t
Nitroprusside
    for aortic regurgitation, 138
    for hypertensive crisis, 314, 314t
    for mitral regurgitation, 144
Noninvasive vascular testing, 78-80
Nonpenetrating cardiac trauma, 264, 264t
Nonsteroidal anti-inflammatory drugs (NSAIDs)
    in acute pericarditis, 242

O

Opening snap, 38
Oral contraceptives
    blood pressure increase caused by, 310
Orthodromic atrioventricular reentrant tachycardia, 214
Orthopnea, 20-22
Oxygen consumption, myocardial, 12

P

P wave, 46
PAI-I. See Plasminogen activator inhibitor-1
Pain
    of angina, 18
Palpitation, 22
Papillary muscles, 4
Percutaneous left ventricular assist devices, 266-268, 266t
Percutaneous mechanical circulatory support, 266-268, 266t

室间隔缺损，111
肌肉
    心肌，9-15，9f
心肌疾病，249-257
    心肌病，251-257，251t，255f，257t
    心肌炎，249
心肌梗死
    心导管和无创性检查，191
    并发症，187-191
    心电监测，191
    左束支传导阻滞，51
    机械并发症，189
    患者教育和康复治疗，193
    心肌梗死后心源性猝死的预测因子，235t
    心肌梗死后风险分层，191
    二级预防，191-193
    ST 段和 T 波异常，51-53，55f，57t
    血栓栓塞并发症，189-191
心肌缺血
    阻塞性 CAD 引起，19
心肌氧耗量，13
心肌灌注成像，73
心肌炎，249
心肌，7-9
    结构，7-9
肌细胞
    解剖学，7-9
    收缩，9
肌原纤维，心脏，7-9
肌球蛋白，心肌细胞，9，9f

N

高血压肾硬化症，305
神经心源性晕厥，23
纽约心脏协会心功能分级，25
尼卡地平，治疗高血压危象，315，315t
硝酸盐
    心力衰竭，97
一氧化氮
    冠状动脉血管扩张剂，15
硝酸甘油
    高血压危象，315，315t
硝普钠
    主动脉瓣反流，139
    高血压危象，315，315t
    二尖瓣反流，145
无创血管检查，79-81
非穿透性心脏创伤，265，265t
非甾体抗炎药（NSAID）
    急性心包炎，243

O

开瓣音，39
口服避孕药
    引起血压升高，311
顺向型房室折返性心动过速，215
端坐呼吸，21-23
心肌氧耗量，13

P

P 波，47
PAI-I 参见纤溶酶原激活物抑制物-1
胸痛
    心绞痛，19
心悸，23
乳头肌，5
经皮左心室辅助装置，267-269，267t
经皮机械循环支持，267-269，267t

Pericardial disease, 242-248
    acute pericarditis, 242, 244t
    cardiac tamponade, 242-244
    constrictive pericarditis, 246, 246f, 256t
    effusive constrictive pericarditis, 248
    pericardial effusion, 242-244, 246f
Pericardial effusion, 242-244, 246f
Pericardial fluid
    normal properties of, 4
Pericardial knock, 38
Pericardial rubs, 42
Pericardiocentesis, in pericardial effusions, 244
Pericarditis
    acute, 242, 244t
    constrictive, 246, 246f, 256t
    effusive constrictive, 248
    pain of, 18-20
    traumatic, 264
Pericardium, 242
    anatomy and physiology of, 4
    lipomas of, 264
    trauma to, 264-266, 264t
Peripartum cardiomyopathy, in pregnancy, 260
Peripheral arterial disease, 16, 274-278, 274t, 276f
    diagnosis of, 274, 274t
    prospects for future of, 316
Pheochromocytoma, 298-304
Physical examination, for ST elevation myocardial infarction, 182
Physiologic murmurs, 34
Poiseuille's law, 14
Positron emission tomography (PET), 62
Post-thrombotic syndrome, upper extremity, 286
PR interval, 44
Precordial leads, 46, 48f
Precordium, examination of, 32
Preeclampsia, 310-312
Preexcitation syndromes, 214
Pregnancy
    cardiac disease in, 258-262, 260t
        arising during, 260-262
        congenital heart disease, 260
        Marfan syndrome, 258-260
        peripartum cardiomyopathy, 260
        spontaneous coronary artery dissection (SCAD), 262, 262f
        valvular heart disease, 258
    hypertension in, 260, 310-312
Preload, 10-12, 12t
Premature beats, 22
Prinzmetal angina, electrocardiography in, 52
Prostacyclin, for pulmonary arterial hypertension, 284
Prostacyclin analog
    in Buerger's disease, 280-282
    for pulmonary arterial hypertension, 284
Pseudoinfarction, 52
Pulmonary artery
    Takayasu's arteritis of, 282
Pulmonary capillary wedge pressure, 76
    as measure of preload, 10
    in pulmonary arterial hypertension, 284
Pulmonary circulation
    physiology of, 14
Pulmonary embolism, 288-290, 288f-290f, 290t
    dyspnea in, 22
    pain in, 20
Pulmonary hypertension, 282
    arterial, 284
    atrial septal defects and, 106
    classification of, 284t
    definition of, 282

心包疾病，243-249
    急性心包炎，243，245t
    心脏压塞，243-245
    缩窄性心包炎，247，247f，257t
    渗出性缩窄性心包炎，249
    心包积液，243-245，247f
心包积液，243-245，247f
心包液
    正常性质，5
心包叩击音，39
心包摩擦音，43
心包穿刺术，治疗心包积液，245
心包炎
    急性，243，245t
    缩窄性，247，247f，257t
    渗出性缩窄性，249
    疼痛，19-21
    创伤性，265
心包，243
    解剖学和生理学，5
    脂肪瘤，265
    创伤，265-267，265t
围产期心肌病，妊娠，261
周围动脉疾病，17，275-279，275t，277f
    诊断，275，275t
    未来展望，317
嗜铬细胞瘤，299-305
体格检查，ST 段抬高型心肌梗死，183
生理性杂音，35
泊肃叶定律，15
正电子发射断层成像（PET），63
血栓后综合征，上肢，287
PR 间期，45
心前区导联，47，49f
心前区检查，33
先兆子痫，311-313
预激综合征，215
妊娠
    心脏病，259-263，261t
        妊娠引起，261-263
        先天性心脏病，261
        马方综合征，259-261
        围产期心肌病，261
        自发性冠状动脉夹层（SCAD），263，263f
        心脏瓣膜病，259
    高血压，261，311-313
前负荷，11-13，13t
早搏，23
变异型心绞痛，心电图，53
前列环素，治疗肺动脉高压，285
前列环素类似物
    血栓闭塞性脉管炎，281-283
    肺动脉高压，285
假性梗死，53
肺动脉
    大动脉炎，283
肺毛细血管楔压，77
    前负荷测量，11
    肺动脉高压，285
肺循环
    生理机制，15
肺栓塞，289-291，289f-291f，291t
    呼吸困难，23
    胸痛，21
肺动脉高压，283
    动脉型，285
    房间隔缺损，107
    分类，285t
    定义，283

Pulmonary regurgitation, pulmonary valve stenosis and, 116
Pulmonary valve stenosis, 114-116
Pulmonic stenosis, 132-136
    clinical presentation of, 134
    definition and etiology of, 132
    diagnosis of, 136
    natural history of, 134
    pathophysiology of, 134
    physical examination for, 134
    treatment of, 136
Pulse, arterial, 28-32
Pulsus bisferiens, 252
Pulsus paradoxus, 32, 244
Pulsus parvus, 124-126
Purkinje cells, 6

Q

Q wave, and myocardial infarction, 52
QRS complex, 44
QT interval, 46
Quincke pulses, in chronic severe regurgitation, 140t
Quinidine, 200t
    side effects of, 200-202, 202t

R

R prime, 44
Raynaud's phenomenon, 282
Reciprocating atrioventricular tachycardia, 214
Reentry, 196-198, 196f
Renal artery stenosis
    atherosclerotic, 296, 300f
    hypertension and, 296
Renal insufficiency
    hypertension and, 296
Renovascular hypertension, 296
Reperfusion therapy, for ST elevation myocardial infarction, 184-186
Resistance vessels, 14
Restrictive cardiomyopathy, 250t, 254
    constrictive pericarditis vs., 256t
Retinopathy
    hypertensive, 312, 312f
Revascularization
    percutaneous or surgical, 276, 276f
    of renal artery, 296
Rhabdomyoma, cardiac, 264
Rheumatic fever, criteria for diagnosis of, 130t
Rheumatic valve disease, 124
Right ventricular failure
    pulmonary embolism with, 288
Right ventricular hypertrophy, 48-50
Right ventricular support, 268
Right-dominant circulation, 4
Risk factor modification, in peripheral arterial disease, 274
Rosenbach sign, in chronic severe regurgitation, 140t

S

S_1, 34
S_2, 34
    abnormal splitting of, 36, 36t
S_3, 36
S_4 gallop, 36-38
Salt, dietary, hypertension and, 304
Sarcomeres, 6-8
Sarcoplasmic reticulum, 6-8
Semilunar valves, 8-10
Septal reduction therapy, in hypertrophic cardiomyopathy, 254, 254f
Short RP tachycardia, 214
Shunt lesions, types of, 108f

肺动脉瓣反流，肺动脉瓣狭窄，117
肺动脉瓣狭窄，115-117
肺动脉瓣狭窄，133-137
    临床表现，135
    定义和病因，133
    诊断，137
    自然病程，135
    病理生理学，135
    体格检查，135
    治疗，137
动脉脉搏，29-33
双峰脉，253
奇脉，33，245
细迟脉，125-127
浦肯野细胞，7

Q

Q波，心肌梗死，53
QRS波，45
QT间期，47
Quincke脉搏，见于慢性主动脉瓣反流，141t
奎尼丁，201t
    副作用，201-203，203t

R

R′波，45
雷诺现象，283
房室折返性心动过速，215
折返，197-199，197f
肾动脉狭窄
    动脉粥样硬化，297，301f
    高血压，297
肾功能不全
    高血压，297
肾血管性高血压，297
再灌注治疗，ST段抬高型心肌梗死，185-187
阻力血管，15
限制型心肌病，251t，255
    vs. 缩窄性心包炎，257t
视网膜病变
    高血压性，313，313f
血运重建
    经皮或手术，277，277f
    肾动脉，297
心脏横纹肌瘤，265
风湿热，诊断标准，131t
风湿性瓣膜病，125
右心室衰竭
    肺栓塞，289
右心室肥厚，49-51
右心室支持，269
右优势循环，5
危险因素干预，周围动脉疾病，275
Rosenbach征，见于慢性主动脉瓣反流，141t

S

S_1，35
S_2，35
    异常分裂，37，37t
S_3，37
S_4奔马律，37-39
盐，饮食，高血压，305
肌节，7-9
肌质网，7-9
半月瓣，9-11
室间隔减容治疗，肥厚型心肌病，255，255f
短RP间期心动过速，215
分流病变，类型，109f

Sick sinus syndrome, 206
Silent myocardial ischemia, 170
Sinoatrial exit block, 206, 208f
Sinoatrial (SA) node, 4-6
Sinus bradycardia
   myocardial infarction and, 186
   resting, 206
Sinus node
   action potential in, 194
   dysfunction of, 206-208, 208f
Sinus pauses/arrest, 206
Sinus rhythm, restoration of, 224
Sinus venosus atrial septal defects, 106
Sinuses of Valsalva, 4
Sleep apnea
      hypertension secondary to, 300t
Sodium-channel blockers, 200
Sotalol, 202t, 204
Spinal canal stenosis, lumbar degenerative, 274
Spironolactone
   for resistant hypertension, 312
ST elevation myocardial infarction (STEMI), acute, 180-186
   clinical presentation of, 180-182
   definition and epidemiology of, 180, 182f
   differential diagnosis of, 182-184
   pathology of, 180
   treatment for, 184-186
ST segment, 46
ST segment abnormalities
   in myocardial infarction, 50-52, 54f, 56t
   in myocardial ischemia, 50-52, 54f, 56t
Statins
   in peripheral arterial disease, 276
Stress cardiac magnetic resonance imaging, 72
Stress echocardiography, 72
Stress electrocardiography, 72
Stroke, 16
   blood pressure lowering for secondary prevention of, 310
   risk factors for
      hypertension, 292, 296f
Stroke volume, 10
Subaortic stenosis, atrioventricular septal defects and, 112
Sudden cardiac death
   causes of, 234t
   in hypertrophic cardiomyopathy, 254
   predictors of, after myocardial infarction, 234t
   prevention of, 230-234
   ventricular arrhythmias and, 228-238
Supraventricular tachycardias, 212-218
   ventricular tachycardia vs., 232t
Surgery
   noncardiac
      cardiovascular disease and, 268-270
         arrhythmias, 270
         conduction defects, 270
         heart failure, 270
         ischemic heart disease, 270
         valvular heart disease, 270
Swan-Ganz catheter, 76, 78f
   diagnosis using, 80t
Sympatholytics, central, 302t
   contraindications to, 306t-308t
   side effects of, 306t-308t
Syncope, 22, 228
   causes of, 230t
   evaluation of, 232f
   in hypertrophic cardiomyopathy, 252
Syndrome of apparent mineralocorticoid excess, 298
Systemic circulation, physiology of, 14

病态窦房结综合征，207
无症状性心肌缺血，171
窦房传出阻滞，207，209f
窦房（SA）结，5-7
窦性心动过缓
   心肌梗死，187
   静息，207
窦房结
   动作电位，195
   功能障碍，207-209，209f
窦性停搏，207
窦性心律，恢复，225
静脉窦型房间隔缺损，107
主动脉窦，5
睡眠呼吸暂停
      继发性高血压，301t
钠通道阻滞剂，201
索他洛尔，203t，205
椎管狭窄，腰椎退行性，275
螺内酯
   难治性高血压，313
急性ST段抬高型心肌梗死（STEMI），181-187
   临床表现，181-183
   定义和流行病学，181，183f
   鉴别诊断，183-185
   病理学，181
   治疗，185-187
ST段，47
ST段异常
   心肌梗死，51-53，55f，57t
   心肌缺血，51-53，55f，57t
他汀类药物
   周围动脉疾病，277
负荷心脏磁共振成像，73
负荷超声心动图，73
负荷心电图，73
卒中，17
   降低血压对卒中的二级预防，311
   危险因素
      高血压，293，297
每搏输出量，11
主动脉瓣下狭窄，房室间隔缺损，113
心源性猝死
   病因，235t
   肥厚型心肌病，255
   心肌梗死后心源性猝死的预测因子，235t
   预防，231-235
   室性心律失常和心源性猝死，229-239
室上性心动过速，213-219
   vs. 室性心动过速，233t
外科手术
   非心脏手术
      心血管疾病，269-271
         心律失常，271
         传导障碍，271
         心力衰竭，271
         缺血性心脏病，271
         心脏瓣膜病，271
Swan-Ganz导管，77，79f
   使用Swan-Ganz导管进行鉴别诊断，81t
中枢交感神经阻滞剂，303t
   禁忌证，307t-309t
   副作用，307t-309t
晕厥，23，229
   原因，231t
   评估，233f
   肥厚型心肌病，253
表象性盐皮质激素过多综合征，299
体循环，生理机制，15

Systemic vascular resistance, 14
Systemic venous flow, in transposition of great arteries, 118
Systole, 4, 8-10
Systolic murmurs, 38-42
    in aortic coarctation, 112
    in aortic valve stenosis, 116
    in atrial septal defects, 106-108
    in atrioventricular septal defects, 112

T

T tubules, 6-8
T wave, 46
    inversion, 50
Tachycardia, 212-228, 216f-218f, 226f
Takayasu's arteritis, 282
Takotsubo (stress-induced) cardiomyopathy, 250t
Tamponade, cardiac
    malignant tumors and, 264
    trauma with, 264-266
TandemHeart, 268
Temporal arteritis, 282
Tetralogy of Fallot, 118, 120f
Thiazide diuretics
    for hypertension, 302t, 304, 308
Third-degree atrioventricular blocks, 210f, 212
Thoracic outlet obstruction, 286
Thrills, 32
Thrombolytic therapy
    for acute limb ischemia, 276-278
    for pulmonary embolism, 288-290
Tobacco
    abstinence, Buerger's disease and, 280-282
Transannular patch, for tetralogy of Fallot, 118
Transcatheter closure, for atrial septal defects, 108
Transesophageal echocardiography (TEE), 60
    in mitral regurgitation, 142-144
Transposition of great arteries, 118-122
Transthoracic echocardiography (TTE)
    in aortic stenosis, 126
    in constrictive pericarditis, 246
    in mitral regurgitation, 142-144
    in pericardial effusions, 244
    in pulmonic stenosis, 136
    in tricuspid regurgitation, 146
Traube sign, in chronic severe regurgitation, 140t
Trauma
    cardiac
        nonpenetrating, 264, 264t
        penetrating, 264-266, 264t
Treadmill, stress testing in, 68
Tricuspid regurgitation, 146
    jugular venous pulse and, 26, 28f
Tricuspid stenosis, 136
    jugular venous pulse and, 26-28, 28f
Tricuspid valve
    after arterial switch procedure, 120
    anatomy of, 4
    in auscultation, 32-34
Triggered activity, cardiac, 196
TroponinC, 8
Tumor plop, 38

U

Unstable angina, pain in, 18

V

Valsalva maneuver, 32-34
Valvotomy, for pulmonary valve stenosis, 116

体循环血流阻力，15
体循环静脉血，见于大动脉转位，119
收缩期，5，9-11
收缩期杂音，39-43
    主动脉缩窄，113
    主动脉瓣狭窄，117
    房间隔缺损，107-109
    房室间隔缺损，113

T

T管，7-9
T波，47
    倒置，51
心动过速，213-229，217f-219f，227f
大动脉炎，283
Takotsubo（应激性）心肌病，251t
心脏压塞
    恶性肿瘤，265
    创伤，265-267
TandemHeart，269
颞动脉炎，283
法洛四联症，119，121f
噻嗪类利尿剂
    高血压，303t，305，309
三度房室传导阻滞（完全性心脏传导阻滞），211f，213
胸廓出口梗阻，287
震颤，33
溶栓治疗
    急性肢体缺血，277-279
    肺栓塞，289-291
烟草
    戒烟，血栓闭塞性脉管炎，281-283
跨环补片，治疗法洛四联症，119
经导管封堵，治疗房间隔缺损，109
经食管超声心动图（TEE），61
    二尖瓣反流，143-145
大动脉转位，119-123
经胸超声心动图（TTE）
    主动脉瓣狭窄，127
    缩窄性心包炎，247
    二尖瓣反流，143-145
    心包积液，245
    肺动脉瓣狭窄，137
    三尖瓣反流，147
Traube征，见于慢性主动脉瓣反流，141t
创伤
    心脏
        非穿透性，265，265t
        穿透性，265-267，265t
平板（跑步机），运动负荷试验，69
三尖瓣反流，147
    颈静脉搏动，27，29f
三尖瓣狭窄，137
    颈静脉搏动，27-29，29f
三尖瓣
    动脉调转术后，121
    解剖学，5
    听诊，33-35
触发活动，197
肌钙蛋白C，9
肿瘤扑落音，39

U

不稳定型心绞痛，19

V

Valsalva动作，33-35
瓣膜切开术，治疗肺动脉瓣狭窄，117

Valvular heart disease, 16, 124-148
    aortic regurgitation, 136-138
    aortic stenosis, 124-128, 126f
    mitral regurgitation, 138-144, 140f-142f
    mitral stenosis, 128-132, 130f
    noncardiac surgery inpatient with, 270
    in pregnancy, 258
    pulmonic stenosis, 132-136
    stages of, 126t
    tricuspid regurgitation, 146
    tricuspid stenosis, 136
Variant angina, 170, 170f
Vascular disease
    hypertension and, 274-316
Vasoconstriction
    coronary artery, 12-14
Vasodilators, direct, 302t
    contraindications to, 306t-308t
    side effects of, 306t-308t
Vena cava filter
    in deep vein thrombosis, 286-288
Venous hums, 42
Venous waveforms, 26, 28f
Ventilation-perfusion lung scan, in pulmonary embolism, 288
Ventricular arrhythmias, 228-238, 232f
    myocardial infarction and, 186
Ventricular depolarization, 46
Ventricular fibrillation, without evident heart disease, 234-238
Ventricular flutter, 228-230
Ventricular hypertrophy, electrocardiography in, 48-50, 48f, 50t
Ventricular pressures, 10-12
Ventricular septal defects, 108-110, 108f
Ventricular tachycardia (VT), 228, 234-238
    supraventricular tachycardia *vs.*, 232t
Viral myocarditis, 248

W

Wall stress, 12
    Laplace's law for, 12
    myocardial contraction and, 12
Warfarin
    for venous thromboembolism, 290-292
Water-hammer pulse, 32
Westermark's sign, 288
Wolff-Parkinson-White syndrome, 216-218, 216f
WPW pattern, in ECG, 214-216
Wright test, 286

心脏瓣膜病，17，125-149
    主动脉瓣反流，137-139
    主动脉瓣狭窄，125-129，127f
    二尖瓣反流，139-145，141f-143f
    二尖瓣狭窄，129-133，131f
    非心脏手术患者，271
    妊娠期，259
    肺动脉瓣狭窄，133-137
    进展分期，127t
    三尖瓣反流，147
    三尖瓣狭窄，137
变异型心绞痛，171，171f
血管疾病
    高血压，275-317
血管收缩
    冠状动脉，13-15
直接血管扩张剂，303t
    禁忌证，307t-309t
    副作用，307t-309t
腔静脉滤器
    深静脉血栓形成，287-289
静脉营营音，43
静脉波形，27，29f
V̇/Q̇扫描，肺栓塞，289
室性心律失常，229-239，233f
    心肌梗死，187
心室除极，47
心室颤动，无心脏基础病，235-239
心室扑动，229-231
心室肥厚，心电图，49-51，49f，51t
心室压力，11-13
室间隔缺损，109-111，109f
室性心动过速（VT），229，235-239
    vs. 室上性心动过速，233t
病毒性心肌炎，249

W

壁应力，13
    拉普拉斯定律，13
    心肌收缩，13
华法林
    静脉血栓栓塞，291-293
水冲脉，33
韦斯特马克征，289
WPW综合征，217-219，217f
WPW现象，心电图，215-217
过度外展试验，287